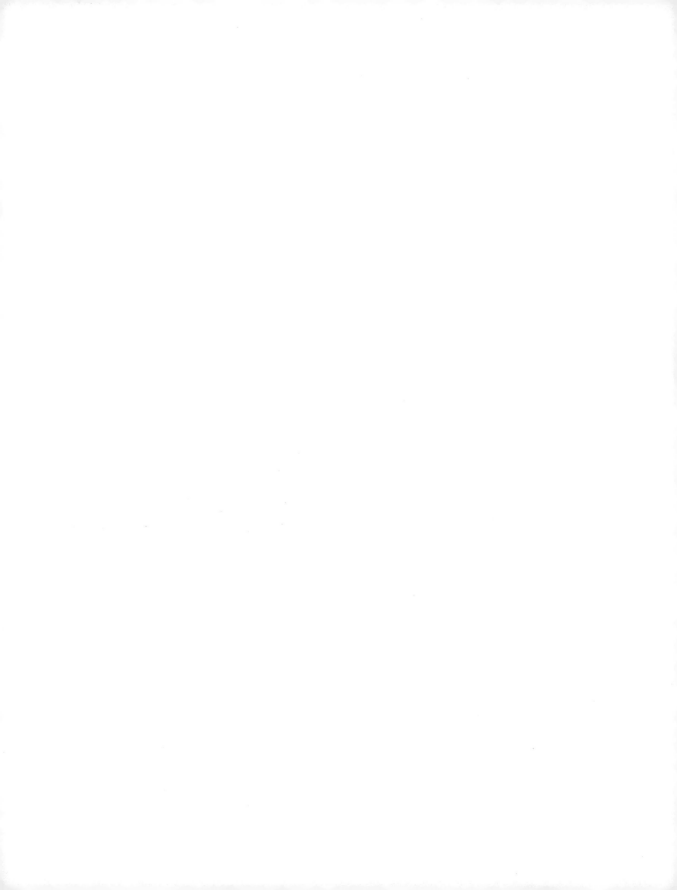

A Comprehensive Guide to Sports Physiology and Injury Management

An Interdisciplinary Approach

A Comprehensive Guide to Sports Physiology and Injury Management

An Interdisciplinary Approach

First Edition

Dr Stuart Porter

PhD, BSc(Hons), SFHEA, PGCAP, GradDipPhys, MCSP, SRP, CertMHS, MLACP

Lecturer in Physiotherapy, University of Salford, Manchester, UK;
Visiting Lecturer, Corpus Christi College, Cambridge, UK;
Senior Fellow of the Higher Education Academy;
Visiting Lecturer, Universidade Paulista, Sao Paulo, Brazil

Johnny Wilson

MSc, PGCE, BSc(Hons)

Clinical Director, 108 Harley Street;
Managing Director, Nottingham Physio;
MSC Sport & Exercise Medicine;
MACP Advanced Manual Therapy Practitioner

ELSEVIER   London   New York   Oxford   Philadelphia   St Louis   Sydney   2021

ISBN: 978-0-7020-7489-9

Content Strategist: Poppy Garraway Smith
Content Development Specialist: Helen Leng
Project Manager: Julie Taylor
Design: Ryan Cook
Illustration Manager: Paula Catalano

Printed in Scotland

Last digit is the print number: 9   8   7   6   5   4   3   2   1

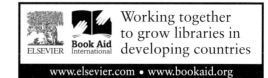

www.elsevier.com • www.bookaid.org

Contents

Contents

Preface

This new textbook will be something that can be used repeatedly, both as a reference work and an education aid, without losing its impact or its relevance. This is a book that comprises over 40 chapters written by authors from all over the globe, each with their own unique expertise and highly respected status in their own fields.

We have divided the book into three sections: the first section deals with key background concepts in sport and performance of the human body; the second section focuses on clinical applications, adopting a regional and sometimes a pathological approach; the final section engages with psychology and first aid for sport. The book contains brand new illustrations using state-of-the-art graphics and is evidence-based throughout.

We recognize that everyone needs a solid platform from which they can develop new skills and the material set out in this book enables this. However, we also challenge readers to draw their own conclusions using their own clinical reasoning skills. The book should appeal to undergraduate and postgraduate students alike, and we truly hope that we will also appeal to an international audience, particularly in those countries where sport is now being embraced more holistically.

Embarking on this project was exciting and daunting in equal measure. We would like to thank Elsevier for entrusting this major responsibility to us; we hope that we have produced something of value. We would also like to thank the contributors, who always responded to our polite nagging with dignity and professionalism when the clock was ticking down to publication. We would like to thank Helen Leng, Poppy Garraway and Gill Cloke at Elsevier for their support during the editorial process.

Change is the end result of all true learning
Leo Buscaglia

Stuart Porter
Johnny Wilson

List of Contributors

Ademola Adejuwon
Consultant Sports and Exercise Medicine, Institute of Sports, Exercise and Health, London (ISEH). Honorary Consultant University College London Hospitals NHS Foundation Trust. 10 years lead club doctor for English Premiership Rugby Club. Founding member of the multi-disciplinary Complex Concussion Clinic at the Institute of Sports Exercise Health, London.

Nikhil Ahluwalia, MBBS, BSc (Hons), MSc in Sports Cardiology
Cardiology Specialty Registrar at St Bartholomew's Hospital, London, UK. Nikhil's clinical subspecialty interests are in arrhythmias and devices. He has an active research interest in atrial fibrillation and early electrophysiological manifestations associated with exercise in amateur athletes.

Jill Alexander, MSc, BSc (Hons), MSST, MSMA, RFU, FHEA
Senior Lecturer and Course Lead for the BSc Sports Therapy programme and module leads on the MSc Football Science and Rehabilitation course at the University of Central Lancashire. Jill is working towards completing her PhD investigating mechanisms of cryotherapy in elite sport. Jill has worked in semi and professional rugby for several years at national and county level and most recently with the France national team at the U20's World Cup. Jill has publications in the area of cryotherapy and her research focuses around the effects of cryotherapy and whole-body cryotherapy in sport through several performance parameters including biomechanical, physiological, psychological markers. Jill currently supervises postgraduate research students across several scopes of elite sport performance, injury, rehabilitation and decision making. Although not limited to this area she has publications in elite performance and injury recovery; and her research interests include current projects in the remit of elite equine and rider performance through kinematic analysis.

Nick Allen, PhD, MSc (Sports Med), BSc (Hons)
Clinical Director, Birmingham Royal Ballet, Honorary Lecturer for Queen Mary's University London. Nick has over 20 years' experience in elite sports and performance. Alongside his work at the ballet he has worked as an external consultant to various professional and Olympic organizations. Prior to joining Birmingham Royal Ballet he was Head of Medical Services for a premiership rugby club. He lectures on the MSc in Sports Medicine at QMUL and Nottingham University. He is on the Sports Advisory Group for the Centre for Sport, Exercise and Osteoarthritis Research Versus Arthritis.

Brent Arnold, PhD, ATC, FNATA
Professor and Chair, Department of Health Sciences, School of Health and Human Sciences, Indiana University (IUPUI). Prior to Indiana University, Dr. Arnold was the Director of the Sports Medicine Research Laboratory and of Graduate studies in the Department of Kinesiology at Virginia Commonwealth University. He was also on the Kinesiology faculty at the University of Virginia and was a practicing athletic trainer at Princeton University. His research has focused on balance and proprioceptive deficits in individuals with chronic ankle instability.

Marcus Bateman, MSc (Physiotherapy), BSc (Hons) (Physiotherapy)
Consultant physiotherapist at Derby Shoulder Unit, University Hospitals of Derby & Burton NHS Foundation Trust, Derby, UK. Marcus is a Copeland Fellow of the British Elbow and Shoulder Society. He has a special interest in atraumatic shoulder instability and designed the Derby Shoulder Instability Rehabilitation Programme which is now used worldwide. Marcus is involved with numerous clinical research trials and lectures internationally on the subject of the assessment and management of shoulder disorders.

Mike Beere, MSc, BSc, ASCC (Accredited Strength and Conditioning Coach with UKSCA)
Senior Strength and Conditioning Coach at Cardiff City Football Club. Mike is focused on the performance enhancement and preparation of football players, and on the role of strength and conditioning practices in rehabilitation, with a key area of interest in hamstring (posterior chain) and calf performance. Mike is currently working for a PhD on strength and conditioning practices in elite football, and how practices can be incorporated into periods of fixture congestion to help maintain and improve performance; and on the use of isometric force testing as a key monitoring and predictive tool for lower limb performance.

Marc Beggs, MSc (Sports and Exercise Medicine), BSc (Hons) Physiotherapy
First Team Physiotherapist, Munster Rugby. Marc has been involved in professional rugby in a range of different roles, including Ulster Rugby, Welsh Rugby and Irish Rugby. Marc's work focuses on the long-term rehabilitation of players as well as the monitoring of previously injured players following their return to play. He has a particular interest in the rehabilitation of upper limb injuries in rugby.

Paco Biosca
Specialist in Orthopaedic Surgery; former President of both the European Federation of Orthopaedic and Sports Trauma and the Spanish Society of Sports Trauma; Professor Titular Anatomia at University of Lleida (INEF-C); Head of Chelsea FC Medical Department.

Lyndsey M. Cannon, BSc, GSR, FAFS
Lecturer in Sport Rehabilitation, School of Sport, Health & Applied Sciences at St Mary's University, Twickenham, London, UK. Lyndsey studied sport rehabilitation at St Mary's, after which she worked in private practice, within professional national sport and taught at St Mary's as a visiting lecturer. Lyndsey has recently become a Fellow of Applied Functional Science after completing her studies with the American functional movement specialists, Gray Institute.

Dean Chatterjee, MBBS, PgDip Clin Ed
Club doctor for Nottingham Rugby and team doctor for the England U18s men's football team. Dean is also an event doctor for England athletics and British gymnastics. He has a keen interest in pitch-side emergency care, sports cardiology and concussion.

David M. Clancy, MSc (Sports Medicine), BSc (Physiotherapy), MISCP
Founder and strategic director of Hauora Ltd., a whole-person wellbeing and healthcare company, based in Dublin, Ireland; Consultant for medical and performance services for the European players of the Brooklyn Nets and the San Antonio Spurs of the NBA. David is the founder and host of the podcast Sleep Eat Perform Repeat, which focuses on what makes high-performing individuals succeed in sport and business. He was involved in research in the Royal College of Surgeons (Dublin, Ireland) as part of a research group investigating injury surveillance and load management in schoolboys rugby in Dublin. He is a guest lecturer at Florida International University. David's work focuses on injury prevention strategies, movement analysis, load management of tendons and the rehabilitation of injuries such as ACL, shoulder instability and hamstring strains. He has written articles in The Times (UK) as a sports medicine opinion expert.

Nicholas Clark, PhD, MSc, MCSP, MMACP, CSCS
Physiotherapy Lecturer and Researcher in the School of Sport, Rehabilitation and Exercise Sciences, University of Essex, UK; External Examiner for masters and doctoral degree programmes in the United Kingdom, Knee Consultant Physiotherapist. As a chartered physiotherapist with more than 21 years of clinical experience, Nick has practiced in London NHS teaching hospitals, at Saracens Rugby Union Football Club, with the British Army Infantry and Parachute Regiments, and in private practice. Nick's teaching roles have included Visiting Lecturer and External Examiner to the MSc Manual Therapy and MSc Sports Physiotherapy degrees at University College London, Clinical Tutor and Examiner for the Musculoskeletal Association of Chartered Physiotherapists (MACP), teaching exercise rehabilitation instructors and physiotherapists for the Ministry of Defence, and teaching on sports medicine masters and doctoral degrees in the United States. Nick also serves as a manuscript reviewer for scientific and clinical journals.

Paul Comfort, BSc (Hons) Sports Science, MSc Exercise and Nutrition Science, PhD in Sports Biomechanics and Strength and Conditioning, PGCAP
Reader in Strength and Conditioning and programme leader for the MSc Strength and Conditioning, University of Salford, UK. Professional Member British Association of Sport and Exercise Sciences (BASES) Certified Strength and Conditioning Coach, recertified with Distinction (CSCS*D) with the National Strength and Conditioning Association (NSCA); Accredited Strength and Conditioning Coach (ASCC) with the United Kingdom Strength and Conditioning Association (UKSCA), Founder Member of the UKSCA. During his time at the University of Salford, Paul has consulted with numerous professional rugby league, rugby union and football teams, in addition to coordinating the sports science support and strength and conditioning for England Men's Lacrosse (2008–2012). He has co-authored >150 peer reviewed journal articles and is on the editorial boards for the Journal of Strength and Conditioning Research, Sports Biomechanics and the European Journal of Sport Science.

Paulina Czubacka, BSc Sport Rehabilitation and Exercise Science, BASRaT-reg.

Paulina graduated from the University of Nottingham in 2017 and following her elective placement at the club, she joined Notts County FC as a First Team Sport Rehabilitator. Currently Paulina works at Nottingham Trent University as a lead therapist for Women's and Men's Football Programme, Men's Basketball Programme, as well as Nottingham Forest Women's Football Club. She is also working in the private sector at a Physiotherapy & Sport Rehabilitation Clinic – Nottingham Physio. Paulina's work is primarily focused around lower limb rehabilitation. She is passionate about end stage and return to play rehab.

Eamonn Delahunt, PhD, BSc, MISCP

Professor, University College Dublin, Dublin, Ireland. Eamonn is recognized nationally and internationally as a leading academic sports physiotherapist. He has published >120 peer-reviewed articles.

Carrie Docherty, PhD, LAT, ATC

Dr. Docherty is the Executive Associate Dean in the School of Public Health – Bloomington at Indiana University. She is also a Professor in the Department of Kinesiology and the Program Director of the Graduate Athletic Training Program. Her research focuses on rehabilitation sciences, specifically how chronic ankle instability affects the ability to participate in physical activity and health related quality of life. She is an internationally recognized scholar and educator in athletic training.

Jon Fearn, MSc, MACP, MCSP

First Team Physiotherapist, Chelsea Football Club. Jon's career in professional football spans over 20 years, with the past 10 years at Chelsea FC. Jon's work is primarily involved in managing the rehabilitation of first team players after injury and overseeing the Medical Department in the Academy. He also speaks on a number of postgraduate MSc courses and occasionally represents the Chelsea medical team at international conferences.

Ian Gatt, MSc, OMT, MAACP, MCSP, SRP, BSc (Hons)

Head of Performance Services and Lead Physiotherapist for GB Boxing. Ian has been a sport physiotherapist for over 20 years, working predominately in Olympic and Professional boxing. He is an Upper Limb Injury specialist with the prestigious English Institute of Sport (EIS), providing an advisory role particularly on Hand-Wrist injuries. Ian has lectured on Sporting Upper Limb biomechanics and injuries through various platforms, as well as collaborating on several publications. He is currently a PhD candidate with Sheffield Hallam University on wrist kinematics in boxing.

Michael Giakoumis, MSc (Exercise Science S&C), MSc (Sports Physiotherapy), BSc (Physiotherapy)

Sports Physiotherapist and Medical Research and Innovation Lead at British Athletics, the Centre for Health and Human Performance (CHHP), and Total Performance UK. Michael's career has involved working across Australian rules and European football, the NBA, and international athletics. His work focuses on the diagnosis, management and rehabilitation of lower limb injuries, with a particular interest in the hip and groin, and lower limb tendon and muscle injuries.

Mark Glaister, BSc, PhD, FACSM

Reader in Exercise Physiology, HEA Senior Fellow, Faculty of Sport, Health and Applied Sciences, St Mary's University, Twickenham, UK. Mark gained his doctorate from the University of Edinburgh and is currently working and researching at St Mary's University, Twickenham. His research interests are in physiological responses to multiple sprint work as well as the effects of various ergogenic aids, particularly caffeine.

Paul Godfrey, MSc, PGDMT(Aus), Grad Dip Phys, MACP, AACP, ACPSEM(Gold), HCPC

Head of Medical & Performance Services at Coventry City FC. Paul is a Chartered Manipulative Physiotherapist and Physiologist with extensive clinical experience of working with individuals and teams across a number of sporting codes and performance genres at national and international levels in the UK and abroad. He has worked with elite athletes in a variety sports for the English Institute for Sport (EIS), UK Athletics (UKA) and a number of professional football teams across all four divisions. Paul has also worked with artistic athletes from Cirque du Soleil and West End productions. Currently, his role involves the management and co-ordination of all the medical, rehabilitation and performance requirements of the club's first team & U23 players.

Neil Greig, PGDip (SEM), BSc (Hons) (Sports Therapy)

Head of the Medical Department, Brentford Football Club. Neil's career within professional sport has spanned 15 years, predominantly within elite football. His work focuses mainly on the rehabilitation of lower limb sports injury, with particular interests in knee pathologies and criteria-guided return to sport.

Tom Hallas, BSc

Tom currently works at Nottingham Forest academy as performance and rehabilitation therapist. In his role Tom liaises with the entire sports science and medicine team to deliver the rehabilitation programmes for injured U16-U23 players. Previously, Tom held the role of first team sports therapist at Notts County FC for five years. Tom has a keen interest in the area of rehabilitation of lower limb sporting injuries and is also a member of BASRAT.

Charlotte Häger, PhD (Neurophysiology), BSc (Physiotherapy)

Professor at the Department of Community Medicine and Rehabilitation, Physiotherapy, Umeå University, Sweden. Charlotte's research spans the study of basic movement functions in health and in pathological conditions to intervention studies and research on how to study and assess human movements reliably. She is head of the U-motion analysis laboratory and has a clinical affiliation to the Orthopaedic Clinic of Umeå University Hospital. Charlotte and her research group have published extensively on ACL injuries, particularly in relation to consequences of injury on movement patterns and strategies.

Kim Hébert-Losier, PhD, BSc (Physiotherapy)

Senior Lecturer for *Te Huataki Waiora* School of Health, Division of Health, Engineering, Computing and Science, University of Waikato, New Zealand. She is the lead biomechanics researcher at the University of Waikato Adams Centre for High Performance. Dr Hébert-Losier's work focuses on the objective quantification of human movement in health and sport, with a particular emphasis on the prevention of musculoskeletal injuries of the lower limb, sports performance, and clinical assessment methods.

Jackie Hindle, MSc, MMACP, MCSP

Senior Lecturer at Manchester Metropolitan University, Manchester, UK. Jackie is also a private practitioner. Jackie has been a member of the Musculoskeletal Association of Chartered Physiotherapists since 2002.

Jonathan Hobbs, BSc (physiotherapy), MSc (acupuncture), MCSP, FHEA

A physiotherapist with over 20 years clinical experience practising acupuncture and dry needling within the NHS, private sector and professional sport. He is a Fellow of the Higher Education Academy and Chairman of the Acupuncture Association of Chartered Physiotherapists. A previous school principal of physiotherapy he currently lectures internationally and consults for physiotherapists from the English Institute of Sport, Sport Wales, Premiership and Championship football clubs as well as the Ministry of Defence and the NHS.

Shivan Jassim, MBBS, BSc (Hons), MRCS, MSc (Sports & Exercise Medicine), FRCS (Tr & Orth)

Senior Orthopaedic Fellow in Melbourne, Australia. Shivan completed his specialist training on the Stanmore Rotation in London. He has worked as a pitch side Rugby Union doctor at International Level in the Men's and Women's games. He has a specialist interest in shoulder and elbow surgery and has just completed the Melbourne Orthopaedic Group Upper Limb Fellowship, which involved the treatment of several elite athletes in Australian Rules Football and Rugby League.

Lester Jones, BSc, MScMed, PGCE

Inaugural Chair of National Pain Group, Australian Physiotherapy Association. Lester is a pain physiotherapist with a wealth of experience spanning 25 years in education and clinical practice. He has worked in a range of clinical settings, including interdisciplinary clinics, with an emphasis on psychologically-informed assessment and treatment of pain. He is coauthor of the Pain and Movement Reasoning Model, a clincial reasoning tool that has been adapted and adopted to assist health practitioners assess pain in a range of settings, including pain associated with the musculoskeletal system, the pelvic region, with breastfeeding and in people who have survived torture or other traumatic experiences.

Paul A. Jones, PhD, MSc, BSc (Hons), CSCS*D, CSci, BASES Accredited

Lecturer in Sports Biomechanics/Strength and Conditioning at the University of Salford, UK. Paul earned a BSc (Hons) and MSc in Sports Science both from Liverpool John Moores University and a PhD in Sports Biomechanics at the University of Salford. He is a Certified Strength and Conditioning Specialist recertified with distinction (CSCS*D) with the National Strength and Conditioning Association (NSCA), an Accredited Sports and Exercise Scientist with the British Association of Sports and Exercise Sciences (BASES) and a Chartered Scientist (CSci) with The Science Council. Paul has over 18 years' experience in Biomechanics and Strength and Conditioning support to athletes and teams, working in sports such as athletics, football and rugby and was a former sports science support co-ordinator for UK disability athletics (2002–2006). Paul has authored/co-authored over 80 peer reviewed journal articles and is a member of the BASES Accreditation committee.

Dimitrios Kalogiannidis, MBBS, FRCEM, MsC SEM
First Team Club Doctor Chelsea Football Club, Emergency Medicine consultant and sport medicine doctor. Has been working at Chelsea FC for the past 6 years and has been involved with Chelsea Women's team, the Academy and Men's First Team. Dimitris's work is primarily now with managing day to day injuries and illnesses of athletes and preparation of Emergency Action plan. He is also currently covering medical care on all home and away games.

Simon Kemp
Associate Professor Simon Kemp is a Specialist Sports Medicine Doctor and the Medical Services Director for the Rugby Football Union, the National Governing Body for the game in England. He worked as a team physician in Rugby, Soccer (Fulham Football Club) and Basketball (English Basketball Team) from 1995 to 2013 and was the England team doctor for the Rugby World Cup campaigns in 2003 and 2007. He was the Tournament Medical Director for the 2015 Rugby World Cup. He has over 20 years of experience from clinical, research and policy perspectives in head injury management. He is a member of World Rugby's Medicine, Science and Research and Concussion working groups and the Football Association Independent Head Injury and Concussion Expert Panel.

Roger Kerry, PhD, MSc, BSc (Hons) Physiotherapy
Associate Professor, Faculty of Medicine and Health Sciences at the University of Nottingham, UK. Roger is a qualified chartered physiotherapist, and an Honorary Fellow of the UK's Musculoskeletal Association of Chartered Physiotherapists. His interests are in adverse events and physiotherapy interventions of the head and neck, particularly on the causal nature of interventions.

Jason Laird, PG Dip (Advanced Musculoskeletal Physiotherapy), MSc (Physiotherapy), BSc (Sport Rehabilitation)
Lead Physiotherapist, British Gymnastics and English Institute of Sport, Lillieshall National Sports Centre, Shropshire, UK. Jason is an experienced sports physiotherapist currently working for the English Institute of Sport as the Lead Physiotherapist for British Gymnastics. Prior to his work in Gymnastics, he worked for British Judo as the Lead Physiotherapist during the Rio 2016 cycle. Jason has extensive experience of elite performance environments having previously worked at the Chelsea FC Academy and the Royal Ballet Company.

Etienne Laverse, MBBS, BSc (Hons), MRCP (UK) (Neurology)
Research Fellow in Traumatic Brain Injury at UCL Institute of Neurology, Queen Square, UK and a Consultant Neurologist in the NHS.

Elaine Lonnemann, PT, DPT, OCS, MTC, FAAOMPT Adv MSC PT
Doctor of Physical Therapy, BS in Physical Therapy; Program Director for the Transitional Doctor of Physical Therapy program, University of Louisville University of St Augustine for Health Sciences; Associate Professor at Bellarmine University in Louisville, Kentucky. Elaine has been involved in teaching in the distance education programme with the University of St Augustine since 1998. She has worked as a physical therapist at Northside Hospital and Sullivan Center in East Tennessee, Flagler Hospital, University of Louisville Hospital, and Roane Physical Therapy in Rockwood, Tennessee. She is a member and a fellow of AAOMPT, and a member of the American Physical Therapy Association (APTA), chair of the AAOMPT's international monitoring and educational standards committee and a member of the board of directors of Physiopedia. She was the 2017 recipient of the John McMillan Mennell Service of AAOMPT.

Tommy Lundberg, PhD Sports Science
Lecturer and researcher at the Division of Clinical Physiology, Karolinska Institutet, Stockholm, Sweden. Tommy's ongoing research project relates to nonsteroidal antiinflammatory drugs and muscle adaptations to exercise regimes. Given the need for effective countermeasures to combat muscle atrophy within the clinical setting (sarcopenia, various muscle disorders, etc.) these studies could have a significant impact on exercise and/or medical prescriptions for maintaining muscle health.

Marc-André Maillet, MSc (Coaching Education & Sports Pedagogy)
Founder and Chief Education Officer at Beyond Pulse in Portland, Oregon USA. Former Ohio University lecturer. Marc-André is dedicated to help improve coaching behavior in youth sports.

Aneil Malhotra, MB BChir, MA, MRCP(UK), MSc, PhD, FESC
Aneil is a Presidential Senior Lecturer, University of Manchester, and Consultant Cardiologist, Wythenshawe Hospital and Manchester Royal Infirmary and Manchester Institute of Heath and Performance.

Simon Marsh, BA, MB BChir, MA, MD, FRCSEng, FRCSGen Surg
Consultant Surgeon and Surgical Director of the Gilmore Groin and Hernia Clinic, London, UK. Simon trained at Trinity College Cambridge and the Clinical School, Addenbrooke's Hospital, and was one of the few students to be awarded the William Harvey Studentship in consecutive years. He qualified in 1987, receiving the London FRCS in 1992. In 1996 he was awarded an MD by the University of Cambridge and received the Intercollegiate Fellowship in General Surgery. In 1999, he joined the Gilmore Groin and Hernia Clinic and has been Surgical Director since 2010. Working with Jerry Gilmore, he has modified, and improved, the original Gilmore's groin repair technique into what is now known as a groin reconstruction (the Marsh modification of the Gilmore technique).

Karen May, MSc Sports Med, PGCE LTHE, FHEA, MCSP, HCPC
Principle Lecturer and Academic Lead for Performance Medicine, the School of Medicine, University of Central Lancashire, UK. Prior to joining the University of Central Lancashire, Karen worked as a lead physiotherapist for both professional and semiprofessional sports covering rugby league Super League in England and Australia, rugby union, club, county and international U21 and England junior women's basketball and UK Athletics multi-events team. She continues to work with Olympic skiers, GB mountain & fell runners, and ultra distance runners. Karen has 25 years of experience of working with musculoskeletal and sports injuries and has focused her clinical research with published papers on whole-body cryotherapy and the effects of localized cryotherapy on joint position sense.

Bruno Mazuquin, PhD, MSc, BSc (Physiotherapy)
Research Fellow in Physiotherapy, Clinical Trials Unit, University of Warwick and Department of Health Professions, Manchester Metropolitan University, UK. Bruno's work is focused on the rehabilitation of musculoskeletal disorders, especially on shoulders. His work also involves the clinical application of biomechanics, evidence-based practice development and epidemiology.

Steve McCaig, BSc Physiotherapy (Hons), MSc Manipulative Therapy
Athlete Health Consultant, English Institute of Sport, Loughborough, UK. Steve has worked as a physiotherapist in elite sport for over 14 years. Previously he was a senior physiotherapist at the England and Wales Cricket Board. He has been involved in research in a number of areas including injury surveillance, workload, bowling biomechanics and low back pain in cricketers. He is currently completing a PhD in throwing arm pain in cricketers.

Christopher J. McCarthy, PhD, PGDs Biomechanics, Man. Therapy, Physiotherapy, FCSP, FMACP
Consultant Physiotherapist and Spinal Fellow, Department of Health Professions, Manchester Metropolitan University, Manchester, UK. After qualifying as a physiotherapist in 1989 Chris undertook postgraduate training in biomechanics and manipulative therapy before undertaking a PhD in rehabilitation within the Faculty of Medicine at Manchester University. Following postdoctoral studies investigating the subclassification of nonspecific low back pain, he joined Imperial College Healthcare. He now teaches and runs the clinical facility of Manchester School of Physiotherapy and teaches internationally on manual therapy, specifically on combined movement theory. He regularly reviews and publishes papers in the academic field of manual therapy. He was awarded a Fellowship of the MACP for advances in manual therapy in 2010 and a Fellowship of the Chartered Society of Physiotherapy in 2011.

Ruth MacDonald
Senior lecturer in physiotherapy at Manchester Metropolitan University, UK. Ruth completed her MSc in Manual Therapy in 2007 and became a member of the MACP in 2004. She continues to work in private practice.

David McKay, B.S. Sports Medicine and Exercise Science, CSCS, USSF A license, UEFA B license
First team assistant coach/performance coach for the Philadelphia Union. He previously served as the director of fitness for Orlando City Soccer Club and assistant fitness coach for Sporting Kansas City.

Jamie McPhee, PGCAP, FHEA, PhD Skeletal Muscle and Exercise Physiology, BSc, Sport and Exercise Science
Deputy Director of University Alliance Doctoral Training Alliance in Applied Biosciences for Health, member of the Management Board at Manchester Interdisciplinary Centre for Research into Ageing (MICRA), Manchester, UK. Jamie is also an expert advisor to several public health groups on falls prevention, Physical Deputy Director of Musculoskeletal Sciences Research, Lead of the Neuromuscular and Skeletal Ageing Research Group, Lead BSc Applied and Environmental Physiology.

Akbar de Medici, MBBS, BSc (Hons), PhD MRCS
Dr de Medici is an Honorary Associate Professor at UCL/UCLH and supported the creation of the Institute of Sport Exercise and Health (ISEH), a major legacy of the 2012 Olympic Games. Akbar has worked closely with the CMO of the NFL, supporting medical provisions for the London games since 2015. He also is the founding partner of Cavendish Health - a leading international health management company.

Said Mekary, PhD in Exercise Physiology
Dr Said Mekary is the Director of the Acadia Active Aging program, an associate professor and exercise physiologist in the School of Kinesiology at Acadia University. He is an emerging scholar with a broad background in the biological and cardiovascular health sciences who has established himself as an up-and-coming leader in the field of exercise physiology, cardiovascular aging and cognition studies in Canada. Dr Mekary was recently awarded the Acadia University Faculty of Professional Studies Outstanding Research Project Award for his work on the role of pulmonary physiology and exercise. Dr Mekary also continues to have applied research interests in the outcomes of exercise interventions in athletes, aging populations, and those with chronic disease and disability.

Claire Minshull, PhD, BSc, PGCHE
Claire is Principal Researcher at the RJAH Orthopaedic Hospital, UK and Director and founder of Get Back To Sport, an education and training company for healthcare professionals. Claire completed her PhD in neuromuscular physiology and exercise science at the University of Wales, Bangor in 2004. She has worked for over 20 years years in academia, research and in practice, including as Senior Lecturer at Nottingham Trent University; collaboration lead between between Universities in Edinburgh and the Royal Infirmary of Edinburgh on physiotherapy-focused clinical trials and, in a rehabilitation role with individual patients and athletes. Claire's research and teaching interests include the influences of exercise and conditioning on rehabilitation endeavours and in the management of osteoarthritis.

James Moore, MPhtySt (Manips), MSc App Biomechanics, BSc (Hons), CSCS
Founder and Director of Sports and Exercise Medicine for the Centre for Health and Human Performance (CHHP), London, UK. James has had an expansive career in sport both as a clinician and a leader. He has worked in cricket for 5 years, with England Rugby Elite Performance Squad in the preparation for the Rugby World Cup 2011, and with Saracens RFC as Head of Medical Services. He has also been involved in four Olympic cycles, culminating in being Deputy Chef De Mission for Performance Services for Team GB at the Olympic Games Rio 2016, the most successful games to date for the British Olympic Association. James has lectured on hip and groin and hamstring injuries, as well as lower limb biomechanics for over 15 years, and is currently a PhD candidate with University College London for modelling the hip.

Puneet Monga, MBBS, MS (Orth.), DNB, MRCS, Dip Sports Med (GB&I), MSc, FRCS (Tr & Orth.), MD
Consultant Orthopaedic Surgeon at Wrightington Hospital, Wigan, UK. Puneet has a specialist clinical practice focusing on shoulder problems. His surgical practice focuses on arthroscopic shoulder surgery, sports injuries and shoulder replacement surgery. His research interests include biomechanics of the shoulder, assessment of surgical outcomes and the application of modern technology, including the use of 3D printing to improve surgical treatment.

Jim Moxon, MB ChB, MRCGP, MSc (MSK ultrasound), MFSEM
Head of Football Medicine and Fitness, Liverpool FC Academy, Liverpool, UK. Jim's research work is focused on the application of shearwave elastography to muscles and tendons.

Ali Noorani, MBBS, BSc (Hons), MRCS, FRCS (Trauma & Orth)
Consultant Trauma & Orthopaedic Surgeon in shoulder, elbow and upper limb surgery at St Bartholomew's and the Royal London Hospital, Barts Health NHS Trust, London, UK. Ali is also the Medical Director of an elite group of surgeons called Orthopaedic Specialists and also the Medical Director of Harley Street Specialist Hospital. He has specialist interests in sports injuries and joint preservation of the shoulder and elbow.

Aidan O'Connell
High Performance Manager with Cork GAA. Formerly Strength and Conditioning Coach with Munster Rugby and the IRFU from 2001–2019. Aidan graduated with a Sport Science Degree from the University of Limerick in 1997 and received his Masters in Coaching Studies from the University of Edinburgh in 2001.

Des O'Shaughnessy
Bachelor of Applied Science (Physiotherapy), Masters of Science Module, ESP for the Allied Health Professional, Masters of Public Health Module. Des works in the Alice Springs Pain Clinic and in private practice, Connections Physical Therapy. Des graduated over 20 years ago from the University of Sydney, and worked in Sydney and Alice Springs. Over half of his clinical experience has been in the UK including as the Clinical Specialist Lead for the Islington Primary Care Trust Musculoskeletal Outpatients Service. He has also worked in the community development field working with indigenous communities of Central Australia addressing their levels of disadvantage.

Jason Palmer, B.H.M.S.(Ed.) Hons., B.Phty.
Jason is an Australian born and trained physiotherapist with more than 25 years' experience working in professional sport. Jason moved to the UK in 2001 to join Fulham Football Club's Medical staff as they entered the English Premiership, before moving to Chelsea Football Club in 2008 where he remains a consultant physiotherapist.

Ioannis Paneris
Ioannis qualified as a physiotherapist in 2006 and completed his MSc in manual therapy in 2013. He has more than 20 years of clinical experience as a physiotherapist in the NHS with the last 19 years in neuro-musculoskeletal care. Since 2008 he has worked as an Advanced Practitioner in central Manchester. He has lectured in manual and neuro-musculoskeletal postgraduate courses for a number of UK universities and he has made chapter contributions in a number of neuro-musculoskeletal physiotherapy and rehabilitation publications. He is an associate lecturer at Manchester Metropolitan University.

Amanda Parry, BSc (Hons) Radiography, PGDip Medical Ultrasound (Aust), PGCert MSK Ultrasound
Amanda is currently studying for MSc in Ultrasound. Amanda is a sonographer with a special interest in musculoskeletal ultrasound; she has been practising for 20 years both in the UK and Australia, in the public and private sector. She currently works within the NHS, alongside sports physicians, orthopaedic surgeons, radiologists and other allied health practitioners.

Nic Perrem, BSc, MSc (Sports Injury Management), BSc (Hons) (Sports Therapy), MSST (Member of the Society of Sports Therapists)
Lecturer in Sport Rehabilitation, St Mary's University, London, UK. Nic is a graduate sports therapist who holds full membership of the Society of Sports Therapists alongside associate membership of the British Association of Sport and Exercise Medicine (BASeM) and professional membership of the British Association of Sport and Exercise Sciences (BASES). Nic holds professional qualifications in manual and manipulative therapy, acupuncture and dry needling, kinesiology taping (RockDoc certified), pitch-side emergency trauma, nutrition and personal training. He has also worked in private practice with varied patient case load. At St Mary's Nic teaches at both undergraduate and postgraduate levels. He is currently engaged in a number of research projects examining factors related to lower limb injury and motor control and is an active member of the Knee Injury Control and Clinical Advancement (KICCA) research group.

Jim Richards, PhD, MSc, BEng
Professor of Biomechanics and Research Lead, Allied Health Research Unit, University of Central Lancashire, UK. Jim's work includes the clinical application of biomechanics, the development of new assessment tools for chronic disease, conservative and surgical management of orthopaedic and neurological conditions and development of evidence-based approaches for improving clinical management and rehabilitation.

James Rowland, PGDip (Sports Physiotherapy), BSc (Hons) Physiotherapy
Senior 1st Team Physiotherapist, Cardiff City Football Club. James has worked in professional football for 10 years, operating from the Premier League to League Two. He has particular interest in the delivery and design of return-to-play protocols, with research interests in isometric posterior chain strength and fatigue-profiling during fixture congested schedules.

Diane Ryding, MSc, BSc (Hons) (Physiotherapy)
Head Physiotherapist for the Foundation and Youth Development Phases at Manchester United FC. Diane has been involved in academy football since 2004. Her role is to ensure that paediatric injuries are managed appropriately whilst considering growth and maturation and ensuring that the long-term athletic development of the player takes precedent over short-term gains. She also teaches on sports trauma management courses.

James Selfe, DSc, PhD, MA, GradDipPhys, FCSP
Professor of Physiotherapy, Manchester Metropolitan University, Manchester, UK. James led the first group to develop an anatomically based method to define a region of interest for thermal imaging analyses. He and his team have used this method to investigate skin temperature response to a variety of low-cost localized cryotherapy interventions which patients and healthcare professionals can apply in domestic environments. They have also used this method to investigate optimum treatment time dosage in whole-body cryotherapy.

Rohi Shah, BMBS, BMedSci, MRCS, MSc SEM
Trauma and Orthopaedic Specialty Registrar at the East Midlands South Deanery. Rohi has been the Club Doctor for Notts County Football Club for 6 years. He has a keen interest in pitch-side emergency care and has been at the forefront of developing and refining the Emergency Action Protocol. His surgical subspecialty interests include soft-tissue reconstruction and trauma surgery.

Adam Sheehan, MSc (Strength & Conditioning) BBUS
Head of Conditioning and Sport Science at Munster Rugby, Munster, Eire. Adam's work is focused on repeated high-intensity efforts in rugby union, specifically at peak game demands and effect on passage duration with respect to repeated high-intensity efforts. His work also involves athletic development and sport science integration.

Natalie Shur, MBChB, BMedSci (Hons), MRes, MRCP(UK)
Sport and Exercise Medicine Registrar and Clinical Research Fellow, University of Nottingham, UK. Dr Shur is currently undertaking a PhD at the University of Nottingham investigating the maintenance of muscle metabolic health in relation to immobilization and injury, before completing her specialty training in sport and exercise medicine.

Graham Smith, GradDipPhys, FCSP, DipTP, CertED
Rehabilitation and Sports Injury Consultant, Fellow of the Chartered Society of Physiotherapy and Chairman of the Society of Sports Therapists (UK). Graham is responsible for setting up and running the Football Association National Rehabilitation Centre at Lilleshall and has worked with British Olympic and representative teams, as well as in professional football. He now runs a clinic and consultancy in Glasgow, and lectures nationally and internationally on the treatment and rehabilitation of musculoskeletal injuries and sports injury management.

Paul Sindall, BSc, MSc, PhD, FHEA
Senior Lecturer at the University of Salford, UK. Paul is a member of the Peter Harrison Centre for Disability Sport and a member of the European Research Group in Disability Sport (ERGiDs). His PhD and masters studies were in exercise physiology, working in the field of disability sports testing and training. Paul has extensive practice-based and managerial experience in the health and fitness industry, and in the provision of sports science support services to athletes in a range of disability and able-bodied sports. He is interested in the role of exercise and physical activity in the prevention and treatment of disease.

Neil Sullivan, MSc, BSc (Hons), chartered physiotherapist, MCSP, MSST
Neil has over 16 years of experience in professional football, leading medical departments at Derby County, Oxford United and Peterborough FC. More recently Neil has focused on private practice and consultancy roles in Elite sports. He has a special interest in pelvic dysfunction and its implications to pain and performance.

Michael Sup, PhD
Michael is a Co-Founder of Beyond Pulse serving as the VP of Sports Education and Research. Michael has a coaching background and has served as an Academy Coach at Luton Town FC as well as a host of different coaching positions in the USA. Michael's research interests involve developing best practices in youth sports development and coaching education.

Richard Sylvester, MB BCh, PhD, FRCP
Consultant Neurologist at the National Hospital of Neurology and Honorary Lecturer at University College London specializing in the management of brain injury and cognitive disorders. Lead of the complex concussion clinic at the Institute of Sport Exercise and Health, UCL. Member of the traumatic brain injury advisory expert group of the Association of British Neurologists and English Football Association's Concussion Expert panel.

Alan J. Taylor, MSc, MCSP, HCPC
Physiotherapy Assistant Professor, Faculty of Medicine and Health Sciences at the University of Nottingham, UK. Alan is a qualified chartered physiotherapist, and a former professional cyclist. He also works as a medico-legal expert witness. His interests are in sports medicine, rehabilitation and haemodynamics. He has written widely on the topic of adverse events linked to physiotherapy interventions of the head and neck.

Mick Thacker, PhD, MSc, GradDipPhys, GradDipMan NMSD, FCSP
Associate Professor, Department of Allied Health Sciences Centre of Human & Aerospace Physiological Sciences, South Bank University, London, UK. Mick is also the director of the Pain: Science and Society MSc course at King's College London.

Keith Thornhill, MSc Exercise Science, BSc (Hons) Physiotherapy
Senior First Team Physiotherapist, Munster Rugby. Since graduating in 2007, Keith has worked in a variety of sporting environments, including Leeds Rhinos and currently Munster Rugby. Keith's current role focuses on the management of acute, short-term and ongoing injuries occurring within the squad. Keith has a particular interest in the promotion of injury reduction strategies and building robustness in a team environment.

Cari Thorpe, BSc, PGcert, MCSP, HCPC
Senior Lecturer in Physiotherapy, Manchester Metropolitan University, UK. Cari has a postgraduate certificate in advanced physiotherapy and is currently working towards her PhD, the focus of which is injury prevention in touch (rugby). This involves reviewing recovery strategies and the use of cryotherapy in the reduction of symptoms and enhancement of performance of elite touch players within a tournament situation. Cari has been the Head of Medical Services of England Touch (Rugby) for the past 5 years. This includes the management of a multidisciplinary team of sport science and physiotherapy staff, updating protocols for preseason screening, injury management and recovery to prevent and minimize the effect of injury.

Tony Tompos, PgDip (Physiotherapy), BSc Hons (Sports Rehabilitation)
Sports Physiotherapist. Tony has worked in professional football for more than 7 years, both in the English Football League and the Scottish Premiership. In 2017 Tony was awarded the Scottish League Award at the Football Medical Association annual awards ceremony for his role in improving the management of concussion protocols during football league matches. Tony has a keen interest in the rehabilitation of hamstring and ACL injuries.

Anna Waters, CPsychol AFBPsS, PhD, MSc, BSc
Director at Chimp Management Ltd., Anna has over 15 years' experience of working within professional and Olympic sports, as well as with performers in the arts, including ballet dancers, actors, singers and classical musicians. Anna's research has focused on understanding the role of psychology in athletic injury and developing psychological interventions to facilitate return to sport.

Tim Watson, PhD, BSc(Hons), FCSP
Professor of Physiotherapy, University of Hertfordshire, Hatfield, UK. Tim trained as a physiotherapist before moving into academic work. He taught at Brunel University before taking up his current post. He is also a freelance consultant and provider of postgraduate education programmes, author and researcher. Tim was honoured with a Fellowship of the Chartered Society of Physiotherapy in 2013. His primary research interests are linked to Tissue Repair and Electrophysical modalities.

Daniel Williams, MBChB BSc (Hons), FRCS (Trauma and Ortho)
Research Fellow, Brisbane Hand and Upper Research Institute, Australia. Daniel completed his specialist training on the Percival Pott Rotation in London. He has a specialist interest in upper limb surgery and is currently undertaking a fellowship with the Brisbane Hand and Upper Research Institute, Australia.

Mark Wilson
UEFA A Licensed Coach, NSCAA DOC Diploma, Co-Founder of Beyond Pulse. Mark is a former professional football player who had a 16 year career. Mark played for Manchester United, Middlesborough, FC Dallas and represented England at U16–U21 levels. Post playing Mark was a Director of coaching for a multi-franchise USA youth soccer club overseeing 500 players and 65 staff. More recently Mark co-founded the Beyond Pulse EDTech platform and product in 2017 which now hosts 7500 players and hundreds of coaches across the USA and Canada. As a keynote speaker and TV football pundit, Mark enjoys sharing his thoughts and perceptions in the public domain.

I hated every minute of training, but I said, 'Don't quit. Suffer now and live the rest of your life as a champion.'

**Muhammad Ali, 1942–2016;
heavyweight champion of the world**

We dedicate this book to sportspeople of every age, ability and orientation who strive to excel, and deserve the best possible support from us medical professionals to achieve their goals.

Chapter | **1** |

Muscle form and function

Jamie McPhee and Tommy Lundberg

Neuromuscular control of movement

The incredible array of voluntary movements that humans can perform is made possible by effective neuromuscular interactions. Control of movements is complex and requires the cooperation of the central nervous system (CNS) and the peripheral nervous system (PNS). The CNS includes the brain and spinal cord, while the PNS includes all the nerve cells outside of the CNS and is further subdivided into sensory and motor portions.

Initiation of voluntary movement starts first with a rough draft of the planned movement created in motivational areas of the brain. The movement plan is sent to the cerebellum and the basal nuclei for conversion of the draft into more precise excitation orders. These motor programs are sent to the motor cortex, then on to the spinal neurons, and are finally transmitted from the CNS to the alpha motor neurons in the PNS. Some modifications are still possible along this command chain in response to subcortical and spinal centre inputs. For example, a planned movement sequence can be adjusted based on afferent sensory feedback from muscle spindles, golgi tendon organs and free nerve endings, known as proprioceptors, sensing pain and muscle stretch, tension and metabolites.

We control movements by increasing numbers of recruited motor units or their individual firing rates. A motor unit consists of a single alpha motor neuron and all of the muscle fibres it innervates. Limb muscles typically have hundreds or thousands of motor units and they range in size, with some small and some very large within the same muscle (Buchthal et al., 1959). In smaller muscles or where fine motor control is needed the numbers of fibres per motor unit (innervation ratio) is small, while in large and powerful muscles the innervation ratio can be as many as 2000 fibres per motor neuron (Buchthal et al., 1959). The 'size principle' describes a highly organized recruitment of motor units in order of their size, from the smallest progressively through to the largest, so that forces produced appropriately match the task demands (Henneman et al., 1965).

Skeletal muscle structure

Whole muscles

There are over 600 skeletal muscles in the human body and their combined mass accounts for 40–50% of total body weight in healthy adults (Al-Gindan et al., 2014) and over 60% for many athletes. Skeletal muscles generate the forces needed for voluntary movements and postural control, contribute to thermoregulation by generating heat from contractions, play a key role in whole-body metabolism and serve endocrine and paracrine functions by releasing growth hormones and other factors that regulate the function of other body organs.

Whole muscles are composed of lots of individual muscle cells, known as *muscle fibres*. They are characteristically long, generally cylindrical and enclosed by a layer of connective tissue known as the *endomysium*. A connective tissue layer called the *perimysium* surrounds groups of fibres organizing them into *fascicles*. Surrounding the whole muscle is the outermost layer of connective tissue called the *epimysium* and a connective tissue *fascia* separates muscles from one another. Several other cell and tissue types are also found within whole muscles, including (but not limited to) blood vessels, capillaries, immune cells and other blood components, as well as sensory and motor nerves.

The individual muscle fibres and associated connective tissue connect to tendons at both ends. The proximal tendon is known as the *origin* and the distal tendon is the *insertion*. A basic principle is that when activated, skeletal muscles shorten to produce force (note that muscles can also lengthen under tension by controlling the process of 'derecruitment' of muscle fibres). As the whole muscle shortens during contraction, the origin remains relatively fixed in position anchored to a bone, while the insertion is connected to a proximal region of a bone positioned distal to the rotating joint and is pulled by the tendon to cause movement.

Muscle arrangements

Muscles are arranged into opposing muscle groups: those that reduce a joint angle are known as *flexors* and those that extend a joint angle are *extensors*. For example, during knee extension the quadriceps muscle group increases the knee joint angle while the hamstrings passively lengthen to allow the knee extension to occur. The active muscle group is known as the *agonist* (quadriceps), while the inactive group is the *antagonist* (hamstrings). Other muscles can help to stabilize the joints during movements and are called *synergists*.

The fascicle arrangement varies from muscle to muscle. Some muscles have a *fusiform* arrangement where the individual muscle fibres are almost parallel and are directly in series with the origin and insertion tendons, for example the biceps brachii. Many of the large limb muscles have *pennate* fascicle arrangement where the fascicles are oblique to the tendon. For example, the vasti muscles of the quadriceps have pennate fascicles that intercept with the muscle's deep layer of connective tissue at angles of around 10–20 degrees. *Bipennate* muscles such as the rectus femoris of the quadriceps have a central strand of thick connective tissue running through the muscle belly and fascicles extend outwards from it obliquely (a bit like the barbs of a bird's feather extending out from the quill). Other more complex fascicle arrangements are also present, including *triangular* (such as pectoralis), *circumpennate* or cylindrical (tibialis anterior) and some *multipennate* muscles appear compartmentalized, with different pennation arrangements depending on the region being looked at, such as the deltoid. The fascicular orientation can influence the force and rate of contractions (Narici et al., 2016).

Microstructure and contractile proteins

Regardless of the fascicular arrangements, all skeletal muscle fibres share the same microstructure (Fig. 1.1). They are generally cylindrical, thin, elongated and can span the full length of the whole muscle or may start or terminate within the fascicle. The fibre cell membrane is called the *sarcolemma* and the inside of the cell is the *sarcoplasm* where all the contractile proteins and organelles are located. Fibres have very many nuclei that contain the entire gene pool and express genes needed to maintain the muscle fibre structure and function. Specialized types of stem cells called *satellite cells* contribute to growth, development and repair of muscle fibres (Pallafacchina et al., 2013).

The proteins regulating muscle contraction are the most abundant proteins and account for about 85% of the fibre volume. Other sarcoplasmic proteins and mitochondrial proteins account for about 10% and 5% of the fibre volume, respectively (Lüthi et al., 1986). Contractile proteins are arranged along *myofibrils* that appear as long, repetitive strands of smaller functional units in series and in parallel known as *sarcomeres*. Sarcomeres are the smallest contractile units and are primarily composed of the contractile proteins *actin* and *myosin* organized along *thin* and *thick filaments*, respectively, and have a striated appearance. The thin filament also includes tropomyosin and troponin. One end of each thin filament is anchored to a Z-disc, which joins successive sarcomeres in series.

Muscle contraction and energy for movement

The sliding filament theory of muscle contraction

The sliding filament theory describes our general understanding of how muscle contraction occurs. When a muscle fibre is activated by the nervous system, calcium ions are released into the sarcoplasm and the myosin on the thick filament can form a *cross bridge* with actin on the thin filament. The myosin head 'pivots' to produce the *power stroke* causing thin filaments to 'slide' across the thick filaments towards the centre of the sarcomere. This process uses energy liberated from the high-energy bonds of adenosine triphosphate (ATP) to leave behind an inorganic phosphate (Pi) and adenosine diphosphate (ADP).

Energy for movement

ATP is synthesized from chemical energy in the form of fats, carbohydrates and proteins that are consumed as part of the diet, and muscles turn this chemical energy into mechanical energy during contractions. Fat is the most abundant energy store and a gram contains approximately 9 kcal of energy, compared with carbohydrate and proteins that contain about 4 kcal of energy per gram. Carbohydrates are stored as glucose chains called *glycogen* in the liver and other cells, with the largest stores in skeletal muscles. The liver glycogen reserves are

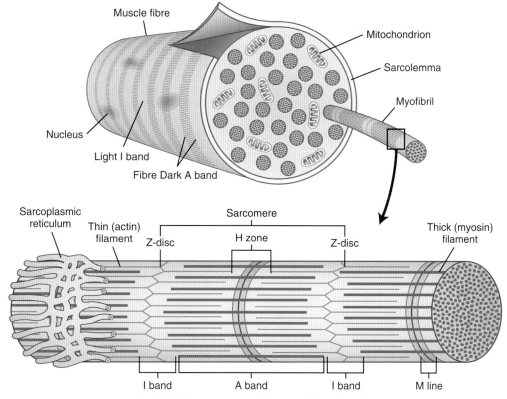

Muscle fibre
Mitochondrion
Sarcolemma
Myofibril
Nucleus
Light I band
Fibre Dark A band

Sarcoplasmic reticulum
Thin (actin) filament
Z-disc
Sarcomere
H zone
Z-disc
Thick (myosin) filament

I band
A band
I band
M line

Fig. 1.1 Microstructure of human skeletal muscle.

used to replenish blood glucose levels when they are low and the muscle glycogen provides large local reserves of glucose immediately available to fuel contractions. Protein makes a smaller direct contribution to overall energy stores, but the constituent amino acids are important metabolic intermediates during energy metabolism and in times of need the amino acid alanine can be converted to glucose in the liver.

There are three main metabolic pathways that synthesize ATP, described as anaerobic (not requiring oxygen) or aerobic (requiring oxygen).

1. The anaerobic *phosphocreatine (PCr) reaction* is the simplest and fastest way to resynthesize ATP. It is catalysed by the enzyme creatine kinase and can be thought of as taking a phosphate from a high-energy creatine–phosphate bond and giving it to ADP, resulting in a free creatine molecule and ATP:

$$ADP + PCr \rightarrow ATP + Cr$$

2. Anaerobic *glycolysis* is the conversion of glucose into 2 pyruvate + 2 ATP. The pyruvate can enter mitochondria to be used for aerobic ATP production during steady-state muscle contractions, or when energy demands are very high, pyruvate accepts hydrogen ions to form lactate. Lactate appearance in the blood is commonly used as a marker of high metabolic rate and fatigue.

3. Aerobic ATP production takes place in specialized organelles called *mitochondria* that convert pyruvate (the product of glycolysis) and fatty acids into ATP needed for prolonged low or moderate intensity activities. Although not a primary energy source in healthy humans, some amino acids (the constituent parts of proteins) can also be used by mitochondria to produce ATP. The aerobic process involves two chemical pathways, the citric acid cycle (also called the Krebs cycle) and the electron transport chain. When pyruvate passes through aerobic respiration the net ATP gain is 32 or 33, depending on whether glucose was formed as glycogen in the first instance. When a typical fatty acid such as palmitate passes through aerobic respiration the net ATP yield is 129.

Contractile properties of muscle

The existence of different fibre types in skeletal muscle has long been recognized. The original basis for classification of

Table 1.1 Characteristics of the different muscle fibre types

	Type 1	Type 2A	Type 2X
Shortening velocity	Slow	Fast	Very fast
Power production	Low	High	Highest
Recruitment threshold	Low	Higher	Highest
Motor units	Small	Larger	Largest
Mitochondrial content	High	Less	The least
Glycolytic capacity	Moderate	High	High
Fatigue resistance	Very high	Moderate	Low

fibre types as red, white or intermediate arose from visual inspection of animal muscle tissue. Since the 1960s, when the percutaneous muscle biopsy procedure was reintroduced, it has been possible to obtain muscle samples from volunteers and studies have revealed differences in the composition and biochemical properties of muscle fibres that can be distinguished using gel electrophoresis or different histochemical staining techniques. By incubating muscle samples at different pH levels, the fibre type composition can be determined enzymatically according to their myosin ATPase activity. Alternatively, muscle fibre types can be determined by staining them with specific antibodies against the slow and fast myosin heavy chain isoforms.

There are three main fibre types found in skeletal muscle, usually known as type 1, type 2A and type 2X. Most skeletal muscles contain these three pure fibre types, but so-called 'hybrid' fibres with mixed characteristics are also present. The muscle fibres of a single motor unit all share the same phenotypic characteristics (i.e., slow or fast) and will contract or relax at the same time in an 'all or none' manner.

The major functional difference between the fibre types is the speed of contraction and relaxation. The slow type 1 fibres have a long time to peak force and the relaxation time is correspondingly long. Fast-twitch fibres, on the other hand, are fast contracting and the relaxation time is shorter. For example, the fastest fibres have a maximum shortening velocity that is about four times greater than type 1 fibres (Bottinelli et al., 1996). Since power is the product of force and velocity, the differences in peak power between fibre types are greater than for force and velocity alone. The typical characteristics of the different fibre types are further outlined in Table 1.1. The slow fibres also possess higher numbers of mitochondria and high capillary-to-fibre ratio than the fast

fibres and these features give a higher capacity for aerobic ATP production and fatigue resistance. The fastest 2X fibres are generally, but not always, larger than the type 1 fibres and apart from the different myosin heavy chain composition and the faster speed of contraction, they contain rapidly acting myosin ATPases (enzymes responsible for splitting the high-energy bonds in ATP) and show a greater glycolytic capacity than the slow fibres. The type 2A fibres are generally seen as intermediate fibres with faster rates of contraction than the type 1 fibres, intermediate mitochondria and capillary densities, and they are less fatigable than type 2X but fatigue more than type 1 (see Table 1.1).

Muscle mechanics and their application for force, speed and power

Excitation–contraction coupling

Signals instructing muscle recruitment are relayed along motor neurons as *action potentials* at more than 50 m/s and can discharge at 5–30 times per second (Enoka and Fuglevand, 2001). An action potential arriving at the motor nerve terminal triggers release of the specialized neurotransmitter *acetylcholine*, which attaches to its receptors on the muscle fibre membrane and stimulates an action potential along the muscle fibre and the release of Ca^{2+} into the sarcolemma, which is needed for the cross-bridge function underpinning muscle contraction. Thus, arrival of action potentials from the motor neuron on to the muscle fibre dictates muscle contractions. This process is known as *excitation–contraction coupling*.

Stretch–shortening cycle

In addition to neural control, there are also several mechanical factors that affect the muscle's force-producing capacity. One of the more important of those factors is the type of muscle action used. Muscle actions can be divided into isometric actions and dynamic actions. In isometric actions the muscle remains at the same length whilst under tension. For example, the elbow flexors perform isometric contractions when holding a weight in the hand with the elbow flexed at 90 degrees and remaining at the same angle. Dynamic actions can be further divided into concentric and eccentric muscle actions. In concentric actions muscles shorten while producing tension, causing the joint angle to change (remember that extensors increase joint angles and flexors decrease joint angles). For instance, concentric elbow flexor contractions progressively decrease the joint angle when lifting a weight. Conversely, the muscle lengthens under tension during eccentric contractions, such as lowering a weight using eccentric elbow flexor contractions. The majority of everyday activities involve successive combinations of eccentric and concentric muscle actions, such as walking, running, jumping or lifting/lowering objects, and this is termed the *stretch–shortening cycle*.

Muscle force is highest in isometric and eccentric muscle actions, compared with concentric actions. This is because at any given time, more actin and myosin cross-bridges are in the attached position during an isometric and eccentric action compared with a concentric action where more time of the cross-bridge cycle is spent in the loose state. There is also consensus that muscle force and power is enhanced in movements involving the stretch–shortening cycle. Although the precise mechanisms for this effect are still under debate, it appears to be due to *potentiation*, which is a term used to describe a process by which initial muscle activation 'primes' the muscles for further contractions, of both contractile and elastic elements.

Length–tension and force–velocity relationships

There is an optimal length of each muscle fibre relative to its ability to generate force. This is termed the *length–tension relationship* (Fig. 1.2). The optimal sarcomere length is where there is optimal overlap of thick and thin filaments (Gordon et al., 1966). Force production is impaired when sarcomere lengths are too short because there is overlap of the actin filaments from opposite ends of the sarcomere. There is also a reduced force capacity when the sarcomere is stretched beyond the optimal length because this also reduces the overlap between actin and myosin filaments. The optimal sarcomere length occurs when muscles are slightly stretched beyond their natural resting length. For example, in the knee extensors and elbow flexors, optimal angle occurs at joint angles of around 80 degrees (taking full extension as 0 degrees).

The so-called *force–velocity relationship* also determines the muscle's ability to produce force and power. As the velocity of muscle action is increased, less force can be generated during the contraction (Hill, 1938). In simple words, the maximal force that can be produced by a muscle is lower during fast movements than it is for slower movements. This is explained at the myofilament level by the time taken for cross-bridges to attach and detach. Specifically, the total number of cross-bridges attached at any given time decreases with increased velocity of muscle shortening, and since the amount of force produced by the muscle is related to the number of cross-bridges formed, force production decreases with increased speed.

Muscle power is different from muscle force. Power is determined by the interaction between force and speed of contraction, and is calculated simply as force × velocity (it can also be expressed as work divided by time). Hence,

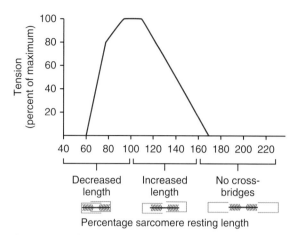

Fig. 1.2 Length–tension relationship of skeletal muscle. Note maximum force is reached during ideal sarcomere length.

muscle peak-power production occurs where the product of force and velocity is the greatest. Single fibres dissected out of a muscle biopsy tend to reach their peak power when the fibre generates only about 20% of peak force. In isolated movements such as seated knee extensions, peak power is typically achieved at speeds corresponding to about one-third of the maximal contraction velocity. However, the velocity at which peak power occurs will differ markedly depending on the type of exercise or loading strategy used.

The moment arm influences joint biomechanics

A muscle's ability to produce force will also vary depending upon the anatomical features of the joint being moved. The *moment arm* is the perpendicular distance from the point of application of muscle force (this is usually the tendon passing over a joint) to the point of joint rotation (which is usually close to the centre of the joint). Taking the knee joint as an example during knee extension, the patella tendon on the anterior aspect of the joint is the application of muscle force, while the centre of joint rotation occurs deep towards the centre of the knee joint: the distance between the centre of rotation and the patella tendon is the moment arm. The larger the moment arm, the larger the maximal possible moment force (or torque, which is a force that causes rotation). Thus, a muscle that is positioned with a large moment arm has a biomechanical advantage to a muscle with similar contractile force but with a smaller moment arm (Narici et al., 2016).

Twitches, summation and tetanus

If only a single action potential triggers Ca^{2+} release into the sarcoplasm to initiate cross-bridge function, then only a single *twitch* of the muscle will result. This twitch has a very brief latency period lasting only a few milliseconds, followed by a period of contraction generally lasting around 40 ms and then relaxation generally lasting around 50 ms. The timings of these phases depend on the fibre types, as slow type 1 fibres contract and relax slowly and the fast type 2 fibres have fast rates of contraction and relaxation due to faster Ca^{2+} release and myosin ATPase activity.

If a second action potential arrives before the muscle has fully relaxed, further Ca^{2+} is released and the resultant force builds upon the first in a process known as *summation*. Summation continues progressively with increasing rates of action potential arrival (motor unit firing rates) until a point is reached where no further summation is possible (usually at around 30–50 Hz in whole muscles), which is known as a *tetanus*. Muscle actions during whole-body movements result from this process of summation and the general principle is that higher motor unit firing rates produce higher muscle forces (Enoka and Fuglevand, 2001).

References

Al-Gindan, Y.Y., Hankey, C., Govan, L., Gallagher, D., Heymsfield, S.B., Lean, M.E., 2014. Derivation and validation of simple equations to predict total muscle mass from simple anthropometric and demographic data. The American Journal of Clinical Nutrition 100, 1041–1051.

Bottinelli, R., Canepari, M., Pellegrino, M.A., Reggiani, C., 1996. Force-velocity properties of human skeletal muscle fibres: myosin heavy chain isoform and temperature dependence. The Journal of Physiology 1 (495), 573–586.

Buchthal, F., Erminio, F., Rosenfalck, P., 1959. Motor unit territory in different human muscles. Acta physiologica Scandinavica 45, 72–87.

Enoka, R.M., Fuglevand, A.J., 2001. Motor unit physiology: some unresolved issues. Muscle & Nerve 24, 4–17.

Gordon, A.M., Huxley, A.F., Julian, F.J., 1966. The variation in isometric tension with sarcomere length in vertebrate muscle fibres. The Journal of Physiology 184, 170–192.

Henneman, E., Somjen, G., Carpenter, D.O., 1965. Functional significance of cell size in spinal motoneurons. Journal of Neurophysiology 28, 560–580.

Hill, A.V., 1938. The heat of shortening and the dynamic constants of muscle. Proceedings Biological Sciences 126 (843), 136–195.

Lüthi, J.M., Howald, H., Claassen, H., Rösler, K., Vock, P., Hoppeler, H., 1986. Structural changes in skeletal muscle tissue with heavy-resistance exercise. International Journal of Sports Medicine 7 (3), 123–127.

Narici, M., Franchi, M., Maganaris, C., 2016. Muscle structural assembly and functional consequences. The Journal of Experimental Biology 219, 276–284.

Pallafacchina, G., Blaauw, B., Schiaffino, S., 2013. Role of satellite cells in muscle growth and maintenance of muscle mass. Nutrition, Metabolism, and Cardiovascular Diseases: NMCD 23 (Suppl. 1), S12–S18.

Further reading

Jones, D.A., Round, J., de Haan, A., 2004. Skeletal Muscle from Molecules to Movement: A textbook of Muscle Physiology for Sport, Exercise, Physiotherapy and Medicine. Churchill Livingstone/Elsevier Ltd, London.

Scott Powers, Edward Howley, 2017. Exercise Physiology: Theory and application of fitness and performance, Tenth ed. McGraw-Hill Education, New York.

Roger Enoka, 2015. Neuromechanics of Human Movement, fifth ed. Human Kinetics, Leeds, UK.

Chapter 2

Muscle adaptations and fatigue

Tommy Lundberg and Jamie McPhee

Introduction

The body quickly adapts to new patterns of use, or disuse. This chapter sets out typical adaptations that occur with regular aerobic training and regular resistance training, focusing mainly on skeletal muscles. However, we also wish to point out that there is considerable interindividual variability in training adaptations, meaning that two people performing the same type and relative intensity of training may not experience the same physiological adaptations. The variability in exercise capacity and adaptation responses has a large heritable genetic component, but we still do not know which combinations of genes interact to create the potential to reach elite athlete status.

Muscle adaptations to endurance training

Important concepts related to endurance exercise

The maximal rate of oxygen uptake ($\dot{V}O_{2max}$) is important for endurance performance because it represents the maximal capacity for oxygen to be used to make energy during whole-body exercise such as running or cycling (Bassett and Howley, 2000). The workload, or exercise intensity, at which $\dot{V}O_{2max}$ occurs is also known as the peak aerobic power. This aerobic power is substantially lower than the maximal power that muscles can produce in very short-term efforts (Zoladz et al., 2000). For example, a trained cyclist might reach $\dot{V}O_{2max}$ at 450 W on a cycle ergometer, but if asked to produce a maximal effort lasting just 5 s the same cyclist might reach >1600 W, but performance would then plummet due to fatigue. Interestingly, even the

most motivated athletes can only work at $\dot{V}O_{2max}$ for short periods before fatigue forces them to slow down, because although the rate of aerobic respiration is high at $\dot{V}O_{2max}$, the flux through glycolysis is also very high and metabolites accumulate to cause fatigue (discussed below). Therefore, endurance sports such as long-distance running, road cycling and cross-country skiing are performed at intensities lower than $\dot{V}O_{2max}$ and rely primarily on aerobic adenosine triphosphate (ATP) production (Coyle, 1995; Faria et al., 2005).

Two other notable features also influence endurance performance: the lactate threshold and the peak rate of fat oxidation. The lactate threshold represents the workload at which lactate concentrations over a certain threshold (often 4 mmol/L) appears in the blood. This appearance signifies high rates of glycolysis beyond the ability for pyruvate (a product of glycolysis) to enter mitochondria. The pyruvate is transformed to lactate by accepting hydrogen (another product of glycolysis) and is released by the muscle. In untrained individuals, lactate threshold can be between 50–60% $\dot{V}O_{2max}$, but in trained individuals it can be as high as 80% $\dot{V}O_{2max}$. The peak rate of fat oxidation is the workload at which the aerobic breakdown of fatty acids to make energy reaches its peak, after which any further requirements for ATP must be met by glucose (Lundsgaard et al., 2018). It occurs at lower intensity than the lactate threshold, usually between 50–60% $\dot{V}O_{2max}$ and it is higher in trained athletes than nonathletes (Venables et al., 2005).

The endurance training stimulus

Exercise at or below the peak rate of fat oxidation will incur very little fatigue and can be maintained for hours, or days should the motivation be there. Exercise at the lactate threshold can be sustained for hours in trained people and is the intensity that a long-distance race is mostly completed. Exercise above the lactate threshold but below $\dot{V}O_{2max}$ can be sustained for relatively long periods of time. The average recreational runner maintains a pace just below the lactate threshold, but serious athletes deliberately include intervals above the lactate threshold and even above $\dot{V}O_{2max}$ to cause a higher training stimulus. The training presents a variety of physiological challenges, such as the need to replenish ATP and fuel stores, eliminate metabolites such as CO_2 and lactate, dissipate heat, maintain blood flow around the body and cope with sensory feedback that may be interpreted as unpleasant or painful.

The adaptation responses

The training stimulus leads to physiological adaptations that enhance the supply of oxygen to working skeletal muscles and the maximal aerobic metabolism of the active muscles. These adaptations increase $\dot{V}O_{2max}$, lactate threshold and the peak rate of fat oxidation (Jones and Carter, 2000). The important thing to keep in mind is that acute exercise is the stimulus, but the biochemical processes underpinning the long-term adaptations take place for several hours in the recovery period after exercise cessation. Therefore, long-term adaptations are triggered by summation of physiological responses to individual training sessions and the adaptations occur in the muscles that were active during exercise (Atherton et al., 2015).

$\dot{V}O_{2max}$ is improved mainly through increased capacity to transport oxygen through the cardiovascular system to the working muscles, not only those in the active limbs but also the respiratory and postural muscles. This in turn is linked to higher plasma and total blood volumes, increased haemoglobin content (red blood cells responsible for carrying oxygen in the blood) and increased contractility of cardiac muscles, especially of the left ventricle. Together, these adaptations increase stroke volume (the amount of blood pumped out of the heart) and thus, cardiac output (the product of stroke volume × heart rate) (Bassett and Howley, 2000). The maximal heart rate changes little with training and if anything, it may even decrease.

Peripheral muscle adaptations include increased muscle mitochondrial enzyme activity, mitochondrial and capillary densities, and intracellular lipid and glycogen stores (Gollnick et al., 1973; Hoppeler et al., 1985). Interestingly, the same stimuli responsible for initiating muscle contractions or those accumulating as a consequence of muscle contractions, including calcium, high-energy compounds – adenosine diphosphate (ADP) and adenosine monophosphate (AMP) – and fatty acid intermediates, alongside hormones and growth factors that circulate in the blood, also trigger cellular signalling processes. They activate secondary protein messengers and signalling molecules such as mitogen-activated protein kinase (MAPK) and AMP-activated protein kinase (AMPK) that in turn increase the expression of genes encoding the precise proteins needed to adapt (Hoppeler, 2016).

Mitochondrial biogenesis

Mitochondria increase in size and number in all three fibre types within just a few weeks of endurance training. The enzymes that coordinate ATP production within mitochondria also increase their activity so that each mitochondrion improves at utilizing any available oxygen and at using fatty acids as an energy source, which has the advantage of sparing glucose (Hoppeler and Fluck, 2003). Hence, the increase in mitochondrial volume is linearly related to increased muscle aerobic potential and endurance performance. A key signalling molecule regulating mitochondrial improvements is peroxisome proliferator-activated receptor gamma coactivator receptor 1-alpha (PGC-1α). PGC-1α activates various other signalling molecules that upregulate the expression of mitochondrial genes (mitochondria contain 37 genes held separate from the nucleus) and the nuclear genes. Single exercise bouts upregulate PGC-1α levels, priming muscles to respond even faster to the next exercise bout. Thus, PGC-1α can be thought of as a master regulator of mitochondrial biogenesis in response to aerobic training (Lin et al., 2005).

Angiogenesis

Endurance training leads to an increase in the numbers of capillaries surrounding each muscle fibre. This process is known as *angiogenesis* and it serves to increase the supply of oxygen to individual muscle fibres that most need it as well as slowing the transit time of blood through the muscle to give more time for oxygen to be extracted from erythrocytes and taken into muscle fibres. The expansion of the capillary network occurs in parallel with increased mitochondria and maximal oxygen uptake (Klausen et al., 1981). Increased capillarity is mainly accomplished by 'sprouting' new capillaries from existing capillary networks. The main stimuli driving angiogenesis are increased blood flow *per se*, shear stress as blood pushes against capillary walls and increases in metabolites from muscle contractions. Vascular endothelial growth factor (VEGF) is a main regulator of angiogenesis. VEGF levels increase in response to acute exercise and signal to increase the local expression of genes involved in capillary growth.

Muscle adaptations to resistance training

The main goal of resistance training is to promote increased maximal voluntary strength. This is primarily mediated through increases in muscle size (i.e., hypertrophy) and neural adaptations favouring greater muscle use (Folland and Williams, 2007). Neural factors such as enhanced neural drive and intermuscular coordination contribute to the rapid strength increases during the first weeks to months of a resistance training programme. Later, muscle size and strength appear to increase in parallel even though there is not necessarily a correlation between the degree of muscle growth (hypertrophy) and the degree of strength gains. Athletes exposed to long-term vigorous resistance training show extraordinary muscle hypertrophy, which could reflect both genetic selection and the adaptive response to long-term training, but most likely a combination of both. There is still considerable debate regarding the most effective training programme to improve strength. The American College of Sports Medicine advocates heavy loading (85–100% of one-repetition maximum (1RM)) and multiple sets to promote increased force; however, these recommendations have rightfully been challenged as recent studies show substantial increases in muscle size and strength when low loads are lifted to voluntary failure (Schoenfeld et al., 2017).

Neural adaptations

Indirect examples of neural adaptations are the large discrepancy in the magnitude between strength gains and muscle hypertrophy seen in the beginning of an exercise programme, and the common observation that the increase in strength is very specific to the particular exercise performed (principle of specificity) (Folland and Williams, 2007). An example of this is the fact that the increase in dynamic strength (1RM) is significantly greater than the increase in isometric strength if the training is performed dynamically. Another example is the so-called crossover or cross-education effect, meaning that strength gains can be observed in the arm or leg contralateral to the extremity that was involved in the actual training (Carroll et al., 2006).

The most concrete evidence of neural adaptation is the increased electromyographic (EMG) signal that can be measured after only one or a few weeks of strength training. An increase in the electrical signal across the muscle simply shows that it is more activated by the nervous system. However, it is important to emphasize that standard EMG measurements cannot determine whether the increased signal is due to increased recruitment of more motor units, increased firing frequency (i.e., increased rate coding) or even due to muscle hypertrophy since the electrical potential is related to fibre cross-sectional area. Nonetheless, the main purpose of the neural adaptation is to increase the activation of the agonists (the muscles that primarily perform the movement). Another challenge is to appropriately activate synergists while antagonists should be minimally active. At the same time, the system must learn to handle the sensory feedback that occurs from muscles and joints (proprioception). Although it is somewhat difficult to measure motor unit recruitment reliably, the collective body of evidence indicates that resistance training is capable of increasing the capacity to more efficiently recruit the highest threshold motor units (i.e., increased recruitment and firing rates).

Muscle hypertrophy

In theory, any increase in muscle cross-sectional area (CSA) could be due to increases in fibre size and/or fibre number (hyperplasia). It is generally agreed that adult muscle hypertrophy predominantly occurs through an increased CSA of individual fibres (Tesch, 1988). In particular, resistance training increases the area of the fast-twitch type 2 fibres. Fibre hypertrophy occurs through synthesis and accumulation of new myofilaments, with concomitant expansion of the fibre volume. Even though the process of muscle hypertrophy starts immediately after the first training session, reflected as an increased net muscle protein turnover, it takes at least a few weeks before muscle hypertrophy can be reliably measured noninvasively by modern imaging techniques (e.g., magnetic resonance imaging), or invasively through assessment of fibre area from muscle biopsies.

Other morphological adaptations

Although the muscle fibre type is largely genetically determined, the fibres quickly adapt metabolically and functionally to specific under- or overloading stimuli, such as specific training programmes. The muscle fibre make-up of different elite athletes has been explored and, in general, it appears athletes relying on high-endurance capacity have a high proportion of type 1 fibres, whereas power athletes such as sprint runners have a high proportion of type 2 fibres (Costill et al., 1976). The reason for this marked difference is likely due to selection bias towards a sport that fits with an individual's genetic make-up rather than the effect of the specific training regimens carried out.

Whether or not, and to what extent, fibre type transformations occur due to training has been a matter of debate for many years (Pette and Staron, 1997; Schiaffino and Reggiani, 2011). The consensus is that long-term exercise training in humans leads to a reduction in hybrid fibres and the type 2X isoform, and an increased proportion of type 2A fibres (Klitgaard et al., 1990; Schiaffino and Reggiani, 2011). Although this at first may appear contradictory to the overall goal of increasing force production where strength training athletes are concerned, this shift is compensated for by neural adaptations, architectural changes and preferential hypertrophy of type 2 fibres.

Other morphological changes that may occur in response to resistance training include an increase in fibre pennation angle, increased fascicle lengths and connective tissue remodelling (Folland and Williams, 2007). An increase in the fascicle pennation angle signifies increased muscle fibre CSA due to addition of sarcomeres in parallel (and thus, contractile proteins) and this enhances the muscle force. If the fascicle length increases, it indicates addition of sarcomeres in series has occurred, and this is generally beneficial for muscle-shortening velocity. Resistance training also leads to adaptations in the muscle–tendon complex to increase tendon stiffness and the rate of force development. Altogether, these morphological factors contribute to the increase in muscle force production seen with chronic resistance training.

Regulation of muscle protein turnover

The ratio of protein synthesis and degradation determines overall muscle protein balance. When muscle protein synthesis exceeds breakdown, the net protein turnover is positive and accretion of muscle proteins occurs. During acute resistance exercise, both protein synthesis and breakdown are stimulated such that the net balance is negative (Kumar et al., 2009). However, when essential amino acids are consumed postexercise, the net protein balance turns positive. Thus the quantity of contractile proteins reaches a new steady-state level through the cumulative effect of repeated exercise bouts and feeding. When repeated over an extended period, this summates into muscle hypertrophy.

Mechanotransduction

It is apparent that the skeletal muscle must possess sensors that transduce active or passive tension into a cellular event favouring increased protein synthesis, termed *mechanotransduction*. Although the understanding of these mechanisms is limited to date, it has been shown that acute loading disturbs sarcolemma integrity and induces phosphatidic acid, which leads to the activation of signalling cascades that regulates protein synthesis (You et al., 2014). Also, an important signalling molecule called focal adhesion kinase (FAK) increases in response to high-force contractions and decreases after unloading, suggesting that FAK senses mechanical loading (Crossland et al., 2013). Collectively, it appears that phosphatidic acid and FAK convert mechanical strain into an appropriate intracellular response initiating protein synthesis and muscle growth.

Transcriptional regulation

It is well established that resistance exercise alters the expression of genes involved in diverse functions such as cell growth, differentiation, inflammation and proteolysis. Although increased messenger RNA (mRNA) translation is the chief regulatory step for increasing protein synthesis,

the gene expression response (including transcriptional coregulators) is also implicated in controlling muscle protein turnover. Notably, the transcription of several hundreds of genes is altered by acute resistance exercise both in untrained and training-accustomed states (Raue et al., 2012).

Among markers exerting transcriptional control is myostatin, a transforming growth factor-β family member functioning as a negative regulator of muscle size. Acute resistance exercise diminishes myostatin expression and aids in promoting muscle hypertrophy by reverting its inhibitory effect on muscle protein synthesis and satellite cell activity (Coffey and Hawley, 2007). Another example is the ubiquitin ligase proteins atrogin-1 and MuRF-1, regulated through FOXO transcription factors. While MuRF-1 and atrogin-1 are linked to muscle atrophy in response to disuse by targeting contractile proteins for degradation, it seems these markers facilitate tissue remodelling in favour of muscle growth in healthy skeletal muscle (Hwee et al., 2014).

New research has demonstrated important roles for microRNAs (miRNA) in the muscle adaptive response to resistance exercise. These noncoding sequences of mRNA degrade target transcripts by binding to complementary sequences. Several miRNAs increase in response to resistance exercise and may take part in regulating training-induced changes in the muscle (Hitachi and Tsuchida, 2013).

Intracellular signalling responses

Translating mRNA into protein includes the processes of initiation, elongation and termination. Of particular importance for this process is the initiation step, which is coordinated by the mechanistic target of rapamycin (mTOR) complex. mTOR integrates signals from mechanical stimuli, energy status and nutrients, to coordinate downstream signalling events. Indeed, activation of mTOR elicits increased protein synthesis after acute resistance exercise, and is crucial for the muscle hypertrophic response (Coffey and Hawley, 2007). Downstream effector targets of mTOR include p70S6 kinase (p70S6K) and eukaryotic initiation factor 4E binding protein 1 (4E-BP1). Translational control of protein synthesis is generally held as a crucial molecular event regulating muscle size.

Hypertrophy, driven by net protein synthesis, also requires increased ribosomal function (Bamman et al., 2017). Ribosomes are the organelle where amino acids are linked together to form the newly built protein from the mRNA blueprint. Apart from the increased ribosomal efficiency, i.e., greater translation of mRNA per ribosome, enhanced protein translation can also occur through elevated ribosomal capacity, i.e., ribosome biogenesis. Interestingly, this energetically expensive process also seems to be largely regulated by mTOR activity.

Satellite cells and myonuclei addition

During hypertrophy, myonuclei addition could aid in maintaining the myonuclei-to-cytoplasmic ratio intact and hence protect the capacity for transcription. The addition of new nuclei to existing fibres is mediated through the proliferation of satellite cells, which are located between the basal lamina and the sarcolemma of the fibre. The importance of satellite cell activity and myonuclei addition in the hypertrophic process is not well understood (Bamman et al., 2017). In support for their role, however, myonuclei content has been shown to be greater in powerlifters than in untrained controls, and fibre hypertrophy induced by resistance training has, in some studies, been paralleled by increased myonuclei content and satellite cell number.

Muscle fatigue

Muscle fatigue is the failure to maintain a given muscle output over time and/or over successive contractions. It is characterized by loss of force, slowing of the velocity of contraction and rate of relaxation, which leads to substantial loss of power (remember that power is the product of force × velocity of contraction) and reduced accuracy of movement (Enoka and Duchateau, 2008). The muscle output is recovered after a period of rest, from as little as a few seconds to as long as a few hours, depending upon circumstances, and any residual loss of force or power will be the result of damage or injury and not fatigue.

The mechanisms of fatigue are complex and not fully understood. They depend on the type and intensity of exercise, but can be classified as 'central' or 'peripheral' in origin. *Central fatigue* describes all aspects of the motor command that determine motor unit recruitment, from the brain through to the motor neuron axon terminal. *Peripheral fatigue* describes all aspects occurring between acetylcholine exchange at the neuromuscular junction and the actin–myosin cross-bridge kinetics. Central and peripheral mechanisms of fatigue both occur during exercise, but their relative importance differs depending on intrinsic characteristics of the motor units and the period of relaxation between contractions allowing for metabolic recovery as well as exercise intensity and duration (Enoka and Duchateau, 2008; Hunter, 2009). Fatigability is strongly influenced by the person's fitness levels and external factors including environmental temperature and humidity.

Fatigue during very intense exercise

Very high–intensity exercise such as sprinting or lifting weights recruits the largest and fastest motor units and is heavily reliant on anaerobic processes to provide ATP. There is a central component of fatigue relating to central nervous system (CNS) 'arousal' and evidence for this comes from studies providing strong verbal encouragement or other stimulation showing it can increase motor unit recruitment and muscle output (Ikai and Steinhaus, 1961). However, this typically accounts for only about 10% of the overall fatigue in very well-motivated individuals and, instead, the main component of fatigue is due to peripheral factors.

The main sites of peripheral fatigue are the propagation of action potentials along the sarcolemma; the release of Ca^{2+} from the sarcoplasmic reticulum; and cross-bridge function (Allen et al., 2008). There is normally an influx of Na^+ and outflux of K^+ along the sarcolemma as the action potential propagates. During sustained, intense muscular activity, K^+ can accumulate in the t-tubules and restrict membrane potential recovery and thus limit any further muscle fibre activation. Another mechanism of fatigue is that the Pi liberated from ATP during cross-bridge cycles enters the sarcoplasmic reticulum and binds with Ca^{2+} (forming calcium phosphate), which diminishes the free calcium available for release into the sarcoplasm and thus reduces the numbers of cross-bridges that can form. Pi may also interfere directly with cross-bridge function to slow their kinetics. Other metabolic byproducts of intense contractile activity including lactate, hydrogen ions and ADP may also inhibit muscle fibre contractions and there is a possibility of localized depletion of ATP that would restrict sarcolemma ion transporter ATPase activity or myosin ATPase activity along sarcomeres. Accumulation of these metabolites within muscles can additionally stimulate muscle chemoreceptors, triggering proprioceptor feedback along type III/IV afferent (sensory) nerves that synapse with alpha motor neurons in the CNS to inhibit motor unit recruitment (Garland and Kaufman, 1995; Taylor and Gandevia, 2008).

Fatigue during prolonged endurance exercise

The ATP needed to fuel intense exercise lasting 2 or 3 min comes equally from aerobic and anaerobic sources and the intensity is typically >90% $\dot{V}O_{2max}$, but prolonged exercise lasting 20 min and longer is performed at 'submaximal' intensity <80% $\dot{V}O_{2max}$ and progressively lower than that when duration is progressively increased to several hours. ATP derived almost entirely from mitochondrial aerobic respiration powers these longer duration activities. Mechanisms of fatigue during prolonged exercise are different from those occurring during high-intensity exercise due to the clear differences in the motor unit recruitment, fibre metabolism and sum of proprioceptor and other sensory inputs. There is evidence to show an important role for central fatigue as well as peripheral factors to do with fuel substrates.

11

Central fatigue leads to a reduction in the numbers of motor units recruited and/or motor unit firing rates. These decreases are due to afferent feedback from proprioceptors causing inhibition of motor unit recruitment as well as decreased motor drive from the brain and CNS (Carroll et al., 2017). The CNS continually receives sensory inputs and during prolonged endurance exercise, factors such as core body temperature, dehydration, muscle tension, pain and damage are associated with increased brain serotonin levels and reduced motor drive. Applying a cold stimulus, such as water, to the forehead and forearms, or swilling a glucose solution around the mouth, or providing strong verbal or visual encouragement, can temporarily overcome the central fatigue to enable higher motor unit recruitment and muscle output, but any effects last only a few minutes and marginal (though important for elite athletes) improvements in performance are seen (Carter et al., 2004; Jensen et al., 2018).

Muscle and liver glycogen stores as well as fatty acids provide most of the fuel for aerobic respiration. However, glycogen reserves are limited and there are reports of muscle glycogen depletion during long-distance endurance running (Bergstrom and Hultman, 1967). This may correspond with 'hitting the wall', which is a term used to describe the marked decrement in exercise intensity and very strong feelings of fatigue and exhaustion in marathon and other distance events. However, we point out that the scientific evidence for glycogen depletion is very mixed and some studies have demonstrated substantial glycogen reserves in athletes showing typical signs of fatigue (Costill et al., 1971; Madsen et al., 1990). Glycogen depletion or any other factor reducing glucose use without any additional glucose intake would slow the resynthesis of ATP by increasing reliance on beta oxidation (use of fatty acids in the mitochondria to make energy). Fat oxidation is a relatively slow process and the peak rate occurs at about 50–60% $\dot{V}O_{2max}$ (Venables et al., 2005). Exercise intensities higher than 60% $\dot{V}O_{2max}$ must use glucose and can, in fact, inhibit fat oxidation (Lundsgaard et al., 2018). An important adaptation of endurance training is to increase use of fatty acids and increase the intensity at which fats continue to supply fuel so that glycogen can be spared and performance enhanced. Taking practical steps to increase carbohydrate intake in the days before a long-distance event and to consume carbohydrates and fluids during the events help to prolong glucose stores and delay fatigue.

References

Allen, D.G., Lamb, G.D., Westerblad, H., 2008. Skeletal muscle fatigue: cellular mechanisms. Physiological Reviews 88, 287–332.

Atherton, P.J., Phillips, B.E., Wilkinson, D.J., 2015. Exercise and regulation of protein metabolism. Progress in Molecular Biology and Translational Science 135, 75–98.

Bamman, M.M., Roberts, B.M., Adams, G.R., 2017. Molecular regulation of exercise-induced muscle fiber hypertrophy. Cold Spring Harbor Perspectives in Medicine.

Bassett Jr., D.R., Howley, E.T., 2000. Limiting factors for maximum oxygen uptake and determinants of endurance performance. Medicine & Science in Sports & Exercise 32, 70–84.

Bergstrom, J., Hultman, E., 1967. A study of the glycogen metabolism during exercise in man. Scandinavian Journal of Clinical and Laboratory Investigation 19, 218–228.

Carroll, T.J., Herbert, R.D., Munn, J., Lee, M., Gandevia, S.C., 2006. Contralateral effects of unilateral strength training: evidence and possible mechanisms. Journal of Applied Physiology 101, 1514–1522.

Carroll, T.J., Taylor, J.L., Gandevia, S.C., 2017. Recovery of central and peripheral neuromuscular fatigue after exercise. Journal of Applied Physiology 122, 1068–1076.

Carter, J.M., Jeukendrup, A.E., Jones, D.A., 2004. The effect of carbohydrate mouth rinse on 1-h cycle time trial performance. Medicine & Science in Sports & Exercise 36, 2107–2111.

Coffey, V.G., Hawley, J.A., 2007. The molecular bases of training adaptation. Sports Medicine 37, 737–763.

Costill, D.L., Daniels, J., Evans, W., Fink, W., Krahenbuhl, G., Saltin, B., 1976. Skeletal muscle enzymes and fiber composition in male and female track athletes. Journal of Applied Physiology 40, 149–154.

Costill, D.L., Sparks, K., Gregor, R., Turner, C., 1971. Muscle glycogen utilization during exhaustive running. Journal of Applied Physiology 31, 353–356.

Coyle, E.F., 1995. Integration of the physiological factors determining endurance performance ability. Exercise and Sport Sciences Reviews 23, 25–63.

Crossland, H., Kazi, A.A., Lang, C.H., Timmons, J.A., Pierre, P., Wilkinson, D.J., et al., 2013. Focal adhesion kinase is required for IGF-I-mediated growth of skeletal muscle cells via a TSC2/mTOR/S6K1-associated pathway. American Journal of Physiology. Endocrinology and Metabolism 305, E183–E193.

Enoka, R.M., Duchateau, J., 2008. Muscle fatigue: what, why and how it influences muscle function. Journal of Physiology 586, 11–23.

Faria, E.W., Parker, D.L., Faria, I.E., 2005. The science of cycling: physiology and training – part 1. Sports Medicine 35, 285–312.

Folland, J.P., Williams, A.G., 2007. The adaptations to strength training : morphological and neurological contributions to increased strength. Sports Medicine 37, 145–168.

Garland, S.J., Kaufman, M.P., 1995. Role of muscle afferents in the inhibition of motoneurons during fatigue. Advances in Experimental Medicine and Biology 384, 271–278.

Gollnick, P.D., Armstrong, R.B., Saltin, B., Saubert , C.W., Sembrowich, W.L., Shepherd, R.E., 1973. Effect of training on enzyme activity and fiber composition of human skeletal muscle. Journal of Applied Physiology 34, 107–111.

Hitachi, K., Tsuchida, K., 2013. Role of microRNAs in skeletal muscle hypertrophy. Frontiers in Physiology 4, 408.

Hoppeler, H., Fluck, M., 2003. Plasticity of skeletal muscle mitochondria: structure and function. Medicine & Science in Sports & Exercise 35, 95–104.

Hoppeler, H., Howald, H., Conley, K., Lindstedt, S.L., Claassen, H., Vock, P., et al., 1985. Endurance training in humans: aerobic capacity and structure of skeletal muscle. Journal of Applied Physiology 59, 320–327.

Hoppeler, H., 2016. Molecular networks in skeletal muscle plasticity. Journal of Experimental Biology 219, 205–213.

Hunter, S.K., 2009. Sex differences and mechanisms of task-specific muscle fatigue. Exercise and Sport Sciences Reviews 37, 113–122.

Hwee, D.T., Baehr, L.M., Philp, A., Baar, K., Bodine, S.C., 2014. Maintenance of muscle mass and load-induced growth in Muscle RING Finger 1 null mice with age. Aging Cell 13, 92–101.

Ikai, M., Steinhaus, A.H., 1961. Some factors modifying the expression of human strength. Journal of Applied Physiology 16, 157–163.

Jensen, M., Klimstra, M., Sporer, B., Stellingwerff, T., 2018. Effect of carbohydrate mouth rinse on performance after prolonged submaximal cycling. Medicine & Science in Sports & Exercise 50, 1031 -1038.

Jones, A.M., Carter, H., 2000. The effect of endurance training on parameters of aerobic fitness. Sports Medicine 29, 373–386.

Klausen, K., Andersen, L.B., Pelle, I., 1981. Adaptive changes in work capacity, skeletal muscle capillarization and enzyme levels during training and detraining. Acta Physiologica Scandinavica 113, 9–16.

Klitgaard, H., Bergman, O., Betto, R., Salviati, G., Schiaffino, S., Clausen, T., et al., 1990. Co-existence of myosin heavy chain I and IIa isoforms in human skeletal muscle fibres with endurance training. Pflügers Archiv 416, 470–472.

Kumar, V., Atherton, P., Smith, K., Rennie, M.J., 2009. Human muscle protein synthesis and breakdown during and after exercise. Journal of Applied Physiology 106, 2026–2039.

Lin, J., Handschin, C., Spiegelman, B.M., 2005. Metabolic control through the PGC-1 family of transcription coactivators. Cell Metabolism 1, 361–370.

Lundsgaard, A.M., Fritzen, A.M., Kiens, B., 2018. Molecular regulation of fatty acid oxidation in skeletal muscle during aerobic exercise. Trends in Endocrinology and Metabolism 29, 18–30.

Madsen, K., Pedersen, P.K., Rose, P., Richter, E.A., 1990. Carbohydrate supercompensation and muscle glycogen utilization during exhaustive running in highly trained athletes. European Journal of Applied Physiology and Occupational Physiology 61, 467–472.

Pette, D., Staron, R.S., 1997. Mammalian skeletal muscle fiber type transitions. International Review of Cytology 170, 143–223.

Raue, U., Trappe, T.A., Estrem, S.T., Qian, H.R., Helvering, L.M., Smith, R.C., et al., 2012. Transcriptome signature of resistance exercise adaptations: mixed muscle and fiber type specific profiles in young and old adults. Journal of Applied Physiology 112, 1625–1636.

Schiaffino, S., Reggiani, C., 2011. Fiber types in mammalian skeletal muscles. Physiological Reviews 91, 1447–1531.

Schoenfeld, B.J., Grgic, J., Ogborn, D., Krieger, J.W., 2017. Strength and hypertrophy adaptations between low- vs. high-load resistance training: a systematic review and meta-analysis. Journal of Strength and Conditioning Research 31, 3508–3523.

Taylor, J.L., Gandevia, S.C., 2008. A comparison of central aspects of fatigue in submaximal and maximal voluntary contractions. Journal of Applied Physiology 104, 542–550.

Tesch, P.A., 1988. Skeletal muscle adaptations consequent to long-term heavy resistance exercise. Medicine & Science in Sports & Exercise 20, S132–S134.

Venables, M.C., Achten, J., Jeukendrup, A.E., 2005. Determinants of fat oxidation during exercise in healthy men and women: a cross-sectional study. Journal of Applied Physiology 98, 160–167.

You, J.S., Lincoln, H.C., Kim, C.R., Frey, J.W., Goodman, C.A., Zhong, X.P., et al., 2014. The role of diacylglycerol kinase zeta and phosphatidic acid in the mechanical activation of mammalian target of rapamycin (mTOR) signaling and skeletal muscle hypertrophy. Journal of Biological Chemistry 289, 1551–1563.

Zoladz, J.A., Rademaker, A.C., Sargeant, A.J., 2000. Human muscle power generating capability during cycling at different pedalling rates. Experimental Physiology 85, 117–124.

Chapter | 3 |

The physiology of disuse, immobilization and low-load environments

Nicholas C. Clark, Mark Glaister, Lyndsey M. Cannon and Nic Perrem

Introduction

Sports injuries occur to all parts of the body (Boyce and Quigley, 2004; Tirabassi et al., 2016), with peripheral joint injuries consistently being most frequent (Hootman et al., 2007; Tirabassi et al., 2016). Traumatic peripheral joint injuries, in particular, often present with tissue damage (Atef et al., 2016; Olsson et al., 2016; Roemer et al., 2014) and impairments such as pain (Aarnio et al., 2017; Alaia et al., 2015), effusion (Luhmann, 2003; Man et al., 2007) and muscle weakness (Hohmann et al., 2016; Punt et al., 2015). Therefore, sports injuries frequently result in short-term physical activity (PA) limitations and time loss from sports participation in order to facilitate the healing process and undertake rehabilitation (Hootman et al., 2007). The PA limitations that manifest as a result of sports injuries are part of a 'spectrum of disuse' (Fig. 3.1). For this chapter, the term 'disuse' refers to decreased use of a body part relative to an individual's habitual PA levels because of traumatic or overuse injury. The term 'immobilize' (*v.* (immobilization *n.*)) means to prevent all movement of a body part because of injury. The term 'load' is defined as the application of force to a body part (Whiting and Zernicke, 2008); 'low-load environments' (LLE), therefore, are defined here as when loads lower than those habitually applied to an individual's body part exist due to postinjury disuse. Because injury results in some level of disuse, multiple body tissues and body systems are affected by the ensuing decreased PA levels (Bloomfield, 1997; Convertino, 1997).

To develop efficacious clinical interventions that limit the sequelae of disuse, it is necessary for clinicians to possess an understanding of the secondary effects of injury on the body tissues and systems, and how such effects influence rehabilitation practice (Clark, 2015). The purpose of this chapter, therefore, is to review the physiological effects of disuse, immobilization and LLE. Our research group operates using the analogy of an automobile: you cannot condition the engine (cardiorespiratory system) if the chassis (musculoskeletal (MSK) system) breaks down first (Clark, 2008); this is an important analogy because common clinical observation reveals how many athletes cannot perform, for example, long slow distance running until postinjury knee pain has resolved. Further, MSK disorders are associated with the onset and progression of medical disease mitigated by endurance-type PA (Hawker et al., 2014; Toomey et al., 2017). Consequently, we will review the physiological effects of disuse, immobilization and LLE with an emphasis on the skeletal, muscular and cardiorespiratory systems. Due to current limitations in knowledge and science, it is not ethical or technologically possible to study some effects of disuse with human *in vivo* paradigms because of the likelihood of harming study participants. Therefore, research has employed a variety of scientific paradigms to help answer clinical questions; for example, animal *in vitro* and *in vivo*, human *in vitro*, and *in silico* paradigms (Huang and Wikswo, 2006; Maglio and Mabry, 2011). A holistic approach to evidence-informed clinical practice involves integrating different research models to answer complex clinical questions (Drolet and Lorenzi, 2011; Mabry et al., 2008) and results in a rich translation of research to the clinical context (Drolet and Lorenzi, 2011; Rubio et al., 2010). We will, subsequently, employ multiple mammalian research paradigms (e.g., human, primate, dog, rabbit, rat) and study types (*in vitro*, *in vivo*, *in silico*) to review the physiological effects of disuse in a way that highlights to the clinician important clinical considerations beyond the primary injury site and type for athletes with noncontractile tissue sports injuries.

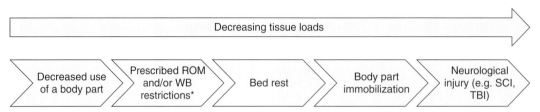

Fig. 3.1 Spectrum of disuse following sports injury. *ROM*, range of motion; *SCI*, spinal cord injury; *TBI*, traumatic brain injury; *WB*, weight-bearing; *, typically enforced by use of a brace and/or crutches. Modified from Bloomfield, S., 1997. Changes in musculoskeletal structure and function with prolonged bed rest. *Medicine and Science in Sports and Exercise,* 29 (2), 197–206.

Bone

Bones form the skeleton which functions to provide support and protection for other body tissues, a lever system to facilitate movement, a reservoir for minerals and a store for haematopoietic cells (Weiner and Wagner, 1998; Whiting and Zernicke, 2008). The cellular constituents of bone are osteoblasts and osteoclasts, which are responsible for the continuous remodelling of bone by the secretion of new bone extracellular matrix (ECM) and the erosion of old bone ECM, respectively (Crockett et al., 2011; Feng and McDonald, 2011; Weiner and Wagner, 1998). The ECM of bone includes fibrous (type I collagen), ground substance (hydroxyapatite, calcium, nonstructural proteins) and water components (Crockett et al., 2011; Feng and McDonald, 2011; Weiner and Wagner, 1998). Bone homeostasis and health is controlled by coordinated actions of hormones (Harada and Rodan, 2003), the sympathetic nervous system (Elefteriou et al., 2014) and mechanotransduction (Ehrlich and Lanyon, 2002; Liedert et al., 2006; Oftadeh et al., 2015; Pavalko et al., 2003; Rosa et al., 2015). Intermittent tension and compression loads are particularly important for influencing bone homeostasis through multiple cell-stimulating pathways including physical deformation of the bone ECM, induction of canalicular fluid flow and generation of lacunocanalicular electrical streaming (Bonewald, 2006; Oftadeh et al., 2015; Turner and Pavalko, 1998).

Decreased osteoblast and increased osteoclast activity can be observed soon after limb disuse or immobilization, resulting in a net decrease in bone volume (Weinreb et al., 1989; Wronski and Morey, 1983; Young et al., 1986). Evidence of bone collagen breakdown has been reported after prolonged periods of disuse (Fiore et al., 1999; Uebelhart et al., 2000), and postinjury and postsurgery disuse can result in osteopenia both local to, proximal from and distal from the primary injury site (Ceroni et al., 2012; Ejerhed et al., 2004; Leppälä et al., 1999; Reiman et al., 2006; Smith et al., 1992). On magnetic resonance imaging (MRI), bone marrow signal abnormalities have also been reported after periods of limb disuse and immobilization (Elias et al., 2007; Nardo et al., 2013).

Limb disuse and immobilization are consistently observed to result in changes in bone physiology and structure, both local to and remote from the primary injury site or location of immobilization. With decreasing volumetric bone mineral density and/or change in bone structure (geometry) comes a decrease in direction-specific bone ultimate strength and a lower threshold for bone fracture (Bach-Gansmo et al., 2016; Guo and Kim, 2002; Lepola et al., 1993; Mosekilde et al., 2000; Peng et al., 1994). Following periods of limb disuse and immobilization, clinicians should be conscious of potential negative changes in both local and remote bone strength and how this may influence both short- and long-term rehabilitation from the preceding primary sports injury.

Articular cartilage

Articular cartilage (AC) covers the ends of bones forming synovial joints and facilitates the transmission of loads across articular surfaces whilst permitting almost friction-free movement and minimizing pressure on the underlying subchondral bone (Bhosale and Richardson, 2008). Chondrocytes are the active cells in AC, being responsible for secreting the tissue's ECM which contains a network of collagen (predominantly type II) and noncollagenous proteins within a viscous water-like substance (Lafont, 2010; Poole et al., 2001). The ECM is also composed of large proteoglycans with the core protein, aggrecan, predominating (Fox et al., 2009). Articular cartilage is avascular, and so intermittent loading is important for altering intraarticular hydrostatic pressure and facilitating oxygen and nutrient diffusion from the synovial fluid to the AC (Bhosale and Richardson, 2008; Carter et al., 1987; Fermor et al., 2007; Vanwanseele et al., 2002b), thereby maintaining chondrocyte health and AC morphology and function (Milner et al., 2012; Vanwanseele et al., 2002b).

Peripheral joint immobilization can result in changes in chondrocyte size, shape and metabolic activity (Palmoski and Brandt, 1981; Roy, 1970). A hypoxic environment can result from immobilization and, in turn, reduced diffusion of oxygen from the synovial fluid (Sakamoto et al., 2009). Hypoxic environments that result from immobilization have been reported to show increased expression of vascular endothelial growth factor (VEGF) within AC, which can lead to angiogenesis and vascular ingrowth from the subchondral bone (Garcia-Ramirez et al., 2000; Sakamoto et al., 2009). Joint immobilization can also trigger chondrocyte apoptosis (Mutsuzaki et al., 2017), a reduced number of chondrocytes in AC (Hagiwara et al., 2009; Iqbal et al., 2012; Palmoski and Brandt, 1981) and a reduction in proteoglycan concentration (Jortikka et al., 1997). Cellular responses to disuse and immobilization may be different across the zones of AC, with the deep and calcified zones being less affected than the superficial zone (Sood, 1971). A decrease in, or absence of, intermittent hydrostatic pressure changes due to disuse or immobilization is associated with advancement of the ossification front into the AC zones (Carter et al., 1987). Thinning of AC consistent with that in primary osteoarthritis (OA) can be observed after joint immobilization (Nomura et al., 2017; Vanwanseele et al., 2002b). In addition to the local effects of joint immobilization on AC, disuse of a body part due to injury elsewhere in the body can affect AC. Partial weight-bearing due to ankle fracture can induce a reduction in AC thickness in all compartments of the knee joint (Hinterwimmer et al., 2004). Paralysis due to spinal cord injury has been reported to demonstrate thinning of AC in both the patello-femoral and tibiofemoral joints (Vanwanseele et al., 2002a).

The full effects of disuse, immobilization and LLE on AC are not currently well understood. The removal of intermittent load appears to have a negative impact on the physiological functioning of AC (Carter et al., 1987; Milner et al., 2012; Smith et al., 1992; Vanwanseele et al., 2002b). An important consideration for clinical practice may be that the changes observed in AC after periods of disuse may impair the tissue's future ability to tolerate load, making it more prone to 'overload' and, consequently, an abnormal stress response and further injury following a return to PA.

Ligament

Ligaments are bands of collagenous tissue that cross joints, attaching directly to the periarticular region of the bones that form the joint (Frank, 2004). The mechanical functions of ligaments include augmenting mechanical joint stability, guiding joint movement and restraining excessive joint motion (Bray et al., 2005). Fibroblasts are the predominant cells found in ligamentous tissue, synthesizing the ECM which includes collagen (predominantly type I), proteoglycans, elastin and other proteins and glycoproteins, including lactin and laminin (Frank, 2004). Fibroblast proliferation and activation specifically occurs in response to controlled tensile loads (Gehlsen et al., 1999; Neidlinger-Wilke et al., 2001),

and activated fibroblasts then align themselves to lay collagen down along the lines of tensile stress (Eastwood et al., 1998; Mudera et al., 2000; Neidlinger-Wilke et al., 2001).

Immobilization has been reported to result in disruption of the normal attachment of ligaments to bone, with increased attachment site and periarticular osteoclastic activity and bone resorption (Klein et al., 1982; Noyes, 1977; Woo et al., 1987). Within ligaments, immobilization can result in changes in the number, size and shape of fibroblasts (Chen et al., 2007; Kanda et al., 1998; Newton et al., 1995; Newton et al., 1990). Ligament enzyme activity changes in favour of collagen degradation are evident after joint immobilization (Gamble et al., 1984). Ligament turnover is represented by the rate and balance between collagen synthesis and degradation, both of which are altered following immobilization (Amiel et al., 1982; 1983; Harwood and Amiel, 1992). Subsequently, ligament composition and structure can alter, with a shift from smaller to larger diameter collagen fibrils being observed (Binkley and Peat, 1986), along with irregular collagen fibre patterns and alignment (Chen et al., 2007). Changes in collagen turnover rate do not appear to be coupled with a change in total collagen mass, although there is a shift towards more immature collagen and a reduced density of collagen fibrils (Amiel et al., 1982; Binkley and Peat, 1986).

Cellular responses to immobilization are consistently linked with changes in the mechanical properties of ligament tissue (Amiel et al., 1982; Newton et al., 1990; 1995; Noyes, 1977). Decreases in habitual, or complete removal of, ligament tensile loads consistently results in negative adaptations in ligament and joint mechanical characteristics (Amiel et al., 1982; Larsen et al., 1987; Newton et al., 1995; Noyes, 1977). Immobilization has been reported to result in a decrease in ligament stiffness (Amiel et al., 1982; Larsen et al., 1987; Woo et al., 1987), meaning that greater strain or deformation of ligamentous tissue is observed following the application of a fixed load. Periods of disuse or immobilization may also result in a reduction in the ultimate strength of ligaments (Binkley and Peat, 1986; Larsen et al., 1987; Noyes, 1977; Woo et al., 1987), meaning that tissue failure can occur when lower levels of external load are experienced. A variety of research study findings report that periods of immobilization lead to negatively altered ligament physiology and mechanical behaviour. Following periods of disuse and immobilization, careful consideration should be given to the inferior mechanical properties of ligaments and how this may impact clinical interventions directed at a safe and effective return to PA.

Joint capsule

Joint (articular) capsules are sleeves of connective tissue that enclose synovial joints, attaching adjacent to the margins of the articular surfaces via fibrocartilaginous attachment zones (Neumann, 2002; Ralphs and Benjamin, 1994). The joint capsule is composed of two histologically distinct layers of tissue: a dense superficial fibrous layer ('capsule') and a relatively thin deep membranous layer ('synovium') (Neumann, 2002; Ralphs and Benjamin, 1994). The mechanical functions of the capsule include augmenting mechanical joint stability and containing the contents of the joint space (Neumann, 2002; Ralphs and Benjamin, 1994). The synovium is a thin membrane that has a negligible mechanical function in joint stability, but instead provides a sterile barrier against the extrasynovial space and secretes synovial fluid to lubricate and nourish the intrasynovial environment (Neumann, 2002; Ralphs and Benjamin, 1994; Simkin, 1991). As for ligaments, fibroblasts are the predominant cells found in capsular tissue, synthesizing the ECM which includes predominantly type I collagen, although type II and III collagen can also be evident (Amiel et al., 1980; Gay et al., 1980; Matsumoto et al., 2002; Ralphs and Benjamin, 1994). The capsule is composed of irregularly organized collagen fibres, with specific thickenings or expansions evident around some joints that function as 'capsular ligaments' (Neumann, 2002; Ralphs and Benjamin, 1994). The synovium contains two predominant cell types; type A and type B synoviocytes (Ando et al., 2010). Type A synoviocytes are macrophage-like in nature whilst type B synoviocytes display fibroblast-like characteristics (Ando et al., 2010). Type A synoviocytes are mainly located in the superficial layer of the synovium, whilst type B synoviocytes are predominantly found in the deep layer of the synovial membrane producing hyaluronic acid and collagen fibres (Ando et al., 2010). Collagen fibres in the synovium are typically of type I, III, IV and V (Gay et al., 1980; Ralphs and Benjamin, 1994). Tensile loads are important for stimulating appropriate fibroblast activity and collagen synthesis along the lines of mechanical stress (Eastwood et al., 1998; Gehlsen et al., 1999; Mudera et al., 2000; Neidlinger-Wilke et al., 2001), whilst normal physiological joint motion is critical for ensuring cellular homeostasis and capsular health (Kaneguchi et al., 2017; Lee et al., 2010; Yabe et al., 2013).

Periods of immobilization appear to be associated with a progressive decrease in cell density over time in both the capsule and the synovium (Lee et al., 2010). Peripheral joint immobilization has demonstrated a decrease in capsular blood vessel density, progressive hypoxia and an increased presence of inflammatory mediators (Kaneguchi et al., 2017; Yabe et al., 2013). In some research work, fibroblast proliferation and increased collagen synthesis has been observed (Kaneguchi et al., 2017), with others reporting increased disorganization of capsular collagen fibrils and a relative increase in type I collagen and decrease in type III collagen after disuse and immobilization (Lee et al., 2010; Matsumoto et al., 2002; Yabe et al., 2013). Adhesions between synovial villi and resultant shortening of the synovium can be seen to occur after immobilization (Trudel et al., 2000). Following peripheral joint immobilization, adhesion of the synovium to AC has also been reported (Ando et al., 2010; Evans et al., 1960), as has proliferation of fibrofatty intraarticular tissue that demonstrates subsequent infiltration of the joint space (Schollmeier et al., 1994).

As for ligaments, cellular responses and tissue adaptations to immobilization are consistently linked with changes in the mechanical behaviour of capsular tissue and joints (Ando et al., 2012; Lee et al., 2010; Trudel et al., 2000; 2014). Joint hypomobility due to capsular stiffening or contracture is a consistent observation following disuse and immobilization: the longer the duration of disuse and immobilization, the less frequently original joint mobility is regained (Ando et al., 2012; Lee et al., 2010; Trudel et al., 2000; 2014). The location of adhesions and capsular stiffening is associated with the direction of restricted joint mobility (Ando et al., 2010; Lobenhoffer et al., 1996; Mariani et al., 1997). As for ligaments, a range of research study findings report that periods of disuse and immobilization lead to negatively altered capsular physiology and mechanical behaviour. For joint capsules, the principal clinical concern is with regard to how to limit capsular stiffening and contracture in situations of disuse and immobilization.

Skeletal muscle

The most abundant tissue in the human body is skeletal muscle (Neumann, 2002). Skeletal muscle functions to stabilize bones, move bones, shield the noncontractile tissues from excessive forces, absorb shock and generate heat (Clark and Lephart, 2015; MacIntosh et al., 2006; Neumann, 2002). Skeletal muscles can be found in many different shapes and sizes, the principal cells of a single muscle being the muscle fibres themselves and surrounding satellite cells (MacIntosh et al., 2006). The connective tissue (ECM) of skeletal muscle is identified as the epimysium, perimysium and endomysium, all of which are principally composed of collagen (types I–V) with some elastin also being present (MacIntosh et al., 2006). A muscle fibre is composed of many myofibrils, each myofibril containing contractile proteins (actin, myosin) and stabilizing proteins (titin, nebulin) (MacIntosh et al., 2006). Stimulation of muscle fibres by the nervous system initiates the actin–myosin cross-bridge cycle and the generation of force; force is ultimately transmitted through the stabilizing proteins and muscle connective tissue to the muscle's tendons and the bones to which the tendons attach (MacIntosh et al., 2006). Repeated stimulation of muscle fibres and satellite cells is important for maintaining muscle fibre health and force-generating capability (MacIntosh et al., 2006).

Following peripheral joint injury and resultant disuse, the cross-sectional area (CSA) of individual muscle fibres can reduce, the phenotype of muscle fibres can change, the number of satellite cells can reduce and the number of muscle fibroblasts can increase (Fry et al., 2014; 2017; Noehren et al., 2016). Because the number of satellite cells can reduce and the number of muscle fibroblasts can increase after limb disuse, an expansion of the ECM can occur within skeletal muscle with postinjury disuse (Fry et al., 2014; 2017; Noehren et al., 2016); this means there is a relative decrease in the space available for regenerating skeletal muscle contractile elements to occupy. As well as intramuscular tissue changes, the intermuscular space fills with adipose tissue with limb disuse and immobilization (Clark, 2009). Because the CSA of individual muscle fibres reduces with postinjury disuse, the CSA of a whole muscle can also be seen to significantly reduce as muscle atrophy (Norte et al., 2019; Perry et al., 2015; Stevens et al., 2006). With limb immobilization, significant losses of skeletal muscle CSA and volume can be apparent after just 5 days (Wall et al., 2014). The rate and magnitude of muscle atrophy is greater in the lower limb antigravity and lumbar spine muscles when compared to the upper limb muscles (Clark, 2009).

Physiological and structural changes rapidly occur in skeletal muscle after disuse or immobilization. Structural changes in skeletal muscle occur in such a way that there is a proliferation of connective tissue and atrophy of contractile tissue, with the lumbar spine and lower limb skeletal muscles being most affected. Following disuse or immobilization for noncontractile tissue sports injuries, careful consideration is warranted for how to minimize periods of body part disuse or immobilization and ensure frequent, intermittent activation of skeletal muscle fibres.

Cardiorespiratory system

The cardiorespiratory system contributes to the transport of oxygen, nutrients and hormones around the body and the removal of metabolic byproducts (Wilmore et al., 2015). The cardiorespiratory adaptations to exercise are well established, leading to improvements in the integration of various central and peripheral oxygen transport mechanisms (Wilmore et al., 2015). In contrast, the removal of the training stimulus leads to a reversal of those adaptations, the extent of which depends on the extent and duration of disuse, immobilization and reduced overall PA (Convertino, 1997). The effects of reduced PA on the principal measure of aerobic fitness, namely maximal oxygen uptake ($\dot{V}O_{2max}$), are reported to depend on the duration of immobilization and the training status of the individual. In a recent meta-analysis, Ried-Larsen et al. (2017) reported that

$\dot{V}O_{2max}$ decreased linearly during bed rest at a mean rate of 0.43% per day when expressed relative to body mass. Moreover, the rate of decline in $\dot{V}O_{2max}$ was inversely related to training status, such that well-trained individuals experienced the fastest rates of decline (Ried-Larsen et al., 2017). The main reasons for the initial decline (within the first 2 weeks) in $\dot{V}O_{2max}$ are largely due to changes in central oxygen transport mechanisms resulting from reductions in blood volume (hypovolaemia) and cardiac output (Ade et al., 2015; Convertino, 1997; 2007). In the case of the former, reduced loading is associated with an increase in renal sodium excretion leading to an increase in diuresis and a concomitant reduction in central venous pressure (Convertino, 2007). Indeed, bed rest has been shown to induce a 10–30% reduction in blood volume, the majority of which occurs within the first 72 hours (Convertino, 1997; 2007). Although the decrease in blood volume accounts for most of the decline in cardiac output, inactivity also results in a reduction (approximately 1% per week) in cardiac mass; although not, in most instances, to an extent where it appears to have any measurable influence on myocardial contractility (Ade et al., 2015). Although central adaptations to reduced PA are dominant in the early stages of the process, peripheral limitations to $\dot{V}O_{2max}$ are reported to increase as the duration of inactivity increases; accounting for approximately 27% of the decline after 42 days and 40% of the decline after 90 days (Ade et al., 2015). The main reasons for the peripheral changes in $\dot{V}O_{2max}$ are a decrease in intracellular oxidative metabolism due to a reduction in mitochondrial content and oxidative enzyme activity (Mujika and Padilla, 2001; Ringholm et al., 2011) and a reduction in capillary volume leading to a decline in peripheral oxygen delivery and a reduced oxygen diffusion capacity (Ade et al., 2015). These changes are concomitant with a reduction in slow-twitch muscle fibre isoforms and are reported to lead to an increased reliance on energy from carbohydrate metabolism (Mujika and Padilla, 2001).

Following disuse and immobilization, cardiorespiratory function is clearly compromised relative to preinjury levels because of reduced use of the MSK system (Convertino, 2007; Frangolias et al., 1997; Widman et al., 2007). Clinical consideration is for how function of the cardiorespiratory system can be optimized during the rehabilitation process and when the volume of training targeted specifically at enhancing cardiorespiratory performance can safely be increased after an initial period of injury rehabilitation.

Summary

Traumatic peripheral joint injuries are consistently the most frequent type of injury across multiple sports. The tissue damage and postinjury impairments that follow traumatic peripheral joint injuries frequently result in PA limitations and temporary sports participation restrictions. The PA limitations that manifest as a result of sports injuries are part of a 'spectrum of disuse' (see Fig. 3.1).

Bone, AC, ligament, joint capsule and skeletal muscle are all complex tissues with cellular, ECM and fluid components. Frequent, intermittent movement and loading of tissues is important for nurturing good tissue physiology and mechanics. Disuse and immobilization of body parts consistently demonstrates negative alterations in bone, AC, joint capsule and skeletal muscle physiology; the alterations in physiology then appear to consistently and negatively affect tissue mechanics and function. Alterations in tissue physiology and mechanics can be evident both local to and remote from the primary injury site (Fig. 3.2). Cardiorespiratory function and aerobic fitness are also negatively altered as a result of body part disuse and immobilization. Although disuse and immobilization negatively alters skeletal and muscle tissue physiology and function, as well as cardiorespiratory system physiology and function, subsequent exercise interventions have been reported as potentially able to mitigate the negative physiological and mechanical tissue alterations that follow from disuse (Bloomfield, 1997; Convertino, 1997; Iqbal et al., 2012; Kaneguchi et al., 2017; Noyes, 1977; Perry et al., 2015; Vanwanseele et al., 2002b; Woo et al., 1987). Clinicians should,

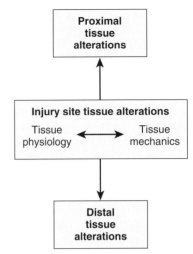

Fig. 3.2 Locations of potential tissue alterations following disuse.

therefore, consider the local and remote effects of body part disuse, immobilization and LLE following a primary injury, and which interventions are best suited for positively altering a particular tissue's physiology and mechanical function within a clinically reasoned rehabilitation process.

References

Aarnio, M., Appel, L., Fredrikson, M., Gordh, T., Wolf, O., Sörensen, J., et al., 2017. Visualization of painful inflammation in patients with pain after traumatic ankle sprain using [11C]-D-deprenyl PET/CT. Scandinavian Journal of Pain 17, 418–424.

Ade, C.J., Broxterman, R.M., Barstow, T.J., 2015. $\dot{V}O_{2max}$ and microgravity exposure: convective versus diffusive O_2 transport. Medicine and Science in Sports and Exercise 47 (7), 1351–1361.

Alaia, M.J., Khatib, O., Shah, M., Bosco, J.A., Jazrawi, L.M., Strauss, E.J., et al., 2015. The utility of plain radiographs in the initial evaluation of knee pain amongst sports medicine patients. Knee Surgery, Sports Traumatology, Arthroscopy 23 (8), 2213–2217.

Amiel, D., Akeson, W., Harwood, F., Mechanic, G., 1980. The effect of immobilization on the types of collagen synthesized in periarticular connective tissue. Connective Tissue Research 8 (1), 27–32.

Amiel, D., Akeson, W.H., Harwood, F.L., Frank, C.B., 1983. Stress deprivation effect on metabolic turnover of the medial collateral ligament collagen. A comparison between nine-and 12-week immobilization. Clinical Orthopaedics and Related Research (172), 265–270.

Amiel, D., Woo, S.L., Harwood, F.L., Akeson, W.H., 1982. The effect of immobilization on collagen turnover in connective tissue: a biochemical–biomechanical correlation. Acta Orthopaedica Scandinavica 53 (3), 325–332.

Ando, A., Hagiwara, Y., Onoda, Y., Hatori, K., Suda, H., Chimoto, E., et al., 2010. Distribution of type A and B synoviocytes in the adhesive and shortened synovial membrane during immobilization of the knee joint in rats. The Tohoku Journal of Experimental Medicine 221 (2), 161–168.

Ando, A., Suda, H., Hagiwara, Y., Onoda, Y., Chimoto, E., Itoi, E., et al., 2012. Remobilization does not restore immobilization-induced adhesion of capsule and restricted joint motion in rat knee joints. The Tohoku Journal of Experimental Medicine 227 (1), 13–22.

Atef, A., EL-Tantawy, A., Gad, H., Hefeda, M., 2016. Prevalence of associated injuries after anterior shoulder dislocation: a prospective study. International Orthopaedics 40 (3), 519–524.

Bach-Gansmo, F.L., Wittig, N.K., Brüel, A., Thomsen, J.S., Birkedal, H., 2016. Immobilization and long-term recovery results in large changes in bone structure and strength but no corresponding alterations of osteocyte lacunar properties. Bone 91, 139–147.

Bhosale, A.M., Richardson, J.B., 2008. Articular cartilage: structure, injuries and review of management. British Medical Bulletin 87, 77–95.

Binkley, J.M., Peat, M., 1986. The effects of immobilization on the ultrastructure and mechanical properties of the medial collateral ligament of rats. Clinical Orthopaedics and Related Research 203, 301–308.

Bloomfield, S., 1997. Changes in musculoskeletal structure and function with prolonged bed rest. Medicine and Science in Sports and Exercise 29 (2), 197–206.

Bonewald, L.F., 2006. Mechanosensation and transduction in osteocytes. Bonekey Osteovision 3 (10), 7–15.

Boyce, S., Quigley, M., 2004. Review of sports injuries presenting to an accident and emergency department. Emergency Medicine Journal 21 (6), 704–706.

Bray, R.C., Salo, P.T., Lo, I.K., Ackermann, P., Rattner, J., Hart, D.A., et al., 2005. Normal ligament structure, physiology and function. Sports Medicine and Arthroscopy Review 13 (3), 127–135.

Carter, D., Orr, T., Fyhrie, D., Schurman, D., 1987. Influences of mechanical stress on prenatal and postnatal skeletal development. Clinical Orthopaedics and Related Research 219, 237–250.

Ceroni, D., Martin, X., Delhumeau, C., Rizzoli, R., Kaelin, A., Farpour-Lambert, N., et al., 2012. Effects of cast-mediated immobilization on bone mineral mass at various sites in adolescents with lower-extremity fracture. Journal of Bone and Joint Surgery America 94 (3), 208–216.

Chen, C.-H., Liu, X., Yeh, M.-L., Huang, M.-H., Zhai, Q., Lowe, W.R., et al., 2007. Pathological changes of human ligament after complete mechanical unloading. American Journal of Physical Medicine and Rehabilitation 86 (4), 282–289.

Clark, B.C., 2009. In vivo alterations in skeletal muscle form and function after disuse atrophy. Medicine and Science in Sports and Exercise 41 (10), 1869–1875.

Clark, N., Lephart, S., 2015. Management of the sensorimotor system: the lower limb. In: Jull, G., Moore, A., Falla, D., Lewis, J., McCarthy, C., Sterling, M. (Eds.), Grieve's Modern Musculoskeletal Physiotherapy. Elsevier, Edinburgh.

Clark, N.C., 2008. Strength training programme design in physiotherapy practice: what you need to know. Association of Chartered Physiotherapists in Exercise Therapy (ACPET) Study Day. University of Hertfordshire.

Clark, N.C., 2015. (vii) The role of physiotherapy in rehabilitation of soft tissue injuries of the knee. Orthopaedics and Trauma 29 (1), 48–56.

Convertino, V., 1997. Cardiovascular consequences of bed rest: effect on maximal oxygen uptake. Medicine and Science in Sports and Exercise 29 (2), 191–196.

Convertino, V.A., 2007. Blood volume response to physical activity and inactivity. The American Journal of the Medical Sciences 334 (1), 72–79.

Crockett, J.C., Rogers, M.J., Coxon, F.P., Hocking, L.J., Helfrich, M.H., 2011. Bone remodelling at a glance. Journal of Cell Science 124 (Pt 7), 991–998.

Drolet, B.C., Lorenzi, N.M., 2011. Translational research: understanding the continuum from bench to bedside. Translational Research 157 (1), 1–5.

Eastwood, M., Mudera, V., McGrouther, D., Brown, R., 1998. Effect of precise mechanical loading on fibroblast populated collagen lattices: morphological changes. Cell Motility and the Cytoskeleton 40 (1), 13–21.

Ehrlich, P., Lanyon, L., 2002. Mechanical strain and bone cell function: a review. Osteoporosis International 13 (9), 688–700.

Ejerhed, L., Kartus, J., Nilsén, R., Nilsson, U., Kullenberg, R., Karlsson, J., et al., 2004. The effect of anterior cruciate ligament surgery on bone mineral in the calcaneus: a prospective study with a 2-year follow-up evaluation. Arthroscopy 20 (4), 352–359.

Elefteriou, F., Campbell, P., Ma, Y., 2014. Control of bone remodeling by the peripheral sympathetic nervous system. Calcified Tissue International 94 (1), 140–151.

Elias, I., Zoga, A.C., Schweitzer, M.E., Ballehr, L., Morrison, W.B., Raikin, S.M., et al., 2007. A specific bone marrow edema around the foot and ankle following trauma and immobilization therapy: pattern description and potential clinical relevance. Foot and Ankle International 28 (4), 463–471.

Evans, E.B., Eggers, G., Butler, J.K., Blumel, J., 1960. Experimental immobilization and remobilization of rat knee joints. Journal of Bone and Joint Surgery America 42 (5), 737–758.

Feng, X., McDonald, J.M., 2011. Disorders of bone remodeling. Annual Review of Pathology: Mechanisms of Disease 6, 121–145.

Fermor, B., Christensen, S., Youn, I., Cernanec, J., Davies, C., Weinberg, J., et al., 2007. Oxygen, nitric oxide and articular cartilage. European Cells and Materials 13, 56–65.

Fiore, C., Pennisi, P., Ciffo, F., Scebba, C., Amico, A., Di Fazzio, S., et al., 1999. Immobilization-dependent bone collagen breakdown appears to increase with time: evidence for a lack of a new bone equilibrium in response to reduced load during prolonged bed rest. Hormone and Metabolic Research 31 (1), 31–36.

Fox, A., Bedi, A., Rodeo, S., 2009. The basic science of articular cartilage: structure, composition, and function. Sports Health 1 (6), 461–468.

Frangolias, D., Taunton, J., Rhodes, E., McConkey, J., Moon, M., 1997. Maintenance of aerobic capacity during recovery from right foot Jones fracture: a case report. Clinical Journal of Sport Medicine 7 (1), 54–57.

Frank, C., 2004. Ligament structure, physiology and function. Journal of Musculoskeletal and Neuronal Interactions 4 (2), 199–201.

Fry, C.S., Johnson, D.L., Ireland, M.L., Noehren, B., 2017. Acl injury reduces satellite cell abundance and promotes fibrogenic cell expansion within skeletal muscle. Journal of Orthopaedic Research 35 (9), 1876–1885.

Fry, C.S., Lee, J.D., Jackson, J.R., Kirby, T.J., Stasko, S.A., Liu, H., et al., 2014. Regulation of the muscle fiber microenvironment by activated satellite cells during hypertrophy. The Faseb Journal 28 (4), 1654–1665.

Gamble, J., Edwards, C., Max, S., 1984. Enzymatic adaptation in ligaments during immobilization. American Journal of Sports Medicine 12 (3), 221–228.

Garcia-Ramirez, M., Toran, N., Andaluz, P., Carrascosa, A., Audi, L., 2000. Vascular endothelial growth factor is expressed in human fetal growth cartilage. Journal of Bone and Mineral Research 15 (3), 534–540.

Gay, S., Gay, R.E., Miller, E.J., 1980. The collagens of the joint. Arthritis and Rheumatism 23 (8), 937–941.

Gehlsen, G.M., Ganion, L.R., Helfst, R., 1999. Fibroblast responses to variation in soft tissue mobilization pressure. Medicine and Science in Sports and Exercise 31 (4), 531–535.

Guo, X., Kim, C., 2002. Mechanical consequence of trabecular bone loss and its treatment: a three-dimensional model simulation. Bone 30 (2), 404–411.

Hagiwara, Y., Ando, A., Chimoto, E., Saijo, Y., Ohmori–Matsuda, K., Itoi, E., et al., 2009. Changes of articular cartilage after immobilization in a rat knee contracture model. Journal of Orthopaedic Research 27 (2), 236–242.

Harada, S.-I., Rodan, G.A., 2003. Control of osteoblast function and regulation of bone mass. Nature 423 (6937), 349–355.

Harwood, F., Amiel, D., 1992. Differential metabolic responses of periarticular ligaments and tendon to joint immobilization. Journal of Applied Physiology 72 (5), 1687–1691.

Hawker, G.A., Croxford, R., Bierman, A.S., Harvey, P.J., Ravi, B., Stanaitis, I., et al., 2014. All-cause mortality and serious cardiovascular events in people with hip and knee osteoarthritis: a population based cohort study. Plos One 9 (3), e91286.

Hinterwimmer, S., Krammer, M., Krötz, M., Glaser, C., Baumgart, R., Reiser, M., et al., 2004. Cartilage atrophy in the knees of patients after seven weeks of partial load bearing. Arthritis and Rheumatism 50 (8), 2516–2520.

Hohmann, E., Bryant, A., Tetsworth, K., 2016. Strength does not influence knee function in the ACL-deficient knee but is a correlate of knee function in the and ACL-reconstructed knee. Archives of Orthopaedic and Trauma Surgery 136 (4), 477–483.

Hootman, J.M., Dick, R., Agel, J., 2007. Epidemiology of collegiate injuries for 15 sports: summary and recommendations for injury prevention initiatives. Journal of Athletic Training 42 (2), 311–319.

Huang, S., Wikswo, J., 2006. Dimensions of systems biology. Reviews of Physiology, Biochemistry and Pharmacology 157, 81–104.

Iqbal, K., Khan, M., Minhas, L., 2012. Effects of immobilisation and re-mobilisation on superficial zone of articular cartilage of patella in rats. Journal of the Pakistan Medical Association 62 (6), 531–535.

Jortikka, M.O., Inkinen, R.I., Tammi, M.I., Parkkinen, J.J., Haapala, J., Kiviranta, I., et al., 1997. Immobilisation causes longlasting matrix changes both in the immobilised and contralateral joint cartilage. Annals of the Rheumatic Diseases 56 (4), 255–261.

Kanda, T., Ochi, M., Ikuta, Y., 1998. Adverse effects on rabbit anterior cruciate ligament after knee immobilization: changes in permeability of horseradish peroxidase. Archives of Orthopaedic and Trauma Surgery 117 (6–7), 307–311.

Kaneguchi, A., Ozawa, J., Kawamata, S., Yamaoka, K., 2017. Development of arthrogenic joint contracture as a result of pathological changes in remobilized rat knees. Journal of Orthopaedic Research 35 (7), 1414–1423.

Klein, L., Player, J., Heiple, K., Bahniuk, E., Goldberg, V., 1982. Isotopic evidence for resorption of soft tissues and bone in immobilized dogs. Journal of Bone and Joint Surgery America 64 (2), 225–230.

Lafont, J.E., 2010. Lack of oxygen in articular cartilage: consequences for chondrocyte biology. International Journal of Experimental Pathology 91 (2), 99–106.

Larsen, N.P., Forwood, M.R., Parker, A.W., 1987. Immobilization and retraining of cruciate ligaments in the rat. Acta Orthopaedica Scandinavica 58 (3), 260–264.

Lee, S., Sakurai, T., Ohsako, M., Saura, R., Hatta, H., Atomi, Y., et al., 2010. Tissue stiffness induced by prolonged immobilization of the rat knee joint and relevance of AGEs (pentosidine). Connective Tissue Research 51 (6), 467–477.

Lepola, V., Väänänen, K., Jalovaara, P., 1993. The effect of immobilization on the torsional strength of the rat tibia. Clinical Orthopaedics and Related Research (297), 55–61.

Leppälä, J., Kannus, P., Natri, A., Pasanen, M., Sievänen, H., Vuori, I., et al., 1999. Effect of anterior cruciate ligament injury of the knee on bone mineral density of the spine and affected lower extremity: a prospective one-year follow-up study. Calcified Tissue International 64 (4), 357–363.

Liedert, A., Kaspar, D., Blakytny, R., Claes, L., Ignatius, A., 2006. Signal transduction pathways involved in mechanotransduction in bone cells. Biochemical and Biophysical Research Communications 349 (1), 1–5.

Lobenhoffer, H., Bosch, U., Gerich, T., 1996. Role of posterior capsulotomy for the treatment of extension deficits of the knee. Knee Surgery, Sports Traumatology, Arthroscopy 4 (4), 237–241.

Luhmann, S., 2003. Acute traumatic knee effusions in children and adolescents. Journal of Pediatric Orthopedics 23 (2), 199–202.

Mabry, P.L., Olster, D.H., Morgan, G.D., Abrams, D.B., 2008. Interdisciplinarity and systems science to improve population health: a view from the nih office of behavioral and social sciences research. American Journal of Preventive Medicine 35 (Suppl. 2), S211–S224.

MacIntosh, B., Gardiner, P., McComas, A., 2006. Skeletal Muscle. Form and Function, second ed. Human Kinetics, Illinois.

Maglio, P.P., Mabry, P.L., 2011. Agent-based models and systems science approaches to public health. American Journal of Preventive Medicine 40 (3), 392–394.

Man, I., Morrissey, M., Cywinski, J., 2007. Effect of neuromuscular electrical stimulation on ankle swelling in the early period after ankle sprain. Physical Therapy 87 (1), 53–65.

Mariani, P.P., Santori, N., Rovere, P., Della Rocca, C., Adriani, E., 1997. Histological and structural study of the adhesive tissue in knee fibroarthrosis: a clinical–pathological correlation. Arthroscopy 13 (3), 313–318.

Matsumoto, F., Trudel, G., Uhthoff, H.K., 2002. High collagen type I and low collagen type Iii levels in knee joint contracture. Acta Orthopaedica Scandinavica 73 (3), 335–343.

Milner, P., Wilkins, R., Gibson, J., 2012. Cellular physiology of articular cartilage in health and disease. In: Rothschild, B. (Ed.), Principles of Osteoarthritis – Its Definition, Character, Derivation, and Modality-Related Recognition. InTech, London.

Mosekilde, L., Thomsen, J.S., Mackey, M., Phipps, R.J., 2000. Treatment with risedronate or alendronate prevents hind-limb immobilization-induced loss of bone density and strength in adult female rats. Bone 27 (5), 639–645.

Mudera, V., Pleass, R., Eastwood, M., Tarnuzzer, R., Schultz, G., Khaw, P., et al., 2000. Molecular responses of human dermal fibroblasts to dual cues: contact guidance and mechanical load. Cell Motility and the Cytoskeleton 45 (1), 1–9.

Mujika, I., Padilla, S., 2001. Cardiorespiratory and metabolic characteristics of detraining in humans. Medicine and Science in Sports and Exercise 33, 413–421.

Mutsuzaki, H., Nakajima, H., Wadano, Y., Furuhata, S., Sakane, M., 2017. Influence of knee immobilization on chondrocyte apoptosis and histological features of the anterior cruciate ligament insertion and articular cartilage in rabbits. International Journal of Molecular Sciences 18 (2), 253.

Nardo, L., Sandman, D.N., Virayavanich, W., Zhang, L., Souza, R.B., Steinbach, L., et al., 2013. Bone marrow changes related to disuse. European Radiology 23 (12), 3422–3431.

Neidlinger-Wilke, C., Grood, E., Wang, J.C., Brand, R., Claes, L., 2001. Cell alignment is induced by cyclic changes in cell length: studies of cells grown in cyclically stretched substrates. Journal of Orthopaedic Research 19 (2), 286–293.

Neumann, D., 2002. Kinesiology of the Musculoskeletal System. Mosby, St Louis.

Newton, P., Woo, S.-Y., Kitabayashi, L., Lyon, R., Anderson, D., Akeson, W., et al., 1990. Ultrastructural changes in knee ligaments following immobilization. Matrix 10 (5), 314–319.

Newton, P., Woo, S., MacKenna, D., Akeson, W., 1995. Immobilization of the knee joint alters the mechanical and ultrastructural properties of the rabbit anterior cruciate ligament. Journal of Orthopaedic Research 13 (2), 191–200.

Noehren, B., Andersen, A., Hardy, P., Johnson, D.L., Ireland, M.L., Thompson, K.L., et al., 2016. Cellular and morphological alterations in the vastus lateralis muscle as the result of ACL injury and reconstruction. Journal of Bone and Joint Surgery America 98 (18), 1541–1547.

Nomura, M., Sakitani, N., Iwasawa, H., Kohara, Y., Takano, S., Wakimoto, Y., et al., 2017. Thinning of articular cartilage after joint unloading or immobilization. An experimental investigation of the pathogenesis in mice. Osteoarthritis and Cartilage 25 (5), 727–736.

Norte, G.E., Knaus, K.R., Kuenze, C., Handsfield, G.G., Meyer, C.H., Blemker, S.S., et al., 2018. MRI-based assessment of lower extremity muscle volumes in patients before and after Acl reconstruction. Journal of Sport Rehabilitation 27 (3), 201–212.

Noyes, F.R., 1977. Functional properties of knee ligaments and alterations induced by immobilization: a correlative biomechanical and histological study in primates. Clinical Orthopaedics and Related Research (123), 210–242.

Oftadeh, R., Perez-Viloria, M., Villa-Camacho, J.C., Vaziri, A., Nazarian, A., 2015. Biomechanics and mechanobiology of trabecular bone: a review. Journal of Biomechanical Engineering 137 (1), 0108021–01080215.

Olsson, O., Isacsson, A., Englund, M., Frobell, R., 2016. Epidemiology of intra- and peri-articular structural injuries in traumatic knee joint hemarthrosis – data from 1145 consecutive knees with subacute MRI. Osteoarthritis and Cartilage 24 (11), 1890–1897.

Palmoski, M., Brandt, K., 1981. Running inhibits the reversal of atrophic changes in canine knee cartilage after removal of a leg cast. Arthritis and Rheumatism 24 (11), 1329–1337.

Pavalko, F.M., Norvell, S.M., Burr, D.B., Turner, C.H., Duncan, R.L., Bidwell, J.P., et al., 2003. A model for mechanotransduction in bone cells: the load–bearing mechanosomes. Journal of Cellular Biochemistry 88 (1), 104–112.

Peng, Z., Tuukkanen, J., Zhang, H., Jämsä, T., Väänänen, H., 1994. The mechanical strength of bone in different rat models of experimental osteoporosis. Bone 15 (5), 523–532.

Perry, B.D., Levinger, P., Morris, H.G., Petersen, A.C., Garnham, A.P., Levinger, I., et al., 2015. The effects of knee injury on skeletal muscle function, Na^+, K^+–ATPase content, and isoform abundance. Physiological Reports 3 (2), e12294.

Poole, A., Kojima, T., Yasuda, T., Mwale, F., Kobayashi, M., Laverty, S., et al., 2001. Composition and structure of articular cartilage: a template for tissue repair. Clinical Orthopaedics and Related Research (Suppl. 391), S26–33.

Punt, I., Ziltener, J., Laidet, M., Armand, S., Allet, L., 2015. Gait and physical impairments in patients with acute ankle sprains who did not receive physical therapy. PM R. 7 (1), 34–41.

Ralphs, J., Benjamin, M., 1994. The joint capsule: structure, composition, ageing and disease. Journal of Anatomy 184 (Pt 3), 503–509.

Reiman, M.P., Rogers, M.E., Manske, R.C., 2006. Interlimb differences in lower extremity bone mineral density following anterior cruciate ligament reconstruction. Journal of Orthopaedic and Sports Physical Therapy 36 (11), 837–844.

Ried-Larsen, M., Aarts, H.M., Joyner, M.J., 2017. Effects of strict prolonged bed rest on cardiorespiratory fitness: systematic review and meta-analysis. Journal of Applied Physiology 123 (4), 790–799.

Ringholm, S., Biensø, R.S., Kiilerich, K., Guadalupe-Grau, A., Aachmann-Andersen, N.J., Saltin, B., et al., 2011. Bed rest reduces metabolic protein content and abolishes exercise-induced mrna responses in human skeletal muscle. American Journal of Physiology-Endocrinology and Metabolism 301 (4), E649–E658.

Roemer, F.W., Jomaah, N., Niu, J., Almusa, E., Roger, B., D'hooghe, P., et al., 2014. Ligamentous injuries and the risk of associated tissue damage in acute ankle sprains in athletes: a cross-sectional MRI study. American Journal of Sports Medicine 42 (7), 1549–1557.

Rosa, N., Simoes, R., Magalhães, F.D., Marques, A.T., 2015. From mechanical stimulus to bone formation: a review. Medical Engineering and Physics 37 (8), 719–728.

Roy, S., 1970. Ultrastructure of articular cartilage in experimental immobilization. Annals of the Rheumatic Diseases 29 (6), 634–642.

Rubio, D.M., Schoenbaum, E.E., Lee, L.S., Schteingart, D.E., Marantz, P.R., Anderson, K.E., et al., 2010. Defining translational research: implications for training. Academic Medicine 85 (3), 470–475.

Sakamoto, J., Origuchi, T., Okita, M., Nakano, J., Kato, K., Yoshimura, T., et al., 2009. Immobilization-induced cartilage degeneration mediated through expression of hypoxia-inducible factor-1alpha, vascular endothelial growth factor, and chondromodulin-I. Connective Tissue Research 50 (1), 37–45.

Schollmeier, G., Uhthoff, H.K., Sarkar, K., Fukuhara, K., 1994. Effects of immobilization on the capsule of the canine glenohumeral joint. A structural functional study. Clinical Orthopaedics and Related Research (304), 37–42.

Simkin, P.A., 1991. Physiology of normal and abnormal synovium. Seminars in Arthritis and Rheumatism 21 (3), 179–183.

Smith, R., Thomas, K., Schurman, D., Carter, D., Wong, M., Van Der Meulen, M., et al., 1992. Rabbit knee immobilization: bone remodeling precedes cartilage degradation. Journal of Orthopaedic Research 10 (1), 88–95.

Sood, S., 1971. A study of the effects of experimental immobilisation on rabbit articular cartilage. Journal of Anatomy 108 (Pt 3), 497–507.

Stevens, J.E., Pathare, N.C., Tillman, S.M., Scarborough, M.T., Gibbs, C.P., Shah, P., et al., 2006. Relative contributions of muscle activation and muscle size to plantarflexor torque during rehabilitation after immobilization. Journal of Orthopaedic Research 24 (8), 1729–1736.

Tirabassi, J., Brou, L., Khodaee, M., Lefort, R., Fields, S., Comstock, R., et al., 2016. Epidemiology of high school sports-related injuries resulting in medical disqualification: 2005–2006 through 2013–2014 academic years. American Journal of Sports Medicine 44 (11), 2925–2932.

Toomey, C., Whittaker, J., Nettel-Aguirre, A., Reimer, R., Woodhouse, L., Ghali, B., et al., 2017. Higher fat mass is associated with a history of knee injury in youth sport. Journal of Orthopaedic and Sports Physical Therapy 47 (2), 80–87.

Trudel, G., Laneuville, O., Coletta, E., Goudreau, L., Uhthoff, H.K., 2014. Quantitative and temporal differential recovery of articular and muscular limitations of knee joint contractures; results in a rat model. Journal of Applied Physiology 117 (7), 730–737.

Trudel, G., Seki, M., Uhthoff, H., 2000. Synovial adhesions are more important than pannus proliferation in the pathogenesis of knee joint contracture after immobilization: an experimental investigation in the rat. Journal of Rheumatology 27 (2), 351–357.

Turner, C.H., Pavalko, F.M., 1998. Mechanotransduction and functional response of the skeleton to physical stress: the mechanisms and mechanics of bone adaptation. Journal of Orthopaedic Science 3 (6), 346–355.

Uebelhart, D., Bernard, J., Hartmann, D., Moro, L., Roth, M., Uebelhart, B., et al., 2000. Modifications of bone and connective tissue after orthostatic bedrest. Osteoporosis International 11 (1), 59–67.

Vanwanseele, B., Eckstein, F., Knecht, H., Stüssi, E., Spaepen, A., 2002a. Knee cartilage of spinal cord–injured patients displays progressive thinning in the absence of normal joint loading and movement. Arthritis and Rheumatism 46 (8), 2073–2078.

Vanwanseele, B., Lucchinetti, E., Stüssi, E., 2002b. The effects of immobilization on the characteristics of articular cartilage: current concepts and future directions. Osteoarthritis and Cartilage 10 (5), 408–419.

Wall, B.T., Dirks, M.L., Snijders, T., Senden, J.M., Dolmans, J., Loon, L.V., et al., 2014. Substantial skeletal muscle loss occurs during only 5 days of disuse. Acta Physiologica 210 (3), 600–611.

Weiner, S., Wagner, H.D., 1998. The material bone: structure–mechanical function relations. Annual Review of Materials Science 28, 271–298.

Weinreb, M., Rodan, G., Thompson, D., 1989. Osteopenia in the immobilized rat hind limb is associated with increased bone resorption and decreased bone formation. Bone 10 (3), 187–194.

Whiting, C., Zernicke, F., 2008. Biomechanics of Musculoskeletal Injury. Human Kinetics, Illinois.

Widman, L., Abresch, R., Styne, D., McDonald, C., 2007. Aerobic fitness and upper extremity strength in patients aged 11 to 21 years with spinal cord dysfunction as compared to ideal weight and overweight controls. Journal of Spinal Cord Medicine 30 (Suppl. 1), S88–96.

Wilmore, J., Costill, D., Kenney, W., 2015. Physiology of Sport and Exercise. Human Kinetics, Illinois.

Woo, S., Gomez, M., Sites, T., Newton, P., Orlando, C., Akeson, W., et al., 1987. The biomechanical and morphological changes in the medial collateral ligament of the rabbit after immobilization and remobilization. Journal of Bone and Joint Surgery America 69 (8), 1200–1211.

Wronski, T., Morey, E., 1983. Inhibition of cortical and trabecular bone formation in the long bones of immobilized monkeys. Clinical Orthopaedics and Related Research (181), 269–276.

Yabe, Y., Hagiwara, Y., Suda, H., Ando, A., Onoda, Y., Tsuchiya, M., et al., 2013. Joint immobilization induced hypoxic and inflammatory conditions in rat knee joints. Connective Tissue Research 54 (3), 210–217.

Young, D., Niklowitz, W., Brown, R., Jee, W., 1986. Immobilization-associated osteoporosis in primates. Bone 7 (2), 109–117.

Chapter | 4 |

Strength and conditioning: scientific aspects including principles of rehabilitation

Paul Jones and Paul Comfort

Introduction

Strength and conditioning is the application of strength training and various other conditioning methods to physically prepare athletes for all aspects of sporting performance. Effective physical preparation of athletes should maintain their health status and reduce the risk of non-contact sports injuries, whilst enhancing their sporting performance.

Whilst the role of a strength and conditioning coach is to utilize information from all members of the sports science and medicine team in developing such programmes, physiotherapists should utilize principles of strength and conditioning to design more effective rehabilitation programmes to better prepare athletes for return to full training and competition. To achieve this a progressive training programme must be implemented that adheres to the principles of progressive overload, by effectively manipulating both the volume and intensity of training/rehabilitation, to result in the appropriate adaptations to the desired physiological tissues and structure, while restoring function. This chapter outlines basic scientific principles of strength and conditioning that must be considered in designing effective training or rehabilitation programmes. Whilst strength and conditioning may involve a range of training modalities to prepare athletes for competition – such as resistance training, plyometric training, endurance training, flexibility training, and speed, change of direction and agility training methods – it is beyond the scope of this chapter to cover all conditioning methods. Therefore, this chapter focuses on the importance of strength and factors that influence the expression of strength, the basic principles for developing strength, the development of specific strength qualities,

and it provides an overview with worked examples of how to design 'strength' workouts and periodize training using the concept of phase potentiation.

The importance of muscle strength

Muscular strength is defined as the ability to exert force on an external resistance. Within sports, an athlete may be required to manipulate their own body mass against gravity (e.g., sprinting, jumping), both their body mass and an opponent's body mass (e.g., rugby), or that of an external object (e.g., shot put, weightlifting). Ultimately, the force exerted will change, or tend to change, the motion of a body in space. This is based on Newton's second law of acceleration whereby force (f) is equal to the product of mass (m) and acceleration (a). Based on this principle, the acceleration of a given mass is directly proportional to, and in the same direction as, the force applied. Therefore, muscular strength is the primary factor for producing an effective and efficient movement of an athlete's body or an external object. This concept is supported by several studies that have found a relationship between muscular strength and performance in a range of motor skills such as sprinting (Comfort et al., 2014; Kirkpatrick and Comfort, 2012; Styles et al., 2015; Seitz et al., 2014a; Wisloff et al., 2004), jumping (Hori et al., 2008; Wisloff et al., 2004), and change of direction (Hori et al., 2008; Nimphius et al., 2010).

Previous literature has indicated that both rate of force development (RFD; change in force divided by the change in time) and power output (rate of work performed) are two of the most important characteristics regarding an athlete's performance (Baker et al., 2001; Morrissey et al., 1995 Stone et al., 2002). RFD is critical given the time constraints of various sporting tasks. For instance, evidence suggests that it takes individuals a longer period of time (>300 ms) to produce their maximum force (Aagaard et al., 2002; Aagaard, 2003) compared to the duration of jumping and ground contact time during sprinting (Andersen and Aagaard, 2006). Furthermore, athletes have limited time to perform the mechanical work involved with typical sporting tasks and thus, it would seem beneficial to complete the work as fast as possible. For example, an athlete who completes the required work of a given task more quickly may be given a competitive edge compared to their opponent (e.g., beating an opponent in a sprint to the ball in soccer). Given that muscular strength serves as the foundation upon which other abilities can be enhanced, improvements in RFD and power output can result from increases in strength (Suchomel and Comfort, 2017). Furthermore, unless athletes are strong (maximal back squat ≥1.9 × body mass), increasing strength appears to result in greater improvements in performance than ballistic or plyometric training using lighter loads, but with a focus on the velocity of movement (Cormie et al., 2007; 2010a; 2010b; 2011).

Factors affecting muscle force

There are three basic forms of muscle actions: concentric, eccentric and isometric (Table 4.1). During each, forces are generated within the muscle that pull the muscle ends toward each other depending on the magnitude of the external resistance. Furthermore, often during sporting movements an eccentric action is preceded by a concentric action, which enhances the resulting concentric action known as the stretch–shorten cycle (SSC) (see Table 4.1). Several factors are involved in the expression of human strength during such actions including aspects of neural control, morphological factors, muscle length and contraction velocity.

Motor unit recruitment

The recruitment of muscle fibres is directly related to the size of the motor neuron (Milner-Brown et al., 1973). Initially small motor neurons are recruited followed by large motor neurons as more force is required (Henneman et al., 1965; Henneman and Olson 1965). This has been referred to as the Henneman size principle, where small motor units (type I) are recruited first and then large motor units (type II). The greater the stimulus, the greater the number of muscle fibres stimulated and the greater the strength of the muscle action. The fact that all muscles contain both type I and II muscle fibres enables graded levels of muscle contraction to occur. In order for a motor unit to be trained, it must be recruited; therefore to recruit high-threshold motor units, heavy loads are required, along with the 'intention' to accelerate them

Table 4.1 Summary of common muscle actions

Muscle action	Description
Isometric	An isometric muscle action results when the moment generated by a muscle or group of muscles is equal to the resistive moment. No movement occurs
Concentric	A concentric action results when the moment generated by the muscle or group of muscles is greater than the resistive moment. This leads to shortening of the muscle–tendon complex
Eccentric	An eccentric action results when the moment generated by the muscle or group of muscles is less than the resistive moment. This leads to lengthening of the muscle–tendon complex
Stretch–shorten cycle (SSC)	The SSC is when the force of a concentric action is enhanced by a preceding eccentric muscle action due to (a) stretch reflex through stimulation of the muscle spindle during the eccentric phase and (b) storage and release of elastic energy. Both actions are separated by a brief amortization phase, with shorter amortization phases taking advantage of both mechanisms, leading to greater potentiation in the concentric phase. SSC movements may therefore be subdivided into short (<250 ms) and long (>250 ms) response SSC

rapidly. Furthermore, to train RFD and power preferential, recruitment of high-threshold motor units are required. However, whilst orderly recruitment of motor units exists following ballistic-type training, motor units are recruited at lower force thresholds (van Cutsem et al., 1998). Therefore, it would appear that training modalities that are ballistic in nature (weightlifting, jump squats, etc.) will allow recruitment of larger, type II motor units at lower thresholds, using lower external loads, thus allowing for positive strength and power adaptations to occur.

Firing frequency

The frequency of the neural stimulation affects the force of the muscular action. A single neural stimulus will result in a muscle twitch. A muscle twitch consists of a brief latent period followed by a muscle contraction and then a relaxation period. The force of the action and the total time will depend on the type of muscle fibre, with fast-twitch fibres contracting more quickly and with more force than slow-twitch fibres. If a series of neural stimuli are used (1–3 ms apart) (Ghez, 1991), the muscle has not had time to relax and so an increase in muscle tension is produced due to the summation of each twitch. If the frequency of the neural stimuli is increased still further, individual contractions are blended together in a single sustained contraction known as fused tetanus (Ghez, 1991). This action will continue until the neural stimulus is stopped or the muscle fatigues. Research has demonstrated that again ballistic-type training may enhance motor unit firing frequency (van Cutsem et al., 1998), leading to enhanced strength–power performance.

Modification by muscle and tendon receptors

The nervous system has many mechanisms for providing feedback in the form of information on the forces applied, joint position and muscle length changes. This allows movement to be monitored, controlled and to prevent injury by limiting the contraction force of the muscles. The stretch reflex is mediated by receptors in the muscle (muscle spindle), which allows muscle to produce more force when it has suddenly been stretched through an eccentric muscle action. This is one mechanism of the SSC, whereby concentric muscle force is enhanced following a prior eccentric muscle action (providing only a very short delay occurs between each muscle action). Plyometric training is a method to enhance this muscle phenomenon (Table 4.2).

In contrast, the golgi tendon organ has a role in inhibiting the force produced by the muscle to prevent forces being produced that could tear muscle and tendon. However, heavy strength training may downregulate Ib afferent feedback to the spinal motor neuron pool, ultimately reducing neuromuscular inhibition and increasing force production (Aagaard et al., 2000). Thus, heavy resistance training may lead to decreased neuromuscular inhibition, leading to potential enhanced strength and power of athletes.

Cross-sectional area

Greater muscle fibre cross-sectional area (CSA) results in a greater size of the overall muscle. From a physiological perspective, greater muscle CSA enhances force production due to an increased number of sarcomeres in parallel (greater spatial summation). An increase in the number of sarcomeres (i.e., smallest contractile unit within a muscle cell) increases the number of potential interactions between

actin and myosin microfilaments (i.e., cross-bridges), which ultimately increases the force a muscle can produce.

Muscle architecture

Architectural properties of skeletal muscle have also been shown to affect both force and velocity of muscle actions. A decrease in pennation angle or an increase in fascicle length results in an increase in velocity of contraction due to an increased length of the contractile component (Blazevich, 2006; Earp et al., 2010). In contrast, an increase in pennation angle results in an increase in the number of fibres for a given cross-sectional area, which increases force-generation capacity (Blazevich, 2006; Manal et al., 2006; Earp et al., 2010).

Muscle length and the mechanical model of muscle

When a muscle is at its resting length, the actin and myosin filaments lie next to each other, so that a maximal number of potential cross-bridge sites are available. This allows a greater level of force to be generated at resting length. When the muscle shortens, the actin filaments overlap and the number of cross-bridge sites is reduced, decreasing force-generating potential. When the muscle is stretched, a reduced proportion of actin and myosin filaments lie next to each other, again reducing force-generating potential. This phenomenon describes the length–tension relationship of muscle (Fig. 4.1). Due to the nature of many sports it is essential to train muscles across their entire range, where possible.

Fig. 4.2 illustrates the mechanical model of muscle, composed of the contractile component, parallel and series elastic components. When the muscle–tendon complex is stretched during an eccentric muscle action, tension 'passively' increases in the muscle–tendon complex due to the elastic properties of the tendon and tissues surrounding muscle fibres (see Fig. 4.1), particularly with increasing velocity. During SSC movements, stored elastic energy, primarily in the tendon, is utilized during the subsequent concentric phase, leading to enhanced force production providing a short delay between eccentric and concentric muscle actions (in addition to the stretch reflex mentioned earlier). Furthermore, the length–tension relationship of muscle (see Fig. 4.1) has implications for eccentric training in that greater loads (i.e., 110% one-repetition maximum (1RM) for novice trainers) are required (compared to concentric actions only) during the eccentric phases of exercises (e.g., descent of a back squat).

Contraction velocity

Based on the classic work on isolated animal muscle of Hill (1970), the force capability of muscle declines as the velocity of contraction increases, perhaps due a decline in formed

Table 4.2 Overview of different strength–power training methods

Modality	Rationale and benefits	Disadvantages
Bodyweight exercise	Bodyweight exercise is one of the most basic forms of resistance training and has several advantages including a focus on improving relative strength and greater accessibility and versatility compared to other training methods (Harrison, 2010)	The most obvious limitation of bodyweight exercises is the inability to continue to provide an overload stimulus to the athlete, preventing significant development of absolute strength (Harrison, 2010). Practitioners may prescribe a greater number of repetitions or modify the movement (i.e., push-up variations) in order to progress each exercise. However, a continual increase in repetitions leads to the development of strength–endurance instead of strength–power necessary for enhanced sport performance
Machine weight training	Machine-based exercises allow for the isolation of specific muscle groups, which may be useful for rehabilitation from injury	Machine-based exercise may lack movement specificity. For example, athletic movements rarely include isolated muscle actions (Behm and Anderson, 2006). Therefore, transfer from isolation exercises to athletic performance maybe somewhat limited (Augustsson et al., 1998; Blackburn and Morrissey, 1998)
Free-weight training	Free-weight training incorporates multiple muscle groups and provides superior training stimulus than isolation exercises performed on a machine (Anderson and Behm, 2005). Free-weight exercises may recruit muscle stabilizers to a greater extent than machine-based exercises (Haff, 2000) and thus, greater strength–power adaptations as they relate to sport performance	Free-weight exercises require a greater level of technique development compared to machine weights. Utilizing free-weight exercises to develop power is limited without modifying the exercise, as exercises such as the bench press and squat result in deceleration during the later stages of the concentric phase (Lake et al., 2012; Newton et al., 1996). These exercises could be modified (ballistic) to ensure acceleration throughout the concentric phase such as bench press throws or jump squats (Newton et al., 1996)
Weightlifting	Weightlifting exercises produce the greatest power outputs compared to other types of exercise. Weightlifting movements are unique in they exploit both the force and velocity aspects of power output by moving moderate-to-heavy loads with ballistic intent (Suchomel and Comfort, 2017). A major advantage of weightlifting is that the athlete aims to accelerate throughout the concentric phase, unlike traditional free-weight exercises (i.e., bench press and squat)	Weightlifting exercises require time spent developing lifting technique competency. However, simpler weightlifting derivatives (i.e., pulling actions – mid-thigh clean pull, clean from the knee) require less technical competency than full clean and snatch lifts and, thus, are useful approaches to rate of force development and power development (Suchomel et al., 2015)

Table 4.2 Overview of different strength–power training methods—cont'd

Modality	Rationale and benefits	Disadvantages
Plyometric training	Plyometric movements may be defined as quick, power movements that use a prestretch resulting in utilization of the stretch–shortening cycle (see Table 4.1). Several meta-analyses have shown that plyometric training can enhance vertical jump ability (Sáez de Villarreal et al., 2009), sprint performance (Sáez de Villarreal et al., 2012) and change of direction ability (Asadi et al., 2016). Furthermore, plyometric training has been shown to improve running economy (Spurrs et al., 2002; Turner et al., 2003) and address poor landing mechanics (Hewett et al., 1996)	Most plyometric exercises are implemented using the athlete's body mass as the resistance. Using only the athlete's body mass as a resistance may be limited in terms of strength–power development. Practitioners are able to prescribe small additional loads to increase the loading stimulus on the athlete; however, a more sensible approach would be to increase the plyometric exercise intensity via changing the plyometric exercise, changing drop height or changing coaching instruction, while simultaneously adjusting the volume to meet the needs of each athlete
Eccentric training	Eccentric muscle actions are those that lengthen the muscle as a result of a greater force being applied to a muscle than the muscle itself can produce. Although not well understood, eccentric muscle actions possess unique molecular and neural characteristics that may produce similar or greater adaptations in muscle function, morphological adaptations, neuromuscular adaptations, and performance compared to concentric, isometric and traditional (eccentric/concentric) training (Douglas et al., 2016a; 2016b). However, little is known about how to best implement eccentric training. Accentuated eccentric training involves performing the eccentric phase of a lift with a heavier load than the concentric phase by removing a portion of the load, and this has some support in the literature. Methods include using a weight-release system (Ojasto and Häkkinen, 2009), spotters (Brandenburg and Docherty, 2002), the athlete dropping it (Sheppard et al., 2008), or flywheel (de Hoyo et al., 2015) at the end of the eccentric phase	Eccentric training can lead to high levels of delayed onset muscle soreness (DOMS) initially, but after a few bouts of eccentric training the muscle should attain a protective effect from further DOMS
Complex/ contrast training (CT)	CT is a training modality that involves completing a resistance training exercise prior to performing a ballistic exercise that is biomechanically similar. For example, back squats may be paired with countermovement jumps. CT appears to take advantage of postactivation potentiation (PAP), which is an acute enhancement in muscular performance as a result of the muscle's contractile history (Robbins, 2005). Numerous studies have demonstrated such a performance improvement in a training context (see Jones et al., 2013a; 2013b for a review)	Whilst the implementation of CT to take advantage of PAP in training is appealing, there is limited research on the longitudinal effects. Furthermore, attempting to elicit PAP with weaker individuals maybe limited as greater muscular strength may lead to faster and greater potentiation (Seitz et al., 2014b; Suchomel et al., 2016). Given that research has shown that >8 min recovery between exercises maybe required to take advantage of PAP, this may lead to logistical issues, as much more training time is spent in recovery (Jones et al., 2013b)

Continued

Part | 1 | Important background concepts in sports

Table 4.2 Overview of different strength–power training methods—cont'd

Modality	Rationale and benefits	Disadvantages
Variable resistance training	Variable resistance training refers to a training method that alters the external resistance through the use of chains or elastic bands during the exercise in order to maximize muscle force throughout the range of motion (Fleck and Kraemer, 2014). The addition of chains or elastic bands alters the loading profile of an exercise (Israetel et al., 2010), allowing the athlete to match changes in joint leverage (Zatsiorsky and Kraemer, 2006) and overcome mechanical disadvantages at various joint angles (Ebben and Jensen, 2002; Wallace et al., 2006). It appears to be an effective training tool for developing muscular strength and power	Determining and adjusting the amount of load off-set by bands and chains during free-weight exercises requires preparation time
Kettlebell training	Kettlebells are implements that consist of a weighted ball and handle. A range of exercises can be performed with kettlebells including swings, goblet squats, accelerated swings and modified weightlifting exercises (i.e., snatch) for the purposes of developing strength and power. Previous research has indicated that kettlebell training may improve various measures of muscular strength and explosive performance (Lake and Lauder, 2012; Otto III et al., 2012)	Although research suggests that kettlebell training may provide an effective strength–power training stimulus, traditional methods such as weightlifting may provide superior adaptations when it comes to developing maximal strength and explosiveness (Otto III et al., 2012), perhaps due to difficulty in generating progressive overload (i.e., size of kettlebell vs. a loaded bar)

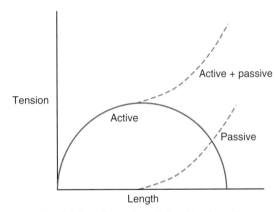

Fig. 4.1 Length–tension relationship of muscle.

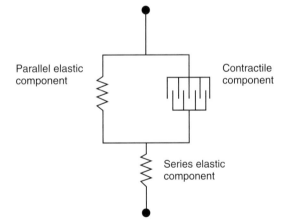

Fig. 4.2 Mechanical model of muscle. 'Contractile component' refers to actin–myosin filaments, the primary source of generating muscle force during concentric actions. 'Series elastic component' (i.e., tendon) stores elastic energy when stretched, increasing force production. 'Parallel elastic component' (i.e., epimysium, perimysium, endomysium and sarcolemma) exerts 'passive' tension when the muscle is stretched. Hill, A.V. (1970). *First and Last Experiments in Muscle Mechanics*. London: Cambridge University Press.

cross-bridges as the speed of shortening increases. The relationship is curvilinear, with the decline in force capability steepest over the lower range of movement speeds (Fig. 4.3). As mentioned above, athletes are required to work against a range of resistances in sport (i.e., their own body, an opponent or sports object) and thus, depending on specific sport demands, athletes may be required to develop different portions of the force–velocity curve (the high- or low-velocity end, or both). This requires manipulation of load and exercise selection (Suchomel et al., 2017).

30

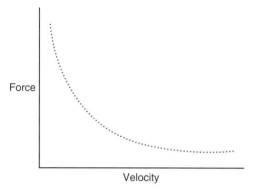

Fig. 4.3 Force–velocity relationship of muscle.

Basic principles for increasing muscle strength and power

There is a variety of exercise regimes to increase muscle strength and power. A summary is given in Table 4.2. The important principles for development of strength and power are overload, specificity, individuality, reversibility and diminishing returns.

Overload

For any of the systems within the body to adapt, the stimuli must be sufficient to create overload, that is, it is necessary to expose the tissue to a load greater than one to which it has recently been subjected. To improve the strength (or other fitness qualities) of a muscle it must be *progressively* and appropriately overloaded (Bruton, 2002). To create overload when strengthening a muscle, the resistance (load) must be greater than the muscles are accustomed to during everyday activities; and as the muscle gains strength the resistance must be progressively increased. Overload in this case can be achieved initially through a slight increase in repetitions (2–6) or sets (3–6), but once the maximum number of repetitions is achieved at a given resistance, the resistance (external load) must be increased (usually ≥85% of maximum). To further increase repetitions alters the focus from muscular strength to muscular endurance. When increasing muscle endurance, there must be a progressive increase in volume of exercise, again via an increase in repetitions (10–20) of sets (2–3), although as with strength, if the maximum number of repetitions can be achieved with a given resistance, the resistance must be increased. It is this progressive nature which ensures that overload continues across rehabilitation/training sessions.

Specificity

This principle relates to the specific adaptation of muscle to the imposed demands (SAID principle) (DiNubile, 1991). The effect on muscle is specific to the nature of the exercise (see Development of specific qualities). The implication of specificity is that the prescribed exercise does not need to mirror the movement pattern of the functional activity it aims to improve (i.e., directly copy the movement patterns of the sports action). The activity needs to target the appropriate musculature, and the loading and/or velocity of movement needs to be specific so that appropriate overload, relative to the aim, is achieved. For example, strengthening the quadriceps should involve high resistance and low repetition, but the exercise could be a squat (e.g., front squat, back squat, box squat), a lunge variation (e.g., forward lunge, reverse lunge, rear foot elevated split squat) or a simple knee extension exercise. However, the transfer from knee extension to, for example, a typical sit to stand will be much less effective than from a squat or lunge variation (Augustsson et al., 1998; Blackburn and Morrissey, 1998).

Individuality

Individuals will respond differently to the same exercise; this response is determined by genetics, cellular growth rates, metabolism and neural and endocrine regulation. For example, an exercise given to an 80-year-old and a 26-year-old will have different effects, as over the age of 60 years the number of fast-twitch fibres diminishes. Differences in strength levels between middle-aged and older men are partly explained by the decrease in anabolic hormones associated with aging (Izquierdo et al, 2001), although these decreases in strength are somewhat reversible with appropriate strength training (Suetta et al, 2004). Training status based on strength levels also determines the response to subsequent training, with individuals who are already strong progressing at a slower rate (Cormie et al, 2010a) due to the law of diminishing returns.

Diminishing returns

An exercise regime will produce a greater improvement in people in poor physical condition than in those already in a good physical condition (Fig. 4.4). It is worth noting, however, that few athletes are really near their genetic ceiling for strength or aerobic capacity, especially in team-based sports.

Reversibility

When training stops, any strength (or other quality) gains will be progressively lost (Bruton, 2002), for instance,

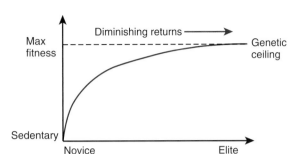

Fig. 4.4 The concept of diminishing returns. All individuals have a genetic ceiling with regard to the development of a specific fitness quality. The impact of an exercise regime will reduce with fitness gain.

when a limb is immobilized the strength and size of the muscles of the limb declines. The rate of decline is slower in well-trained and more experienced athletes.

Development of specific qualities

The above principles need to be borne in mind when aiming to develop strength of an individual. The resistance required to develop strength can be provided through numerous methods (see Table 4.2). During the first 6–8 weeks of strength training, adaptations are largely neural with increases in force production observed (Enoka, 1988). These changes include increased neural activation to the muscle (e.g., increased recruitment and synchronization of motor units) (Sale et al., 1983; Komi, 1986), which parallels the increase in muscle strength, increased activation of prime movers (Sale, 1988), improved intermuscular coordination (Sale, 1988) and decreased activation of antagonists.

After the initial neurological adaptations, subsequent increases in strength are attributable to muscle architectural adaptations and increases in cross-sectional area (hypertrophy). The changes include an increase in the cross-sectional area of the muscle (Housh et al., 1992; Narici et al., 1996) and muscle fibres (Andersen and Aagaard, 2000; Melissa et al., 1997); an increase in the proportion of type IIa fibres and a decrease in type IIx fibres (Andersen and Aagaard, 2000; Hortobagyi et al., 1996); alteration in pennation angles (Kawakami et al., 1993; 1995); alteration in metabolic capacity of muscle (Simoneau et al., 1986); alteration in myosin heavy-chain (MHC) isoforms (Andersen and Aagaard, 2000; Gea, 1997); and an increase in the connective tissue found in muscle structures proportional to muscle hypertrophy.

Muscular endurance refers to the ability of a muscle to produce a specific force repetitively or to sustain an isometric action for a period of time (Bruton, 2002). To increase muscle endurance low loads are used for multiple repetitions (2–3 sets of 10–20 repetitions). Such intensity and repetition ranges help to increase the work capacity of the muscles, but due to the high volume (sets × repetitions × load lifted) associated with such training a hypertrophic response is likely. In addition, initially increasing strength should increase muscular endurance, as activities carried out by the individual are no longer near maximal intensity.

A high number of repetitions of muscle actions against a moderate resistance increases muscle endurance by effecting a change in the muscle (e.g., increased cross-sectional area, increased glycolytic enzymes, increased glycogen storage). The stimulus is the metabolic demand and tensile stress on the muscle and this is reflected in the nature of the changes, including increases in the number of type I and IIa fibres (Demirel et al., 1999; Ingjer, 1979), cross-sectional area of type I and IIx fibres (Ingjer, 1979), number of capillaries surrounding each muscle fibre (Ingjer, 1979), blood flow in muscle (Rohter et al., 1963; Vanderhoof et al., 1961), myoglobin content (Holloszy, 1976); and a decrease in type IIx fibres (Demirel et al., 1999; Ingjer, 1979).

Muscle power is a function of muscle force and velocity; improvement in either or both of these aspects will result in an increase in muscle power. Additionally, repeated practice of the movement, or a component of the movement, at speed, is thought to produce an improvement in muscle power, likely due to improved efficiency of movement and decreased antagonist activation (deVries and Housh, 1994).

Force production (strength) is the key determinant of power; as mentioned earlier increased force production results in an increased ability to accelerate an object (Newton's second law). If acceleration of an object increases from an increase in force production there is a resultant increase in velocity of movement. Therefore increasing both force and velocity results in a greater improvement in power (power = force × velocity).

It has been suggested that movement should be carried out as fast as possible against a resistance of 30% maximal *isometric* force, although exercises performed with low loads result in improvement in power at low loads, whereas exercises using moderate or heavy loads increase power across all loads (Kaneko et al., 1983; Toji and Kaneko, 2004). In line with the principle of specificity, the load and resultant velocity results in the greatest increases in power at those loads and velocities. However, heavy-load training results in greater improvements in power across a range of loads (Harris et al., 2008; Kaneko et al., 1983; Toji et al., 1997; Toji and Kaneko, 2004). The key factor in power development appears to be the ability to rapidly produce force, which is best training with a focus on strength development rather than power, unless the individual is already strong (Cormie et al., 2010b).

Designing a 'strength' workout

Needs analysis

An important first step in developing a 'strength' programme is to conduct a 'needs analysis'. The needs analysis should evaluate the demands of the sport, common injuries and their causes, and the athlete against an agreed profile of the sport. In evaluating the demands of the sport, the following should be considered:

1. *Biomechanical/movement analysis* is required. In order to select exercises with some degree of movement 'transferability', the important movement actions (sprinting, jumping, etc.) of the sport need to first be identified. Once these movements have been identified then the biomechanical characteristics of these actions need to be understood. For example: What forces are generated and absorbed and over what duration? What are the speeds, ranges of motion and muscle actions of the body segments involved in the movement? Biomechanical literature should be considered in order to identify these characteristics. However, if such data is not available from the literature, then a 'qualitative' evaluation of the common sports movements should be performed to understand these characteristics.

2. *Physiological analysis* is required to identify the important physical qualities required for success in that sport. This usually forms the primary training goal (i.e., power development for a shot putter). Here the practitioner needs to consider any physiological (e.g., mean and peak heart rate), time–motion or global positioning systems (GPS) data from competition, in order to identify typical distances covered at different speeds of locomotion, number of changes of direction, typical work:rest ratios, for example. In addition, normative data from high-level athletes should be considered in order to decide what physical factors are important to success and to discriminate between elite and subelite levels of performer.

3. *Injury analysis* is required to identify the common sites for joint and muscle injury pertaining to the sport. Epidemiological literature should be consulted to identify the common injuries associated with the sport. Furthermore, it is important to understand the underlying mechanisms of these injuries and whether they are modifiable by training intervention. Prospective/screening and biomechanical studies of injury mechanisms should be consulted here.

The evaluation of the athlete needs to consider the following: training status and experience, retrospective analysis of previous season(s), injury history of the athlete, and results from performance/*objective* prescreening tests (i.e., any tests performed are based on the evaluated demands of the sport).

The needs analysis allows appropriate training goals to be set with regard to the strength training programme. For instance, a sprinter's primary training goal (Box 4.1) might be the development of power; however, as already alluded to, development of a strength base is required, as the ability to produce force (strength) underpins power. Therefore, the training needs to be periodized (see Periodization of training) in order to allow 'phase potentiation' (i.e., the development of strength in a prior training block allows enhanced development of power in the subsequent block due to the increased ability to produce force). See Table 4.3 for an example.

Training frequency

Training frequency refers to the number of training sessions performed in a given period of time, typically a week. When determining training frequency, the athlete's training status, sports season, projected exercise loads, types of exercises and other concurrent training or activities should be considered.

Typically, three 'strength' sessions per week is recommended, which allows athletes a minimum day recovery between workouts (a general rule is to allow 1 day of rest between workouts, but no more than 3 between sessions that stress the same body part). As an athlete adapts to training, then further workouts may be performed. Athletes could augment their training by using *split routines* in which different muscle groups are trained on different days. Note that using maximal or near-maximal loads may require more recovery between workouts, thus impacting training frequency. However this could be managed by alternating heavy and light loads within the training week. The use of the terms 'heavy' and 'light' in the literature is somewhat misleading, as the appropriate manipulation of training sessions within a week should maintain intensity and alter the total volume of work performed, usually through alterations in the sets and repetition ranges performed within a training session.

The athlete's sports season also influences training frequency. For instance, in-season there are increased demands from games and sports-specific practice, which leads to a decrease in time available for 'conditioning' activities. Furthermore, training frequency is influenced by the overall amount of physical stress. Thus, if an athlete's strength programme runs concurrently with other training (i.e., aerobic or anaerobic), and specific sports practice, then the effects from other forms of training should be considered to avoid negative effects on the strength workouts. Thus, manipulation of training frequency maybe used to reduce the overall weekly training volume.

Exercise selection

In order to select the most appropriate exercises for the athlete's programme, the practitioner must understand the

Box 4.1 **Application of exercise prescription principles in designing strength–power training sessions for a sprinter (100 and 200 m)**

Needs analysis

The duration of 100- and 200-m events for top-level sprinters range from approximately 10 s (100 m) to 21 s (200 m). Therefore, for such athletes there is greater emphasis on 'anaerobic' conditioning and a need to rapidly produce high forces under high velocity conditions (i.e., power). Resistance training programmes for sprinters should primarily focus on the goal of developing power; however, this should be after developing a strength base (see Table 4.3) as maximum strength underpins power. The 100-m sprint can be subdivided into an acceleration phase (0–40 m), a maximum velocity phase (40–70 m), with the remainder of the sprint focused on maintaining velocity (i.e., speed endurance). Both acceleration and maximum velocity phases involve distinctly different biomechanics, which has implications for training exercise selection. The acceleration phase involves short (0.12–0.2 s) ground contacts (Atwater, 1982; Salo et al., 2005), with the emphasis on generating horizontal propulsion force and impulse (Hunter et al., 2005), whilst minimizing braking forces. The lower limb joints extend during ground contact with emphasis on concentric power generation at the ankle and knee (Buckley et al., 2001). Greater trunk lean is required (approx. 45 degrees) to help generate horizontal propulsive force (Kugler and Janssen, 2010). Therefore, exercises with greater emphasis on horizontal concentric (or long response plyometrics) force generation should be incorporated (i.e., standing long jumps; see Table 4.3). The maximum velocity phase is characterized by shorter ground contacts (0.09–0.12 s) (Atwater, 1982; Kuitenen et al., 2002; Mann and Herman, 1985) again highlighting the importance of *rate of force development* to sprint performance. However, optimum vertical force production is required to preserve the flight phase (Weyland et al., 2000), whilst aiming to minimize contact time and braking forces. During ground contact of the maximum velocity phase, greater emphasis is placed on eccentric power absorption (Bezodis et al., 2008) at the ankle and knee, as a sprinter makes greater use of the *stretch–shorten cycle* (fast/short response) during this phase, hence the need for plyometric exercises in the programme (single and bilateral drop jumps, hurdle bounds, etc., see Table 4.3). The lower limb joints extend during the later phase of ground contact, hence the need for similar movements to be incorporated in the programme (i.e., squats, cleans, pulls). However, an optimum level of extension of the hip is required to avoid increasing ground contact time and thus, reducing step frequency (Mann and Herman, 1985). The unilateral nature of sprint running would suggest that unilateral exercises should be incorporated in the programme once the athlete is adequately conditioned to perform them safely and effectively. Finally, hamstring strain injuries are common in sprinters (Lynsholm and Wiklander, 1987), which could be a result of eccentric hamstring weakness making the muscle group more susceptible to strain injury during late swing (Schache et al., 2012). Therefore, exercises dedicated to developing eccentric hamstring strength (i.e., Nordic hamstring lowers) should be included in the programme.

Example of 'power' focused sessions assuming an advanced training status

Example session 1				Example session 2			
Exercise	Load (% 1RM)	Reps	Sets	Exercise	Load (% 1RM)	Reps	Sets
Mid-thigh clean	70%[c]	3	3	Mid-thigh clean pull	60%[c]	3	3
Back Squat[a]	90%	4	3	Split jerk	80%	3	4
Forward lunge[a]	85%	6	2	Front squat[a]	90%	4	3
Nordic hamstring lowers[b]	BW	4	3	Romanian deadlift[b]	87%	5	2

[a]Included to preserve maximum strength, while the programme focuses on power.
[b]Included for injury prevention.
[c]1 RM power clean.
BW, bodyweight; RM, repetition maximum

Atwater, A., 1982. Kinematic analyses of sprinting. Track and Field Quarterly Review 82, 12–16.

Bezodis, I., Kerwin, D., Salo, A., 2008. Lower-limb mechanics during support phases of maximum-velocity sprint running. Med. Sci. Sports Exerc. 40, 707–715.

Hunter, J., Marshall, R., Mcnair, P., 2005. Relationships between ground reaction force impulse and kinematics of sprint-running acceleration. J. Appl. Biomech. 21, 31–43.

Johnson, M., Buckley, J., 2001. Muscle power patterns in the mid-acceleration phase of sprinting. J. Sports Sci. 19, 263–272.

Kugler, F., Janshen, L., 2010. Body position determines propulsive forces in accelerated running. J. Biomech. 43, 343–348.

Kuitenen, S., Komi, P., Kyrolainen, H., 2002. Knee and ankle joint stiffness in sprint running. Med. Sci. Sports Exerc. 34, 166–173.

Lysholm, J., Wiklander, J., 1987. Injuries in runners. American Journal of Sports Medicine 15, 168–171.

Mann, R., Herman, J., 1985. Kinematic analysis of olympic sprint performance: men's 200 meters. Int. J. Sport Biomech. 1, 151–162.

Salo, A., Keranen, T., Viitasalo, J., 2005. Force production in the first four steps of sprint running. In: Wang, Q. (Ed.). XXIII International Symposium on Biomechanics on Sport. The China Institute of Sports Science, Beijing, pp. 313–317.

Schache, A.G., Dorn, T.W., Blanch, P.D., Brown, N.A.T., Pandy, M.G., 2012. Mechanics of the human hamstring muscles during sprinting. Medicine and Science in Sports and Exercise 44 (4), 647–658.

Weyland, P.G., Sternlight, D.B., Bellizzi, M.J., Wright, S., 2000. Faster top running speeds are achieved with greater ground forces not more rapid leg movements. Journal of Applied Physiology 89, 1991–1999.

Table 4.3 Example of periodization for a track sprinter (100 and 200 m)

MACROCYCLE	PREPARATION				COMPETITION	
	General preparation		Specific preparation		Precompetitive	Competitive
Phase of training	Anatomical adaptation[a] (ME/technique)	General strength (hyp./strength)[a]	Maximum Strength[a,b]	Power[b]	Speed	Peaking
Example sessions 1	Clean pull (60–70% 1RM[d] x 10 x 3)[c] Back squat (65–70% 1RM x 10–15 x 3) Split squat (67% 1RM x 12 (6 each leg) x 3) RDL (75% 1RM x 10 x 3)	Clean pull (70–80% 1RM[d] x 10 x 3)[c] Back squat (67–80% 1RM x 8–12 x 3) Forward lunge (80% 1RM x 8 x 4) RDL (80% 1RM x 8 x 4)	Power clean (80% 1RM[d] x 2–4 x 4) Back squat (85–87% 1RM x 5–6 x 3) Walking lunge (80–85% 1RM x 6–8 x 3–4 per leg) RDL (87–90% 1RM x 4–5 x 3)	Hang clean (60% 1RM[d] x 5 x 4) Jump squat (20–40% 1RM[e] x 5 x 3) Walking lunges (87% 1RM x 5 x 2 per leg)/alternated with single leg bounds 5–6 x 2 each leg RDL (87–90% 1RM x 4–5 x 3)	Mid-thigh clean (40% 1RM[d] x 5 x 3) Jump squat (0% 1RM[e] x 5 x 3) Single leg horizontal drop jump (BW x 4 x 4) RDL (87% 1RM x 5 x 2)	Mid-thigh clean (60% 1RM[d] x 3 x 3) Split jerk (60% 1RM x 3 x 2) Maintenance prior to peaking may incorporate strength exercise (i.e., back squat) with high load/low volume (i.e., 90% 1RM x 3–4 x 2)
Example sessions 2	Deadlift (65–70% 1RM x 10–15 x 3) Split squat (65–75% 1RM x 8–12 x 3) Nordic hamstring lower (BW x 3 x 3) Calf raise (65% 1RM x 15 x 3)	Deadlift (80% 1RM x 8 x 3) Bulgarian squat/split squat (80% 1RM x 8 x 4) Nordic hamstring lower (BW x 4–6 x 3–4) Calf raise (67–80% 1RM x 12–8 x 3)	Deadlift (90% 1RM x 4 x 3) Single leg squat (85% 1RM x 6 x 2 (each leg)) Nordic hamstring lower (BW + weight vest x 5–6 x 3–4) Calf raise (85% 1RM x 6 x 3)	Clean from the knee (80–90% 1RM[d] x 2–4 x 2–4) Single leg hops (BW + 6 x 2 (each leg)) Nordic hamstring lower (BW + weight vest x 5–6 x 3–4) Calf raise (90% 1RM x 4 x 2)	Mid-thigh clean pull (60% 1RM[d] x 5 x 3) Split jerk (60% 1RM x 4 x 3) Standing long jump (BW x 5 x 4) Nordic hamstring lowers (BW x 3 x 3) (maintenance)	Mid-thigh pull (40% 1RM[d] x 3 x 2) Split jerk (60% 1RM x 3 x 2) Maintenance prior to peaking may incorporate strength exercise (i.e., back squat) with high load/low volume (i.e., 90% 1RM x 3–4 x 2)

[a] Upper body exercises incorporated for whole-body conditioning (i.e., bent-over row, shoulder press) in these phases.
[b] Phases may be repeated: maximum strength – power – maximum strength – power, to provide greater training variation over this phase of training.
[c] Cluster sets used to maintain technique and velocity (e.g., 15 repetitions divided in to 3 clusters of 5 repetitions with a 20–30 s intra-set rest).
[d] % 1RM power clean.
[e] % 1RM back squat.

BW, bodyweight; Hyp., hypertrophy; ME, muscular endurance; RDL, Romanian deadlift; RM, repetition maximum.

biomechanical characteristics of the various types of training exercises, the movement and muscular requirements of the sport, and the athlete's exercise technique experience. Furthermore, training resources and time available may be additional aspects to consider prior to designing the programme. Exercise can be classified as 'core', 'assistance' or 'power'. *Core exercises* are essentially multi-joint exercises (e.g., squats, deadlifts, power cleans) that recruit one or more muscle area, involve a minimum of two primary joints and demonstrate similarity to the athlete's sport movement patterns. *Assistance exercises* are essentially single-joint exercises (e.g., knee flexion, knee extension), targeting one muscle group and may be included into the programme for 'assistive' or injury-prevention purposes. *Power exercises* are structural exercises (i.e., exercises that load the spine directly) performed quickly with the emphasis on power development. Weightlifting exercises and their derivatives fall into this category, along with ballistic exercises (i.e., jumps, squats, bench press, throws).

Based on the specificity principle stated earlier, exercises selected within a programme need to have relevance to the activities associated with the sport with regard to the muscles and muscle actions involved, loads (intensity), velocity and range of motion. For instance, in Box 4.1 a sprinter may adopt mid-thigh clean pulls during a power phase of their training. Although the exercise may not replicate the exact movement pattern of sprinting the exercise does satisfy the principle of specificity. This is because the mid-thigh clean pull (a) uses the same lower limb muscles, (b) involves triple extension of the lower limb joints from a knee angle similar to the mid-stance phase of the gait cycle, (c) involves a high-velocity of movement (dependent on the load used), and (d) involves rapid force production.

Exercises should also be included in the programme to address any unwanted muscle imbalances from developing. For instance, in Box 4.1 and Table 4.3 the sprinter needs to include exercises to target hamstring strength development (i.e., Nordic hamstring lowers, Romanian deadlifts), as other exercises in the programme alongside the running programme may have too much focus on the quadriceps and, thus, lead to muscle imbalances and potential injury. Hamstring-focused exercises are required to prevent such imbalances from developing, while exercises such as the Romanian deadlift may assist with forceful hip extension, essential to sprinting.

Exercise prescription

Exercise order

Once the athlete's training goal for a session is decided, the practitioner needs to determine the correct exercise order, load and repetition range, number of sets and recovery. With regard to exercise order, generally speaking the session should be designed as follows: power exercises first (i.e., power clean), followed by other multi-joint strength exercises (i.e., back squat) and then single-joint 'assistance' exercises. The rationale for this order is that power exercises require the highest level of skill and concentration of all exercises and may be affected by fatigue, increasing the risk of injury (Fleck and Kraemer, 2014). Furthermore, weightlifting movements that are often performed as the power exercise results in the greatest energy expenditure and are technically the most demanding compared to other exercises (Stone et al., 2006). Therefore, these exercises are performed first in the session when the athlete is 'fresh'. If power exercises are not performed, then multi-joint 'core' exercises are performed followed by 'assistance' exercises.

One method of facilitating the athlete's recovery during a training session and make most efficient use of training time is to alternate lower and upper body exercises throughout the session (Sheppard and Triplett, 2016). Another method is to alternate between pushing (i.e., bench press) and pulling (i.e., bent-over row) exercises; this ensures that the same muscle group is not used on successive exercises and facilitates recovery during the session (Sheppard and Triplett, 2016).

Training load and repetitions

Load simply refers to the amount of load assigned to an exercise set and is the most critical aspect of a resistance training programme. The number of repetitions performed is inversely related to the load lifted (i.e., the heavier the load, the lower number of repetitions performed). The training goal directly influences the selection of load and accompanying repetitions:

Maximum strength

High resistance and low repetition (usually 2–6 repetitions) result in an increase in muscle strength (Hakkinen et al., 1998; Staron et al., 1994). Training to the point of momentary muscle failure (i.e., no further repetitions can be performed within the set) is not necessary (Izquierdo et al., 2006) as long as exercise is performed with sufficient load (usually ≥80% 1RM). Typically, 2–6 sets may be performed.

Hypertrophy

Typically this is achieved through a high volume of work (moderate to high number of repetitions per set, with a high number of sets performed (i.e., 3–6)) completed with moderate to moderately high intensities (60–80% 1RM) (Suchomel and Comfort, 2017).

Muscular endurance

Low resistance (60–75% 1RM) and high repetition (10–20 repetitions) will result in an increase in muscular endurance. Only small increases in strength are associated with the hypertrophic response to muscular endurance training, resulting in an increased cross-sectional area of a muscle. Training to momentary muscle failure appears to be advantageous (Izquierdo et al., 2006). Commonly 2–3 sets are performed to avoid overly inflating the overall volume load.

Power

Low resistances (≤40% 1RM) moved at a high velocity will increase muscle power, that is, an increase in fascicle shortening velocity. Power can also be increased with higher loads (≥60% 1RM) as long as the intention is to move quickly, even if the level of resistance results in a relatively low movement velocity (Behm and Sale, 1993); although such loads are usually used during weightlifting exercises and their derivatives (Suchomel et al., 2017). In order to maximise the quality of the exercise, typically 3–5 sets are performed. Fatigue can also be managed by utilization of cluster sets (short recoveries of <30 s between repetitions within a set) (Haff et al., 2003; 2008; Lawton et al., 2006).

Prior to assigning the training loads, the practitioner needs to evaluate the athlete's strength level for the exercise(s) performed in the programme. This is commonly achieved by evaluating the athlete's 1RM for the exercise. However, this may be unsafe for less experienced individuals and it may not be practical to use this method for all exercises. Alternative strategies can be used in order to assign training loads (Table 4.4).

Recovery

Maximal or near-maximal repetitions involved with strength and power exercise usually require long inter-set rest intervals to allow recovery of the phosphocreatine system. When training for muscle hypertrophy, short-to-moderate inter-set recoveries are used (30–90 s), as it is recommended that the athlete begins the subsequent set before full recovery has been achieved. In order to satisfy the principle of specificity, short recovery periods (30 s) are often utilized when targeting muscular endurance (Sheppard and Triplett, 2016).

Table 4.5 summarizes guidelines for the prescription of resistance exercise based on the training goal with a worked example illustrating the application of this in Box 4.1.

Periodization of training

Periodization can be defined as 'planned distribution or variation in training methods' and means on a 'cyclic or periodic basis' (Plisk and Stone, 2003, p. 19). The goals of periodization are (1) to exploit complementary training effects at optimal times, (2) to manage fatigue and (3) to prevent stagnation or overtraining. An abundance of periodization models exist within the strength and conditioning field such as traditional (often mistakenly termed 'linear'), undulating and conjugate (Plisk and Stone, 2003). Much of the existing literature supports the notion that block periodization may provide superior results compared to other models (DeWeese et al., 2015a; 2015b; Insurrin, 2008; 2010). Block periodization is based on the idea that a concentrated load may be used to train one specific characteristic during each training phase while maintaining the previously developed characteristic(s), rather than develop multiple physiological characteristics or motor abilities simultaneously, which may be counterproductive.

As alluded to above, *progressive overload* is vital in all aspects of physical training, whether the aim is to improve sports performance or rehabilitate an athlete. During a periodized model the athlete progresses through phases (blocks), with each phase targeting a specific fitness quality, culminating in the athlete peaking sports-specific fitness at the exact time of the major competition. For example, the training may begin with a general foundational focus before shifting to sports-specific conditioning. This shift in emphasis requires alterations in training volume and intensity (usually for a power athlete from high volume/ low intensity to low volume/ high intensity) and training specificity (i.e., training becomes more specific in relation to mechanical and metabolic demands of the sport; see Table 4.3).

An important aspect of periodizing strength training is to manage fatigue. Fig. 4.5 illustrates the fitness–fatigue model, whereby following a workout the fatigue effect is large, but short lasting, whilst any fitness gain is small, but lasts longer. Thus, after a period of recovery when fatigue subsides, the specific fitness quality supercompensates. The implication of this is that training needs to be carefully structured within microcycles (1 week of training) and mesocycles (block of training), as fitness gains are not realized until after a period of recovery. With regard to mesocycles, most coaches plan training in 4-week blocks (Fig. 4.6), whereby training increases over a 3-week period followed by an unloading week to allow full recovery; this is usually achieved through reducing volume, whilst maintaining intensity. Please note that 3-week blocks maybe used for young or novice athletes as they may not possess the required training background to tolerate a 3-week increase in volume load; in this way a 2:1 paradigm is used, where training is progressed for 2 weeks followed by an unloading week.

The overall training year is often referred to as a macrocycle (Bompa and Haff, 2009), which consists of the separate micro- and mesocycles. The training year may be

Table 4.4 Methods to determine training load

1RM testing		Multiple RM
Directly measure 1RM	Estimate 1RM from multiple RM test (i.e., 5RM)	Multiple RM based on the number of repetitions planned for that exercise during the training block (i.e., 5 repetitions per set)
Warm-up with light resistance. Estimate a warm-up load to allow the athlete to complete 3–5 repetitions 2 min recovery Estimate a conservative near-maximal load to allow the athlete to perform 2–3 repetitions 2–4 min rest Attempt 1RM and repeat until 1RM achieved (this should be achieved within 2 or 3 attempts). Allow 2–4 min between attempts Note: If athlete fails first attempt, provide 2–4-min recovery and then reattempt with lighter load ((i.e., 2.5–5% lower [upper body] to 5–10% [lower body])	Select target repetitions (i.e., 10RM) Warm-up with light resistance. Estimate a warm-up load to allow the athlete to complete desired number of repetitions 2 min recovery Estimate a conservative near-maximal load to allow the athlete to perform desired number of repetitions Attempt RM and repeat until RM achieved (this should be achieved within 2 or 3 attempts) Once RM load is achieved, 1RM can be estimated via regression equations or conversion tables (see Sheppard and Triplett, 2016)	Select target repetitions (i.e., 5RM) Warm-up with light resistance; estimate a warm-up load to allow the athlete to complete desired number of repetitions 2 min recovery Estimate a conservative near-maximal load to allow the athlete to perform desired number of repetitions 2–4 min rest Attempt RM and repeat until RM achieved (this should be achieved within 2 or 3 attempts) Once RM load is achieved, this load can be used in the subsequent training block for that exercise. Load should be progressed accordingly across the training block (progressive overload)
Appropriate for experienced trainers only	Appropriate for experienced and less-experienced trainers	Appropriate for experienced and less-experienced trainers Can be used to estimate training load for all exercises used in the subsequent training block – assessment takes place in unloading week
Logistically difficult to perform for all exercises within a programme Only core exercises (i.e., back squat, bench press, deadlift, power clean) should be used for safety	Logistically difficult to perform for all exercises within a programme Accuracy of predicting 1RM reduced with increasing number of test repetitions Perhaps not appropriate for power exercises such as the power clean	Care should be taken in using exercises that are more metabolically challenging (i.e., power clean)

RM, repetition maximum.

divided into preparation and competition phases separated by a transition phase, usually precompetition (end of preparation) and active recovery (end of competitive season). As mentioned above, the preparation phases may be further divided into general and specific preparation (see Table 4.3). Usually the general conditioning phase is more focused on hypertrophy/muscular endurance and basic strength, whilst specific preparation may focus on maximum strength and power for a typical strength–power athlete.

The example shown in Table 4.3 illustrates a blocked periodization approach for a sprinter following on from

the example in Box 4.1. Here the athlete begins the training year with high-volume and low-intensity resistance training (general conditioning). This provides a foundation for the later maximum strength and power phases (specific conditioning). Each block of training here would follow a 3:1 paradigm (i.e., 3 weeks of training with increasing volume load, followed by a 1-week unloading period when the athlete's volume decreases to facilitate adaptation). Here the exercises are fairly general and become more 'sports specific' as the training year develops towards major competition. The preseason for such an athlete is generally long,

Table 4.5 Summary of exercise prescription guidelines

	Strength	Muscular endurance	Hypertrophy	Power
Exercise order	• More technical lifts first • Core • Assistance	• Core • Assistance	• Core • Assistance	• Power • Other core • Assistance
Load	High: ≥85% 1RM	Low: ≤67% 1RM	Moderate: 67–85% 1RM	0–80% 1RM[a]
Repetitions	≤6	12–20	6–12	1–6[b]
Sets	2–6	2–3	3–6	3–5
Recovery	2–5 min	≥30 s	30–90 s	2–5 min

[a]Dependent on specific training goals (i.e., low vs. high velocity) and training exercise (see Suchomel et al., 2017).
[b]Power output can deteriorate during a set of 3–6 repetitions, but can be minimized and overload maximized using cluster sets (Haff et al., 2003; 2008; Lawton et al., 2006) For example, 6 repetitions performed as 3 clusters of 2 repetitions, with a 15-s intrarepetition rest between each of the 2 repetitions.
Source: Adapted from Sheppard, J.M., Triplett, N.T., 2016. Program design for resistance training. In: Haff, G.G., Triplett N.T. (Eds.) Essentials of Strength Training and Conditioning, fourth ed. Human Kinetics, Champaign, IL. pp. 439–469.

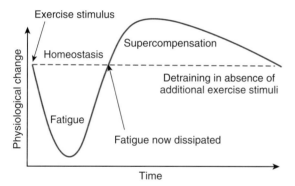

Fig. 4.5 Fitness–fatigue paradigm on which periodization is based.

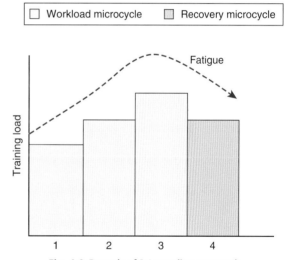

Fig. 4.6 Example of 3:1 paradigm mesocycle.

and therefore to prevent monotony and stagnation once a strength base is established the athlete cycles 'blocks' with a focus on maximum strength (70% strength/30% power) or power (70% power/30% strength) to further develop each quality whilst allowing maintenance of the previously acquired physical quality. Once the athlete reaches the competitive season, they maintain both qualities prior to peaking for power just prior to competition. Box 4.2 illustrates using a periodization approach for rehabilitation of a soccer player from a hamstring strain injury.

The block periodization approach is highly appropriate for athletes in sports whereby a single competition peak is required. Difficulties lie in sports where there are long competitive seasons that require the maintenance of physical qualities throughout the season. Here

a blocked periodization approach may be used in the preseason prior to the competitive season to develop key physical qualities, before shifting to a summated microcycles approach (Baker, 1998; 2001) during the in-season in order to preserve the physical qualities developed. It is beyond the scope of this chapter to provide an in-depth examination of the different periodization approaches available to practitioners or discuss other issues such as concurrent training and tapering. The interested reader is directed to Bompa and Haff (2009) for more information on periodization.

Box 4.2 Example periodized hamstring reconditioning programme for a soccer player

Hamstring strain injuries (HSI) are common in soccer (Ekstrand et al., 2011; 2013; Hawkins et al., 2001). A wide range of extrinsic risk factors (e.g., fixture congestion, sharp increases in volume of high-speed running (HSR)) and intrinsic risk factors (e.g., reduced fascicle length) are associated with HSI (Bengtsson et al., 2013; Duhig et al., 2016; Timmins et al., 2015). Previous injury is the most common factor implicated due to strength losses and morphological changes. HSR results in high-velocity eccentric loading (Schache et al., 2012), as during the late swing phase of the gait cycle the hamstrings work eccentrically to decelerate both the thigh and lower leg in preparation for ground contact; HSIs have been linked to this phase (Heidercheit et al., 2005; Schache et al., 2012; Thelen et al., 2005). Thus, hamstring muscle strength characteristics, particularly low eccentric strength (Jonhagen et al., 1994; Opar et al., 2015), have also been associated with HSI. An understanding of *periodization* is essential to complete an effective rehabilitation programme before being considered for team selection. Prior to this example below, the player has suffered a grade 2 hamstring tear and is embarking on a 12-week rehabilitation programme before being considered for team selection. Prior to this example the player underwent initial treatment (rest, ice, compression and elevation) followed by some restoration of range of motion (stretches, 30–45 s per stretch, performed 3–4 times per day, along with pain-free weight-bearing and isometric exercises).

Example of rehabilitation programme for hamstring injury

	General preparation		*Specific preparation*	
	Mesocycle 1 3 week (2:1 paradigm)	Mesocycle 2 3 week (2:1 paradigm)	Mesocycle 3 3 week (2:1 paradigm)	Mesocycle 4 3 week (2:1 paradigm)
	Initial strengthening	General strength (Low-velocity eccentric)	Specific strength/power (High-velocity eccentric)	Precompetitive
	Strengthening focusing on hamstring-specific exercises (i.e., leg curl; Romanian deadlift). Gradual increases in range of motion (ROM). Lumbopelvic exercises (i.e., planks, single and bilateral straight and bent knee bridges, glute ham raise) should be performed in separate sessions	Begin low-velocity eccentric activities: modified Romanian deadlifts, Nordic hamstring lowers, split squats/lunges. Lumbopelvic exercises (i.e., planks, single and bilateral straight and bent knee bridges, glute ham raise) should be performed in separate sessions	High-velocity eccentric exercises (i.e., plyometrics) incorporated to develop high-velocity eccentric strength. Lumbopelvic exercises (i.e., planks, single and bilateral straight and bent knee bridges, glute ham raise) should be performed in separate sessions	Progress to sports-specific sprint, change of direction drills. Plyometric drills and weightlifting exercises emphasizing deeper 'catch' positions to increase eccentric hamstring loading form the basis of gym sessions (detailed below). Strength and ROM should be maintained. Lumbopelvic exercises (i.e., planks, single and bilateral straight and bent knee bridges, glute ham raise) should be performed in separate sessions
Session 1	Back squat (70–75% 1RM × 10 × 3) Romanian deadlift (70–75% 1RM × 10 × 3)	Split squat (85% 1RM × 6 × 3) Eccentric Romanian deadlifts (RDL)/ concentric deadlift (110% 1RM RDL × 3–4 × 2–3)	Hang clean (40–60% 1RM clean × 5 × 3) Eccentric lunge drops (3 × 5 each leg) Single-leg RDL (50% RDL 1RM × 6 × 3)	Hang squat clean (80% 1RM clean × 3 × 3) Bilateral or single-leg forward and lateral barrier hops (4 × 10)

Box 4.2 Example periodized hamstring reconditioning programme for a soccer player —cont'd

	General preparation		Specific preparation	
	Mesocycle 1 3 week (2:1 paradigm)	Mesocycle 2 3 week (2:1 paradigm)	Mesocycle 3 3 week (2:1 paradigm)	Mesocycle 4 3 week (2:1 paradigm)
	Initial strengthening	General strength (Low-velocity eccentric)	Specific strength/power (High-velocity eccentric)	Precompetitive
Session 2	Front squat (70–75% 1RM × 10 × 3) Swiss ball leg curl (10–12 × 3)	Forward lunge (85% 1RM × 6 × 3) Nordic hamstring lowers (BW × 3 × 2–4)	Hang snatch pulls (40–60% 1RM snatch × 5 × 3) Walking lunges (85% 1RM × 5 × 2 each leg) Eccentric box drops (3 × 6)	Hang squat snatch (70% 1RM snatch × 3 × 3) Depth jumps (3 × 6)

Bengtsson, H., Ekstrand, J., & Hägglund, M., 2013. Muscle injury rates in professional football increase with fixture congestion: an 11-year follow-up of the UEFA Champions League injury study. Brit. J. Sports Med. 47, 743–747.

Duhig, S., Shield, A.J., Opar, D., Gabbett, T.J., Ferguson, C., Williams, M., 2016. Effect of high-speed running on hamstring strain injury risk. British Journal of Sports Medicine 50, 1536–1540.

Ekstrand, J., Hägglund, M., Walden, M., 2011. Epidemiology of muscle injuries in professional football (soccer). The American Journal of Sports Medicine 39, 1226–1232.

Ekstrand, J., Hägglund, M., Kristenson, K., Magnusson, H., Waldén, M., 2013. Fewer ligament injuries but no preventive effect on muscle injuries and severe injuries: an 11-year follow-up of the UEFA champions league injury study. British Journal of Sports Medicine 47, 732–737.

Hawkins, R.D., Hulse, M.A., Wilkinson, C., Hodson, A., Gibson, M., 2001. The association football medical research programme: an audit of injuries in professional football. British Journal of Sports Medicine 35, 43–47.

Heiderscheit, B.C., Hoerth, D.M., Chumanov, E.S., Swanson, S.C., Thelen, B.J., Thelen, D.G., 2005. Identifying the time of occurrence of a hamstring strain injury during treadmill running: a case study. Clinical Biomechanics 20, 1072–1078.

Jonhagen, S., Nemeth, G., Eriksson, E., 1994. Hamstring injuries in sprinters. the role of concentric and eccentric hamstring muscle strength and flexibility. The American Journal of Sports Medicine 22, 262–266.

Opar, D.A., Williams, M.D., Timmins, R.G., Hickey, J., Duhig, S.J., Shield, A.J., 2015. Eccentric hamstring strength and hamstring injury risk in Australian footballers. Medicine and Science in Sports and Exercise 47 (4), 857–865.

Schache, A.G., Dorn, T.W., Blanch, P.D., Brown, N.A.T., Pandy, M.G., 2012. Mechanics of the human hamstring muscles during sprinting. Medicine and Science in Sports and Exercise 44 (4), 647–658.

Thelen, D.G., Chumanov, E.S., Best, T.M., Swanson, S.C., Heiderscheit, B.C., 2005. Simulation of biceps femoris musculo-tendon mechanics during the swing phase of sprinting. Medicine and Science in Sports and Exercise 37, 1931–1938.

Timmins, R.G., Bourne, M.N., Shield, A.J., Williams, M.D., Lorenzen, C., Opar, D.A., 2015. A short biceps femoris long head fascicle length and eccentric knee flexor weakness increase risk of hamstring injury: a prospective cohort study in 152 elite professional football players. British Journal of Sports Medicine 50 (24), 1524–1535.

Summary

Strength and conditioning is the application of strength training and other conditioning methods to physically prepare athletes for sporting performance. Therapists should utilize principles of strength and conditioning in order to design effective rehabilitation programmes that better prepare athletes for return to play/competition. Muscular strength is the ability to exert force and is the cornerstone of RFD, power, athletic performance and injury prevention. The ability to express force (strength) is dependent on modifiable neural and morphological factors. In order to evoke such adaptations, strength training programmes should seek to provide overload and take into account the specificity of the stimulus, as well as the individuality and training status of the athlete. The periodization model, modality of resistance training and exercise prescription may further affect muscular strength and power adaptations and training emphasis. The training programmes of weaker individuals should focus on improving muscular strength before specifically focusing on power. In contrast, stronger athletes may use advanced training strategies to enhance power whilst maintaining or improving their strength level.

References

Aagaard, P., Simonsen, E.B., Andersen, J.L., Magnusson, P., Dyhre-Poulsen, P., 2002. Increased rate of force development and neural drive of human skeletal muscle following resistance training. Journal of Applied Physiology 93, 1318–1326.

Aagaard, P., 2003. Training-induced changes in neural function. Exercise and Sport Sciences Reviews 31, 61–67.

Aagaard, P., Simonsen, E.B., Andersen, J.L., Magnusson, S.P., Halkjaer-Kristensen, J., Dyhre-Poulsen, P., 2000. Neural inhibition during maximal eccentric and concentric quadriceps contraction: effects of resistance training. Journal of Applied Physiology 89, 2249–2257.

Andersen, L.L., Aagaard, P., 2006. Influence of maximal muscle strength and intrinsic muscle contractile properties on contractile rate of force development. European Journal of Applied Physiology 96, 46–52.

Anderson, K., Behm, D.G., 2005. Trunk muscle activity increases with unstable squat movements. Canadian Journal of Applied Physiology 30, 33–45.

Asadi, A., Arazi, H., Young, W.B., Sáez de Villarreal, E., 2016. The effects of plyometric training on change of direction ability: A meta-analysis. International Journal of Sports Physiology and Performance 11, 563–573.

Augustsson, J., Esko, A., Thomee, R., Sventesson, U., 1998. Weight training of the thigh muscles using closed vs. open kinetic chain exercises: a comparison of performance enhancement. Journal of Orthopaedic Sports Physical Therapy 27, 3–8.

Baker, D., 1998. Applying the in-season periodisation of strength and power training to football. Strength & Conditioning 20 (2), 18–27.

Baker, D., 2001. The effects of an in-season of concurrent training on the maintenance of maximal strength and power in professional and college-aged rugby league players. Journal of Strength and Conditioning Research 15 (2), 172–177.

Baker, D., 2001. Comparison of upper-body strength and power between professional and college-aged rugby league players. Journal of Strength and Conditioning Research 15, 30–35.

Blazevich, A.J., 2006. Effects of physical training and detraining, immobilisation, growth and aging on human fascicle geometry. Sports Medicine 36, 1003–1017.

Bruton, A., 2002. Muscle plasticity: response to training and detraining. Physiotherapy 88 (7), 398–408.

Behm, D.G., Anderson, K.G., 2006. The role of instability with resistance training. Journal of Strength and Conditioning Research 20, 716–722.

Behm, D.G., Sale, D.G., 1993. Intended rather than actual movement velocity determines velocity-specific training response. Journal of Applied Physiology 74, 359–368.

Blackburn, J.R., Morrissey, M.C., 1998. The relationship between open and closed kinetic chain strength of the lower limb and jumping performance. Journal of Orthopaedic Sports Physical Therapy 27 (6), 430–435.

Bompa, T.O., Haff, G., 2009. Periodization: Theory and Methodology of Training. Human Kinetics, Champaign, IL.

Brandenburg, J.E., Docherty, D., 2002. The effects of accentuated eccentric loading on strength, muscle hypertrophy, and neural adaptations in trained individuals. Journal of Strength and Conditioning Research 16, 25–32.

Comfort, P., Stewart, A., Bloom, L., Clarkson, B., 2014. Relationships between strength, sprint, and jump performance in well-trained youth soccer players. Journal of Strength & Conditioning Research 28 (1), 173–177.

Cormie, P., McCaulley, G.O., McBride, J.M., 2007. Power versus strength–power jump squat training: influence on the load–power relationship. Medicine and Science in Sports and Exercise 39 (6), 996–1003.

Cormie, P., McGuigan, M.R., Newton, R.U., 2010a. Influence of strength on magnitude and mechanisms of adaptation to power training. Medicine and Science in Sports and Exercise 42 1566-158.

Cormie, P., McGuigan, M.R., Newton, R.U., 2010b. Adaptations in athletic performance after ballistic power versus strength training. Medicine and Science in Sports and Exercise 42 (8), 1582–1598.

Cormie, P., McGuigan, M.R., Newton, R.U., 2011. Developing maximal neuromuscular power: Part 2 – training considerations for improving maximal power production. Sports Medicine 41 (2), 125–146.

De Hoyo, M., Pozzo, M., Sañudo, B., Carrasco, L., Gonzalo-Skok, O., Domínguez-Cobo, S., et al., 2015. Effects of a 10-week in-season eccentric-overload training program on muscle-injury prevention and performance in junior elite soccer players. International Journal of Sports Physiology and Performance 10, 46–52.

Demirel, H.A., Powers, S.K., Naito, H., Hughes, M., Coombes, J.S., 1999. Exercise-induced alterations in skeletal muscle myosin heavy chain phenotype: dose–response relationship. Journal of Applied Physiology (1985) 86 (3), 1002–1008.

Devries, H.A., Housh, T.J., 1994. Physiology of Exercise for Physical Education, Athletics and Exercise Science, fifth ed. Brown & Benchmark, Madison, WI.

Deweese, B.H., Hornsby, G., Stone, M., Stone, M.H., 2015a. The training process: planning for strength–power training in track and field. Part 1: theoretical aspects. The Journal of Sport and Health Science 4, 308–317.

Deweese, B.H., Hornsby, G., Stone, M., Stone, M.H., 2015b. The training process: planning for strength–power training in track and field. Part 2: practical and applied aspects. The Journal of Sport and Health Science 4, 318–324.

Dinubile, N.A., 1991. Strength training. Clinics in Sports Medicine 10 (1), 33–62.

Douglas, J., Pearson, S., Ross, A., McGuigan, M.R., 2016a. Chronic adaptations to eccentric training: a systematic review. Sports Medicine 47 (5), 917–941.

Douglas, J., Pearson, S., Ross, A., McGuigan, M.R., 2016b. Eccentric exercise: physiological characteristics and acute responses. Sports Medicine 47 (4), 663–675.

Earp, J.E., Kraemer, W.J., Newton, R.U., Comstock, B.A., Fragala, M.S., Dunn-Lewis, C., et al., 2010. Lower-body muscle structure and its role in jump performance during squat, countermovement, and depth drop jumps. Journal of Strength and Conditioning Research 24, 722–729.

Ebben, W.P., Jensen, R.L., 2002. Electromyographic and kinetic analysis of traditional, chain, and elastic band squats. Journal of Strength and Conditioning Research 16, 547–550.

Enoka, R.M., 1988. Muscle strength and its development: new perspectives. Sports Medicine 6, 146–168.

Fleck, S.J., Kraemer, W.J., 2014. Designing Resistance Training Programs, fouth ed. Human Kinetics, Champaign, IL.

Gea, J.G., 1997. Myosin gene expression in the respiratory muscles. The European Respiratory Journal 10, 2404–2410.

Ghez, C., 1991. Muscles: effectors of the motor systems. In: Kandel, E.R., Schwartz, J.H., Jessell, T.M. (Eds.), Principles of Neural Science, third ed. Elsevier, New York, pp. 548–563.

Haff, G.G., 2000. Roundtable discussion: machines versus free weights. Strength and Conditioning Journal 22, 18–30.

Haff, G.G., Whitley, L.B., McCoy, H.S., O'Bryant, J.L., Kilgore, E., Haff, E.,K., et al., 2003. Effects of different set configurations on barbell velocity and displacement during a clean pull. Journal of Strength and Conditioning Research 17, 95–103.

Haff, G.G., Hobbs, R.T., Haff, E., Sands, W.A., Pierce, K.C., Stone, M.H., 2008. Cluster training: a novel method for introduction training program variation. Strength and Conditioning Journal 30, 67–76.

Hakkinen, K., Newton, R.U., Gordon, S.E., McCormick, M., Volek, J.S., Nindl, B.C., et al., 1998. Changes in muscle morphology, electromyographic activity, and force production characteristics during progressive strength training in young and older men. The Journals of Gerontology 53A (6), B415–B423.

Harris, N.K., Cronin, J.B., Hopkins, W.G., Hansen, K.T., 2008. Squat jump training at maximal power loads vs. heavy loads: effect on sprint ability. Journal of Strength and Conditioning Research 22, 1742–1749.

Harrison, J.S., 2010. Bodyweight training: a return to basics. Strength and Conditioning Journal 32, 52–55.

Henneman, E., Olson, C.B., 1965. Relations between structure and function in the design of skeletal muscles. Journal of Neurophysiology 28, 581–598.

Henneman, E., Somjen, G., Carpenter, D.O., 1965. Functional significance of cell size in spinal motoneurons. Journal of Neurophysiology 28, 560–580.

Hewett, T.E., Stroupe, A.L., Nance, T.A., Noyes, F.R., 1996. Plyometric training in female athletes. decreased impact forces and increased hamstring torques. The American Journal of Sports Medicine 24 (6), 765–773.

Hill, A.V., 1970. First and Last Experiments in Muscle Mechanics. Cambridge University Press, London.

Holloszy, J.O., 1976. Adaptations of muscular tissue to training. Prog. Cardiovasc. Dis. 18 (6), 445–458.

Hori, N., Newton, R.U., Andres, W.A., Kawamori, N., McGuigan, M.R., Nosaka, K., 2008. Does performance of hang power clean differentiate performance of jumping, sprinting, and changing of direction? Journal of Strength & Conditioning Research 22 (2), 412–418.

Hortobagyi, T., Hill, J.P., Houmard, J.A., Fraser, D.D., Lambert, N.J., Israel, R.G., 1996. Adaptive responses to muscle lengthening and shortening in humans. Journal of Applied Physiology (1985) 80 (3), 765–772.

Housh, D.J., Housh, T.J., Johnson, G.O., Chu, W.K., 1992. Hypertrophic response to unilateral concentric isokinetic resistance training. Journal of Applied Physiology (1985) 73 (1), 65–70.

Jones, P.A., Bampouras, T., Comfort, P., 2013a. A review of complex and contrast training: implications for practice. Part 1. Professional Strength & Conditioning 29, 11–20.

Jones, P.A., Bampouras, T., Comfort, P., 2013b. A review of complex and contrast training: implications for practice. Part 2. Professional Strength & Conditioning 30, 27–30.

Ingjer, F., 1979. Capillary supply and mitochondrial content of different skeletal muscle fiber types in untrained and endurance-trained men. A histochemical and ultrastructural study. European Journal of Applied Physiology and Occupational Physiology 40, 197–209.

Israetel, M.A., McBride, J.M., Nuzzo, J.L., Skinner, J.W., Dayne, A.M., 2010. Kinetic and kinematic differences between squats performed with and without elastic bands. Journal of Strength and Conditioning Research 24, 190–194.

Issurin, V.B., 2008. Block periodization versus traditional training theory: a review. The Journal of Sports Medicine and Physical Fitness 48, 65–75.

Issurin, V.B., 2010. New horizons for the methodology and physiology of training periodization. Sports Medicine 40, 189–206.

Izquierdo, M., Hakkinen, K., Anton, A., Garrues, M., Ibanez, J., Ruesta, M., et al., 2001. Maximal strength and power, endurance performance, and serum hormones in middle-aged and elderly men. Medicine and Science in Sports and Exercise 33, 1577–1587.

Izquierdo, M., Ibanez, J., Gonzalez-Badillo, J.J., Hakkinen, K., Ratamess, N.A., Kraemer, W.J., et al., 2006. Differential effects of strength training leading to failure versus not to failure on hormonal responses, strength, and muscle power gains. Journal of Applied Physiology (1985) 100, 1647–1656.

Kaneko, M., Fuchimoto, T., Toji, H., Suei, K., 1983. Training effect of different loads on the force–velocity relationship and mechanical power output in human muscle. Scandinavian Journal of Medicine & Science in Sports 5, 50–55.

43

Kawakami, Y., Abe, T., Fukunaga, T., 1993. Muscle-fiber pennation angles are greater in hypertrophied than in normal muscles. Journal of Applied Physiology 74 (6), 2740–2744.

Kawakami, Y., Abe, T., Kuno, S.-Y., Fukunaga, T., 1995. Training-induced changes in muscle architecture and specific tension. European Journal of Applied Physiology 72 (1-2), 37–43.

Kirkpatrick, J., Comfort, P., 2012. Strength, power, and speed qualities in English junior elite rugby league players. Journal of Strength and Conditioning Research 27 (9), 2414–2419.

Komi, P.V., 1986. Training of muscle strength and power: interaction of neuromotoric, hypertrophic, and mechanical factors. Journal of Strength and Conditioning Research 7 (Suppl.), 10–15.

Lake, J.P., Lauder, M.A., 2012. Kettlebell swing training improves maximal and explosive strength. Journal of Strength and Conditioning Research 26, 2228–2233.

Lake, J.P., Lauder, M.A., Smith, N.A., Shorter, K.A., 2012. A comparison of ballistic and non-ballistic lower-body resistance exercise and the methods used to identify their positive lifting phases. Journal of Applied Biomechanics 28, 431–437.

Lawton, T.W., Croin, J.B., Lindsell, R.P., 2006. Effect of inter-repetition rest intervals on weight training repetition power output. Journal of Strength and Conditioning Research 20, 172–176.

Manal, K., Roberts, D.P., Buchanan, T.S., 2006. Optimal pennation angle of the primary ankle plantar and dorsiflexors: variations with sex, contraction intensity, and limb. Journal of Applied Biomechanics 22, 255–263.

Melissa, L., MacDougall, J.D., Tarnopolsky, M.A., Cipriano, N., Green, H.J., 1997. Skeletal muscle adaptations to training under normobaric hypoxic versus normoxic conditions. Medicine and Science in Sports and Exercise 29 (2), 238–243.

Milner-Brown, H.S., Stein, R.B., Yemm, R., 1973. The orderly recruitment of human motor units during voluntary isometric contractions. Journal of Physiology (London) 230, 359–370.

Morrissey, M.C., Harman, E.A., Johnson, M.J., 1995. Resistance training modes: specificity and effectiveness. Medicine and Science in Sports and Exercise 27, 648–660.

Narici, M.V., Hoppeler, H., Kayser, B., Landoni, L., Claassen, H., Gavardi, C., et al., 1996. Human quadriceps cross-sectional area, torque and neural activation during 6 months strength training. Acta Physiologica Scandinavica 157 (2), 175–186.

Newton, R.U., Kraemer, W.J., Häkkinen, K., Humphries, B., Murphy, A.J., 1996. Kinematics, kinetics, and muscle activation during explosive upper body movements. Journal of Applied Biomechanics 12, 31–43.

Nimphius, S., McGuigan, M.R., Newton, R.U., 2010. Relationship between strength, power, speed, and change of direction performance of female softball players. Journal of Strength and Conditioning Research 24 (4), 885–895.

Ojasto, T., Häkkinen, K., 2009. Effects of different accentuated eccentric load levels in eccentric-concentric actions on acute neuromuscular, maximal force, and power responses. Journal of Strength and Conditioning Research 23, 996–1004.

Otto III, W.H., Coburn, J.W., Brown, L.E., Spiering, B.A., 2012. Effects of weightlifting vs. kettlebell training on vertical jump, strength, and body composition. Journal of Strength and Conditioning Research 26, 1199–1202.

Plisk, S.S., Stone, M.H., 2003. Periodization strategies. Strength & Conditioning Journal 25 (6), 19–37.

Robbins, D.W., 2005. Postactivation potentiation and its practical applicability: a brief review. Journal of Strength and Conditioning Research 19, 453–458.

Rohter, F.D., Rochelle, R.H., Hyman, C., 1963. Exercise blood flow changes in the human forearm during physical training. Journal of Applied Physiology 18 (4), 789–793.

Sáez de Villarreal, E., Kellis, E., Kraemer, W.J., Izquierdo, M., 2009. Determining variables of plyometric training for improving vertical jump height performance: a meta-analysis. Journal of Strength and Conditioning Research 23 (2), 495–506.

Sáez de Villarreal, E., Requena, B., Cronin, J.B., 2012. The effects of plyometric training on sprint performance: a meta-analysis. Journal of Strength and Conditioning Research 26 (2), 575–584 2012.

Sale, D.G., 1988. Neural adaptation to resistance training. Medicine and Science in Sports and Exercise 20 (5), S135–S145.

Sale, D.G., MacDougall, J.D., Upton, A.R.M., McComas, A.J., 1983. Effect of strength training upon motor neurone excitability in man. Medicine and Science in Sports and Exercise 15 (1), 57–62.

Seitz, L.B., Reyes, A., Tran, T.T., Sáez de Villarreal, E., Haff, G.G., 2014a. Increases in lower-body strength transfer positively to sprint performance: a systematic review with meta-analysis. Sports Medicine 44 (12), 1693–1702.

Seitz, L.B., Sáez de Villarreal, E., Haff, G.G., 2014b. The temporal profile of postactivation potentiation is related to strength level. Journal of Strength and Conditioning Research 28, 706–715.

Sheppard, J., Hobson, S., Barker, M., Taylor, K., Chapman, D., McGuigan, M., et al., 2008. The effect of training with accentuated eccentric load counter-movement jumps on strength and power characteristics of high-performance volleyball players. The International Journal of Sports Science & Coaching 3, 355–363.

Sheppard, J.M., Triplett , N.T., 2016. Program design for resistance training. In: Haff, G.G., Triplett, N.T. (Eds.), Essentials of Strength Training and Conditioning, fourth ed. Human Kinetics, Champaign, IL, pp. 439–469.

Simoneau, J.A., Lortie, G., Boulay, M.R., Marcotte, M., Thibault, M.C., Bouchard, C., 1986. Inheritance of human skeletal muscle and anaerobic capacity adaptation to high-intensity intermittent training. International Journal of Sports Medicine 7 (3), 167–171.

Spurrs, R.W., Murphy, A.J., Watsford, M.L., 2002. The effect of plyometric training on distance running performance. European Journal of Applied Physiology 89, 1–7.

Staron, R.S., Karapondo, D.L., Kraemer, W.J., Fry, A.C., Gordon, S.E., Falkel, J.E., et al., 1994. Skeletal muscle adaptations during early phase of heavy-resistance training in men and women. Journal of Applied Physiology 76 (3), 1247–1255.

Stone, M.H., Moir, G., Glaister, M., Sanders, R., 2002. How much strength is necessary? Physical Therapy in Sport 3, 88–96.

Stone, M.H., Pierce, K.C., Sands, W.A., Stone, M.E., 2006. Weightlifting: a brief review. Strength and Conditioning Journal 28 (1), 50–66.

Styles, W.J., Matthews, M.J., Comfort, P., 2015. Effects of strength training on squat and sprint performance in soccer players. Journal of Strength & Conditioning Research 30 (6), 1534–1539.

Suchomel, T.J., Comfort, P., 2017. Developing strength and power. In: Tuner, A., Comfort, P. (Eds.), Advanced Strength and Conditioning. Routledge, Oxon, pp. 13–38.

Suchomel, T.J., Comfort, P., Lake, J.P., 2017. Enhancing the force–velocity profile of athletes using weightlifting derivatives. Strength & Conditioning Journal 39 (1), 10–20.

Suchomel, T.J., Comfort, P., Stone, M.H., 2015. Weightlifting pulling derivatives: rationale for implementation and application. Sports Medicine 45 (6), 823–839.

Suchomel, T.J., Sato, K., Deweese, B.H., Ebben, W.P., Stone, M.H., 2016. Potentiation following ballistic and non-ballistic complexes: the effect of strength level. Journal of Strength and Conditioning Research 30, 1825–1833.

Suetta, C., Aagaard, P., Rosted, A., Jakobsen, A.K., Duus, B., Kjaer, M., et al., 2004. Training-induced changes in muscle CSA, muscle strength, EMG, and rate of force development in elderly subjects after long-term unilateral disuse. Journal of Applied Physiology (1985) 97, 1954–1961.

Toji, H., Suei, K., Kaneko, M., 1997. Effects of combined training loads on relations among force, velocity, and power development. Canadian Journal of Applied Physiology 22, 328–336.

Toji, H., Kaneko, M., 2004. Effect of multiple-load training on the force–velocity relationship. Journal of Strength and Conditioning Research 18, 792–795.

Turner, A.M., Owings, M., Schwane, J.A., 2003. Improvements in running economy after 6 weeks of plyometric training. Journal of Strength and Conditioning Research 17, 60–67.

Van Cutsem, M., Duchateau, J., Hainaut, K., 1998. Changes in single motor unit behaviour contribute to the increase in contraction speed after dynamic training in humans. The Journal of Physiology 513, 295–305.

Vanderhoof, E.R., Imig, C.J., Hines, H.M., 1961. Effect of muscle strength and endurance development on blood flow. Journal of Applied Physiology 16 (5), 873–877.

Wallace, B.J., Winchester, J.B., McGuigan, M.R., 2006. Effects of elastic bands on force and power characteristics during the back squat exercise. Journal of Strength and Conditioning Research 20, 268–272.

Wisloff, U., Castagna, C., Helgerud, J., Jones, R., Hoff, J., 2004. Strong correlation of maximal squat strength with sprint performance and vertical jump height in elite soccer players. British Journal of Sports Medicine 38 (3), 285–288.

Zatsiorsky, V.M., Kraemer, W.J., 2006. Science and Practice of Strength Training, second ed. Human Kinetics, Champaign, IL.

Chapter | 5 |

Biomechanics of sports injuries, their management and clinical considerations

Jim Richards, Carrie Docherty, Brent Arnold, Kim Hébert-Losier, Charlotte Häger, Bruno Mazuquin and Puneet Monga

Introduction

This chapter will focus on the biomechanical factors associated with different sports injuries and the clinical considerations in their management. This chapter will focus on three of the most common injury sites: lateral ankle, anterior cruciate ligament in the knee and the shoulder.

Ankle injuries

Carrie Docherty, Brent Arnold

Epidemiology

The lateral ankle sprain is the most common injury that occurs during physical activity (Hootman et al., 2007). In the United States, the incidence of ankle sprains in physically active individuals is 0.68 to 3.85 ankle sprains per 1000 person-days or 5 to 7 sprains per 1000 person-years. This equates to approximately 2 million acute ankle sprains each year in the United States alone (Waterman et al., 2010). Disparities exist between the incidence of ankle sprains between men and women, with women sustaining ankle sprains at a higher rate of 13.6 per 1000 compared with 6.9 per 1000 for men (Doherty et al., 2014).

Mechanism and clinical presentation

Lateral ankle sprains can be caused by both contact and noncontact mechanisms. Noncontact injuries are typically the result of uncontrolled inversion and internal rotation following initial foot contact (Gehring et al., 2013).

It appears that this mechanism can occur with or without the presence of plantar flexion. Conversely, contact injuries are most frequently the result of either (1) player-to-player contact on the medial aspect of the leg just before or at foot strike causing an inversion mechanism or (2) forced plantar flexion where the injured player hit the opponent's foot when attempting to shoot or clear the ball. These injuries are most commonly seen in field and court sports, with the ankle sprain accounting for 15% of all injuries in organized collegiate athletics (Hootman et al., 2007).

When evaluating the anatomy of the ankle it is critical to realize the important role that the tibia and fibula play in the occurrence of ankle injuries. The medial side of the ankle is not commonly injured because the fibula creates a bony block that reduces range of motion during eversion movements. However, the lateral side of the ankle lacks this bony infrastructure making it easier for the lateral structures to become damaged. When an inversion ankle sprain occurs, it has the potential to cause damage to the ligaments, as well as the muscles and nerves which cross the ankle joint. Therefore, all of these structures should be considered in the management of this injury.

Not only is the initial injury an area of concern but the incidence of reinjury, recurrent instability and long-term consequences of a lateral ankle sprain is recognized as a major healthcare burden. Epidemiological studies have found that recurrence rates of ankle sprains among national, competitive and recreational athletes is as high as 73%, with 22% sustaining five or more injuries to the same ankle over the course of their lifetime (Yeung et al., 1994). Many individuals will go on to describe recurrent feelings of instability for months and even years after their initial injury. This phenomenon is referred to as chronic ankle instability. These recurrent issues are creating a financial burden through increased healthcare costs as well as health burdens. Individuals with a history of ankle injuries are less physically active as they age and may experience early onset of ankle osteoarthrosis. It has been reported that almost 90% of patients 19 years or older with an acute lateral ankle sprains have osteochondral lesions (Taga et al., 1993). One potential explanation for these long-term consequences is the expedited return to play following an injury.

The majority of individuals return to sport participation after a first-time ankle sprain in 3 days while individuals who suffer from a recurrent ankle sprain return in 1 day (McKeon et al., 2014). This expedited return to play occurs even though individuals will experience mechanical laxity for up to a year after the initial injury (Hubbard and Hicks-Little, 2008). Therefore, management of ankle sprains should incorporate long-term rehabilitation which may decrease the chances of reinjury.

Ankle rehabilitation protocols

Ankle rehabilitation protocols can be divided into three broad areas: balance training as the sole intervention (Lee and Lin, 2008; Matsusaka et al., 2001), strength training (Docherty et al., 1998; Sekir et al., 2007) and neuromuscular training (Coughlan and Caulfield, 2007; Ross et al., 2007). Rehabilitation studies have used a variety of measures that span a continuum to assess efficacy including physiological, impairment, functional limitation and disability.

Physiological measures of neuromuscular performance in rehabilitation have included reflex latencies and proprioception. Impairment can be represented by changes at the organ level (McLeod et al., 2008; Snyder et al., 2008). This includes measures associated with performance of the lower extremity and are represented as balance measures and physical performance tests such as hopping. Self-reported function includes assessment of activities of daily living including sports activities. These may be measured by the Foot and Ankle Disability Index (FADI); FADI Sport; Foot and Ankle Ability Measure (FAAM); and the Ankle Joint Functional Assessment Tool (AJFAT), whereas disability is often measured as general health-related quality of life (HRQoL).

Strength training protocols

One of the most common methods of ankle strength training is elastic band or tube exercises. Docherty et al. (1998) found that elastic band exercises improve dorsiflexor and evertor strength and also improved active joint reposition sense in the inversion and plantar flexion directions. Similarly, Hall et al. (2015) concluded that elastic band training improves strength in the invertors, evertors, plantar flexors, and dorsiflexors. However, in contrast (Wright et al., 2016) found that elastic band training failed to improve strength. These discrepancies may be explained by the fact that different levels of resistance were used during the training protocols.

As an alternative to elastic band exercise, Sekir et al. (2007) demonstrated that isokinetic exercise improved strength in unstable ankles. Both inversion and eversion concentric peak torque were significantly greater following training. This functional deficit is supported by a meta-analysis of ankle strength in unstable ankles by Arnold et al. (2009), who found that unstable ankles were weaker than uninjured ankles, and Feger et al. (2016) who identified a decreased muscle volume with chronic instability. This suggests that injured ankles are indeed weaker, but perhaps ankle strength measures have limited responsiveness to rehabilitation-induced changes.

Balance training
Alterations in pathophysiology

Balance training is a common treatment used for ankle instability and is often combined with other therapies. Several studies have reported on the effects of balance training (Lee and Lin, 2008; Wright et al., 2016).

Use of trapdoor devices to measure peroneus longus and tibialis anterior latencies has shown that balance training decreases latency times in both muscles by as much as 30% compared to controls. This indicates that the response to unexpected perturbation is faster after training. However, how this translates to patient improvement is unknown.

It has also been demonstrated that active and passive joint reposition sense are improved following balance training. Again, it is unknown whether these changes are related to patient improvement. However, there is some evidence that balance training improves pathophysiologic deficiencies at the ankle.

Effects on measures of impairment

Ankle measures of impairment include measures of balance and performance-based measures such as hopping. These measures can be further broken down into laboratory and clinic-based measures.

As we have defined them, laboratory-based methods include those procedures that require equipment typically found in the laboratory setting. That is not to say that this equipment could not be available to the clinician, but rather, is not typically available to the clinician. For ankle rehabilitation research this has been limited to instrumented balance measures from either force plates or use of stability systems such as the Biodex. In both cases improvements have been found in these measures following balance training. For force plate measures, a variety of dependent measures have been found responsive to balance training including: centre of pressure velocity, medial/lateral sway path length, centre of pressure radius, time to boundary, and centre of pressure area. Measures collected with the Biodex Stability System also produced a substantial effect, which clearly indicates that balance training has a potent effect on these measures. However, it is currently unknown whether these changes translate into meaningful improvements for the patient.

Clinic-based methods include those assessments that require minimal equipment and are easily used in the clinical setting. Depending on the measure, these simple clinical measures have been shown to improve with rehabilitation. The star excursion balance test (SEBT) is one of the most frequently used clinic-based measures, and improvement in balance following ankle rehabilitation has been reported (Linens et al., 2016; Wright et al., 2016). Other equally simple clinic-based measures have also been shown to be responsive to ankle rehabilitation. These include the foot lift test, time-in-balance test, figure-of-eight hop and side hop.

In summary, laboratory-based measures of impairment are improved following balance training and may be useful when the equipment is available. More recent research has demonstrated clinic-based measures may be as responsive as laboratory-based tests and have the benefit of needing minimal equipment.

Effect on measures of self-reported function

Measures of self-reported function include questionnaire-based measures that assess the patient's ability to perform activities of daily living and sport-related activities, e.g. FADI and FADI Sport. Although the previous measures may be conceptually linked by clinicians and patients to measures of pathophysiology and impairment, these measures most directly assess the functional tasks that are important to patients. Several studies have shown significant improvements to these measures after balance training (Cruz-Diaz et al., 2015; Linens et al., 2016; Wright et al., 2016). This provides clear evidence that balance training improves function important to the patient. It is not clear which measure is the most responsive as direct comparisons have not been made.

Multiple treatments and training mode protocols

Studies using multiple therapies are those studies that combine different treatment modes into a single overall treatment plan. For example, these therapies have included multiple elastic band kick exercises (Han et al., 2009), multiple hopping tasks combined with balance tasks (McKeon et al., 2008) and balance tasks combined with standard range-of-motion and strength exercises (Hale et al., 2007). From a scientific perspective the variety of measures, exercises and their dosage (both daily and weekly) within the protocols, and variation in the rehabilitation duration, which has included 4 weeks, 6 weeks, 8 weeks and 36

weeks, complicates comparisons among studies. However, treatment plans have been shown to be efficacious on at least one of the measured dependent variables (Hale et al., 2007; McKeon et al., 2009; Ross et al., 2007).

Effects on measures of impairment

Similar to balance training protocols, performance on the SEBT has been shown to improve following treatment protocols that included balance, functional tests, strength exercises and range-of-motion exercises (Hale et al., 2007). Similarly, rehabilitation consisting of hop and balance tasks has also shown improvement in SEBT reach distance (McKeon et al., 2008). However, the difficulty with these studies is that it is not possible to know whether these effects were enhanced by the use of multiple treatments or were the sole product of balance training, with the other components being superfluous.

Effects on measures of functional limitation

Two randomized control trials have assessed multiple treatment protocols on measures of functional limitations. Hale et al. (2007) used balance, functional tests, strength exercises and range-of-motion exercises and demonstrated significant improvements in FADI and FADI Sport scores. Similarly, using hopping and balance tasks McKeon et al. (2008) also demonstrated improvements in the FADI and FADI Sport. Clearly, based on these studies and those previously described, ankle rehabilitation protocols can improve patients' functional limitations, perhaps regardless of training mode.

Summary

In summary, these protocols are efficacious but complex. They typically involve many exercises and often mix different modes of exercise or treatment. The frequency and duration of treatment also vary significantly, making comparison among studies difficult. Finally, the complexity of the treatment protocols and the per-session time needed to complete the treatment may place an impractical time burden on the patient and clinician.

Patient disability resulting from ankle disease

The Short Form (36) Health Survey (SF-36) has been used to assess HRQoL in patients with ankle pathologies such as ankle arthrosis, osteoarthritis, fractures and sprains (Bhandari et al., 2004; Ponzer et al., 1999; Saltzman et al., 2006). In ankle sprains it has been reported that compared to uninjured subjects, subjects with ankle injury had lower scores on the 'General Health' scale and 'Physical Component

Summary' (PCS) of the SF-36. A more recent rehabilitation study has demonstrated that balance board training, but not strength training, can produce improvements in the PCS at levels that are associated with improved ability to work and less risk of job loss (Wright et al., 2016). These studies indicate that ankle sprains lead to a reduced HRQoL and that balance board training can be efficacious in improving HRQoL.

Rehabilitation effects on incidence and recurrence

In addition to the measures previously described, some studies (Emery et al., 2007; Mohammadi, 2007) have reported epidemiological measures of incidence/recurrence. All but one of these studies have shown that balance training decreases the risk of ankle sprain by 2–8 times, with Mohammadi (2007) also showing that strength training can reduce risk by two-fold and demonstrating that balance training was superior to strength training.

Take-home message

Based on the available research, balance training improves ankle function across the disability continuum and reduces sprain recurrence. Combining balance training with other forms of rehabilitation is also efficacious but it is unclear if this combined approach is better than balance training alone. The efficacy of strength training is currently unclear.

Anterior cruciate ligament injuries

Kim Hébert-Losier, Charlotte Häger

Introduction

Anterior cruciate ligament (ACL) ruptures are one of the most common knee injuries, with annual incidence rates of 0.05 to 0.08% (Moses and Orchard, 2012). In the United States alone, there are approximately a quarter of a million new ACL injuries per year (Silvers and Mandelbaum, 2011) Based on a Multicentre Database cost-utility analysis (Mather et al., 2013), preventing one ACL injury in someone under 25 years old leads to lifetime societal and economic savings of US$50,000–95,000. The majority of ACL injuries occur during sporting activities, which not only affect the function of individuals in the short term, but may also do so several decades after injury (Hébert-Losier et al., 2015).

Anatomy

The ACL is an intra-articular extrasynovial ligament oriented obliquely from the posteromedial aspect of the intercondylar femoral condyle notch to a triangular space on the tibia between the medial intercondylar eminence and the anterior horns of the menisci (Fig. 5.1). The bony femoral insertion of the ACL is in continuity with the posterior femoral cortex. The tibial insertion of the ACL is C-shaped and blends with the lateral meniscus insertions. The ACL is frequently described as containing two bundles (anteromedial and posterolateral) named according to their tibial insertion sites in the intercondylaris anterior area. The main role of the ACL is to prevent anterior translation of the tibia with respect to the femur. The ACL also restrains excessive internal tibial rotation, knee hyperextension and knee valgus and varus, especially in weight-bearing.

Injury mechanisms and risk factors

Understanding injury mechanisms is a key component in injury prevention. Most ACL injuries occur in pivoting sports, especially soccer, with up to 85% of ACL injuries occurring during noncontact or indirect contact situations. In particular these occur during deceleration, side-cutting, landing and balancing manoeuvres (Waldén et al., 2015). Although the absolute incidence of ACL injuries and surgeries is greater in men (Gornitzky et al., 2016), the relative risk of sustaining an ACL injury is overall three times greater in women (Agel et al., 2005; Prodromos et al., 2007). Other than soccer, American football, gymnastics, basketball, lacrosse and wrestling have relatively high rates of ACL injuries (Hootman et al., 2007) as do rugby, handball, floorball and skiing. ACL injuries and surgeries are less common in prepubescence, and it has been suggested to peak between 14 to 19 years of age in women and 15 to 34 years in men (Sanders et al., 2016).

ACL injuries occur when loading exceeds the capacity of the biological tissue. Injuries are suspected to occur between 20–50 ms after initial strain (Koga et al., 2010), with multi-plane knee loading in weight-bearing being the most common mode of noncontact ACL injury. The knee is often in hyperextension or slight flexion and undergoes a valgus motion with either an internal or external rotation (Shimokochi and Shultz, 2008), with a 'knee-in and toe-out' position (Fig. 5.2). The terms *dynamic valgus* or *dynamic lower extremity valgus* are commonly used in the literature to describe the multi-plane and multi-joint motion characterizing the ACL injury mechanism, which involves hip adduction and internal rotation, knee abduction, tibial external rotation and anterior translation, and ankle eversion (Hewett et al., 2006). In fact, explanations for ACL injury mechanisms should consider the entire kinematic chain. For instance, a low degree of ankle plantar flexion, large hip flexion (Carlson et al., 2016), a low degree of knee flexion, trunk lateral bending and little trunk flexion are all movements that have been observed during ACL ruptures (Hewett et al., 2009; Hewett et al., 2011).

Other than participating in pivoting sports and *dynamic valgus* movement patterns (Hewett et al., 2006) predisposing

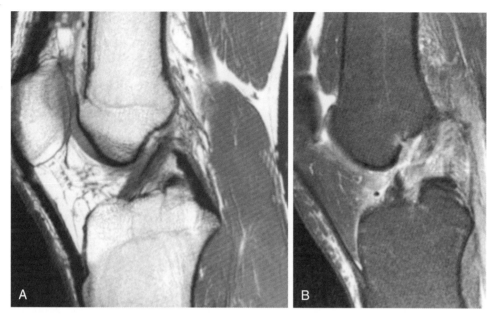

Fig. 5.1 Magnetic resonance images of (A) an intact and (B) a ruptured anterior cruciate ligament of the knee.

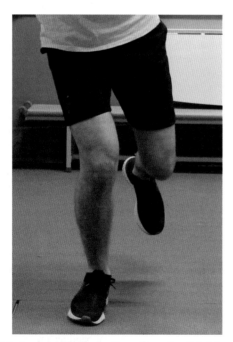

Fig. 5.2 A schematic illustration of a potential risk position of the lower extremity with regard to anterior cruciate ligament injury, where the knee is in valgus motion and the foot externally rotated, the so called 'knee-in and toe-out' configuration.

factors to noncontact ACL injuries common to both sexes include: generalized and/or knee joint laxity (Vacek et al., 2016), previous ACL injury (Arden et al., 2014), restricted hip rotation (VandenBerg et al., 2017), family history of ACL injuries (Vacek et al., 2016) and anatomical factors such as a narrow intercondylar notch (Zeng et al., 2013) and/or steep tibial slope (Hashemi et al., 2010). Evidence emerging over the last decade suggests the involvement of hereditary factors, where genetics may play a role both in anatomical risk factors, such as bone geometry and collagen structure (O'Connell et al., 2015) including risk behaviours. Other risk factors proposed as being more specific to males include decreased ankle dorsiflexion, decreased hip internal rotation and increased hip anteversion. Those specific to females include decreased hamstring-to-quadriceps muscular capacities (Myer et al., 2009), increased body mass index (Uhorchak et al., 2003) and being in the first half of the menstrual cycle (preovulatory and ovulary phases) (Herzberg et al., 2017) due to interrelated variations in ACL laxity (Zazulak et al., 2006). It is unclear whether ACL injuries are more frequent on the dominant or nondominant side, which might depend on differences between sexes, sports, injury mechanisms and definition of side dominance between studies (Ruedl et al., 2012).

Screening and prevention

Screening tests aim to identify athletes at high risk of sustaining an injury and justify the implementation of targeted injury-prevention strategies. The screening tests should be sensitive (i.e., correctly identify high-risk individuals) and specific (i.e., correctly identify low-risk individuals), as well as cost-effective. Screening with regard to potentially injurious movement patterns during drop vertical jumps, wall jumps or tuck jumps (Padua et al., 2015), and impaired postural stability (Dingeman et al., 2016) has received some attention over the years with regard to ACL injury prediction. However, there is some concern involving the reliability, validity, practicality, efficiency and sport-specificity of such screening methods, with only one study demonstrating an ability of field-based measures to prospectively identify youth soccer athletes who sustained an ACL injury through drop vertical jumps (Padua et al., 2015). There is a need for the further development and validation of screening tests that can be used in the primary and secondary prevention of ACL injuries that consider the sensorimotor system and movement quality (van Melick et al., 2016; Dingenen and Gokeler, 2017).

Given the challenges associated with predicting injury risk through mass screening initiatives, the systematic implementation of ACL injury-prevention programmes has been recommended, particularly for individuals who are young, female, participating in high-risk sports and present with a history or family history of ACL injury. Several prevention programmes are available and target modifiable risk factors for noncontact ACL injuries. These programmes typically include one or several of the following components: plyometrics, balance, proprioception, strengthening, core and trunk control, agility, technique correction with feedback, body awareness, education and stretching (Alentorn-Geli et al., 2009; Bien et al., 2011). Programmes targeting several components seem the most effective in preventing ACL injuries, particularly when integrating strengthening, proximal control, plyometrics and feedback exercises. Programmes are also more effective when performed in-season rather than preseason (Michaelidis and Koumantakis, 2014), with compliance and dosage being key factors to successful reduction of ACL injury incidence. The current recommendation is three sessions per week preseason and two sessions per week in-season, with each session lasting at least 20 min (Sugimoto et al., 2014). Similar to screening initiatives, there is concern regarding the cost-effectiveness of injury-prevention programmes, whereby approximately 100 to 120 athletes need to follow an effective programme to prevent one noncontact ACL injury (Noyes et al., 2014). Other strategies advocated in the primary and secondary prevention of ACL injuries include the use of knee braces (Ewing et al., 2016), taping (Harput et al., 2016) or foot orthoses (Jenkins et al., 2008), although more evidence is required to support the effectiveness of such interventions.

Treatment

ACL ruptures are treated either conservatively using a physiotherapy-based rehabilitation approach often with activity modifications as a major concept, or surgically in conjunction with preoperative and postoperative physiotherapy. Bone–patellar tendon–bone and hamstring–tendon autografts are the most commonly harvested autologous tissues used in surgical reconstructions, with the quadriceps tendon also showing promising results. Other graft choices include allografts and synthetic grafts (Kay et al., 2017).

Choosing nonoperative versus operative management is a complex decision, with a lower threshold for offering surgery in the presence of ACL injuries with associated meniscal tears or multi-ligament injuries compared to isolated ACL tears or ruptures.

There is still a lack of conclusive evidence for which treatment approach is best (i.e., non-surgical vs. surgical) at an individual level. Research indicates comparable outcomes in relation to return to sport, need for secondary surgery, development of osteoarthritis, limb symmetry and patient-reported outcomes and satisfaction (Frobell et al., 2013; Grindhem et al., 2014; Smith et al., 2014; Tengman et al., 2014). In addition, there is evidence that following a structured rehabilitation programme may lead to the recuperation of physical performance and muscle strength with or without surgical intervention in young active adults (Ericsson et al., 2013). Directly comparing results between nonoperative and operative approaches is challenging given the lack of, and difficulty conducting, randomized control trials in this area, as well as the continuous evolution of conservative and surgical approaches. Independent of treatment approach, cross-sectional studies on the topic indicate the presence and persistence of compensatory mechanisms and altered biomechanical strategies (Roos et al., 2014; Tengman et al., 2015), with not all individuals successfully returning to preinjury physical activity levels.

Independent of primary management choice, the undertaking of a structured physiotherapy and rehabilitation programme is recommended and should last a minimum of 24 weeks if nonoperative (Frobell et al., 2010) and between 9 and 12 months postoperatively (van Melick et al., 2016). Several factors should be considered during the rehabilitation process, including the type and targeted level of physical activity, tissue healing stages, ability to tolerate load, pain and effusion, self-rated function, and psychological readiness (Arden et al., 2011). Rehabilitation programmes generally focus on the management of symptoms (pain, swelling, giving-way episodes), range of motion, muscle strength, gait, balance, proprioception, neuromuscular control, dynamic knee stability, movement quality, sport-specific exercises and graduated return to play. The use of functional knee bracing during rehabilitation offers a resistance against the anterior translation of the tibia and protection against full extension, and if partaking in high-risk activities (e.g., downhill skiing and pivoting sports) their use is prevalent in both operative and nonoperative management of ACL ruptures. However, currently there is a lack of definitive evidence of improved treatment outcomes, and the prescription of functional bracing in ACL rupture treatment is not routine (Lowe et al., 2017). Taping in the early stages of rehabilitation has also been examined (Balki et al., 2016), but has not been consistently associated with superior outcomes.

Outcome measures

There is no current gold standard in terms of evaluating ACL treatment outcomes (Ahmad et al., 2017) or establishing when an athlete is ready to return to sport (Dingeman and Gokeler, 2017). Highly cited level I ACL clinical trials commonly report knee joint laxity, patient-reported subjective scores, graft failure and range of motion data (Ahmad et al., 2017). More rarely are direct measures of sensorimotor function or movement quality included in clinical studies, which is a shortcoming in the empirical literature given the persistence of deficits seen long term. To assess readiness to return to play, the main guidelines used are time postsurgery, clinical measures relating to mobility and strength, functional performance tests and patient-reported outcomes (Gokeler et al., 2017).

Clinical measures used to objectively quantify outcomes include range-of-motion, strength, and ligament integrity (pivot shift and Lachman) tests. Some of the key patient-reported outcomes available are the Lysholm score, Tegner activity scale, Activities of Daily Living, International Knee Documentation Scores, Knee Injury and Osteoarthritis Outcome Score (KOOS), ACL Return to Sports after Injury (ACL-RSI) questionnaire, and the Injury Psychological Readiness to Return to Sport scale. Increasing evidence indicates that psychological factors (e.g., motivation, fear of movement) play a role in rehabilitation, patient satisfaction and return to preinjury physical activity levels (Arden et al., 2011). Scales that address fear of movement (e.g., Tampa Scale for Kinesiophobia) are being increasingly used in practice and research.

In terms of functional performance, hop tests (e.g., for distance, height or side hops, cross-over, triple hop, and 6-m timed) are the most frequently used. One of the most used criteria for assessing return to 'normal' or 'abnormal' function has been the limb symmetry index (LSI; involved limb/ uninvolved limb × 100%), where a LSI of >90% is considered satisfactory (Thomeé et al., 2011). However, there are several concerns regarding the use of LSI as an outcome measure or sole return-to-play criterion. The LSI can mask the presence of bilateral deficits, conceal individual results, fail to consider absolute performance and overestimate knee function after an ACL injury (Wellsandt et al., 2017). Functional performance tests should not be used as sole return-to-sport criteria and a comprehensive test battery should be employed (van Melick et al., 2016) in combination with psychological readiness scales (Arden et al., 2016), time post surgery, and level of return to sport (Grindem et al., 2020).

Consequences

There is no clear definition of what timeframe constitutes a short-, mid-, and long-term outcome in the ACL literature, with 6, 9, 12, 18, and 24 months being benchmark follow-up timeframes. There is an increasing number of studies with follow-ups of 2–10 years, 10–20 years and beyond 20 years. All these studies provide insights into the potential consequences of ACL injuries, which include short-term, mid-term and long-term alterations in gait (i.e., walking, running and stair negotiation), balance, proprioception, knee joint position sense, joint awareness, lower extremity loading patterns, movement strategies, injury risk, sport participation and physical activity levels and the increased risk of developing ostheoarthitis.

In synthesizing the literature, Ardern et al. (2014) determined that 81% of individuals returned to some form of sport following ACL reconstruction, but only 65% returned to their preinjury levels and 55% to competitive sport. There appears to be no clear difference in the rates of return to sport between operative and nonoperative treatment approaches (Kessler et al., 2008), except for in children and adolescents where operative treatment has been linked to higher rates of return to sport and better functional outcomes (Fabricant et al., 2016), at least in the short term.

Combining information from several sources places second ACL injury rates in the 5 years following an ACL reconstruction at 17.6%, 5.8% on the ipsilateral side and 11.8% on the contralateral side (Wright et al., 2011), with rates reaching 32% in the 15 years post-reconstructive surgery (Leys et al., 2012). The relative risk of sustaining a new knee injury is more than three times greater in athletes with an ACL reconstructed knee than those without (Waldén et al., 2006). The risk of rerupture appears to be greater in younger individuals, and within the first 2 years following reconstruction (Schlumberger et al., 2017). Less information is available for nonoperated individuals, with studies indicating that knee surgery is required in approximately 25% of cases in 14-year follow-ups (Chalmers et al., 2014).

In the very long term (>20 years), ACL-injured individuals tend to report lower levels of knee-specific physical activity based on Tegner and Lysholm scores when compared to matched controls, especially in the presence of knee osteoarthritis. Osteoarthritis is observed in 50–90% of ACL-injured individuals (Tengman et al., 2014), a three to four times greater relative risk compared to noninjured individuals (Suter et al., 2017) irrespective of treatment approach. Furthermore, research provides evidence of altered dynamic knee joint stability during functional tasks, jump capacity, balance and strength in comparison to controls, not only on the injured leg but also on the noninjured leg (Grip et al., 2015; Hébert-Losier et al., 2015; Tengman et al., 2014; 2015). These findings indicate that it might be advisable to continue performing some form of rehabilitation throughout life to limit the long-term sequelae resulting from ACL injuries.

Take-home message

ACL injuries are of great concern in sports and orthopaedic medicine. Biomechanics play a central role in understanding and addressing ACL injuries and their management. There is, however, no current gold standard for detecting individuals at high risk of injuries, prescribing injury prevention programmes, selecting operative versus non-operative treatment, assessing ACL treatment outcomes, returning individuals to sport, reducing reinjury and osteoarthritis rates, and addressing long-term functional deficits. The absence of definitive guidelines is due to the multifactorial and multidimensional nature of ACL injuries, and lack of consensus despite a continuously growing research field. Therefore, ACL injuries should be addressed on a case-by-case basis using the most up-to-date information available to ensure best practice management.

Shoulder injuries

Bruno Mazuquin, Puneet Monga

Introduction

The shoulder has inherent characteristics integrating anatomical structures to allow the greatest range of motion among all joints in the human body. Its mobility is responsible for supporting spatial displacement of the arms, permitting an ample scope of activities of the upper limbs. However, the anatomical shape of the glenohumeral joint, with a much larger humeral head than the glenoid fossa, increases the risk of instability. In order to perform a smooth and controlled movement, the muscles around the shoulder need to provide balanced forces; this relies on information from mechanoreceptors within the muscles themselves and from other adjacent structures such as ligaments and capsule. This important information ensures the safety of the structures, specifically as the joint reaches the limits of a movement. When parts of the shoulder structures do not work correctly, or when the dynamic stabilizers, i.e., rotator cuff muscles (supraspinatus, infraspinatus, teres minor and subscapularis), are not able to control the humeral head, damage may occur and disrupt the inherent biomechanics of the joint. In turn, this may impair sports performance and cause disabling symptoms such as pain. In this section we review the three most commonly observed sports injuries affecting the shoulder: internal impingement, rotator cuff tears and instability.

Internal impingement

Internal impingement is a condition observed commonly in overhead athletes, especially throwers. The classic scenario when this occurs is when throwing a ball – shoulder elevation and rotation are required. Internal impingement occurs mainly during the cocking phase, which is the moment in time when the humerus is over 90 degrees of abduction combined with over 90 degrees of external rotation. In this position, the articular side of the supraspinatus may be compressed between the humeral head and the posterosuperior labrum. Such a contact itself is not of major concern as this is a relatively normal event when the arm is positioned at 90 degrees of abduction and 90 degrees of external rotation. However, due to the repetitive nature of sports activities, the continuous and cumulative overloading of the rotator cuff muscles can lead to injuries to the labrum and tendon (Burkhart et al, 2003).

The main symptoms related to internal impingement are pain during maximal abduction and external rotation, progressive decrease in movement velocity, loss of control and sports performance deterioration. Generally, the athlete shows signs of posterior glenohumeral joint-line tenderness, loss of internal rotation and excessive external rotation. In addition, complementary imaging exams may reveal further potential structural problems such as rotator cuff tears and labral tears.

Rotator cuff tears

By definition, rotator cuff tears are a rupture of one or more tendons of the rotator cuff muscles due to trauma or a degenerative process (Opsha et al., 2008). These are one of the main causes of shoulder pain, and are a common disorder that affects approximately 30% of people older than 60 years; it has an increasing rate associated with ageing (Yamaguchi et al., 2006; Yamamoto et al., 2010). In the sports population, rotator cuff tears are common in overhead athletes; partial tears have been observed in 48% and full-thickness tears in 21% (McMahon et al., 2014). As a result, rotator cuff tears are responsible for approximately 450,000 operations a year in the USA alone (Thigpen et al., 2016).

Considering the stabilizer role of the rotator cuff, the presence of a tear in one of the four tendons may potentially disrupt the shoulder biomechanics and movement control. For instance, if the subscapularis or supraspinatus is impaired, the force pulling the humeral head downwards during elevation will be deficient. Therefore the humeral head will migrate towards the acromion direction, due to the unopposed pull of the deltoid, which will compress the structures under the subacromial space and consequently may provoke pain and discomfort.

Injury mechanism

The mechanisms leading to failure of the rotator cuff tendons in athletes are related to trauma or overuse. Traumatic rotator cuff tear events in sports are more likely to happen in a fall or with traction; in contrast, chronic processes are common in overhead athletes such as baseball pitchers and tennis players. In these sports, movement repetition is required, which demands prolonged use of the rotator cuff muscles as a dynamic stabilizer in high-load positions. The continuous stress applied to the cuff tendons may cause microtrauma, which over time may result in tissue failure.

Management of internal impingement and rotator cuff tears

The first treatment option for internal impingement and chronic rotator cuff tears is often physiotherapy. Performing exercises aimed at improving motor control and rotator cuff recruitment have been shown to be effective in resolving pain symptoms and improving function (Kuhn et al., 2013). In addition, focusing on exercises that involve the whole kinetic chain are also strongly recommended. This type of exercise comprises training the power and energy generated from the lower limbs to be transferred more efficiently through the trunk until reaching the upper limbs, therefore, reducing the stress imposed on the shoulder when performing sports-related movements (McMullen and Uhl, 2000). The majority of patients show a positive response in reducing symptoms when such physiotherapy is carried for about 12 weeks (Kuhn et al., 2013). Another conservative option is corticosteroid injections, which are used to reduce inflammation. However, the evidence shows that this treatment has good short-term effects but does not have long-lasting benefits. Furthermore, there are concerns that the use of corticosteroids may jeopardize the tendon and cartilage tissues by negatively impacting collagen expression (Abdul-Wahab Taiceer et al., 2016).

When conservative approaches do not achieve a satisfactory result, surgery is considered. For rotator cuff tears, surgery involves repairing the damaged tendons by reinserting them to their attachment on the humerus. Depending on the tear size and tissue quality, different techniques may be used to provide greater stability to the footprint. However, studies have shown no statistically significant differences in patient-reported outcome measures comparing single-row or double-row methods (McCormick et al., 2014; Trappey and Gartsman, 2011).

In contrast to chronic rotator cuff tears, surgery is considered as the first treatment option for acute tears. Early surgery, up to 3 months after the event, has been shown to significantly improve patient outcomes and has been shown to increase the probability of return to play. Klouche et al. (2016) performed a systematic review with meta-analysis to determine the rate of return to sport after rotator cuff repairs. The authors found an overall rate of return of 84.7% for recreational athletes, of which 65.4% returned to a similar level of play, whereas 49.9% of the

professional and competitive individuals returned to sport to similar level prior to surgery. In addition, Antoni et al. (2016) reported good results for recreational athletes; this included individuals who had a rotator cuff repair and a minimum of 2 years' follow-up. Of these, 88.2% of the athletes returned to sports activities with an average time to return of 6 months (SD = 4.9 months).

Physiotherapy after rotator cuff repair is currently an area of considerable debate, particularly regarding the length of time for sling usage after surgery. Previously, a 6-week period of immobilization after surgery was recommended to avoid re-tear episodes. However, using a sling for long periods of time may cause stiffness and has been shown to change activity in the motor and somatosensory cortices (Berth et al., 2009; Huber et al., 2006). An overview of systematic reviews has demonstrated that using a sling for less than 6 weeks is not the main cause of higher re-tear rates (Mazuquin et al., 2018). With acute tears in the young population, the tendon and muscle tissue are generally of good quality, which allows a good repair that has a better chance of good stability and potentially lower tension. For these repairs, starting mobilization before the 6-week period may bring greater benefits and reduce the time to return to sport, although a individualized approach and consensus between the surgeon and therapist is important.

Instability

Shoulder instability is an abnormal symptomatic motion of the humerus on the glenoid fossa that may cause pain, subluxation or dislocation (Lewis et al., 2004). There are various methods to classify shoulder instability. One of the most common is the Stanmore classification system, which classifies patients into three main polar groups that differ according to the cause of the instability (Lewis et al., 2004) (Fig. 5.3). Although three distinct groups are defined, some patients may also present mutual characteristics from more than one polar type and therefore be positioned between two poles of the triangle.

- Polar I: Caused by a traumatic event that damages anatomical structures responsible for shoulder stability, mainly the static stabilizers (labrum, capsule, ligaments).
- Polar II: Caused by structural defects that may not be consequence of trauma.
- Polar III: Nonstructural and mainly caused by abnormal muscle activity.

The main symptoms of patients who are under the polar I instability classification will be apprehension of dislocation when testing for anterior instability with the apprehension test. There is usually a history of injury and, in addition, they may present internal rotation weakness if the subscapularis is affected. For subscapularis weakness the Gerber's lift-off test can be used (Monga and Funk,

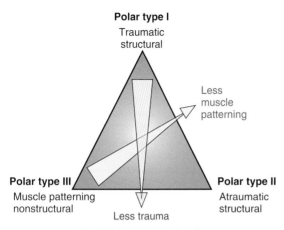

Polar type I
Traumatic
structural

Less
muscle
patterning

Polar type III
Muscle patterning
nonstructural

Less trauma

Polar type II
Atraumatic
structural

Fig. 5.3 Stanmore triangle.

Table 5.1 Common structures affected in shoulder instability

Injury	Structure
SLAP	Superior labrum
Bankart	Anteroinferior labrum
Hill–Sachs	Bone loss over humeral head
HAGL	Avulsion of the humeral attachment of the glenohumeral ligament

HAGL, humeral avulsion of the glenohumeral ligament; *SLAP* superior labrum anterior–posterior.

2017). The polar type II patient will also present apprehension, which may be associated with internal rotation deficit and increased external rotation, and this may be associated with joint hyperlaxity. Polar type III generally will show less apprehension; instead poor muscle control is observed, especially for the rotator cuff when performing various shoulder movements.

For those patients who present instability due to structural involvement, imaging exams such as magnetic resonance imaging (MRI) and X-ray are beneficial to observe what structures are compromised and for planning the surgical intervention.

Injury mechanism

In sports such as rugby and American football, the vast majority of shoulder instability is caused by traumatic events which consequently compromise the shoulder anatomical structure integrity (Crichton et al., 2012; Gibbs et al., 2015). The most common game situation that exposes athletes to shoulder instability injury is when going for a tackle (shoulder abducted) or when trying to reach the ball and landing with the arm flexed over 90 degrees. In both situations, a high-energy impact generates forces towards the anterior or posterior direction which is applied on the distal end of the limb; consequently this force produces a levering effect on the glenohumeral joint moving the humerus head anteriorly or posteriorly respectively (Crichton et al., 2012). The most common injuries and the respective shoulder structures affected in each are described in Table 5.1.

Management of instability

The management will depend on what kind of instability the patient presents. Those with a polar type I, less than 20

years of age and who intend to return to sport have a greater benefit from surgery (Jaggi and Lambert, 2010). In this scenario, surgery has been shown to avoid recurrence and a high percentage of patients return to sport at the same level and often in about 4 months (Gibson et al., 2016; Kim et al., 2003).

In contrast, patients with instability which is nontraumatic in origin may benefit from conservative treatment such as physiotherapy first. In these cases, physiotherapy has been demonstrated to be effective at avoiding surgery in up to 80% of individuals (Jaggi and Lambert, 2010). Rehabilitation programmes should prioritize exercises aiming to improve their interrelated muscle activity deficits of the rotator cuff. In addition, exercises aiming to strengthen other shoulder muscles should be considered. Moreover, similar to the rehabilitation programme for internal impingement and rotator cuff tears, these patients also benefit from exercises incorporating the kinetic chain to develop movement efficiency. For patients classified as polar type II, surgery would be recommended after a period of 6 months of trying physiotherapy (Jaggi and Lambert, 2010).

The first stage after surgery requires caution to allow good healing of the repaired structures. At this stage, physiotherapy needs to find the balance between mobilizing the joint to avoid stiffness but without exceeding the limits that may cause damage to the repaired tissues. Therefore, closed-chain exercises are a good option in the initial rehabilitation phase as the range of motion can be controlled and at the same time the muscles are already starting to be stimulated and recruited. As patients progress and pain levels improve, exercises may advance to improve strength, endurance and range of motion, moving from closed chain to open chain and adjusting lever arms and resistance accordingly.

The return-to-play rates after instability surgery is high. Elsenbeck and Dickens (2017) demonstrated in their review that the rate of return to sport varies from 63% to 100%, with the majority of the studies showing a rate of over 80%, which has been confirmed by Robins et al. (2017).

Take-home message

Due to its great mobility, the shoulder is exposed to injuries and relies on the integrity of static and dynamic stabilizers working in synergy to maintain the joint biomechanics fluidity. Overhead athletes are more prone to internal impingement and rotator cuff tears, while athletes participating in contact sports may be more susceptible to instability. Surgical interventions have demonstrated positive results regarding return to play, and physiotherapy plays a major role in athletes' recovery, either as a first treatment option or after surgical procedures.

References

Ankle injuries

Arnold, B.L., Linens, S.W., de la Motte, S.J., Ross, S.E., 2009. Concentric evertor strength differences and functional ankle instability: A meta-analysis. Journal of Athletic Training 44 (6), 653–662.

Bhandari, M., Sprague, S., Hanson, B., Busse, J.W., Dawe, D.E., Moro, J.K., et al., 2004. Health-related quality of life following operative treatment of unstable ankle fractures: A prospective observational study. Journal of Orthopaedic Trauma 18 (6), 338–345.

Coughlan, G., Caulfield, B., 2007. A 4-week neuromuscular training program and gait patterns at the ankle joint. Journal of Athletic Training 42 (1), 51–59.

Cruz-Diaz, D., Lomas-Vega, R., Osuna-Perez, M.C., Contreras, F.H., Martinez-Amat, A., 2015. Effects of 6 weeks of balance training on chronic ankle instability in athletes: A randomized controlled trial. International Journal of Sports Medicine 36 (9), 754–760.

Docherty, C.L., Moore, J.H., Arnold, B.L., 1998. Effects of strength training on strength development and joint position sense in functionally unstable ankles. Journal of Athletic Training 33 (4), 310–314.

Doherty, C., Delahunt, E., Caulfield, B., Hertel, J., Ryan, J., Bleakley, C., et al., 2014. The incidence and prevalence of ankle sprain injury: a systematic review and meta-analysis of prospective epidemiological studies. Journal of Sports Medicine 44, 123–140.

Emery, C.A., Rose, M.S., McAllister, J.R., Meeuwisse, W.H., 2007. A prevention strategy to reduce the incidence of injury in high school basketball: A cluster randomized controlled trial. Clinical Journal of Sport Medicine 17 (1), 17–24.

Feger, M.A., Snell, S., Handsfield, G.G., Blemker, S.S., Wombacher, E., Fry, R., et al., 2016. Diminished foot and ankle muscle volumes in young adults with chronic ankle instability. Orthopaedic Journal of Sports Medicine 4 (6), 2325967116653719.

Gehring, D., Wissler, S., Mornieux, G., Gollhofer, A., 2013. How to sprain your ankle – a biomechanical case report of an inversion trauma. Journal of Biomechanics 46 (1), 175–178.

Hale, S.A., Hertel, J., Olmsted-Kramer, L.C., 2007. The effect of a 4-week comprehensive rehabilitation program on postural control and lower extremity function in individuals with chronic ankle instability. Journal of Orthopaedic & Sports Physical Therapy 37 (6), 303–311.

Hall, E.A., Docherty, C.L., Simon, J., Kingma, J.J., Klossner, J.C., 2015. Strength-training protocols to improve deficits in participants with chronic ankle instability: A randomized controlled trial. Journal of Athletic Training 50 (1), 36–44.

Han, K., Ricard, M.D., Fellingham, G.W., 2009. Effects of a 4-week exercise program on balance using elastic tubing as a perturbation force for individuals with a history of ankle sprains. Journal of Orthopaedic & Sports Physical Therapy 39 (4), 246–255.

Hootman, J., Dick, R., Agel, J., 2007. Epidemiology of collegiate injuries for 15 sports: summary and recommendations for injury prevention initiatives. Journal of Athletic Training 42, 311–319.

Hubbard, T.J., Hicks-Little, C.A., 2008. Ankle ligament healing after an acute ankle sprain: an evidence-based approach. Journal of Athletic Training 43 (5), 523–529.

Lee, A.J.Y., Lin, W., 2008. Twelve-week biomechanical ankle platform system training on postural stability and ankle proprioception in subjects with unilateral functional ankle instability. Clinical Biomechanics 23, 1065–1072.

Linens, S.W., Ross, S.E., Arnold, B.L., 2016. Wobble board rehabilitation for improving balance in ankles with chronic instability. Clinical Journal of Sport Medicine 26 (1), 76–82.

Matsusaka, N., Yokoyama, S., Tsurusaki, T., Inokuchi, S., Okita, M., 2001. Effect of ankle disk training combined with tactile stimulation to the leg and foot on functional instability of the ankle. American Journal of Sports Medicine 29 (1), 25–30.

McKeon, J.M., Bush, H.M., Reed, A., Whittington, A., Uhl, T.L., McKeon, P.O., 2014. Return-to-play probabilities following new versus recurrent ankle sprains in high school athletes. Journal of Science and Medicine in Sport 17 (1), 23–28.

McKeon, P.O., Ingersoll, C.D., Kerrigan, D.C., Saliba, E., Bennett, B.C., Hertel, J., et al., 2008. Balance training improves function and postural control in those with chronic ankle instability. Medicine and Science in Sports and Exercise 40 (10), 1810–1819.

McKeon, P.O., Paolini, G., Ingersoll, C.D., Kerrigan, D.C., Saliba, E.N., Bennett, B.C., et al., 2009. Effects of balance training on gait parameters in patients with chronic ankle instability: A randomized controlled trial. Clinical Rehabilitation 23 (7), 609–621.

McLeod, T.C.V., Snyder, A.R., Parsons, J.T., Bay, R.C., Michener, L.A., Sauers, E.L., et al., 2008. Using disablement models and clinical outcomes assessment to enable evidence-based athletic training practice, part II: Clinical outcomes assessment. Journal of Athletic Training 43 (4), 437–445.

Mohammadi, F., 2007. Comparison of 3 preventive methods to reduce the recurrence of ankle inversion sprains in male soccer players. American Journal of Sports Medicine 35 (6), 922–926.

Ponzer, S., Nasell, H., Bergman, B., Tornkvist, H., 1999. Functional outcome and quality of life in patients with type B ankle fractures: A two-year follow-up study. Journal of Orthopaedic Trauma 13 (5), 363–368.

Ross, S.E., Arnold, B.L., Blackburn, J.T., Brown, C.N., Guskiewicz, K.M., 2007. Enhanced balance associated with coordination training with stochastic resonance stimulation in subjects with functional ankle instability: An experimental trial. Journal of Neuroengineering and Rehabilitation 4, 47.

Saltzman, C.L., Zimmerman, M.B., O'Rourke, M., Brown, T.D., Buckwalter, J.A., Johnston, R., et al., 2006. Impact of comorbidities on the measurement of health in patients with ankle osteoarthritis. Journal of Bone and Joint Surgery. American Volume 88 (11), 2366–2372.

Sekir, U., Yildiz, Y., Hazneci, B., Ors, F., Aydin, T., 2007. Effect of isokinetic training on strength, functionality and proprioception in athletes with functional ankle instability. Knee Surgery, Sports Traumatology, Arthroscopy 15 (5), 654–664.

Snyder, A.R., Parsons, J.T., McLeod, T.C.V., Bay, R.C., Michener, L.A., Sauers, E.L., et al., 2008. Using disablement models and clinical outcomes assessment to enable evidence-based athletic training practice, part I: Disablement models. Journal of Athletic Training 43 (4), 428–436.

Taga, I., Shoni, K., Inoue, M., Nakata, K., Maeda, A., 1993. Articular cartilage lesions in ankles with lateral ligament injury. An arthrocospic study. The American Journal of Sports Medicine 21 (1), 120–126.

Waterman, B.R., Belmont, P.J., Cameron, K.L., DeBerardino, T.M., Owens, B.D., 2010. Epidemiology of ankle sprain at the United States Military Academy. The American Journal of Sports Medicine 38, 797–803.

Wright, C.J., Linens, S.W., Cain, M.S., 2016. A randomized controlled trial comparing rehabilitation efficacy in chronic ankle instability. Journal of Sport Rehabilitation 26 (4), 238–249.

Yeung, M., Chang, K., So, C., 1994. An epidemiological survey on ankle sprain. British Journal of Sports Medicine 28, 112–116.

Anterior cruciate ligament injuries

Agel, J., Arendt, E.A., Bershadsky, B., 2005. Anterior cruciate ligament injury in national collegiate athletic association basketball and soccer. The American Journal of Sports Medicine 33 (4), 524–531.

Ahmad, S.S., Meyer, J.C., Krismer, A.M., Ahmad, S.S., Evangelopoulos, D.S., Hoppe, S., et al., 2017. Outcome measures in clinical ACL studies: An analysis of highly cited level I trials. Knee Surgery, Sports Traumatology, Arthroscopy 25 (5), 1517–1527.

Alentorn-Geli, E., Myer, G.D., Silvers, H.J., Samitier, G., Romero, D., Lázaro-Haro, C., et al., 2009. Prevention of non-contact anterior cruciate ligament injuries in soccer players. Part 2: A review of prevention programs aimed to modify risk factors and to reduce injury rates. Knee Surgery, Sports Traumatology, Arthroscopy 17 (8), 859–879.

Ardern, C.L., Glasgow, P., Schneiders, A., Witvrouw, E., Clarsen, B., Cools, A., et al., 2016. Consensus statement on return to sport from the first world congress in sports physical therapy, Bern. British Journal of Sports Medicine 50 (14), 853–864.

Ardern, C.L., Taylor, N.F., Feller, J.A., Webster, K.E., 2014. Fifty-five per cent return to competitive sport following anterior cruciate ligament reconstruction surgery: an updated systematic review and meta-analysis including aspects of physical functioning and contextual factors. British Journal of Sports Medicine 48 (21), 1543–1552.

Ardern, C.L., Webster, K.E., Taylor, N.F., Feller, J.A., 2011. Return to sport following anterior cruciate ligament reconstruction surgery: A systematic review and meta-analysis of the state of play. British Journal of Sports Medicine 45 (7), 596–606.

Balki, S., Göktaş, H., Öztemur, Z., 2016. Kinesio taping as a treatment method in the acute phase of ACL reconstruction: A double-blind, placebo-controlled study. Acta Orthopaedica et Traumatologica Turcica 50 (6), 628–634.

Bien, D.P., 2011. Rationale and implementation of anterior cruciate ligament injury prevention warm-up programs in female athletes. Journal of Strength and Conditioning Research 25 (1), 271–285.

Carlson, V.R., Sheehan, F.T., Boden, B.P., 2016. Video analysis of anterior cruciate ligament (ACL) injuries: A systematic review. JBJS Rev. 4 (11).

Chalmers, P.N., Mall, N.A., Moric, M., Sherman, S.L., Paletta, G.P., Cole, B.J., et al., 2014. Does ACL reconstruction alter natural history? A systematic literature review of long-term outcomes. The Journal of Bone and Joint Surgery. American volume 96 (4), 292–300.

Dingenen, B., Gokeler, A., 2017. Optimization of the return-to-sport paradigm after anterior cruciate ligament reconstruction: A critical step back to move forward. Journal of Sports Medicine 47 (8), 1487–1500.

Dingenen, B., Malfait, B., Nijs, S., Peers, K.H., Vereecken, S., Verschueren, S.M., et al., 2016. Postural stability during single-leg stance: A preliminary evaluation of noncontact lower extremity injury risk. The Journal of Orthopaedic and Sports Physical Therapy 46 (8), 650–657.

Ericsson, Y.B., Roos, E.M., Frobell, R.B., 2013. Lower extremity performance following ACL rehabilitation in the KANON-trial: Impact of reconstruction and predictive value at 2 and 5 years. British Journal of Sports Medicine 47 (15), 980–985.

Ewing, K.A., Fernandez, J.W., Begg, R.K., Galea, M.P., Lee, P.V., 2016. Prophylactic knee bracing alters lower-limb muscle forces during a double-leg drop landing. Journal of Biomechanics 49 (14), 3347–3354.

Fabricant, P.D., Lakomkin, N., Cruz, A.I., Spitzer, E., Marx, R.G., 2016. ACL reconstruction in youth athletes results in an improved rate of return to athletic activity when compared with non-operative treatment: a systematic review of the literature. Journal of ISAKOS: Joint Disorders & Orthopaedic Sports Medicine 1, 62–69.

Frobell, R.B., Roos, E.M., Roos, H.P., Ranstam, J., Lohmander, L.S., 2010. A randomized trial of treatment for acute anterior cruciate ligament tears. The New England Journal of Medicine 363 (4), 331–342.

Frobell, R.B., Roos, H.P., Roos, E.M., Roemer, F.W., Ranstam, J., Lohmander, L.S., 2013. Treatment for acute anterior cruciate ligament tear: five year outcome of randomised trial. British Medical Journal 346:f232.

Gokeler, A., Welling, W., Benjaminse, A., Lemmink, K., Seil, R., Zaffagnini, S., et al., 2017. A critical analysis of limb symmetry indices of hop tests in athletes after anterior cruciate ligament reconstruction: A case control study. Orthopaedics and Traumatology, Surgery and Research 103 (6), 947–951.

Gornitzky, A.L., Lott, A., Yellin, J.L., Fabricant, P.D., Lawrence, J.T., Ganley, T.J., et al., 2016. Sport-specific yearly risk and incidence of anterior cruciate ligament tears in high school athletes: A systematic review and meta-analysis. The American Journal of Sports Medicine 44 (10), 2716–2723.

Grindem, H., Eitzen, I., Engebretsen, L., Snyder-Mackler, L., Risberg, M.A., 2014. Nonsurgical or surgical treatment of ACL injuries: Knee function, sports participation, and knee reinjury: The Delaware–Oslo ACL Cohort Study. The Journal of Bone and Joint Surgery. American volume 96 (15), 1233–1241.

Grindem, H., Engebretsen, L., Axe, M., Snyder-Mackler, L., Risberg, M.A., 2020. Activity and functional readiness, not age, are the critical factors for second anterior cruciate ligament injury - the Delaware-Oslo ACL cohort study. British Journal of Sports Medicine 54, 1099-1102.

Grip, H., Tengman, E., Hager, C.K., 2015. Dynamic knee stability estimated by finite helical axis methods during functional performance approximately twenty years after anterior cruciate ligament injury. Journal of Biomechanics 48 (10), 1906–1914.

Harput, G., Ulusoy, B., Ozer, H., Baltaci, G., Richards, J., 2016. External supports improve knee performance in anterior cruciate ligament reconstructed individuals with higher kinesiophobia levels. Knee 23 (5), 807–812.

Hashemi, J., Chandrashekar, N., Mansouri, H., Gill, B., Slauterbeck, J.R., Schutt Jr., R.C., et al., 2010. Shallow medial tibial plateau and steep medial and lateral tibial slopes: New risk factors for anterior cruciate ligament injuries. The American Journal of Sports Medicine 38 (1), 54–62.

Hébert-Losier, K., Pini, A., Vantini, S., Strandberg, J., Abramowicz, K., Schelin, L., et al., 2015. One-leg hop kinematics 20 years following anterior cruciate ligament rupture: Data revisited using functional data analysis. Clinical Biomechanics (Bristol, Avon) 30 (10), 1153–1161.

Herzberg, S.D., Motu'apuaka, M.L., Lambert, W., Fu, R., Brady, J., Guise, J.M., et al., 2017. The effect of menstrual cycle and contraceptives on ACL injuries and laxity: A systematic review and meta-analysis. Orthopaedic Journal of Sports Medicine 5 (7), 2325967117718781.

Hewett, T.E., Myer, G.D., Ford, K.R., 2006. Anterior cruciate ligament injuries in female athletes: Part 1, mechanisms and risk factors. The American Journal of Sports Medicine 34 (2), 299–311.

Hewett, T.E., Myer, G.D., 2011. The mechanistic connection between the trunk, hip, knee, and anterior cruciate ligament injury. Exercise and Sport Sciences Reviews 39 (4), 161–166.

Hewett, T.E., Torg, J.S., Boden, B.P., 2009. Video analysis of trunk and knee motion during non-contact anterior cruciate ligament injury in female athletes: Lateral trunk and knee abduction motion are combined components of the injury mechanism. British Journal of Sports Medicine 43 (6), 417–422.

Jenkins, W.L, Raedeke, S.G., Williams 3rd, D.S.B., 2008. The relationship between the use of foot orthoses and knee ligament injury in female collegiate basketball players. Journal of the American Podiatric Medical Association 98 (3), 207–211.

Kay, J., Naji, L., de SA, D., et al., 2017. Graft choice has no significant influence on the rate of return to sport at the preinjury level after revision anterior cruciate ligament reconstruction: A systematic review and meta-analysis. Journal of ISAKOS: Joint Disorders & Orthopaedic Sports Medicine 2 (1), 21–30.

Kessler, M.A., Behrend, H., Henz, S., Stutz, G., Rukavina, A., Kuster, M.S., et al., 2008. Function, osteoarthritis and activity after ACL-rupture: 11 years follow-up results of conservative versus reconstructive treatment. Knee Surgery, Sports Traumatology, Arthroscopy 16 (5), 442–448.

Kiadaliri, A.A., Englund, M., Lohmander, L.S., Carlsson, K.S., Frobell, R.B., 2016. No economic benefit of early knee reconstruction over optional delayed reconstruction for ACL tears:

Registry enriched randomised controlled trial data. British Journal of Sports Medicine 50 (9), 558–563.

Koga, H., Nakamae, A., Shima, Y., Iwasa, J., Myklebust, G., Engebretsen, L., et al., 2010. Mechanisms for noncontact anterior cruciate ligament injuries: Knee joint kinematics in 10 injury situations from female team handball and basketball. The American Journal of Sports Medicine 38 (11), 2218–2225.

Leys, T., Salmon, L., Waller, A., Linklater, J., Pinczewski, L., 2012. Clinical results and risk factors for reinjury 15 years after anterior cruciate ligament reconstruction: A prospective study of hamstring and patellar tendon grafts. The American Journal of Sports Medicine 40 (3), 592–605.

Lowe, W.R., Warth, R.J., Davis, E.P., Bailey, L., 2017. Functional bracing after anterior cruciate ligament reconstruction: A systematic review. The Journal of the American Academy of Orthopaedic Surgeons 25 (3), 239–249.

Mather 3rd, R.C., Koenig, L., Kocher, M.S., Dall, T.M., et al., 2013. Societal and economic impact of anterior cruciate ligament tears. The Journal of Bone and Joint Surgery. American volume 95 (19), 1751.

Michaelidis, M., Koumantakis, G.A., 2014. Effects of knee injury primary prevention programs on anterior cruciate ligament injury rates in female athletes in different sports: A systematic review. Physical Therapy in Sport 15 (3), 200–210.

Moses, B., Orchard, J., 2012. Systematic review: Annual incidence of ACL injury and surgery in various populations. Research in Sports Medicine 20 (3–4), 157–179.

Myer, G.D., Ford, K.R., Barber Foss, K.D., Liu, C., Nick, T.G., Hewett, T.E., et al., 2009. The relationship of hamstrings and quadriceps strength to anterior cruciate ligament injury in female athletes. Clinical Journal of Sport Medicine 19 (1), 3–8.

Noyes, F.R., Barber-Westin, S.D., 2014. Neuromuscular retraining intervention programs: Do they reduce noncontact anterior cruciate ligament injury rates in adolescent female athletes? Arthroscopy 30 (2), 245–255.

O'Connell, K., Knight, H., Ficek, K., Leonska-Duniec, A., Maciejewska-Karlowska, A., Sawczuk, M., et al., 2015. Interactions between collagen gene variants and risk of anterior cruciate ligament rupture. European Journal of Sport Science 15 (4), 341–350.

Padua, D.A., DiStefano, L.J., Beutler, A.I., de la Motte, S.J., DiStefano, M.J., Marshall, S.W., et al., 2015. The Landing Error Scoring System as a screening tool for an anterior cruciate ligament injury-prevention program in elite-youth soccer athletes. Journal of Athletic Training 50 (6), 589–595.

Prodromos, C.C., Han, Y., Rogowski, J., Joyce, B., Shi, K., 2007. A meta-analysis of the incidence of anterior cruciate ligament tears as a function of gender, sport, and a knee injury-reduction regimen. Arthroscopy 23 (12), 1320–1325.e1326.

Roos, P.E., Button, K., Sparkes, V., van Deursen, R.W., 2014. Altered biomechanical strategies and medio-lateral control of the knee represent incomplete recovery of individuals with injury during single leg hop. Journal of Biomechanics 47 (3), 675–680.

Ruedl, G., Webhofer, M., Helle, K., Strobl, M., Schranz, A., Fink, C., et al., 2012. Leg dominance is a risk factor for noncontact anterior cruciate ligament injuries in female recreational skiers. The American Journal of Sports Medicine 40 (6), 1269–1273.

Sanders, T.L., Maradit Kremers, H., Bryan, A.J., Larson, D.R., Dahm, D.L., Levy, B.A., et al., 2016. Incidence of anterior cruciate ligament tears and reconstruction: A 21-year population-based study. The American Journal of Sports Medicine 44 (6), 1502–1507.

Schlumberger, M., Schuster, P., Schulz, M., Immendörfer, M., Mayer, P., Bartholomä, J., et al., 2017. Traumatic graft rupture after primary and revision anterior cruciate ligament reconstruction: retrospective analysis of incidence and risk factors in 2915 cases. Knee Surgery, Sports Traumatology, Arthroscopy 25 (5), 1535–1541.

Shimokochi, Y., Shultz, S.J., 2008. Mechanisms of noncontact anterior cruciate ligament injury. Journal of Athletic Training 43 (4), 396–408.

Silvers, H.J., Mandelbaum, B.R., 2011. ACL injury prevention in the athlete. Sports Orthopaedics and Traumatology 27 (1), 18–26.

Smith, T.O., Postle, K., Penny, F., McNamara, I., Mann, C.J.V., 2014. Is reconstruction the best management strategy for anterior cruciate ligament rupture? A systematic review and meta-analysis comparing anterior cruciate ligament reconstruction versus non-operative treatment. Knee 21 (2), 462–470.

Sugimoto, D., Myer, G.D., Foss, K.D., Hewett, T.E., 2014. Dosage effects of neuromuscular training intervention to reduce anterior cruciate ligament injuries in female athletes: Meta- and sub-group analyses. Journal of Sports Medicine 44 (4), 551–562.

Suter, L.G., Smith, S.R., Katz, J.N., Englund, M., Hunter, D.J., Frobell, R., et al., 2017. Projecting lifetime risk of symptomatic knee osteoarthritis and total knee replacement in individuals sustaining a complete anterior cruciate ligament tear in early adulthood. Arthritis Care & Research 69 (2), 201–208.

Tengman, E., Brax Olofsson, L., Stensdotter, A.K., Nilsson, K.G., Häger, C.K., 2014. Anterior cruciate ligament injury after more than 20 years. II. Concentric and eccentric knee muscle strength. Scandinavian Journal of Medicine & Science in Sports 24 (6), e501–e509.

Tengman, E., Grip, H., Stensdotter, A.K., Hager, C.K., 2015. Anterior cruciate ligament injury about 20 years post-treatment: A kinematic analysis of one-leg hop. Scandinavian Journal of Medicine & Science in Sports 25 (6), 818–827.

Tengman, E., Olofsson, L.B., Nilsson, K.G., Tegner, Y., Lundgren, L., Hager, C.K., et al., 2014. Anterior cruciate ligament injury after more than 20 years: I. Physical activity level and knee function. Scandinavian Journal of Medicine & Science in Sports 24 (6), e491–e500.

Thomeé, R., Kaplan, Y., Kvist, J., Myklebust, G., Risberg, M.A., Theisen, D., et al., 2011. Muscle strength and hop performance criteria prior to return to sports after ACL reconstruction. Knee Surgery, Sports Traumatology, Arthroscopy 19 (11), 1798–1805.

Uhorchak, J.M., Scoville, C.R., Williams, G.N., Arciero, R.A., St Pierre, P., Taylor, D.C., et al., 2003. Risk factors associated with noncontact injury of the anterior cruciate ligament: a prospective four-year evaluation of 859 West Point cadets. The American Journal of Sports Medicine 31 (6), 831–842.

Vacek, P.M., Slauterbeck, J.R., Tourville, T.W., Sturnick, D.R., Holterman, L.A., Smith, H.C., et al., 2016. Multivariate analysis of the risk factors for first-time noncontact ACL injury in high school and college athletes. The American Journal of Sports Medicine 44 (6), 1492–1501.

van Melick, N., van Cingel, R.E., Brooijmans, F., Neeter, C., van Tienen, T., Hullegie, W., et al., 2016. Evidence-based clinical practice update: Practice guidelines for anterior cruciate ligament rehabilitation based on a systematic review and multi-disciplinary consensus. British Journal of Sports Medicine 50 (24), 1506–1515.

VandenBerg, C., Crawford, E.A., Sibilsky Enselman, E., Robbins, C.B., Wojtys, E.M., Bedi, A., et al., 2017. Restricted hip rotation is correlated with an increased risk for anterior cruciate ligament injury. Arthroscopy 33 (2), 317–325.

Waldén, M., Hägglund, M., Ekstrand, J., 2006. High risk of new knee injury in elite footballers with previous anterior cruciate ligament injury. British Journal of Sports Medicine 40 (2), 158–162.

Waldén, M., Krosshaug, T., Bjørneboe, J., Andersen, T.E., Faul, O., Hägglund, M., et al., 2015. Three distinct mechanisms predominate in non-contact anterior cruciate ligament injuries in male professional football players: A systematic video analysis of 39 cases. British Journal of Sports Medicine 49 (22), 1452–1460.

Wellsandt, E., Failla, M.J., Snyder-Mackler, L., 2017. Limb symmetry indexes can overestimate knee function after anterior cruciate ligament injury. The Journal of Orthopaedic and Sports Physical Therapy 47 (5), 334–338.

Wright, R.W., Magnussen, R.A., Dunn, W.R., Spindler, K.P., 2011. Ipsilateral graft and contralateral ACL rupture at five years or more following ACL reconstruction: A systematic review. The Journal of Bone and Joint Surgery. American volume 93 (12), 1159–1165.

Zeng, C., Gao, S.G., Wei, J., Yang, T.B., Cheng, L., Luo, W., et al., 2013. The influence of the intercondylar notch dimensions on injury of the anterior cruciate ligament: a meta-analysis. Knee Surgery, Sports Traumatology, Arthroscopy 21 (4), 804–815.

Shoulder injuries

Abdul-Wahab, T.A., Betancourt, J.P., Hassan, F., Thani, S.A., Choueiri, H., Jain, N.B., et al., 2016. Initial treatment of complete rotator cuff tear and transition to surgical treatment: systematic review of the evidence. Muscles, Ligaments and Tendons Journal 6 (1), 35–47.

Antoni, M., Klouche, S., Mas, V., Ferrand, M., Bauer, T., Hardy, P., et al., 2016. Return to recreational sport and clinical outcomes with at least 2 years follow-up after arthroscopic repair of rotator cuff tears. Orthopaedics & Traumatology: Surgery & Research 102 (5), 563–567.

Berth, A., Pap, G., Awiszus, F., Neumann, W., 2009. Central motor deficits of the deltoid muscle in patients with chronic rotator cuff tears. Acta Chirurgiae Orthopaedicae et Traumatologiae Cechoslovaca 76 (6), 456–461.

Burkhart, S.S., Morgan, C.D., Kibler, W.B., 2003. The disabled throwing shoulder: Spectrum of pathology part I: Pathoanatomy and biomechanics. Arthroscopy 19 (4), 404–420.

Crichton, J., Jones, D.R., Funk, L., 2012. Mechanisms of traumatic shoulder injury in elite rugby players. British Journal of Sports Medicine 46 (7), 538–542.

Elsenbeck, M.J., Dickens, J.F., 2017. Return to sports after shoulder stabilization surgery for anterior shoulder instability. Current Reviews in Musculoskeletal Medicine 10 (4), 491–498.

Gibbs, D.B., Lynch, T.S., Nuber, E.D., Nuber, G.W., 2015. Common shoulder injuries in american football athletes. Current Sports Medicine Reports 14 (5), 413–419.

Gibson, J., Kerss, J., Morgan, C., Brownson, P., 2016. Accelerated rehabilitation after arthroscopic Bankart repair in professional footballers. Shoulder & Elbow 8 (4), 279–286.

Huber, R., Ghilardi, M.F., Massimini, M., Ferrarelli, F., Riedner, B.A., Peterson, M.J., et al., 2006. Arm immobilization causes cortical plastic changes and locally decreases sleep slow wave activity. Nature Neuroscience 9 (9), 1169–1176.

Jaggi, A., Lambert, S., 2010. Rehabilitation for shoulder instability. British Journal of Sports Medicine 44 (5), 333–340.

Kim, S.H., Ha, K.I., Jung, M.W., Lim, M.S., Kim, Y.M., Park, J.H., et al., 2003. Accelerated rehabilitation after arthroscopic Bankart repair for selected cases: a prospective randomized clinical study. Arthroscopy 19 (7), 722–731.

Klouche, S., Lefevre, N., Herman, S., Gerometta, A., Bohu, Y., 2016. Return to sport after rotator cuff tear repair. The American Journal of Sports Medicine 44 (7), 1877–1887.

Kuhn, J.E., Dunn, W.R., Sanders, R., An, Q., Baumgarten, K.M., Bishop, J.Y., et al., 2013. Effectiveness of physical therapy in treating atraumatic full-thickness rotator cuff tears: a multicenter prospective cohort study. Journal of Shoulder and Elbow Surgery 22 (10), 1371–1379.

Lewis, A., Kitamura, T., Bayley, J.I., 2004. (ii) The classification of shoulder instability: new light through old windows! Current Orthopaedics 18 (2), 97–108.

Mazuquin, B.F., Wright, A.C., Russell, S., Monga, P., Selfe, J., Richards, J., et al., 2018. Effectiveness of early compared with conservative rehabilitation for patients having rotator cuff repair surgery: An overview of systematic reviews. British Journal of Sports Medicine 52 (2), 111–121.

McCormick, F., Gupta, A., Bruce, B., Harris, J., Abrams, G., Wilson, H., et al., 2014. Single-row, double-row, and transosseous equivalent techniques for isolated supraspinatus tendon tears with minimal atrophy: A retrospective comparative outcome and radiographic analysis at minimum 2-year follow-up. International Journal of Shoulder Surgery 8 (1), 15–20.

McMahon, P.J., Prasad, A., Francis, K.A., 2014. What is the prevalence of senior-athlete rotator cuff injuries and are they associated with pain and dysfunction? Clinical Orthopaedics and Related Research 472 (8), 2427–2432.

McMullen, J., Uhl, T.L., 2000. A kinetic chain approach for shoulder rehabilitation. Journal of Athletic Training 35 (3), 329–337.

Monga, P., Funk, L., 2017. Diagnostic Clusters in Shoulder Conditions. Springer International Publishing, New York.

Opsha, O., Malik, A., Baltazar, R., Primakov, D., Beltran, S., Miller, T.T., et al., 2008. MRI of the rotator cuff and internal derangement. European Journal of Radiology 68 (1), 36–56.

Robins, R.J., Daruwalla, J.H., Gamradt, S.C., McCarty, E.C., Dragoo, J.L., Hancock, R.E., et al., 2017. Return to play after shoulder instability surgery in National Collegiate Athletic Association Division I intercollegiate football athletes. The American Journal of Sports Medicine 45 (10), 2329–2335.

Thigpen, C.A., Shaffer, M.A., Gaunt, B.W., Leggin, B.G., Williams, G.R., Wilcox 3rd, R.B., et al., 2016. The American Society of Shoulder and Elbow Therapists' consensus statement on rehabilitation following arthroscopic rotator cuff repair. Journal of Shoulder and Elbow Surgery 25 (4), 521–535.

Trappey, G.J., Gartsman, G.M., 2011. A systematic review of the clinical outcomes of single row versus double row rotator cuff repairs. Journal of Shoulder and Elbow Surgery 20 (Suppl. 2), S14–S19.

Yamaguchi, K., Ditsios, K., Middleton, W.D., Hildebolt, C.F., Galatz, L.M., Teefey, S.A., et al., 2006. The demographic and morphological features of rotator cuff disease – A comparison of asymptomatic and symptomatic shoulders. The Journal of Bone and Joint Surgery. American volume 88 (8), 1699–1704 2006 Aug.

Yamamoto, A., Takagishi, K., Osawa, T., Yanagawa, T., Nakajima, D., Shitara, H., et al., 2010. Prevalence and risk factors of a rotator cuff tear in the general population. Journal of Shoulder and Elbow Surgery 19 (1), 116–120.

Chapter | 6 |

Electrophysical agents: physiology and evidence

Tim Watson

Introduction

There is a general trend to move away from the term 'electrotherapy' towards a more encompassing term 'electrophysical agents' (EPAs). Electrotherapy, in the strictest sense, only applies to those modalities that involve the delivery of electrical and possibly also electromagnetic energies. As a term, 'EPA' is more inclusive and is a more accurate reflection of the wide range of modalities employed in therapy, such as ultrasound, laser and shockwave (Watson, 2010).

Modern EPA use should be evidence based and the modalities used judiciously. When used appropriately, these modalities have an established and demonstrable capacity to achieve significant benefit. Used unwisely, they will either do no good at all, or worse still, aggravate the clinical condition. In addition to the skills needed to deliver each modality, there is skill in making the appropriate clinical decision as to which modality to use and when. There are few, if any, circumstances in which modalities are most effective when used in isolation. Their use as part of an integrated and individually tailored treatment programme is where they are able to achieve maximal benefit. EPAs are not an essential component for all patients and should only be used when and where they are justified and significant benefit can be reasonably expected.

The aim of this chapter is to enable the reader to quickly identify the key modalities that are able to influence tissue repair and recovery from injury. It does not aim to fully examine or explain the evidence for every modality, and there are many modalities that have been excluded. This is a reflection of the complexity of modern EPA evidence and practice. Further details are available in the standard texts (e.g., Bellew et al., 2016; Knight and Draper, 2012; Michlovitz et al., 2012; Watson and Nussbaum, 2020). Key

references are provided at the end of the chapter and the (open access) online resource www.electrotherapy.org has details on all modalities together with an objective summary of the key literature.

Therapeutic ultrasound

Ultrasound (US) therapy is one of the most commonly employed electrophysical treatments (Shah and Farrow, 2012) and has a wide range of applications in soft tissue and sports-related repair and recovery (de Brito Viera et al., 2012; Watson, 2014).

Ultrasound is a form of mechanical energy. The normal human sound range is from 16 Hz to approximately 20,000 Hz. Beyond this upper limit, mechanical vibration is known as ultrasound. The frequencies used in therapy are typically 1.0–3.0 MHz (1 MHz = 1 million cycles per second) and is therefore beyond the human sound range. Some therapy devices offer application frequencies at other rates, e.g., 1.5 MHz, 0.75 MHz and long-wave ultrasound devices that operate in the kilohertz range (e.g., 48 kHz and 150 kHz). The relatively recent development of low-intensity pulsed ultrasound (LIPUS) is used primarily in relation to bone injury, particularly fracture repair, commonly employing a 1.5 MHz application frequency.

Sound waves are longitudinal waves consisting of zones of compression and rarefaction. Particles of a material when exposed to a sound wave will oscillate about a fixed point. Any increase in the molecular vibration in the tissue can result in heat generation, and ultrasound can be used to produce thermal changes in the tissues, although most current usage in therapy does not focus on this phenomenon (Baker et al., 2001; Nussbaum, 1997; ter Haar, 1999; Watson, 2020). The vibration of the tissues has effects that are considered to be 'nonthermal' in nature, although, as

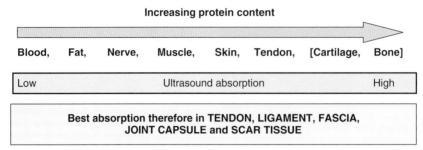

Fig. 6.1 Ultrasound absorption in different tissues.

with other modalities, there must be a thermal component, however small. As the US wave passes through a material (the tissues), the energy levels within the wave will diminish as energy is transferred to the material.

A coupling media is employed to enable transfer of the sound energy to the tissues. At the present time the gel-based media are preferable to the oils and creams. Water is an effective transmission medium and can be used as an alternative. There is no realistic (clinical) difference between the gels in common clinical use (Poltawski and Watson, 2007).

The absorption of US energy follows an exponential distribution. In order for energy to have an effect it must be absorbed. As the US energy penetrates further into the tissues, a greater proportion of the energy will have been absorbed and therefore there is less energy available to achieve therapeutic effects. Ultrasound can be clinically effective to depths of 5–6 cm.

Some tissues are capable of greater absorption of US energy than others. Tissues with a higher protein content absorb US to a greater extent. Thus, tissues with high water content and low protein content absorb little of the energy (e.g., blood and fat), while tissues with a lower water content and a higher protein content will absorb US far more efficiently. It has been suggested that tissues can therefore be ranked according to their tissue absorption (Fig. 6.1).

Although cartilage and bone are at the upper end of this scale, the problems associated with wave reflection mean that the majority of US energy striking the surface of either of these tissues is likely to be reflected. The best absorbing tissues in terms of clinical practice are those with high collagen content; ligament, tendon, fascia, joint capsule, scar tissue (Nussbaum, 1998; ter Haar, 1999; Watson, 2000; 2008; 2020).

Most machines offer the facility for pulsed US output. Typical pulse formats are 1:1 and 1:4, although others are available. In 1:1 mode, the machine offers an output for 2 ms followed by 2 ms rest. In 1:4 mode, the 2 ms output is followed by an 8-ms rest period.

The effects of pulsed US are well documented (Watson, 2020; Watson and Nussbaum, 2020) and this type of output is preferable, especially in the treatment of more acute lesions.

Clinical uses of ultrasound therapy

The therapeutic effects of US are generally divided into *thermal* and *nonthermal* categories. Whilst the application of US energy at sufficient power levels will be capable of generating a thermal change in the tissues (Draper et al., 1995; Draper and Ricard, 1995; Meakins and Watson, 2006; Nussbaum, 1998), in soft tissue and sports-related therapy, low-dose, pulsed applications with a nonthermal intent dominate the evidence. Higher doses with thermal potential do have a place in the longer term and for more chronic presentations.

Ultrasound nonthermal effects and uses

The nonthermal effects of US are now attributed primarily to a combination of *cavitation* and *acoustic streaming* (Baker et al., 2001; ter Haar, 1999; Watson and Nussbaum, 2020). Details of these primary physical effects of ultrasound are detailed in appropriate texts and papers (Robertson et al., 2006; Watson, 2020).

The result of the combined effects of stable cavitation and acoustic streaming is that the cell membrane becomes 'excited' (i.e., it upregulates), increasing its activity levels. US energy acts as a trigger for this process, but it is the increased cellular activity which is in effect responsible for the therapeutic benefits of the modality (Izadifar et al., 2017; Watson, 2000; 2008; 2020). Recent evidence strongly identifies that the applied mechanical energy results in cellular upregulation and as a result stimulates the release/synthesis/expression of various chemical mediators, growth factors and cytokines, which are responsible for the observed physiological and clinical effects (Watson, 2016).

Ultrasound application in relation to tissue repair

The process of tissue repair is a complex series of cascaded, chemically mediated events that lead to the production of scar tissue that constitutes an effective material to restore the continuity of the damaged tissue.

Inflammation

During the inflammatory phase, US has a stimulating effect on the mast cells, platelets, white cells with phagocytic roles and the macrophages (Maxwell, 1992; Nussbaum, 1997; ter Haar, 1999). Ultrasound application induces the degranulation of mast cells, causing the release of arachidonic acid which itself is a precursor for the synthesis of prostaglandins and leukotrienes – which act as inflammatory mediators (Nussbaum, 1997). By increasing the activity of these cells, the overall influence of therapeutic US is *pro-inflammatory* rather than *anti-inflammatory*. The benefit is not to 'increase' the inflammatory response, but rather to act as an 'inflammatory optimizer'. The inflammatory response is essential to the effective repair of tissue, and the more efficiently the process can complete, the more effectively the tissue can progress to the next phase (proliferation). US is effective at promoting the normal inflammatory events, and as such has a therapeutic value in promoting overall repair events. A further benefit is that chemically mediated inflammatory events are associated with stimulation of the proliferative phase, and via this route also promote repair.

The evidence of chemically mediated ultrasound effects is identified in many publications (Bajpai et al., 2018; Kim et al., 2020; Maxwell, 1992; Nakamura et al., 2010; Nussbaum, 1997; Renno et al., 2011; Sahu et al., 2020; ter Haar, 1999; Watson, 2014; 2020; Watson and Nussbaum, 2020; Zhou et al., 2008).

Employed at an appropriate treatment dose, with optimal treatment parameters (intensity, pulsing, time), the benefit of US is to induce the most efficiently achieved earliest repair phase, thus promoting the healing cascade.

Proliferation

During the proliferative phase, US also has a stimulating effect (cellular upregulation), and the primary active targets are fibroblasts, endothelial cells and myofibroblasts (Maxwell, 1992; Nussbaum, 1997; 1998; Ramirez et al., 1997). These are all cells that are normally active during scar production and US is therefore *pro-proliferative*. It does not change the normal proliferative phase, rather it maximizes its efficiency; producing the required scar tissue in an optimal fashion. Harvey et al. (1975) demonstrated that low-dose pulsed ultrasound increases protein synthesis, and several research groups have demonstrated enhanced

fibroplasia and collagen synthesis (Enwemeka et al., 1990; Ramirez et al., 1997; Turner et al., 1989). Recent work has identified the critical role of numerous growth factors in relation to tissue repair, and some accumulating evidence has identified that therapeutic US has a positive role to play in this context (de Oliveira Perrucini et al., 2020; Leung et al., 2006; Lovric et al., 2013; McBrier et al., 2007; Watson, 2016).

Remodelling

During the remodelling phase of repair, the generic scar that is produced during proliferation is refined. This is achieved by a number of processes, mainly related to the orientation of the collagen fibres in the developing scar and also to the change in collagen type, from predominantly type III to predominantly type I collagen (Watson, 2006).

The application of therapeutic ultrasound can influence the remodelling of the scar tissue as it enhances the orientation of the newly formed collagen fibres (Byl et al., 1996) and stimulates collagen change from type III to a more predominantly type I construction, increasing tensile strength and enhancing scar mobility (Nussbaum, 1998; Wang, 1998). Ultrasound applied to tissues enhances the functional capacity of scar tissues (Nussbaum, 1998; Yeung et al., 2006).

The application of ultrasound during the inflammatory, proliferative and repair phases does not change the normal sequence of events; rather it has the capacity to stimulate or enhance these normal events and thus increase the efficiency of the repair phases (ter Haar, 1999; Watson, 2006; 2008; 2014). It has recently been proposed (Watson, 2016) that the mode of action, in keeping with other electrophysical modalities, is primarily by enhancing the chemically mediated inflammatory, proliferative and remodelling events. The effective application of ultrasound to achieve these aims is dose dependent. The details of dose applications are beyond the remit of this text, but are reviewed at www.electrotherapy.org.

Whilst the emphasis of the evidence reviewed in this section has been related to tissue repair, clearly there are circumstances in which inflammation is present without overt injury. The published evidence illustrates that ultrasound has a demonstrable benefit in these inflammatory lesions, for example, osteoarthritis-related changes (Yegin et al., 2017; Zeng et al., 2014; Zhang et al., 2016); carpal tunnel syndrome (Ahmed et al., 2017; Huisstede et al., 2018); myofascial pain syndrome (Ilter et al., 2015); and epicondylitis (Dingemanse et al., 2014).

Low-intensity pulsed ultrasound (LIPUS) and fracture healing

A number of recent research papers have identified the potential for low-intensity ultrasound to promote tissue

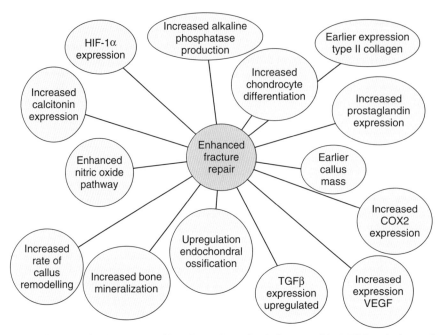

Fig. 6.2 Evidenced mechanisms for the action of low-intensity pulsed ultrasound (LIPUS) in relation to fracture repair. *COX2*, cyclooxygenase-2; *HIF-1α*, hypoxia-inducible factor-1alpha; *TGFβ*, transforming growth factor beta; *VEGF*, vascular endothelial growth factor.

repair, most strongly evidenced in relation to fractures, including both normal, delayed/nonunion and postsurgery clinical scenarios.

A systematic review and meta-analysis (Busse et al., 2009) has considered the evidence for the effect of LIPUS on the time to fracture healing. They conclude that the evidence from randomized controlled trial (RCT) pooled data (three studies, 158 fractures), the time to fracture healing was significantly reduced in the ultrasound-treated groups compared with the control groups and the mean difference in healing time was 64 days. A systematic review (Griffin et al., 2008) evaluating LIPUS for fresh fractures considers seven RCTs and two meta-analyses, and suggests that this body of evidence is supportive.

The mechanism by which LIPUS enhances or stimulates the fracture repair sequence is summarized in Fig. 6.2 and is usefully summarized by Claes and Willie (2007); Della Roca (2009); Jingushi (2009); Lu et al. (2009); Padilla et al. (2014); Zhang et al. (2017); and Zuo et al. (2018). The mechanism is primarily by means of enhanced chemical mediation pathways as is the case for traditional ultrasound.

The machines used for these treatments deliver a very low intensity (0.03 W/cm² or 30 mW/cm²) at 1.5 MHz pulsed at a ratio of 1:4 at 1 kHz, applied for 20 min daily. The intensity of this application is considerably lower than the lowest intensity which is deliverable by the majority of

current ultrasound machines (normally 0.1 W/cm²). At the present time, a conventional therapy ultrasound machine will not deliver a sufficiently controlled low dose to make LIPUS an option. LIPUS-specific devices are marketed, although it is anticipated that future clinical machines are likely to offer a LIPUS option.

The early clinical studies (e.g. Heckman et al., 1994; Kristiansen et al., 1997) demonstrated acceleration in fracture healing rates of 30–38%. Jensen (1998) identifies the beneficial effects of ultrasound in the treatment of stress fractures with an overall success rate of 96%. Mayr et al. (2000) report a series of outcomes when using low-intensity pulsed ultrasound for patients with delayed unions (n = 951) and nonunions (n = 366). The overall success rate for the delayed unions was 91% and for the nonunions 86%.

Numerous recent evidence-based reviews are published (Bayat et al., 2018; Harrison et al., 2016; Mehta et al., 2015; Padilla et al., 2016), all of which are supportive of this intervention. A recent suggestion that the clinical effects of LIPUS are not as pronounced as originally suggested (Schandelmaier et al., 2017) was challenged by Aspenberg (2017) amongst others. The current weight of evidence is in favour of LIPUS applications as a means to enhance repair of fresh fractures and to instigate a response in delayed and nonunion clinical presentations. The use of LIPUS in therapy is likely to increase on this basis.

Pulsed shortwave therapy and other radiofrequency applications

Pulsed shortwave therapy (PSWT) is a widely used modality (Al Mandeel and Watson, 2006). The older term 'pulsed shortwave diathermy' is not really appropriate as the modality is not primarily employed as a diathermy (literally 'through heating').

The output of the shortwave machine (operating at 27.12 MHz) is pulsed such that the 'on' time is considerably shorter than the 'off' time; thus, the mean power delivered to the patient is relatively low even though the peak power (during the 'on' pulses) can be high (typically around 150–200 W with modern machines).

The user can vary (a) the mean power delivered to the patient and (b) the pulsing parameters governing the mode of delivery of the energy. Current evidence suggests that the *mean power* is the most important parameter (Al Mandeel and Watson, 2020; Hill et al., 2002).

When using pulsed shortwave in the clinical environment, there are two 'modes' of application, and the information in this section relates to application using the 'monode' or 'drum' electrode rather than the capacitor plate delivery system which lacks sufficient supportive evidence.

Main parameters. The pulse repetition rate (Hz or pulses/second) controls the number of pulses of shortwave energy that are delivered to the patient in a second. The pulse duration (pulse width) refers to the duration, in microseconds (μs), of each individual pulse of energy.

The combination of pulse rate and duration management enables the user to influence the mean power delivered to the patient, which is the critical treatment parameter.

The peak power is typically around 150–200 W in modern machines. This is the 'strength' of the shortwave whilst the pulse is 'on'. The *mean power* takes account of the fact that there are 'on' and 'off' phases, i.e., the energy delivery is intermittent; it describes the average power output rather than the power output at any one moment in time (which might be maximum or zero).

Clinical applications typically range from 10–20 min at mean power levels of <5 W (acute lesions) up to 48 W (thermal dose, chronic lesions).

The relationship between the pulse parameters and the power levels are illustrated in Fig. 6.3.

Tissue heating. With respect to the effects of pulsed shortwave, there is an element of tissue heating that occurs during the 'on' pulse, but this is dissipated during the prolonged 'off' phase. Therefore, it is possible to give treatment with no net increase in tissue temperature. Fig. 6.4A demonstrates no accumulation of either thermal or nonthermal

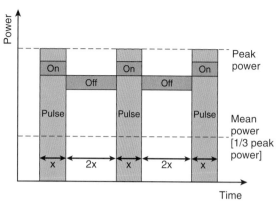

Fig. 6.3 The relationship between pulse parameters and power levels with pulsed shortwave therapy.

effects. In Fig. 6.4B the pulses are sufficiently close to generate an accumulative nonthermal effect and in Fig. 6.4C there is an accumulation of both thermal and nonthermal effects. The settings applied on the machine will determine which of these is achieved in a particular treatment. The 'nonthermal' effects of the modality are generally thought to be of greater significance, especially in soft tissue/sports-related applications. They appear to accumulate during the treatment time and have a significant effect after a latent period, possibly in the order of 6–8 hours. It is suggested (Hayne, 1984) that the energy levels required to produce such an effect in humans is low.

Research has demonstrated that PSWT has a thermal component and that real tissue heating can occur (Bricknell and Watson, 1995). A measurable heating effect can be demonstrated at power levels over 5 W, although on average it will become apparent at 11 W mean power or more.

If a 'nonthermal' treatment is required (in acute injury management for example), the treatment should be delivered at a level below 5 W mean power. If a thermal effect is intended, power levels in excess of 5 W are required, but if undertaken the therapist must ensure that the precautions are taken as for any other thermal intervention.

Pulsed shortwave therapy: clinical effects

The clinical effects of PSWT are primarily related to the inflammatory and repair phases in musculoskeletal tissues. Goldin et al. (1981) lists the effects of the modality (following research in soft tissue repair following skin graft application). The effects are covered in the standard texts (Al Mandeel and Watson, 2020; Robertson et al., 2006; Watson, 2006). It is most effective when employed following tissue injury at low (nonthermal) levels whilst higher-power applications are of benefit in more chronic

Pulses at sufficient 'distance' – no accumulative effect

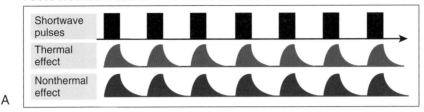

A

Pulses closer together – accumulating nonthermal effect, no thermal accumulation

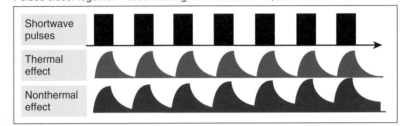

B

Pulses closer still – accumulation of thermal and nonthermal effects

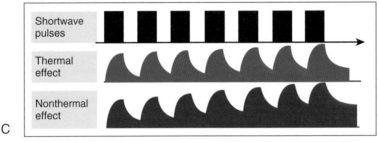

C

Fig. 6.4 Effect of varying the pulse parameters on the accumulated heat generated in the tissues.

presentations. Whereas ultrasound therapy is the modality of choice when treating dense collagenous tissue (ligament, tendon, fascia, joint capsule, scar tissue), pulsed shortwave is optimally employed when the target tissue has a high water content (muscle, nerve, areas of oedema, haematoma). The effects of the two therapy modalities are largely the same; it is the type of tissue in which the effects are achieved which varies between them. The use of pulsed shortwave has been recently reviewed across both acute and chronic conditions (Kumaran and Watson, 2015; 2016) with supportive evidence in both groups.

Higher-dose applications have been reported in the sports literature for managing long-standing injuries (Draper et al., 2017) with apparently good effect. At the other extreme, very low-dose, portable home-use units delivering shortwave through a skin contact loop have potential use in acute lesions (including postsurgery), being used for hours a day rather than tens of minutes (Brook et al., 2012).

Non-shortwave radiofrequency applications (Indiba, Tecar)

The delivery of radiofrequency (RF) energy at non-shortwave frequencies (typically under 1 MHz) is gaining traction, including in the sports medicine arena. The topic was recently reviewed (Kumaran and Watson, 2015; 2016) including RF at both shortwave and non-shortwave frequencies. The treatment is typically delivered with a two-electrode system (one smaller active electrode and a larger return plate) in either a capacitive or resistive mode. The electrodes are in direct contact with the tissues via a conductive cream; thus, a current will flow through the tissues, bringing about a significant thermal effect when applied with sufficient energy.

In addition to tissue temperature changes, physiologically there is a highly significant effect on local blood flow, at both superficial and deep tissue levels. These changes are evident even at low (nonthermal) doses (Kumaran and Watson, 2017). Additionally, these effects are of significantly

Representation of the electromagnetic spectrum

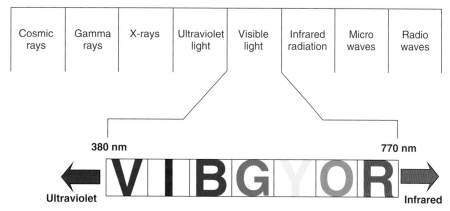

Fig. 6.5 Light energy as a part of the electromagnetic spectrum.

longer duration than equivalent energy levels applied with pulsed shortwave devices (Kumaran and Watson, 2018).

Increased blood flow is an essential tissue reaction during the repair sequence (Watson, 2006) and it is therefore proposed that by enhancing this local response, the tissue repair process will be enhanced. The early clinical evidence supports this proposition (Kumaran and Watson, 2018).

Laser therapy/Photobiomodulation

The term 'laser' is an acronym for *light amplification by stimulated emission of radiation*. In simple terms, the laser can be considered to be a form of light amplifier – it provides enhancement of particular properties of light energy.

Laser light behaves according to the basic laws of light, in that it travels in straight lines at a constant velocity in space. It can be transmitted, reflected, refracted and absorbed. It can be placed within the electromagnetic spectrum according to its wavelength/frequency, which will vary according to the particular generator under consideration (Fig. 6.5).

There are several aspects of laser light that are deemed to be unique and are often referred to in the literature. These include *monochromacity*, *coherence* and *polarization* (see Baxter and Nussbaum, 2020; Hamblin and Huang, 2013; Karu, 1998; Tuner and Hode, 2004 for details of physics and mechanism of interaction).

Terminology. The terms 'low-level laser therapy' (LLLT) and 'low-intensity laser therapy' (LILT) are used with equivalence. Most recently, the terms 'photomodulation' or 'photobiomodulation' have been adopted as the preferred terms for this therapy (Hamblin, 2016).

Therapy lasers have several common characteristics which are briefly summarized below.

Parameters. LLLT apparatus generates light in the red visible and near-infrared bands of the electromagnetic spectrum, with typical wavelengths of 600–1000 nm. The mean power of such devices is generally low (1–100 mW). The treatment device may be a single emitter or a cluster of several emitters. The beam from single probes is usually narrow (Ø 1–7 mm) at the source. A cluster probe will usually incorporate both higher- and lower-power emitters of different wavelengths. The output may be continuous or pulsed, with narrow pulse widths (in the nano- or microsecond ranges) and a wide variety of pulse repetition rates from 2 Hz up to several thousand Hz. It is difficult to identify the evidence for the use of pulsing from the research literature, although it will affect the applied energy and thus impact on dose parameters.

The recent promotion of higher-powered lasers (often described by virtue of their safety classification, class 4 lasers) is on the basis that with higher delivered energy levels, penetration of the light energy into the tissue will be greater (no evidence identified) and treatment times shorter (supported by the evidence based on energy delivery times).

Alternative generators using light-emitting diodes (LEDs) or laser diodes are available. The evidence suggests that these alternative light sources will be able to achieve equivalent effects so long as the energy applied is at the same level (de Abru Chaves et al., 2014; Lima et al., 2017).

Light absorption in the tissues

The absorption of light energy within the tissues is a complex issue but, generally, the shorter wavelengths (ultraviolet and shorter visible) are primarily absorbed in the epidermis by the pigments, amino and nucleic acids. The longer infrared wavelengths (>1300 nm) appear to be rapidly absorbed by water and therefore have a limited penetration into the tissues. The 600–1000 nm band are capable of penetration beyond the superficial epidermis and are available for absorption by deeper tissues.

Although much of the applied laser light is absorbed in the superficial tissues, it is proposed that deeper or more distant effects can be achieved as a secondary consequence via chemical mediator or second messenger systems, although there is limited evidence to fully support this contention. Most of the applied light energy will be absorbed in the first 5 mm of tissue depth when wavelengths in the visible red part of the spectrum are employed. A useful percentage of the light energy available at the surface will be available at 10–15 mm into the tissues with infrared wavelengths (over 770 nm) but clinically effective penetration beyond this level is debatable.

Laser–tissue interaction

Photobiomodulation (or *photobioactivation*) is a commonly used term in connection with laser therapy, and refers to the stimulation of various biological events using light energy but without significant temperature changes. It has now been adopted as the preferred term for this modality (Hamblin, 2016).

The early principles of photobioactivation were proposed by Karu (1987) who reported and demonstrated several key factors. She notes in her paper that some biomolecules change their activity in response to exposure to low-intensity visible light, but that these molecules do not appear to absorb the light directly. The cell and mitochondrial membranes are the primary absorbers of the energy which then generates intracellular effects by means of a second messenger/cascade response. The magnitude of the photoresponse appeared to be determined by the state of the tissues prior to irradiation. The laser light irradiation of the tissues is a trigger for the alteration of cell metabolic processes, via a process of photosignal transduction. Although the Karu research is not recent, it was the first robust demonstration of these effects, which have been confirmed by many authors subsequently. The cellular level targets and achieved effects have been usefully reviewed by Hamblin (2017).

The following list of physiological and cellular level effects is compiled from several reviews and research papers (Baxter, 2002; 2008; Hamblin et al., 2013; Tuner and Hode, 2004):

- altered cell proliferation
- altered cell motility

- activation of phagocytes
- stimulation of immune responses
- increased cellular metabolism
- stimulation of macrophages
- stimulation of mast cell degranulation
- activation and proliferation of fibroblasts
- alteration of cell membrane potentials
- stimulation of angiogenesis
- alteration of action potentials
- altered prostaglandin production
- altered endogenous opioid production.

The effects of laser photobiomodulation on the *inflammatory phase* of repair are very similar to those achieved by ultrasound therapy and almost certainly achieved via chemical mediation and similar system activation (Alves et al., 2013; 2014; Aras et al., 2015; Dos Santos et al., 2014; Hamblin, 2017; Hwang et al., 2015; Moura Júnior et al., 2014; Pires et al., 2011; Silva et al., 2015; Torres-Silva et al., 2015). In the *proliferative phase*, laser effects again largely mirror those achieved by ultrasound-based therapies (Alves et al., 2013; Chen et al., 2015; Colombo et al., 2013; Cury et al., 2013; Dungel et al., 2014; Ginani et al., 2015; Halon et al., 2015; Kuryliszyn-Moskal et al., 2015; Park et al., 2015; Rhee et al., 2016; Solmaz et al., 2017; Staffoli et al., 2017). Laser has less well demonstrated effects on the *remodelling stage* (when compared with ultrasound) although some evidence of efficacy and mechanisms of action have been identified (De Souza et al., 2011).

Treatment doses

Most research groups recommend that the dose delivered to a patient during a treatment session should be based on the *energy density* rather than the power or other measure of dose. Energy density is measured in joules per square centimetre (J/cm^2). It is currently argued that joules (i.e., *energy*) may in fact be the most critical parameter rather than energy density. The debate is not yet resolved, and energy density is used here as the published research almost exclusively cites it.

Most authorities suggest that the energy density per treatment session should generally fall in the range of 0.1–12.0 J/cm^2 although there are some recommendations which go up to 30 J/cm^2. Again, as a generality, lower doses should be applied to the more acute lesions which appear to be more energy sensitive.

Clinical applications

The recent research concentrates on a few key areas. Most dominant amongst these are wound healing, inflammatory arthropathies, soft tissue injury and the relief of pain (which includes laser acupuncture).

Open wounds

There is a growing body of evidence for the use of laser treatment this context, with the majority being positive outcome trials (there are useful sections in Baxter, 1994; Baxter and Nussbaum, 2020; Hamblin, 2013; Tuner and Hode, 2004). Whilst the evidence for these applications remains strong, it is not widely employed in sports medicine practice.

Inflammatory arthropathies

There have been several trials involving the use of LILT for various inflammatory problems in joints. The results are mixed, but the general trend is supportive. The Ottawa Panel (2004) review is supportive of laser therapy in rheumatoid arthritis. There is a relatively small volume of literature relating to inflammatory arthropathy in sports medicine – it is dominated by degenerative (osteoarthritis) and classic inflammatory (rheumatoid arthritis) type presentations (Rayegani et al., 2017).

Soft tissue injury

There is a widespread use of LILT in soft tissue applications. Tuner and Hode (2004) describe multiple examples of effective soft tissue treatments and identify some of the key research in this area. Further material is also included in the Baxter and Nussbaum (2020) review and in the Hamblin (2013) text. Recent work has concentrated on the effect of laser as a preexercise intervention to limit delayed onset muscle soreness (DOMS) and enhance recovery rather than as an injury treatment *per se*. The results have been mixed, but in some cases application of laser before exercise has demonstrated a significant recovery benefit for athletes (De Marchi et al., 2017; de Oliveira et al., 2017; Jowko et al., 2019; Pinto et al., 2016).

Pain

It has been broadly assumed that the effect of laser therapy for pain relief is a secondary effect of dealing with the inflammatory state. Whilst symptomatic pain relief may be beneficial from a patient perspective (de Souza et al., 2018; Izukura et al., 2017), it is argued that the use of laser to affect the underlying injury/pathology has the potential to provide longer lasting effects. There is growing evidence that laser therapy has a direct effect on nerve conduction characteristics and may result in reduced pain as a direct effect (Casale et al., 2013; Chow and Armati, 2016).

In recent years, there have been multiple studies evaluating laser therapy as a means of modifying postexercise pain (DOMS) or enhancing postexercise muscle recovery (Antonialli et al., 2014; de Oliveira et al., 2017). Whilst these are not fully established clinical applications, there is certainly sufficient evidence to identify them as promising applications.

Summary

In terms of enhancing tissue repair and recovery from injury, laser-based therapies have a substantial supportive evidence base. The effects of the therapy are very similar to those achieved by ultrasound therapy, although the target tissue is different – laser being most effective in the superficial tissues, especially those with high vascularity – and its effect predominantly in more acute rather than chronic stages.

Shockwave therapy

Shockwave therapy is a relatively recent development for injury and sports-related applications.

Shockwaves were initially employed as a noninvasive treatment for kidney stones in the 1970s and 1980s, and this has become established as a first-line intervention for these conditions. The animal model experiments associated with this work identified that shockwaves could have an (adverse) effect on bone. This led to a series of experimental investigations evaluating the effect of shockwaves on bone, cartilage and soft tissues (tendon, ligament, fascia) resulting in the current therapy applications.

A succinct history of the development of shockwaves for medical applications can be found in Thiel (2001). The pneumatic (ballistic) shockwave generators are most commonly employed in therapy.

There are essentially two 'modes' of shockwave therapy: *focused* and *radial*. The focused version is 'stronger', i.e., the applied energy reaches a focal point in the tissue, and is generally considered to be the more powerful form of the therapy. It is considered effective down to approximately 12 cm tissue depth. The radial mode is most commonly generated with a compressed-air mechanism, sending a projectile along a cylinder, striking the end plate in the applicator. There are now electromagnetic devices that operate in a similar fashion. The acoustic pressure wave is transmitted to the tissues (normally through a conductive gel, which improves efficacy and comfort). The energy does not reach a point of concentration in the tissue, and thus it is never more 'concentrated' than it is at the surface. It is suggested that this energy is clinically effective to depths of 5–6 cm into the tissue (Eaton and Watson, 2020; Foldager et al., 2012).

When the shockwave enters the tissues, it is reflected, refracted, transmitted and dissipated in the same way as any other energy. The energy content of the wave and the propagation of the wave varies with tissue type.

Shockwaves can be applied at both high and low powers. The high-power treatments (>0.6 mJ/mm^2) are given as a 'one-off' and generate a significant amount of pain. Some form of local anaesthetic is often needed for the patient to be able to tolerate the treatment. The more common approach is to use several (usually three to five) applications at low power (up to 0.08 mJ/mm^2; no anaesthetic is required) with typically 1500–2000 shocks delivered per session using a radial shockwave device.

As the shockwave travels through a medium and comes to an interface, part of the wave is reflected and part is transmitted. The dissipation of the energy at the interface is responsible for the generation of the physical, physiological and therapeutic effects.

Shockwave therapy is at its most effective when employed as part of a treatment programme for chronic tendinopathy-type presentations. This includes plantar fasciitis; Achilles (midportion and insertional), patellar, medial and lateral epicondylar lesions; supraspinatus (calcific and noncalcific) and other rotator cuff lesions. There are myriad developing treatment applications including greater trochanteric pain syndrome, medial tibial stress syndrome, myositis ossificans, local muscle problems, ligament lesions, problematic bone healing and some 20 or 30 others. Whilst some of these are developmental, there is already published research evidence in their support.

The tendinopathy literature is summarized in several key reviews and evidence compilation papers (Aqil et al., 2013; Császár and Schmidt, 2013; Everhart et al., 2017; Hawk et al., 2017; Ioppolo et al., 2013; Korakakis et al., 2018; Leal et al., 2015; Roehrig et al., 2005; Romeo et al., 2014; Santamato et al., 2016; Speed, 2014; Taheri et al., 2017; van der Worp et al., 2013; Verstraelen et al., 2014; Wang et al., 2012; Yin et al., 2014).

This is a provocative intervention and is not intended to 'soothe' the tissue to which it is applied. By provoking the chronic lesion with relatively high energy levels, a more acute lesion will be activated with associated pro-inflammatory mechanisms.

The role of shockwave therapy will stabilize with time (i.e., the clinical presentations for which it is most/least effective will become established), but at present, its use in cases of chronic tendinopathy is recognized and is supported by clinical research and systematic reviews.

Microcurrent therapy

Microcurrent therapy is becoming increasingly employed in the clinical environment as a new and emerging modality,

although strong evidence to support its use dates back several decades.

Interestingly, it appears to break all the classification 'rules' identified earlier in the chapter. It is not delivered with the intention of stimulating nerves, rather it plays to the bioelectric environment of the tissues, and therefore has a primary effect in terms of tissue repair (Poltawski and Watson, 2009; Watson and Nussbaum, 2020). The general characteristics of this type of therapy are that they utilize a direct current (pulsed or continuous), delivered at a very low amplitude (in the microampere (millionths of an ampere) range), which is usually subsensory from the patient perspective. This type of therapy has already been shown the be effective in several clinical areas, most notably fracture repair (Ciombor and Aaron, 2005; Simonis et al., 2003) and healing of open wounds (Evans et al., 2001; Watson, 1996; 2008) Soft tissue repair research is now evolving and shows strong future potential. The use of this therapy in tissue injury treatment has been recently reviewed (Poltawski and Watson, 2009) and some supportive clinical trial results are published (Chapman-Jones and Hill, 2002; Poltawski et al., 2012).

Microcurrent therapy devices appear to be most effectively employed when used for hours a day (rather than minutes a week in the clinic). Therefore, home-based therapy with small, inexpensive, portable devices is a likely way forward.

Conclusion

Electrophysical agents have an evidence-based role in physiotherapy practice. This chapter has attempted to summarize the key modalities in use in the current clinical environment, with focus on those modalities with the strongest role to play in healing and postinjury management. Each modality has a range of specific physiological effects, and these can be employed in turn to bring about therapeutic effects.

The overuse of electrotherapy in the past has resulted in the demise of this area of practice. This chapter has attempted to identify the key issues for relevant modalities, to illustrate their potential clinical applications based on the available evidence and to identify detailed sources for further information.

References

Ahmed, O.F., Elkharbotly, A.M., Taha, N., Bekheet, A.B., 2017. Treatment of mild to moderate carpal tunnel syndrome in patients with diabetic neuropathy using low level laser therapy versus ultrasound controlled comparative study. Biochimica et Biophysica Acta Clinical 8, 43–47.

Al-Mandeel, M., Watson, T., 2020. Pulsed and continuous shortwave and radiofrequency therapies. In: Watson, T. and Nussbaum, N. (Eds.), Electrophysical Agents: Evidence-Based Practice, thirteenth ed. Elsevier, Edinburgh, pp. 132–149.

Al-Mandeel, M., Watson, T., 2006. An audit of patient records into the nature of pulsed shortwave therapy use. International Journal of Therapy and Rehabilitation 13 (9), 414–420.

Alves, A.C., Vieira, R., Leal-Junior, E., dos Santos, S., Ligeiro, A.P., Albertini, R., et al., 2013. Effect of low-level laser therapy on the expression of inflammatory mediators and on neutrophils and macrophages in acute joint inflammation. Arthritis Research & Therapy 15 (5), R116.

Alves, A.N., Fernandes, K.P., Deana, A.M., Bussadori, S.K., Mesquita-Ferrari, R.A., 2014. Effects of low-level laser therapy on skeletal muscle repair: a systematic review. American Journal of Physical Medicine & Rehabilitation 93 (12), 1073–1085.

Antonialli, F.C., De Marchi, T., Tomazoni, S.S., Vanin, A.A., Dos Santos Grandinetti, V., de Paiva, P.R., et al., 2014. Phototherapy in skeletal muscle performance and recovery after exercise: effect of combination of super-pulsed laser and light-emitting diodes. Lasers in Medical Science 29 (6), 1967–1976.

Aqil, A., Siddiqui, M.S., Solan, M., Redfern, D., Gulati, V., Cobb, J., 2013. Extracorporeal shock wave therapy is effective in treating chronic plantar fasciitis: a meta-analysis of RCTs. Clinical Orthopaedics and Related Research 471 (11), 3645–3652.

Aras, M.H., Bozdag, Z., Demir, T., Oksayan, R., Yanik, S., Sokucu, O., 2015. Effects of low-level laser therapy on changes in inflammation and in the activity of osteoblasts in the expanded premaxillary suture in an ovariectomized rat model. Photomedicine and Laser Surgery 33 (3), 136–144.

Aspenberg, P., 2017. Comment to a BMJ Editorial: is LIPUS the baby in the bathwater? Acta Orthopaedica 88 (1), 1.

Bajpai, A., Nadkarni, S., Neidrauer, M., Weingarten, M.S., Lewin, P.A., Spiller, K.L., 2018. Effects of non-thermal, non-cavitational ultrasound exposure on human diabetic ulcer healing and inflammatory gene expression in a pilot study. Ultrasound in Medicine & Biology 44 (9), 2043–2049.

Baker, K.G., Robertson, V.J., Duck, F.A., 2001. A review of therapeutic ultrasound: biophysical effects. Physical Therapy 81 (7), 1351–1358.

Baxter, D., 1994. Therapeutic Lasers: Theory & Practice. Churchill Livingstone, Edinburgh.

Baxter, D., 2002. Low-intensity laser therapy. In: Kitchen, S. (Ed.), Electrotherapy: Evidence Based Practice, eleventh ed. Churchill Livingstone/Elsevier, Edinburgh.

Baxter, D., Nussbaum, E., 2020. Laser/photobiomodulation. In: Watson, T. and Nussbaum, N. (Eds.), Electrophysical Agents: Evidence-Based Practice, thirteenth ed. Elsevier, Edinburgh, pp. 189–207.

Bayat, M., Virdi, A., Rezaei, F., Chien, S., 2018. Comparison of the in vitro effects of low-level laser therapy and low-intensity pulsed ultrasound therapy on bony cells and stem cells. Progress in Biophysics and Molecular Biology 133, 36–48 2018.

Bellew, J.W., Michlovitz, S.L., Nolan, T., 2016. Michlovitz's Modalities for Therapeutic Intervention, sixth ed. F.A. Davis Company, Philadelphia, PA.

Bricknell, R., Watson, T., 1995. The thermal effects of pulsed shortwave therapy. British Journal of Therapy & Rehabilitation 2 (8), 430–434.

Brook, J., Dauphinee, D.M., Korpinen, J., Rawe, I.M., 2012. Pulsed radiofrequency electromagnetic field therapy: a potential novel treatment of plantar fasciitis. The Journal of Foot and Ankle Surgery 51 (3), 312–316.

Busse, J.W., Kaur, J., Mollon, B., Bhandari, M., Tornetta 3rd, P., Schunemann, H.J., et al., 2009. Low intensity pulsed ultrasonography for fractures: systematic review of randomised controlled trials. British Medical Journal 338, b351.

Byl, N.N., Hill Toulouse, L., Sitton, P., Hall, J., Stern, R., 1996. Effects of ultrasound on the orientation of fibroblasts: an invitro study. European Journal of Physical and Rehabilitation Medicine 6 (6), 180–184.

Casale, R., Damiani, C., Maestri, R., Wells, C.D., 2013. Pain and electrophysiological parameters are improved by combined 830-1064 high-intensity LASER in symptomatic carpal tunnel syndrome versus transcutaneous electrical nerve stimulation. A randomized controlled study. European Journal of Physical and Rehabilitation Medicine 49 (2), 205–211.

Chapman-Jones, D., Hill, D., 2002. Novel microcurrent treatment is more effective than conventional therapy for chronic Achilles tendinopathy: randomised comparative trial. Physiotherapy 88 (8), 471–480.

Chen, M.H., Huang, Y.C., Sun, J.S., Chao, Y.H., 2015. Second messengers mediating the proliferation and collagen synthesis of tenocytes induced by low-level laser irradiation. Lasers in Medical Science 30 (1), 263–272.

Chow, R.T., Armati, P.J., 2016. Photobiomodulation: implications for anesthesia and pain relief. Photomedicine and Laser Surgery 34 (12), 599–609.

Ciombor, D.M., Aaron, R.K., 2005. The role of electrical stimulation in bone repair. Foot and Ankle Clinics 10 (4), 579–593 vii.

Claes, L., Willie, B., 2007. The enhancement of bone regeneration by ultrasound. Progress in Biophysics and Molecular Biology 93 (1–3), 384–398.

Colombo, F., Neto Ade, A., Sousa, A.P., Marchionni, A.M., Pinheiro, A.L., Reis, S.R., et al., 2013. Effect of low-level laser therapy (λ660 nm) on angiogenesis in wound healing: a immunohistochemical study in a rodent model. Brazilian Dental Journal 24 (4), 308–312.

Császár, N.B., Schmitz, C., 2013. Extracorporeal shock wave therapy in musculoskeletal disorders. Journal of Orthopaedic Surgery and Research 8 (1), 22.

Cury, V., Moretti, A.I., Assis, L., Bossini, P., Crusca Jde, S., Neto, C.B., et al., 2013. Low level laser therapy increases angiogenesis in a model of ischemic skin flap in rats mediated by VEGF, HIF-1α and MMP-2. Journal of Photochemistry and Photobiology. B, Biology 125, 164–170.

de Abreu Chaves, M.E., de Araújo, A.R., Piancastelli, A.C.C., Pinotti, M., 2014. Effects of low-power light therapy on wound healing: LASER x LED. Anais Brasileiros de Dermatologia 89 (4), 616–623.

de Brito Vieira, W.H., Aguiar, K.A., da Silva, K.M., Canela, P.M., da Silva, F.S., Abreu, B.J., et al., 2012. Overview of ultrasound usage trends in orthopedic and sports physiotherapy. Critical Ultrasound Journal 4 (1), 11.

De Marchi, T., Schmitt, V.M., Danubia da Silva Fabro, C., da Silva, L.L., Sene, J., Tairova, O., et al., 2017. Phototherapy for improvement of performance and exercise recovery: comparison of 3 commercially available devices. Journal of Athletic Training 52 (5), 429–438.

de Oliveira, A.R., Vanin, A.A., Tomazoni, S.S., Miranda, E.F., Albuquerque-Pontes, G.M., De Marchi, T., et al., 2017. Pre-exercise infrared photobiomodulation therapy (810 nm) in skeletal muscle performance and postexercise recovery in humans: what is the optimal power output? Photomedicine and Laser Surgery 35 (11), 595–603.

de Oliveira Perrucini, P.D., Poli-Frederico, R.C., de Almeida Pires-Oliveira, D.A., Dragonetti Bertin, L., Beltrao Pires, F., Shimoya-Bittencourt, W., et al., 2020. Anti-inflammatory and healing effects of pulsed ultrasound therapy on fibroblasts. American Journal of Physical Medicine & Rehabilitation 99 (1), 19–25.

de Souza, R.C., de Sousa, E.T., Scudine, K.G., Meira, U.M., de Oliveira, E.S.E.M., Gomes, A.C., et al., 2018. Low-level laser therapy and anesthetic infiltration for orofacial pain in patients with fibromyalgia: a randomized clinical trial. Medicina Oral, Patologia Oral y Cirugia Bucal 23 (1), e65–e71.

de Souza, T., Mesquita, D., Ferrari, R., dos Santos Pinto, D., Correa, L., Bussadori, S., et al., 2011. Phototherapy with low-level laser affects the remodeling of types I and III collagen in skeletal muscle repair. Lasers in Medical Science 26 (6), 803–814.

Della Rocca, G., 2009. The science of ultrasound therapy for fracture healing. Indian Journal of Orthopaedics 43 (2), 121–126.

Dingemanse, R., Randsorp, M., Koes, B.W., Huisstede, B.M.A., 2014. Evidence for the effectiveness of electrophysical modalities for treatment of medial and lateral epicondylitis: a systematic review. British Journal of Sports Medicine 48 (12), 957–965.

dos Santos, S.A., Alves, A.C., Leal-Junior, E.C., Albertini, R., Vieira Rde, P., Ligeiro, A.P., et al., 2014. Comparative analysis of two low-level laser doses on the expression of inflammatory mediators and on neutrophils and macrophages in acute joint inflammation. Lasers in Medical Science 29 (3), 1051–1058.

Draper, D.O., Ricard, M.D., 1995. Rate of temperature decay in human muscle following 3 MHz ultrasound: the stretching window revealed. Journal of Athletic Training 30 (4), 304–307.

Draper, D.O., Schulthies, S., Sorvisto, P., Hautala, A.M., 1995. Temperature changes in deep muscles of humans during ice and ultrasound therapies: an in vivo study. The Journal of Orthopaedic and Sports Physical Therapy 21 (3), 153–157.

Draper, D.O., Veazey, E., 2017. Pulsed shortwave diathermy and joint mobilizations restore a twice fractured elbow with metal implants to full range of motion. Journal of Novel Physiotherapy and Rehabilitation 1, 020–026.

Dungel, P., Hartinger, J., Chaudary, S., Slezak, P., Hofmann, A., Hausner, T., et al., 2014. Low level light therapy by LED of different wavelength induces angiogenesis and improves ischemic wound healing. Lasers in Surgery and Medicine 46 (10), 773–780.

Dyson, M., Smalley, D., 1983. Effects of ultrasound on wound contraction. In: Millner, R., Rosenfeld, E., Cobet, U. (Eds.), Ultrasound Interactions in Biology & Medicine. Plenum Press, New York, pp. 151–158.

Eaton, C., Watson, T., 2020. Shockwave. In: Watson, T. and Nussbaum, N. (Eds.), Electrophysical Agents: Evidence-Based Practice, thirteenth ed. Elsevier, Edinburgh, pp. 229–246.

Enwemeka, C.S., Rodriguez, O., Mendosa, S., 1990. The miomechanical effects of low intensity ultrasound on healing tendons. Ultrasound in Medicine & Biology 16 (8), 801–807.

Evans, R.D., Foltz, D., Foltz, K., 2001. Electrical stimulation with bone and wound healing. Clinics in Podiatric Medicine and Surgery 18 (1), 79–95 vi.

Everhart, J.S., Cole, D., Sojka, J.H., Higgins, J.D., Magnussen, R.A., Schmitt, L.C., et al., 2017. Treatment options for patellar tendinopathy: a systematic review. Arthroscopy 33 (4), 861–872.

Foldager, C.B., Kearney, C., Spector, M., 2012. Clinical application of extracorporeal shock wave therapy in orthopedics: focused versus unfocused shock waves. Ultrasound in Medicine & Biology 38 (10), 1673–1680.

Ginani, F., Soares, D.M., Barreto, M.P., Barboza, C.A., 2015. Effect of low-level laser therapy on mesenchymal stem cell proliferation: a systematic review. Lasers in Medical Science 30 (8), 2189–2194.

Goldin, J.H., Broadbent, N.R.G., Nancarrow, J.D., Marshall, T., 1981. The effects of Diapulse on the healing of wounds: a double-blind randomised controlled trial in man. British Journal of Plastic Surgery 34 (3), 267–270.

Griffin, X.L., Costello, I., Costa, M.L., 2008. The role of low intensity pulsed ultrasound therapy in the management of acute fractures: a systematic review. The Journal of Trauma 65 (6), 1446–1452.

Halon, A., Donizy, P., Dziegala, M., Dobrakowski, R., Simon, K., 2015. Tissue laser biostimulation promotes post-extraction neoangiogenesis in HIV-infected patients. Lasers in Medical Science 30 (2), 701–706.

Hamblin, M.R., 2016. Photobiomodulation or low-level laser therapy. Journal of Biophotonics 9 (11–12), 1122–1124.

Hamblin, M.R., 2017. Mechanisms and applications of the anti-inflammatory effects of photobiomodulation. American Institute of Mathematical Sciences Biophysics 4 (3), 337–361.

Hamblin, M.R., Huang, Y., 2013. Handbook of Photomedicine. CRC Press, Boca Raton, FL.

Harrison, A., Lin, S., Pounder, N., Mikuni-Takagaki, Y., 2016. Mode & mechanism of low intensity pulsed ultrasound (LIPUS) in fracture repair. Ultrasonics 70, 45–52.

Harvey, W., Dyson, M., Pond, J.B., Grahame, R., 1975. The stimulation of protein synthesis in human fibroblasts by therapeutic ultrasound. Rheumatology & Rehabilitation 14 (4), 237.

Hawk, C., Minkalis, A.L., Khorsan, R., Daniels, C.J., Homack, D., Gliedt, J.A., et al., 2017. Systematic review of nondrug, nonsurgical treatment of shoulder conditions. Journal of Manipulative and Physiological Therapeutics 40 (5), 293–319.

Hayne, C.R., 1984. Pulsed high frequency energy – Its place in physiotherapy. Physiotherapy 70, 459–464.

Heckman, J.D., Ryaby, J.P., McCabe, J., Frey, J.J., Kilcoyne, R.F., 1994. Acceleration of tibial fracture-healing by non-invasive, low-intensity pulsed ultrasound. The Journal of Bone and Joint Surgery. American Volume 76 (1), 26–34.

Hill, J., Lewis, M., Mills, P., Kielty, C., 2002. Pulsed short-wave diathermy effects on human fibroblast proliferation. Archives of Physical Medicine and Rehabilitation 83 (6), 832–836.

Huisstede, B.M.A., Hoogvliet, P., Franke, T.P.C., Randsorp, M.S., Koes, B.W., 2018. Carpal tunnel syndrome: effectiveness of physical therapy and electrophysical modalities. An updated systematic review of randomized controlled trials. Archives of Physical Medicine and Rehabilitation 99 (8), 1623–1634.e23.

Hwang, M.H., Shin, J.H., Kim, K.S., Yoo, C.M., Jo, G.E., Kim, J.H., et al., 2015. Low level light therapy modulates inflammatory mediators secreted by human annulus fibrosus cells during intervertebral disc degeneration in vitro. Photochemistry and Photobiology 91 (2), 403–410.

Ilter, L., Dilek, B., Batmaz, I., Ulu, M.A., Sariyildiz, M.A., Nas, K., et al., 2015. Efficacy of pulsed and continuous therapeutic ultrasound in myofascial pain syndrome: a randomized controlled study. American Journal of Physical Medicine & Rehabilitation 94 (7), 547–554.

Ioppolo, F., Tattoli, M., Di Sante, L., Venditto, T., Tognolo, L., Delicata, M., et al., 2013. Clinical improvement and resorption of calcifications in calcific tendinitis of the shoulder after shock wave therapy at 6 months' follow-up: a systematic review and meta-analysis. Archives of Physical Medicine and Rehabilitation 94 (9), 1699–1706.

Izadifar, Z., Babyn, P., Chapman, D., 2017. Mechanical and biological effects of ultrasound: a review of present knowledge. Ultrasound in Medicine & Biology 43 (6), 1085–1104.

Izukura, H., Miyagi, M., Harada, T., Ohshiro, T., Ebihara, S., 2017. Low Level Laser Therapy in patients with chronic foot and ankle joint pain. Laser Therapy 26 (1), 19–24.

Jensen, J.E., 1998. Stress fracture in the world class athlete: a case study. Medicine and Science in Sports and Exercise 30 (6), 783–787.

Jingushi, S., 2009. [Bone fracture and the healing mechanisms. Fracture treatment by low-intensity pulsed ultrasound]. Clinical Calcium 19 (5), 704–708.

Jowko, E., Plaszewski, M., Cieslinski, M., Sacewicz, T., Cieslinski I., Jarocka, M., 2019. The effect of low level laser irradiation on oxidative stress, muscle damage and function following neuromuscular electrical stimulation. A double blind, randomised, crossover trial. BMC Sports Science, Medicine and Rehabilitation 11, 38.

Karu, T., 1987. Photobiological fundamentals of low-power laser therapy. IEEE Journal of Quantum Electronics 23 (10), 1703–1717.

Karu, T., 1998. The Science of Low-Power Laser Therapy. Gordon & Breach Science Publishers, Amsterdam.

Kim, K.H., Im, H.W., Karmacharya, M.B., Kim, S., Min, B.H., Park, S.R., Choi, B.H., 2020. Low-intensity ultrasound attenuates paw edema formation and decreases vascular permeability induced by carrageenan injection in rats. Journal of Inflammation 17 (1), 7.

Knight, K.L., Draper, D.O., 2012. Therapeutic Modalities: The Art and Science. Lippincott Williams & Wilkins, Baltimore, MD.

Korakakis, V., Whiteley, R., Tzavara, A., Malliaropoulos, N., 2018. The effectiveness of extracorporeal shockwave therapy in common lower limb conditions: a systematic review including quantification of patient-rated pain reduction. British Journal of Sports Medicine 52 (6), 387–407.

Kristiansen, T.K., Ryaby, J.P., McCabe, J., Frey, J.J., Roe, L.R., 1997. Accelerated healing of distal radial fractures with the use of specific, low-intensity ultrasound. A multicenter, prospective, randomized, double-blind, placebo-controlled study. The Journal of Bone and Joint Surgery. American Volume 79 (7), 961–973.

Kumaran, B., Herbland, A., Watson, T., 2017. Continuous-mode 448 kHz capacitive resistive monopolar radiofrequency induces greater deep blood flow changes compared to pulsed mode shortwave: a crossover study in healthy adults. European Journal of Physiotherapy 19 (3), 137–146.

Kumaran, B., Watson, T., 2015. Radiofrequency-based treatment in therapy-related clinical practice – a narrative review. Part I: acute conditions. Physical Therapy Reviews 20 (4), 241–254.

Kumaran, B., Watson, T., 2016. Radiofrequency-based treatment in therapy-related clinical practice – a narrative review. Part II: chronic conditions. Physical Therapy Reviews 20 (5-6), 325–343.

Kumaran, B., Watson, T., 2018. Skin thermophysiological effects of 448 kHz capacitive resistive monopolar radiofrequency in healthy adults: a randomised crossover study and comparison with pulsed shortwave therapy. Electromagnetic Biology and Medicine 37 (1), 1–12.

Kuryliszyn-Moskal, A., Kita, J., Dakowicz, A., Chwiesko-Minarowska, S., Moskal, D., Kosztyla-Hojna, B., et al., 2015. The influence of Multiwave Locked System (MLS) laser therapy on clinical features, microcirculatory abnormalities and selected modulators of angiogenesis in patients with Raynaud's phenomenon. Clinical Rheumatology 34 (3), 489–496.

Leal, C., Ramon, S., Furia, J., Fernandez, A., Romero, L., Hernandez-Sierra, L., et al., 2015. Current concepts of shockwave therapy in chronic patellar tendinopathy. International Journal of Surgery 24 (Pt B), 160–164.

Leung, M.C., Ng, G.Y., Yip, K.K., 2006. Therapeutic ultrasound enhances medial collateral ligament repair in rats. Ultrasound in Medicine & Biology 32 (3), 449–452.

Lima, A.C., Fernandes, G.A., de Barros Araujo, R., Gonzaga, I.C., de Oliveira, R.A., Nicolau, R.A., et al., 2017. Photobiomodulation (laser and LED) on sternotomy healing in hyperglycemic and normoglycemic patients who underwent coronary bypass surgery with internal mammary artery grafts: a randomized, double-blind study with follow-up. Photomedicine and Laser Surgery 35 (1), 24–31.

Lovric, V., Ledger, M., Goldberg, J., Harper, W., Bertollo, N., Pelletier, M.H., et al., 2013. The effects of low-intensity pulsed ultrasound on tendon–bone healing in a transosseous-equivalent sheep rotator cuff model. Knee Surgery, Sports Traumatology, Arthroscopy 21 (2), 466–475.

Lu, H., Qin, L., Lee, K., Cheung, W., Chan, K., Leung, K., et al., 2009. Identification of genes responsive to low-intensity pulsed ultrasound stimulations. Biochemical and Biophysical Research Communications 378 (3), 569–573.

Maxwell, L., 1992. Therapeutic ultrasound: its effects on the cellular and molecular mechanisms of inflammation and repair. Physiotherapy 78 (6), 421–426.

Mayr, E., Frankel, V., Ruter, A., 2000. Ultrasound – an alternative healing method for nonunions? Archives of Orthopaedic and Trauma Surgery 120 (1-2), 1–8.

McBrier, N.M., Lekan, J.M., Druhan, L.J., Devor, S.T., Merrick, M.A., 2007. Therapeutic ultrasound decreases mechano-growth factor messenger ribonucleic acid expression after muscle contusion injury. Archives of Physical Medicine and Rehabilitation 88 (7), 936–940.

Meakins, A., Watson, T., 2006. Longwave ultrasound and conductive heating increase functional ankle mobility in asymptomatic subjects. Physical Therapy in Sport 7, 74–80.

Mehta, S., Long, K., DeKoven, M., Smith, E., Steen, R.G., 2015. Low-intensity pulsed ultrasound (LIPUS) can decrease the economic burden of fracture non-union. Journal of Medical Economics 18 (7), 542–549.

Michlovitz, S.L., Bellew, J.W., Nolan, T.P., 2012. Modalities for Therapeutic Intervention, fifth ed. F. A. Davis Company, Philadelphia, PA.

Moura Júnior, M. de J., Arisawa, E.Â., Martin, A.A., de Carvalho, J.P., da Silva, J.M., Silva, J.F., et al., 2014. Effects of low-power LED and therapeutic ultrasound in the tissue healing and inflammation in a tendinitis experimental model in rats. Lasers in Medical Science 29 (1), 301–311.

Nakamura, T., Fujihara, S., Katsura, T., Yamamoto, K., Inubushi, T., Tanimoto, K., et al., 2010. Effects of low-intensity pulsed ultrasound on the expression and activity of hyaluronan synthase and hyaluronidase in IL-1beta-stimulated synovial cells. Annals of Biomedical Engineering 38 (11), 3363–3370.

Nussbaum, E., 1997. Ultrasound: to heat or not to heat – that is the question. Physical Therapy Reviews 2 (2), 59–72.

Nussbaum, E., 1998. The influence of ultrasound on healing tissues. Journal of Hand Therapy 11 (2), 140–147.

Ottawa Panel, 2004. Ottawa Panel evidence-based clinical practice guidelines for electrotherapy and thermotherapy interventions in the management of rheumatoid arthritis in adults. Physical Therapy 84 (11), 1016–1043.

Padilla, F., Puts, R., Vico, L., Guignandon, A., Raum, K., 2016. Stimulation of Bone Repair with Ultrasound. Advances in Experimental Medicine and Biology 880, 385–427.

Padilla, F., Puts, R., Vico, L., Raum, K., 2014. Stimulation of bone repair with ultrasound: a review of the possible mechanic effects. Ultrasonics 54 (5), 1125–1145.

Park, I.S., Chung, P.S., Ahn, J.C., 2015. Adipose-derived stromal cell cluster with light therapy enhance angiogenesis and skin wound healing in mice. Biochemical and Biophysical Research Communications 462 (3), 171–177.

Pinto, H.D., Vanin, A.A., Miranda, E.F., Tomazoni, S.S., Johnson, D.S., Albuquerque-Pontes, G.M., et al., 2016. Photobiomodulation therapy improves performance and accelerates recovery of high-level rugby players in field test: a randomized, crossover, double-blind, placebo-controlled clinical study. Journal of Strength and Conditioning Research 30 (12), 3329–3338.

Pires, D., Xavier, M., Araujo, T., Silva Jr., J.A., Aimbire, F., Albertini, R., et al., 2011. Low-level laser therapy (LLLT; 780 nm) acts differently on mRNA expression of anti- and pro-inflammatory mediators in an experimental model of collagenase-induced tendinitis in rat. Lasers in Medical Science 26 (1), 85–94.

Poltawski, L., Johnson, M., Watson, T., 2012. Microcurrent therapy in the management of chronic tennis elbow: pilot studies to optimize parameters. Physiotherapy Research International 17 (3), 157–166.

Poltawski, L., Watson, T., 2007. Relative transmissivity of ultrasound coupling agents commonly used by therapists in the UK. Ultrasound in Medicine & Biology 33 (1), 120–128.

Poltawski, L., Watson, T., 2009. Bioelectricity and microcurrent therapy for tissue healing – a narrative review. Physical Therapy Reviews 14 (2), 104–114.

Ramirez, A., Schwane, J.A., McFarland, C., Starcher, B., 1997. The effect of ultrasound on collagen synthesis and fibroblast proliferation in vitro. Medicine and Science in Sports and Exercise 29 (3), 326–332.

Rayegani, S.M., Raeissadat, S.A., Heidari, S., Moradi-Joo, M., 2017. Safety and effectiveness of low-level laser therapy in patients with knee osteoarthritis: a systematic review and meta-analysis. Journal of Lasers in Medical Sciences 8 (Suppl. 1), S12–S19.

Renno, A.C., Toma, R.L., Feitosa, S.M., Fernandes, K., Bossini, P.S., de Oliveira, P., et al., 2011. Comparative effects of low-intensity pulsed ultrasound and low-level laser therapy on injured skeletal muscle. Photomedicine and Laser Surgery 29 (1), 5–10.

Rhee, Y.H., Moon, J.H., Choi, S.H., Ahn, J.C., 2016. Low-level laser therapy promoted aggressive proliferation and angiogenesis through decreasing of transforming growth factor-β1 and increasing of akt/hypoxia inducible factor-1α in anaplastic thyroid cancer. Photomedicine and Laser Surgery 34 (6), 229–235.

Robertson, V.J., Ward, A., Low, J., Reed, A., 2006. Electrotherapy Explained: Principles and Practice, fourth ed. Butterworth-Heinemann/Elsevier, Oxford.

Roehrig, G.J., Baumhauer, J., DiGiovanni, B.F., Flemister, A.S., 2005. The role of extracorporeal shock wave on plantar fasciitis. Foot Ankle Clinics 10 (4), 699–712 ix.

Romeo, P., Lavanga, V., Pagani, D., Sansone, V., 2014. Extracorporeal shock wave therapy in musculoskeletal disorders: a review. Medical Principles and Practice 23 (1), 7–13.

Sahu, N., Viljoen, H.J., Subramanian, A., 2019. Continuous low-intensity ultrasound attenuates IL-6 and TNFalpha-induced catabolic effects and repairs chondral fissures in bovine osteochondral explants. BMC Musculoskeletal Disorders 20 (1), 193.

Santamato, A., Panza, F., Notarnicola, A., Cassatella, G., Fortunato, F., de Sanctis, J.L., et al., 2016. Is extracorporeal shockwave therapy combined with isokinetic exercise more effective than extracorporeal shockwave therapy alone for subacromial impingement syndrome? A randomized clinical trial. The Journal of Orthopaedic and Sports Physical Therapy 46 (9), 714–725.

Schandelmaier, S., Kaushal, A., Lytvyn, L., Heels-Ansdell, D., Siemieniuk, R.A.C., Agoritsas, T., et al., 2017. Low intensity pulsed ultrasound for bone healing: systematic review of randomized controlled trials. British Medical Journal 356, j656.

Shah, S.G.S., Farrow, A., 2012. Trends in the availability and usage of electrophysical agents in physiotherapy practices from 1990 to 2010: a review. Physical Therapy Reviews 17 (4), 207–226.

Silva, G.B., Sacono, N.T., Othon-Leite, A.F., Mendonca, E.F., Arantes, A.M., Bariani, C., et al., 2015. Effect of low-level laser therapy on inflammatory mediator release during chemotherapy-induced oral mucositis: a randomized preliminary study. Lasers in Medical Science 30 (1), 117–126.

Simonis, R.B., Parnell, E.J., Ray, P.S., Peacock, J.L., 2003. Electrical treatment of tibial non-union: a prospective, randomised, double-blind trial. Injury 34 (5), 357–362.

Solmaz, H., Ulgen, Y., Gulsoy, M., 2017. Photobiomodulation of wound healing via visible and infrared laser irradiation. Lasers in Medical Science 32 (4), 903–910.

Speed, C., 2014. A systematic review of shockwave therapies in soft tissue conditions: focusing on the evidence. British Journal of Sports Medicine 48 (21), 1538–1542.

Staffoli, S., Romeo, U., Amorim, R.N.S., Migliau, G., Palaia, G., Resende, L., et al., 2017. The effects of low level laser irradiation on proliferation of human dental pulp: a narrative review. La Clinica Terapeutica 168 (5), e320–e326.

Taheri, P., Emadi, M., Poorghasemian, J., 2017. Comparison the effect of extra corporeal shockwave therapy with low dosage versus high dosage in treatment of the patients with lateral epicondylitis. Advanced Biomedical Research 6, 61.

ter Haar, G., 1999. Therapeutic ultrasound. European Journal of Ultrasound 9 (1), 3–9.

Thiel, M., 2001. Application of shock waves in medicine. Clinical Orthopaedics & Related Research 387, 18–21.

Torres-Silva, R., Lopes-Martins, R.A., Bjordal, J.M., Frigo, L., Rahouadj, R., Arnold, G., et al., 2015. The low level laser therapy (LLLT) operating in 660 nm reduce gene expression of inflammatory mediators in the experimental model of collagenase-induced rat tendinitis. Lasers in Medical Science 30 (7), 1985–1990.

Tuner, J., Hode, L., 2004. The Laser Therapy Handbook. Prima Books, Grangesberg, Sweden.

Turner, S., Powell, E., Ng, C., 1989. The effect of ultrasound on the healing of repaired cockerel tendon: is collagen cross-linkage a factor? The Journal of Hand Surgery 14 (4), 428–433.

van der Worp, H., van den Akker-Scheek, I., van Schie, H., Zwerver, J., 2013. ESWT for tendinopathy: technology and clinical implications. Knee Surgery, Sports Traumatology, Arthroscopy 21 (6), 1451–1458.

Verstraelen, F.U., In den Kleef, N.J., Jansen, L., Morrenhof, J.W., 2014. High-energy versus low-energy extracorporeal shock wave therapy for calcifying tendinitis of the shoulder: which is superior? A meta-analysis. Clinical Orthopaedics and Related Research 472 (9), 2816–2825.

Wang, C.J., 2012. Extracorporeal shockwave therapy in musculoskeletal disorders. Journal of Orthopaedic Surgery and Research 7 (1), 11.

Wang, E.D., 1998. Tendon repair. Journal of Hand Therapy 11 (2), 105–110.

Watson, T., 1996. Electrical stimulation for wound healing. Physical Therapy Reviews 1 (2), 89–103.

Watson, T., 2000. The role of electrotherapy in contemporary physiotherapy practice. Manual Therapy 5 (3), 132–141.

Watson, T., 2006. Electrotherapy and tissue repair. Journal of Sportex Medicine 29, 7–13.

Watson, T., 2010. Narrative review: key concepts with electrophysical agents. Physical Therapy Reviews 15 (4), 351–359.

Watson, T., 2014. Crest of a wave: effectiveness of therapeutic ultrasound in musculoskeletal injury. International Therapist (110), 18–20.

Watson, T., 2016. Expanding our Understanding of the Inflammatory Process and its Role in Pain & Tissue Healing. IFOMPT 2016, Glasgow.

Watson, T., Nussbaum, N., 2020. Electrophysical Agents: Evidence-Based Practice, thirteenth ed. Elsevier, Edinburgh.

Watson, T., 2020. Ultrasound. In: Watson, T. and Nussbaum, N. (Eds.), Electrophysical Agents: Evidence-Based Practice, thirteenth ed. Elsevier, Edinburgh, pp. 164–188.

Williams, R., 1987. Production and transmission of ultrasound. Physiotherapy 73 (3), 113–116.

Yegin, T., Altan, L., Kasapoglu Aksoy, M., 2017. The effect of therapeutic ultrasound on pain and physical function in patients with knee osteoarthritis. Ultrasound in Medicine & Biology 43 (1), 187–194.

Yeung, C.K., Guo, X., Ng, Y.F., 2006. Pulsed ultrasound treatment accelerates the repair of Achilles tendon rupture in rats. Journal of Orthopaedic Research 24 (2), 193–201.

Yin, M.C., Ye, J., Yao, M., Cui, X.J., Xia, Y., Shen, Q.X., et al., 2014. Is extracorporeal shock wave therapy clinical efficacy for relief of chronic, recalcitrant plantar fasciitis? A systematic review and meta-analysis of randomized placebo or active-treatment controlled trials. Archives of Physical Medicine and Rehabilitation 95 (8), 1585–1593.

Zeng, C., Li, H., Yang, T., Deng, Z.H., Yang, Y., Zhang, Y., et al., 2014. Effectiveness of continuous and pulsed ultrasound for the management of knee osteoarthritis: a systematic review and network meta-analysis. Osteoarthritis Research Society 22 (8), 1090–1099.

Zhang, C., Xie, Y., Luo, X., Ji, Q., Lu, C., He, C., et al., 2016. Effects of therapeutic ultrasound on pain, physical functions and safety outcomes in patients with knee osteoarthritis: a systematic review and meta-analysis. Clinical Rehabilitation 30 (10), 960–971.

Zhang, N., Chow, S.K.-H., Leung, K.-S., Cheung, W.-H., 2017. Ultrasound as a stimulus for musculoskeletal disorders. Journal of Orthopaedic Translation 9, 52–59.

Zhou, S., Bachem, M.G., Seufferlein, T., Li, Y., Gross, H.J., Schmelz, A., et al., 2008. Low intensity pulsed ultrasound accelerates macrophage phagocytosis by a pathway that requires actin polymerization, Rho, and Src/MAPKs activity. Cellular Signalling 20 (4), 695–704.

Zuo, J., Zhen, J., Wang, F., Li, Y., Zhou, Z., 2018. Effect of low-intensity pulsed ultrasound on the expression of calcium ion transport-related proteins during tertiary dentin formation. Ultrasound in Medicine & Biology 44 (1), 223–233.

Chapter | 7 |

Cryotherapy: physiology and new approaches

James Selfe, Cari Thorpe, Karen May and Jill Alexander

Introduction

In a chapter that focuses on cryotherapy it is ironic to note that the homeostatic mechanisms for human thermoregulation are actually geared to protect against overheating (Sawka and Wegner, 1988). Humans have a much lower capacity to adapt to prolonged exposure to cold compared to prolonged exposure to heat (Young, 1988). Clinically, hypothermia is more common than hyperthermia (Kelman, 1980).

According to Fu et al. (2016) regulation of human body temperature takes place in a hierarchical order:

- thermal reception by temperature sensitive neurons
- integration of thermal data through neural pathways
- thermoregulatory response through separate branches of the nervous system.

There are two sets of thermal receptors in the body: those mostly located in the skin which monitor the external environmental temperature, and those mostly located in the hypothalamus which monitor the internal core temperature (Kelman, 1980). The majority of the processing and integration of thermal sensory data takes place in the hypothalamus, which then delivers an appropriate thermoregulatory response (Box 7.1). The hypothalamus maintains core body temperature in a narrow range around 37°C (Fu et al., 2016), usually between 36.1°C and 37.8°C (Anderson and Hall, 1995). The anterior hypothalamus controls heat loss through vasodilatation in the skin and sweating when body temperature increases; the posterior hypothalamus stimulates heat production through shivering and increased metabolism when body temperature decreases (Green, 1981).

Human skin temperature is lower than core temperature. Unlike core temperature, skin temperature can fluctuate widely. Heat loss to the environment is reduced when blood flow to the skin is low; conversely when there is high skin blood flow, skin temperature rises, as does heat loss to the environment (Green, 1981). In humans, there is generally a decreasing skin temperature gradient when moving from the trunk along the limbs (Fig. 7.1).

The main exception to the general reduction in skin temperature along the limbs occurs at the knee, where the patella acts as a heat shield and is normally cooler than the more distal shank and calf (Ammer, 2012) (Fig. 7.2). This is important in terms of clinical reasoning and understanding what is normal and what is potentially a sign of pathology, and when applying cryotherapy locally. For example the dose/response may be different when applying cryotherapy to a muscle injury in the lower leg compared to its application to a painful swollen knee. In a clinical environment, whether applying cryotherapy locally or to the whole body, there are also significant psychological factors that may mediate an individual's response. These include understanding the reason for the application of cryotherapy and an individual's unique perception of, and emotional reaction to, cold in terms of thermal sensation and thermal comfort.

Heat transfer

On a microscopic scale, the kinetic energy of molecules is in direct relation to thermal energy. As temperature rises, there is a molecular increase in kinetic energy (thermal agitation) manifested by increased motion and vibration. As temperature decreases, there is less molecular motion and vibration. *Thermal equilibrium* is a condition when two substances in physical contact with each other reach the same temperature – no heat flow occurs between them and they maintain a constant temperature. *Heat transfer* is the

Box 7.1 **Key factors involved in thermal homeostasis**

Thermal stress imposed on the body due to the challenge of cold is highly relative and depends on the following factors (Toner et al., 1984):
- the environmental temperature
- the temperature of the cooling medium
- individual physiological differences
  Fu et al., (2016) lists the following important physiological characteristics influencing an individual's response to thermal stress:
- overall body weight
- surface area
- thermal capacitance
- conductance of fat
- blood flow
- solar absorption for skin colour
- age
- gender
- ability to acclimatize
  The following gender differences in reaction to thermal stress have been observed (Anderson and Hall, 1995; Burse, 1979; Otte et al., 2002):
- there is little difference in heat tolerance between genders
- women have a greater number of heat-activated sweat glands but sweat less

- women commence sweating at higher skin and core temperatures
- women rely on circulatory mechanisms for heat dissipation
- men rely on evaporation for cooling
- females typically have greater levels of adipose tissue therefore demonstrate a higher insulate response to cooling

Anderson, M., Hall, S., 1995. *Sports Injury Management*. Lippincott Williams and Wilkins, Baltimore, MD.

Burse, R.L., 1979. Sex differences in human thermoregulatory response to heat and cold stress. Human Factors 21 (6), 687–699.

Fu, M., Weng, W., Chen, W., Luo, N., 2016. Review on modelling heat transfer and thermoregulatory responses in the human body. Journal of Thermal Biology 62, 189–200.

Otte, J.W., Merrick, M.A., Ingersoll, C.D., Cordova, M.L., 2002. Subcutaneous adipose tissue thickness alters cooling time during cryotherapy. Archives of Physical Medicine and Rehabilitation 83 (11), 1501–1505.

Toner, M.M., Sawka, M.N., Pandolf, K.B., 1984. Thermal responses during arm and leg and combined arm–leg exercise in water. J Appl Physiol Respir Environ Exerc Physiol 56 (5), 1355–1360.

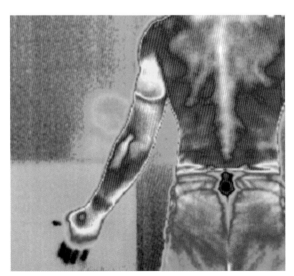

Fig. 7.1 Infrared thermal image showing the upper limb skin temperature gradient (red warmer than blue) in a healthy adult male subject.

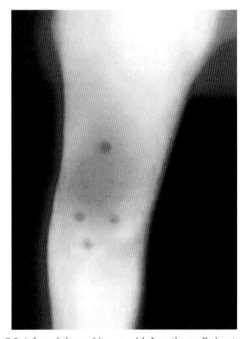

Fig. 7.2 Infrared thermal image with four thermally inert anatomical markers in place showing a cooler (orange) skin temperature over a healthy knee.

physical act of thermal energy exchange between two systems at differing temperatures. Heat transfer is always unidirectional from high to low; therefore regions that contain higher kinetic energy transfer energy to regions with lower kinetic energy (Gonzales, 2015). Merrick et al. (2003) state that cryotherapy modalities do not transfer cold to the tissues as cold (low kinetic energy) is not transferable. It is the tissues that warm the cold modalities by losing heat to them. Put another way, because heat transfer is unidirectional, cryotherapy modalities work by absorbing heat from the skin and superficial tissue. In turn, deeper tissues are cooled by heat loss to more superficial tissues. This relationship is negatively quadratic in nature (see Skin surface and deep tissue temperature relationship). There are five methods of heat transfer applicable to humans; these are described below.

Convection

When a fluid (gas or liquid) is heated, the molecules expand, become less dense, rise and are replaced with denser cooler molecules. These in turn heat up and this repetitive process creates a cycle identifiable as a convection current. In humans, this is probably the most important source of heat loss, as warm air from the surface of the skin rises and is replaced with cooler air, causing a cooling of the skin. This process is enhanced by the movement of air which helps to explain the concept of wind chill (Kelman, 1980). When cryotherapy is applied to the skin, thermal disequilibrium is created. Part of the physiological response attempting to restore thermal equilibrium is the circulation of warm blood in the superficial tissues – this transfers heat to the cooled area of skin in contact with the cryotherapy.

Conduction

Conduction transfers heat via direct molecular collision and is the most common form of heat transfer. Therapeutically this is usually achieved through local cryotherapy. When using cryotherapy modalities, heat is transferred unidirectionally from the patient to the modality. The greater the temperature difference between the cryotherapy and the patient's skin the faster the rate of heat transference (Cameron, 1999). Water has a large specific heat capacity (see Table 7.2), much higher than air, and at 10°C the conductivity of air is only 0.0151 W/mK, compared to that of water which is 0.5846 W/mK (Holmes and Willoughby, 2016). Therefore, cooling takes place rapidly and more efficiently in water or in a wet material placed against the skin. This is one justification for placing a wet towel between a bag of crushed ice and the skin during treatment. LaVelle and Snyder (1985) confirmed this when examining the effect of a variety of barriers on skin temperature when applying 500 g of chipped ice in a plastic bag for 30 min to the right ankle (Table 7.1).

Table 7.1 The effect of different barriers between skin and ice

Type of barrier	Mean skin temperature
Padded bandage	30.5°C
Unpadded bandage	20.5°C
Dry washcloth	17.8°C
No barrier	10.8°C
Damp washcloth	9.9°C

Source: LaVelle, B.E., Snyder, M., 1985. Differential conduction of cold though barriers. Journal of Advanced Nursing 10 (1), 55–61.

Radiation

Thermal radiation is a result of random movements of atoms and molecules in matter. Movement of charged protons and electrons results in the emission of electromagnetic radiation. Emissivity is defined as an object's effectiveness in emitting energy as thermal radiation. The emissivity of thermal radiation is quantified around the theoretical extremes of a perfect emitter (blackbody radiator = 1) and a perfect reflector (= 0). Humans emit significant amounts of infrared radiation and the emissivity of human skin is usually reported as 0.97 or 0.98, similar to the emissivity of ice (0.97). This is due to the high water content of skin. Infrared thermal imaging cameras can therefore be used clinically to measure changes in skin thermal radiation.

Evaporation

In humans, sweat on the skin surface is heated and vaporizes; the remaining water particles in the sweat have a lower average kinetic energy, causing the skin to cool as evaporation occurs. If sweat rolls off the skin and does not evaporate, cooling does not occur. Relative humidity is the most important factor that determines the effectiveness of evaporative heat loss. Humans can stand very high environmental temperatures if the air is dry but temperatures well below body temperature can be uncomfortable if humidity is high (Green, 1981).

Conversion

Heat transfer can also occur when nonthermal forms of energy are converted into heat (Cameron, 1999). The most common therapeutic examples of this are ultrasound and shortwave diathermy that create heat due to friction as a result of molecular agitation. From a cooling perspective, some cold packs work through endothermic chemical reactions driven through conversion of the heat absorbed from the body.

Specific heat capacity

The specific heat capacity of a substance is the amount of energy needed to change the temperature of 1 kg of the substance by 1°C (Cameron, 1999). Tissues with a higher specific heat capacity require more energy to heat them or greater energy removal to cool them. Tissues with a higher specific heat capacity store more energy than materials with a lower specific heat capacity when both are at the same temperature. The human body has a specific heat capacity similar to that of water, which is not surprising considering the average water content of the adult human body is approximately 65% (Watson et al., 1980).

It is interesting to note that, due to their high water content, frozen peas and ice have similar specific heat capacities (Table 7.2). Bags of frozen peas have often been suggested as a form of cryotherapy application. Based on the specific heat capacity, it is therefore reasonable to substitute crushed ice with frozen peas if crushed ice is unavailable. It is also noteworthy that the precise chemical composition of gel packs varies widely – currently there are in excess of 100 different products listed on the FDA devices listing (FDA,

Table 7.2 Specific heat capacity of different materials

Material	Specific heat capacity (J/g/°C)
Average for human body	3.56
Skin	3.77
Muscle	3.75
Fat	2.30
Bone	1.59
Gel pack: silica gel	1.13
Gel pack: hydroxyethyl cellulose	3.85–4.15
Frozen peas	1.98
Water	4.19
Ice	2.11
Air	1.01

Sources: Cameron, M., 1999. Physical Agents in Rehabilitation. From Research to Practice. W.B. Saunders Company. Philadelphia, PA; Moschiano, H., Dabney, W., Johnson, R., Placek, L., 2010. Thermal and electrical characterization of PAA and HEC gel used in MRI testing of active and passive medical implants. Proceedings of International Society for Magnetic Resonance in Medicine 18, Sweden.

2017), and this can have a marked influence on their performance as cooling agents.

Latent heat of fusion

Latent heat of fusion (enthalpy) is the amount of heat required for a material to undergo phase change, e.g., for ice (solid) to melt into water (liquid). When a material undergoes phase change a large quantity of energy is required to break the bonds holding the atoms in place, yet the temperature of the material remains the same. This is one of the reasons why ice is such a good cryotherapy modality, as very large amounts of heat from the body are required to achieve the phase change from solid to liquid.

Evidence base

Cryotherapy is generally inexpensive, easily self-administered, noninvasive and has few side effects (Song et al., 2016). Therefore it is a highly popular and commonly used clinical intervention. Cryotherapy has been considered the standard first-line treatment for the management of acute injury for many years. The main goal of many rehabilitation professionals is to minimize the effects of inflammation and ultimately aid return to function, i.e., work and sport, as quickly as possible (Smith, 2005). However, confusion exists as to what the precise effects of cryotherapy are on injured tissues and what the optimum clinical application protocols for cryotherapy should be, despite significant research on cryotherapy and in contrast to the understanding of the physical principles of thermodynamics (MacAuley, 2001) (Box 7.2).

It is well known that the rate of chemical reactions is temperature dependent. Q10 is the magnitude of change in the rate of a chemical reaction when there is a 10°C change in temperature. It is often suggested that Q10 = 2, i.e., the reaction rate doubles with every 10°C increase in temperature and vice versa. Despite this being an important concept when considering cryotherapy, it is unknown what the Q10 is for specific enzyme reactions following musculoskeletal injuries (Merrick, 2007).

One of the interesting clinical challenges regarding cryotherapy is the choice of temperature. Under most circumstances practitioners actually have very little control over the amount of cooling produced by the majority of commonly available modalities. Baranov and Malyseva (2006) correctly point out that the resultant temperature is usually determined by the cooling properties of the modality rather than the physiological/therapeutic aim.

A number of studies have compared different cryotherapy modalities to try and determine the most effective application. Consistently crushed or wetted ice is reported

Box 7.2 Some of the reasons for controversy in the evidence base for cryotherapy

- Varied experimental methodologies
- Different cryotherapy thermodynamic properties (thermal conductivity and specific heat capacity)
- Variation in thermal gradient, i.e., the difference between starting skin temperature (T_{sk}) and cryotherapy temperature (Fourier's law)
- Differences in size of contact areas: Compression may cause more of the cryotherapy modality to be in closer contact with the skin, resulting in improved cooling
- Variation of duration of application/exposure times
- Differing frequencies of intervention schedules
- Variety of bodily areas (muscle or joint)
- Healthy vs. injured subjects, different injury types and severity of injuries
- Differing levels of subcutaneous fat
- Different genders
- Low sample sizes

Bleakley, C., Costello, J.T., Glasgow, P.D., 2012. Should athletes return to sport after applying ice. A systematic review of the effect of local cooling on functional performance. Sports Medicine 42 (1), 69–87.

Crystal, N.J., Townson, D.H., Cook, S.B., LaRoche, D.P., 2013. Effect of cryotherapy on muscle recovery and inflammation following a bout of damaging exercise. European Journal of Applied Physiology 113 (10), 2577–2586.

Hubbard, T.J., Denegar, C.R., 2004. Does cryotherapy improve outcomes with soft tissue injury? Journal of Athletic Training 39 (3), 278–279.

MacAuley, D.C., 2001. Ice therapy: how good is the evidence? International Journal of Sports Medicine 22 (5), 379–384.

Merrick, M., Jutte, L., Smith, M., 2003. Cold modalities with different thermodynamic properties produce different surface and intramuscular temperatures. Journal of Athletic Training 38 (1), 28–33.

Merrick, M., Knight, K., Ingersoll, C., Potteiger, J., 1993. The effects of ice and compression wraps on intramuscular temperatures at various depths. Journal of Athletic Training 28 (3), 236–245.

Smith, M., 2005. A review of the initial management of soft tissue sports injuries. Journal of Orthopaedic Nursing 9 (2), 103–107.

Von Nieda, K., Michlovitz, S.L., 1996. Cryotherapy. In: Michlovitz, S.L. (Ed.), Thermal Agents in Rehabilitation, third, 3rd ed. F.A. Davies Company, Philadelphia, PA.

White, G.E., Wells, G.D., 2013. Cold-water immersion and other forms of cryotherapy: physiological changes potentially affecting recovery from high-intensity exercise. Extreme Physiology and Medicine 2 (1), 26.

as the most effective and gel packs the least effective in lowering skin temperature (T_{sk}) sufficiently to induce an analgesic response or to reduce intramuscular temperature (T_{im}) (Dykstra et al., 2009; Hardy and Woodall, 1998; Kennet et al., 2007; Selfe et al., 2009). Herrera et al. (2010) reported that the use of cold water immersion (CWI) had the most significant effect on nerve conduction velocity; this is likely to be due to the large surface area of contact.

The most well established clinical guidelines for applying local cryotherapy follow the PRICE acronym, (protection, rest, ice, compression, elevation) (Bleakley et al., 2011). However this has been superseded by the POLICE acronym (protection, optimal loading, ice, compression and elevation) (Bleakley et al., 2012c). Progression from the original PRICE guideline to the POLICE strategy encourages diverse thinking for the additional prescription of effective, controlled loading during the early management of soft tissue injuries (Bleakley et al., 2012c). The regulation of optimal loading through early rehabilitation stages is vital for recovery; Bleakley et al. (2012c) suggest optimal loading should include interventions such as manual techniques and movement regulation through the use of crutches or braces.

Dose–response

There is no consensus on the optimum method of cryotherapy application for injury management (Merrick et al., 2003; Myrer et al., 2001; White and Wells, 2013), or on dose–response relationships. The key variables yet to be understood are:

- optimum temperature
- optimum time (i.e., length of each exposure)
- optimum number of exposures per day and number of sessions per week.

Additionally, there is a growing realization that factors such as gender and adiposity have a significant bearing on the dose–response to cryotherapy, leading researchers to consider these factors more closely in an attempt to 'personalize' or target cryotherapy to the individual.

Pain is often the most obvious symptom of initial injury and the reason most patients seek advice and treatment. The main aim of cryotherapy is to decrease tissue temperature, resulting in a reduction in pain perception, nerve conduction velocity (NCV), cell metabolism and swelling (Algafly and George, 2007; Bugaj, 1975; Jutte et al., 2001; Topp et al., 2003). NCV is seen to significantly reduce in correlation to T_{sk} with an average sensory reduction of 33% demonstrated at a T_{sk} of 10 °C (Algafly and George, 2007). Supporting the concept that reduction in NCV is important in the control of pain, Algafly and George (2007) reported that changes in both pain tolerance and pain threshold were found in areas remote to the area of ice application, challenging the concept that cryotherapy influences pain in relation to the gate control theory.

It is suggested that the earlier the application of cryotherapy the more beneficial the effect, as the earliest reduction in metabolic rate will minimize the effect of secondary damage (Merrick et al., 2003). Cryotherapy is often applied with compression. This has demonstrated lower temperatures, achieved more quickly, and with greater improvements in pain and swelling compared to cryotherapy alone (Song et al., 2016). Evidence also suggests that intermittent cryotherapy application in conjunction with exercise allows patients to return to function earlier (Bleakley et al., 2011).

Skin surface and deep tissue temperature relationship

To determine the effects of cryotherapy modalities, skin surface temperature (T_{sk}) measurement is an effective method (Hardaker et al., 2007; Hildebrandt et al., 2010; Kennet et al., 2007; Selfe et al., 2009). Thermal imaging used in line with the 'Thermographic imaging in sports and exercise medicine' guidelines (Moreira et al., 2017) provides real-time, noninvasive analysis, producing accurate and reliable data (Costello et al., 2012c; Ring and Ammer, 2000; Selfe et al., 2006). Various other devices are available to record clinically relevant measures of T_{sk} including infrared digital handheld thermometers (Fig. 7.3), thermistors and contact thermography devices (Erande et al., 2016; Merrick et al., 2003). The use of tympanic temperature measurement is reported to be of poor accuracy when assessing whole-body cryotherapy applications (Cuttell et al., 2017).

A relationship between T_{sk} and T_{im} exists following the application of cryotherapy, with unidirectional heat transfer occurring from deep to superficial tissue structures. The

effect of blood flow within muscle tissue and the insulation provided by adipose tissue both reduce the effect of cooling (Hardy and Woodall, 1998; Otte et al., 2002). There is a negative quadratic relationship between T_{sk} and T_{im}, i.e., as T_{sk} increases, T_{im} decreases (Hardaker et al., 2007) (Fig. 7.4). This means deeper soft tissue structures continue cooling after the removal of cryotherapy as heat from the deeper tissues is transferred to the superficial tissues to rewarm the skin. Hardaker et al. (2007) report this deep tissue cooling continues after removal of cryotherapy in sub-adipose tissue of 3 cm depth for up to 30–40 min. This highlights the need to consider appropriate rewarming periods for deeper tissues postcryotherapy application, and the effect this is likely to have on muscle function. Clinically this becomes relevant when deciding to return an athlete to functional weight-bearing tasks or to the field of play following cryotherapy.

Effect of cooling on muscle

A variety of physiological changes such as alterations in muscle stiffness (Point et al., 2017), torque output

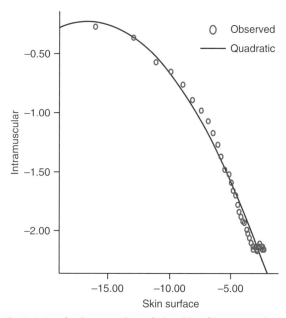

Fig. 7.4 **Quadratic regression relationship of intramuscular temperature and skin surface temperature following cooling of the quadriceps.** (From Hardaker, N., Moss, A., Richards, J., Jarvis., S., McEwan, I., Selfe, J., 2007. The relationship between skin surface temperatures measured via non-contact thermal imaging and intra-muscular temperature of the rectus femoris muscle. Thermology International 17(1), 45–50.)

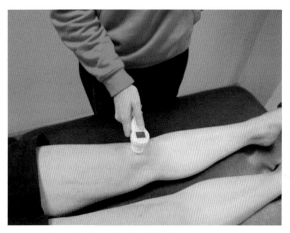

Fig. 7.3 **Handheld digital thermometer.**

(Dewhurst et al., 2010), muscle strength, power (Thornley et al., 2013) and performance recovery (Poppendieck et al., 2013) following local cryotherapy are reported in the literature. Although consensus exists regarding the reduction of NCV mediated through local cryotherapy, which contributes to decrements in muscle strength and function, some authors suggest decreases in receptor firing rates (Knight, 1995) and muscle spindle activity (Oska et al., 2000) causing strength deficits postcryotherapy. However, the magnitude of reported muscle strength reduction varies. Burgh and Ekblom (1979) reported reductions in extension torque and power of around 5% for every 1 °C decrease in T_{im}. Others, however, describe moderate (Thornley et al., 2003) or contradictory changes with increases in isometric muscle strength (Sanya and Bello, 1999) in the lower limb following local cryotherapy. Acute effects of cryotherapy on the upper limb have also demonstrated conflicting results. De Nardi et al. (2017) reported hand-grip strength improved after partial-body cooling at −110 °C in a cryotherapy chamber. In contrast, after local cryotherapy, reductions in maximal voluntary grip strength following CWI of the hand and forearm (Pathak, 2014; Rabelo et al., 2016; Vincent and Tipton, 1988) have been reported. Torres et al. (2017) reported reductions in muscle strength following a local application of cryotherapy at the shoulder.

Evidence of increased muscle stiffness (Point et al., 2017), supports the suggestion that myotatic stretch reflex variance occurs due to reductions in enzymatic activity as a result of the reduced temperatures associated with cryotherapy (Ferretti, 1992; Ranatunga et al., 1987; Rutkove, 2001). This, however, is not universally accepted, with some researchers suggesting changes in muscle activation are due to increases in motor neuron excitability (Oksa et al., 2000; Palmieri-Smith et al., 2007) and more recently that there are global viscoelastic changes following temperature change (Point et al., 2017). Within the extracellular matrix, Point et al. (2017) describe changes in active and passive elastic components that are thought to cause increases in mechanical properties of the soft tissue. It is known that muscle–tendon stiffness relates to incidences of muscle strains (Watsford et al., 2010); therefore an intrinsic inability to effectively monitor the stretch reflex within muscle following cryotherapy may increase risk of injury. This is thought to be due to limitations in the capability of the muscle–tendon unit to sustain strain coupled with increases in the shear modulus of muscle tissue.

Effect of cooling on joint position sense

Alterations in joint position sense (JPS) and proprioception (Alexander et al., 2016; 2018; Costello and Donnelly, 2010) have been reported following cryotherapy. JPS is a complex component of the somatic sensory system. It is a submodality of proprioception, specific to the awareness of a joint within a given space, controlled by mechanoreceptors located in the musculotendinous unit, ligaments and skin (Grob et al., 2002; Lephart et al., 1997). JPS acuity is important, not only for performance but also as a predictor for injury risk (Kaynak et al., 2019). The effect of cryotherapy on JPS is widely debated. There is little consensus on how JPS in the knee, for example, is affected by the application of cryotherapy; recent systematic reviews report varied conclusions (Bleakley et al., 2012a; Bleakley and Costello, 2013). Studies on the ankle (Costello and Donnelly, 2011; Hopper et al. 1997; LaRiviere and Osternig, 1994) and the shoulder (Dover and Powers, 2004; Wassinger et al. 2007) have also demonstrated conflicting results.

Alexander et al. (2015) reported an application of crushed ice to the nondominant limb for 20 min had an immediate adverse effect on weight-bearing knee joint repositioning, in particular the reproduction of knee flexion with reduced control during eccentric loading in a small knee bend. This is consistent with previously published research (Sürenkök et al., 2008; Uchio et al., 2003). Similarly, Alexander et al. (2016) highlighted prolonged adverse responses in weight-bearing knee JPS with significant reductions in rotational control 20 min following ice removal. It is not known if these reported effects on repositioning and dynamic stability occurred in relation to an increase in joint stiffness or to neuromuscular adaptations.

Although the effects of cryotherapy on JPS are not fully understood (Alexander et al., 2015; 2016; Costello and Donnelly, 2010) clinicians and therapists continue to use cryotherapy in clinical and pitch-side settings (Bleakley et al., 2010) during intermittent breaks in play to allow their athletes to continue to train or compete. Potentially this exposes their athletes to a higher risk of injury due to a proprioceptive deficit (Bleakley et al., 2006). Team doctors, clinicians and therapists should consider these findings when deciding to return an athlete to functional weight-bearing tasks or the field of play following cryotherapy, where there is the potential for increased risk of injury both immediately and at 20-min postcryotherapy.

Hindering or optimizing?

Inflammation is a natural and normal component of healing. Why then do we spend so much time and effort using cryotherapy to minimize it? One theory suggests that the reduction of swelling will 'speed up' the healing process, thereby aiding a more timely return to function. However, if we consider that inflammation, along with the components of this process, are the building blocks in the initial stages of healing, then we might question the premise of minimizing it. Physiologically, it is unlikely that healing can be accelerated with the use of cryotherapy. However, the conditions for healing to take place may be optimized. Some clinicians argue that we are using cryotherapy to ensure that the inflammatory process does not become out of control. But how do we know what 'out of control' is and whether it delays return to function? It would seem logical that anything that reduces inflammation would actually slow healing. The evidence for the use of cryotherapy in controlling oedema is also contradictory. In the post–initial injury phase there is secondary tissue death (Merrick, 2002), which has been suggested to be due to the hypoxic nature of the environment and enzymatic activity following the initial injury (Knight, 1995). Merrick (2002) states that the ability to distinguish between primary and secondary cell death is difficult, as there is considerable overlap of the two as well as an inability to determine secondary cell death from the extent of the injury or the hypoxic environment. Merrick (2002) also discussed the ischemic nature of tissue possibly resulting in secondary cell death.

Reducing tissue temperature results in a reduction in cell metabolism, thereby reducing the ischaemic or hypoxic effect and secondary cell death. The application of cryotherapy is also considered to reduce blood flow through vasoconstriction, thereby reducing oedema and further ischaemic effects on tissue (Bleakley et al., 2007). However, the majority of studies related to this have been conducted on healthy tissue and controversy over the perfusion of tissue following cryotherapy remains (Merrick, 2002). Reduction in oedema is found to be useful in reducing blood flow in animal studies, resulting in the minimization of swelling and pressure on surrounding tissues, which would impact on pain and range of movement. However, this has yet to be replicated in human trials (Bleakley et al., 2011).

Whilst cooling of tissues will result in reduced blood flow, and may serve to reduce swelling and pressure, it has been found that the prolonged application of cryotherapy can cause damage to superficial lymph vessels resulting in an increase in limb circumference and an increase in blood flow with application of superficial cold modalities (McMaster and Liddle, 1980; Meeusen and Lievens, 1986). The increase in blood flow during the inflammatory phase of healing needs consideration.

Cryotherapy modalities and methods

Many forms of local cryotherapy modalities exist, with differences in their ability to achieve a clinically therapeutic T_{sk} ranging between 10 and 15°C (Kennet et al., 2007). This makes the choice of modality an important aspect of clinical decision making (Kennet et al., 2007). Cryotherapy modalities include:

- ice (cubed, crushed, flaked and wetted)
- cold water immersion
- gel packs
- cold sprays
- ice massage
- frozen peas
- IceMan
- CryoCuff
- Game Ready
- Swellaway

Ice (crushed/cubed/wetted)

There is consensus that modalities with a higher specific heat capacity and those that pass through phase change are more effective at cooling the skin and reducing intramuscular temperature (Dykstra et al., 2009). Traditionally, the most commonly used and reported as the most effective cryotherapy modality is crushed ice. Dykstra et al. (2009) compared various types of ice used clinically, such as crushed, wetted and cubed; they reported wetted ice was more effective than crushed or cubed ice in lowering T_{sk}. The ability of wetted ice to extract heat from superficial tissues is clear and may be enhanced due to the ability of wetted ice to also conform well to bodily contours, which increases contact surface area.

Cold water immersion

CWI allows lower temperatures to be achieved and maintained compared to other modalities and it is frequently used in sport for recovery – commonly for reduction of delayed onset muscle soreness (DOMS) (Bleakley et al., 2012b; White and Wells, 2013). DOMS is often used as an injury model to assess the effectiveness of CWI, but the generalizability of this approach is in question, as an association between the inflammatory process following injury and that found postexercise has not yet been substantiated (Hawkins, 2016). CWI is commonly used in the management of acute soft tissue injury, most often in the lower limbs (Thain et al., 2015). In particular authors have reported perceived benefits in fatigue and muscle soreness (Crystal et al., 2013; Hohenauer et al., 2015; White and Wells, 2013) as well as enhanced recovery of muscle function, reduced swelling, venous O_2 saturation and plasma myoglobin (Roberts et al., 2014). Following CWI, cold-induced analgesia occurs which facilitates early rehabilitation exercises (Bleakley et al., 2004; Knight et al., 2000).

CWI has also been adopted as a strategy to reduce symptoms that would possibly interfere with competition and or training performance. However, Stephens et al. (2017) point out that there is variability in the current literature on the effectiveness of CWI for recovery and it has recently been reported that regular application of CWI may attenuate long-term adaptations to training, mainly strength gains (Peake et al., 2017). CWI studies that investigate the effect on recovery tend to observe systemic markers of inflammation following eccentric exercise or traditional resistance, but as Roberts et al. (2014) highlighted, research fails to observe changes after resistance exercise from 1–24 hours postsession. Roberts et al. (2014) reported CWI enhanced recovery of submaximal muscle function, although compared with active recovery, CWI did not alter recovery of maximal strength or countermovement jump performance. Pointon et al. (2012) examined the effects of CWI after a simulated sport collision in rugby; they suggested the use of CWI after simulated contact drills reduced perception of soreness in players.

Allan and Mawhinney (2017) report there is a lack of evidence to support the effects of CWI on postexercise inflammatory and cellular stress responses. It has been suggested that CWI used during preseason training for hypertrophic responses lacks justification because of reductions in the adaptive training responses this modality causes. Importantly the discussion highlights that available studies generally support the use of CWI within competition settings, usually in sports with quick tournament turnaround or that are highly damaging in nature. The use of CWI as a recovery strategy seems more promising for short-term recovery, i.e., during the competitive phase to allow quick recovery between events, but long-term use appears detrimental to strength and muscles mass gains (Peake et al., 2017).

Cryotherapy and compression

The PRICE guidelines (Bleakley et al., 2011) reported that there was little evidence of an optimal level of compression. The degree of external compression to hold cryotherapy modalities in place during application varies between devices and among clinicians; therefore differences occur in the magnitude of tissue cooling (Tomchuck et al., 2010).

Studies that investigate compression vs. no compression during cryotherapy suggest deeper cooling of intramuscular tissues occur when compression is applied (Jutte et al., 2001; Merrick et al., 1993). Flex-i-Wrap (Cramer Products Inc., Gardner, KS) and elastic film wraps are commonly used to hold bags of ice in place during pitch-side applications, whilst products such as IceMan or CryoCuff apply a compressive element around the limb during application from the pressure of liquid in the product design. Tomchuck et al. (2010) compared the effects of two common types of external compression on the magnitude of surface and intramuscular cooling in the lower limb during and after a 30-min ice bag treatment and reported that elastic wrap was more effective than Flex-i-Wrap at reducing intramuscular temperature. The elastic wrap probably provides a greater insulating effect (Tomchuck et al., 2010).

Pitch-side applications

Pitch-side application of cryotherapy may be considered as 'nonstandard' compared to its use in the clinical environment. There is great variability in exposure/duration times of many modalities applied during competitive play compared to the traditional PRICE guidelines, which suggest that a 20-min exposure is required to induce physiological changes in the tissues leading to an analgesic effect following acute soft tissue injury (Bleakley et al., 2012a). Specifically, T_{sk} lower than 13°C elicits an optimal analgesic response (Bleakley and Hopkins, 2010; Bugaj, 1975). In a recent review of sports physical therapists' practice, Hawkins and Hawkins (2016) reported wide variability in the application of cryotherapy. Cryotherapy is known to be applied randomly through breaks in play or at half-time in competitive fixtures (Fullam et al., 2015) but the ideal application times to achieve therapeutic responses are unknown, as is the safe period for athletes to return to sport postcooling in these circumstances. A number of studies report concerns regarding athletes returning to play following pitch-side cooling exposures of lower limb peripheral joints (Alexander et al., 2016; Costello and Donnelly, 2010; Fullam et al., 2015) due to risk of further injury. However some studies of short-duration cryotherapy application suggest there are minimal deleterious effects from these exposures (Thain et al., 2015).

Whole-body cryotherapy
Background

Developed in Japan in the 1970s, whole-body cryotherapy (WBC) has, over the last 15–30 years, gained popularity across North America and Europe. Introduced into clinical practice for the management of patients with rheumatoid arthritis (Yamauchi et al., 1981a; 1981b) WBC is becoming more accessible and has grown in use within sporting populations (Bleakley et al., 2014) and in sports medicine despite a lack of empirical evidence. A therapeutic application of cold dry air, WBC is credited anecdotally with the ability to reduce recovery time postexercise, prevent injury and reduce inflammatory responses to pathology or overuse (Furmanek et al., 2014) via a single exposure of temperatures between −110°C and −140°C (Costello et al., 2015) (Fig. 7.5).

The use of WBC is controversial and in 2016 the US Food and Drug Administration (FDA) released a consumer health information statement entitled *Whole Body Cryotherapy (WBC): A 'Cool' Trend that Lacks Evidence, Poses Risks* (FDA, 2016). This warned consumers about misleading medically related claims concerning the use of WBC and

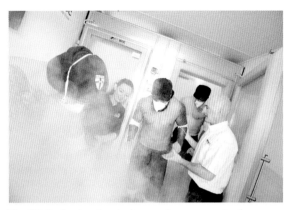

Fig. 7.5 Professional rugby league players emerging from a mobile whole-body cryotherapy unit.

pointed out that no WBC device at that time had received FDA clearance or approval as a safe and effective medical device. However, WBC is not strictly limited to just treating medical conditions; it is also being used in sport to enhance performance and recovery. Nonetheless the concerns expressed by the FDA over the lack of evidence on the safety and effectiveness of WBC remain pertinent for any practitioners involved in the administration of WBC, whether for medical or sport applications.

There are two main types of cryogenic chamber: WBC chambers that include cooling of the head (see Fig. 7.5) and partial-body cryotherapy (PBC) chambers where the design of the chamber excludes the head.

Louis et al. (2015) reported that both WBC and PBC stimulate the autonomic nervous system (ANS), with WBC providing only a slightly greater stimulation than PBC. Therefore, exposure to cooling via cryostimulation of the whole body including the head may not be the main influence of ANS changes (Louis et al., 2015). Some WBC research indicates that it provides improvement in recovery and reduction in muscle soreness, with a specific focus on the physiological and molecular effects (Russell et al., 2017; Ziemann et al., 2014). Optimal WBC protocols for treatment sessions in sporting and clinical environments are still contentious, with considerations for anthropometry and gender influencing duration and exposure times (Cuttell et al., 2017; Hammond et al., 2014). Typically exposure times are quoted as being between 1 and 3 min per single session, although there are known differences in physiological outcomes when comparing single-bout exposure times. Selfe et al. (2014) reported an optimum exposure of 2 min at −135°C, where a 2-min WBC exposure induced potentially beneficial physiological and perceptual changes, greater than those achieved following a 1-min WBC exposure but without any of the negative effects demonstrated

by a 3-min exposure. In contrast, Pournot et al. (2011) observed positive changes following multiple exposures of WBC at 3 min, suggesting positive reductions in inflammatory responses postexercise. A recent Cochrane review highlights that single-session 2–4 min exposures are generally implemented in WBC protocols (Costello et al., 2015).

WBC and physiology

There appear to be significant physiological reactions in response to WBC, including analgesia reactions in both the circulatory and immune systems as well as reductions in swelling (Lombardi et al., 2017). Some authors have highlighted that WBC does not reduce T_{sk} to <13°C to induce analgesia over the patella region (Costello et al., 2014) unlike direct cooling modalities. With regard to determining the depth of cooling achieved by WBC (whether superficial, deep, muscular or core body temperature) there are a very limited number of studies available (Holmes and Willoughby, 2016). Selfe et al. (2014) reported on T_{sk} and core body temperature changes following three randomized exposures of WBC, noting significant reductions in T_{sk} but no changes in core body temperature. It has been suggested that this may be due to vascular shunting to maintain the function of vital organs. Additionally, Costello et al. (2012b) investigated T_{im} pre- and post-WBC exposure and reported comparable decreases in skin, muscle and core temperature to CWI applications after a single WBC exposure of −110°C.

As previously mentioned, body composition can affect WBC cooling efficiency and potentially treatment effectiveness, with a recent study by Cuttell et al. (2017) highlighting the differences noted in mean body temperature between the sexes and local site-specific T_{sk} measurements. This study identified the importance of optimizing WBC treatments by taking into account dimorphism between the sexes. An earlier study by Hammond et al. (2014) noted the relationship between percentage body fat and T_{sk} response after WBC; they found that males presenting with higher levels of adipose tissue cooled significantly more than those with less adipose tissue.

Reductions in inflammatory markers (Banfi et al., 2009; 2010; Lubkowska et al., 2010; Wozniak et al., 2007) and changes to haematological profiles (Twist et al., 2012) are thought to have positive effects on exercise-induced muscle damage (EIMD) and on DOMS (Pournot et al., 2011). A number of papers suggest that inflammation-induced bone resorption may be counteracted post-WBC (Lombardi et al., 2017), therefore the use of WBC may support post-fracture recovery (Galliera et al., 2012).

Most endocrinological studies suggest changes occur in hormone levels with WBC exposure (Lombardi et al., 2017), which is particularly important when considering workloads in athletes. In the majority of studies using sporting populations, levels of hormones such as cortisol associated with psychophysical stress changed; it either decreased (Wozniak et al., 2013) or increased (Ziemann et al., 2012). However some authors reported no change (Russell et al., 2017; Sutkowy et al., 2014). Increases in testosterone levels have also been reported (Grasso et al., 2014; Russell et al., 2017), but other studies demonstrate no change post-WBC exposure (Sutkowy et al., 2014). These inconsistencies in results most likely highlight differences in the stress levels applied across different sports and the different WBC protocols used.

Inflammatory markers have been more commonly investigated (Lombardi et al., 2017) and are a key topic of interest. Suggestions that WBC reduces inflammation are common; however, as mentioned above, comparison between studies is difficult due to protocol variability and heterogeneity of participants from a variety of sporting, nonsporting, normative and systemic pathology populations (Bettoni et al., 2013; Lombardi et al., 2017). Despite this, there still appears to be a dearth of literature on which to form a consensus as to whether levels of inflammation are reduced by WBC and whether this has any positive benefits on performance or recovery.

WBC and recovery

Ziemann et al. (2012; 2014) reported no changes in resting metabolic rates or energy expenditure during exercise following multiple-exposure treatments of WBC. Costello et al. (2015) suggest more studies should compare WBC to known effective modalities such as CWI when assessing its effectiveness in muscle recovery postexercise. A number of studies have investigated the role of WBC in aiding muscle recovery (Fonda and Sarabon, 2013; Markovic et al., 2014; Pournot et al., 2011; Selfe et al., 2014) and in comparison to other cryotherapy modalities (Abaïdia et al., 2017; Holmes and Willoughby, 2016). Bleakley et al. (2014) propose that whilst WBC may achieve reductions in tissue temperature comparable with other methods of cryotherapy, perception of recovery may be diminished by awareness of the weak standard of evidence; this may override or lessen the impact of actual recovery through enhanced performance or function when combatting EIMD. Holmes and Willoughby (2016) attempted to synthesize current WBC data, yet were unable to establish overall guidelines or protocols for use in sporting populations for recovery benefits. This is probably due to the variety of inflammatory markers used across the studies. Holmes and Willoughby (2016) compared WBC to CWI using several markers of physiological change commonly associated with sport recovery (White and Wells, 2013) and reported that WBC was less effective than CWI at reducing tissue temperature. They suggest

this is due to the increased rewarming speed post-WBC exposure.

One of the key biomarkers measured in this field of research is interleukin 6 (IL-6) which is secreted by T cells and macrophages during infection and after trauma. IL-6 is both pro- and antiinflammatory as it assists in initiating the immune response and it plays a role in fighting infection. Lombardi et al. (2017) confirm that an antiinflammatory effect occurs in response to WBC but that differences in reported IL-6 levels occur across studies due to protocol variation. The consensus suggests that single sessions of WBC increase the concentration of Il-6, whereas baseline levels recover following multiple exposures (Lombardi et al., 2017).

The impact of WBC exposures on sports performance with respect to functional recovery requires further study to investigate the full extent of effects. Poppendieck et al. (2013) and Pournot et al. (2011) reported positive effects in elite athletic groups from postexercise cooling, suggesting that WBC accelerates recovery when administered immediately postexercise but overall evidence is limited (Kępińska et al., 2013; Lombardi et al., 2017). Although minimal benefits in functional recovery are reported (Hornery et al., 2005; Zalewski et al., 2014), subjective recovery appears to be sustained (Bleakley et al., 2014). Further studies should investigate similar functional recovery protocols to Kruger et al. (2015) who have reported on postexercise recovery in WBC-treated athletes and noted improvements in working muscle oxygenation alongside cardiovascular strain reductions.

WBC and injury

Pain scores related to soreness perception following strenuous exercise or training are reported to improve following WBC (Pournot et al., 2011; Russell et al., 2017; Ziemann et al., 2014). Many more studies have investigated the effect of WBC on EIMD (Banfi et al., 2009; Ferreira-Junior et al., 2014) compared to its effect on posttraumatic sports injury. Therefore, it is only possible to make theoretical assumptions as to the reported antiinflammatory effects of WBC on acute injuries.

WBC and psychology

The reported impact of WBC exposures on psychological factors is generally positive. Lower fatigue and improvement in mood alongside reduction of clinical depression syndromes, and better sleep and sleep quality are described following repeated WBC treatments (Rymaszewska et al., 2007; Sieroń et al., 2007).

Pournot et al. (2011) found reduced psychological perceptions of pain and muscular tiredness following WBC exposure. This has been supported by Schaal et al. (2015) who found improvements in training load tolerance due to better sleep following daily 3-min WBC treatments at −110°C. This randomized controlled study proposed that the advantageous effects of WBC on duration of sleep and latency was due to postexercise parasympathetic reactivation. In contrast to the above studies, Russell et al. (2017) reported no effect on recovery or soreness perception following a single WBC exposure at −135°C for 2 min. Once again, it is difficult to compare the results of Russell et al. (2017) to Schaal et al. (2015) due to disparities in both the gender of participants and the number of WBC exposures.

Discrepancies in research results appear to be related to the variation in WBC exposure, ranging from multiple exposures within short periods of time, e.g., training camp–like periods (Ziemann et al., 2014) to repeated exposures throughout the off-season training sessions (Russell et al., 2017; Schaal et al., 2015). It is worth noting, however, that WBC has been shown to significantly enhance patient wellbeing and mood; Szczepanska-Gieracha et al. (2014) reported improvements in psychological and somatic aspects resulting in improved quality of life.

WBC and systemic pathologies

The use of cryotherapy in the treatment of a range of inflammatory diseases is widely accepted and well documented. Physiological reactions such as analgesic, anti-inflammatory, vasoconstrictive, anti-oedematous and antioxidative effects have been reported (Demoulin and Vanderthommen, 2012; Guillot et al., 2014; Oosterveld and Rasker, 1994). Whilst cryotherapy can be used in rheumatological disorders such as rheumatoid arthritis (RA), spondyloarthritis and gout (Oosterveld and Rasker, 1994) it is also advocated for painful arthropathies such as osteoarthritis, capsulitis and fibromyalgia (Bettoni et al., 2013; Chatap et al., 2007; Demoulin and Vanderthommen, 2012). WBC has additionally been found to affect bone biomarkers (Galliera et al., 2012) and is useful in neurological disorders including multiple sclerosis (MS) due to its effect on antioxidants. Oxidative stress is a hallmark of many chronic diseases including neurodegenerative and cardiovascular disorders (Miller et al., 2010a; 2012) and has an influence on depressive and anxiety disorders (Rymaszewska et al., 2008). WBC has been utilized as an adjunct to improve pharmacological and rehabilitation protocols in many diseases of the musculoskeletal system. The precise mechanisms of such treatments, especially WBC and the influence of extremely low temperatures on the human body and physiological reactions, are still not fully understood (Lange et al. 2008; Lubkowska et al., 2010; Miller et al. 2010a; 2010b; 2010c; Stanek et al., 2010).

Clinical studies and those on animal models suggest that mild hypothermia has an antiinflammatory effect (Lubkowska et al., 2011) that may inhibit white blood cell infiltrate formation, proinflammatory cytokine gene transcription and enzymatic pathways (Guillot et al., 2014). Elevated levels of inflammatory markers such as serum C reactive protein (CRP), mucoproteins, plasma fibrinogen concentration as well as erythrocyte sedimentation rate (ESR) present in ankylosing spondylitis (AS) were reduced to a statistically significant degree following exposure to a cycle of 10 daily WBC sessions of −120°C for 2 min; similar results were also found in healthy subjects (Stanek et al., 2010). Guillot et al. (2014) substantiated these positive findings in their systematic review where they also noted that WBC tends to decrease serum IL-6 and histamine levels in RA patients.

These findings suggest a potential therapeutic effect for inflammatory rheumatic diseases such as RA, where these molecular pathways are shown to be linked with pain, reduced disease activity scores such as the Disease Activity Score using 28 joint counts (DAS28), biological inflammatory markers and radiographically visible joint changes. WBC has been shown to significantly reduce both pain reports and DAS28 score in RA patients (Guillot et al., 2014).

Miller et al. (2010a; 2010b; 2010c) reported that a series of 10 sessions of WBC had a significant and positive effect in MS patients with neurological deficits in relation to increased muscle strength and levels of antioxidative status, with a reduction in spasticity and disability. As outlined above, hypothermia has antiinflammatory effects and is a neuroprotectant, reducing intracellular acidosis and ischaemia. Hypothermia also inhibits generation of oxygen free radicals involved in secondary damage from reperfusion, linked to inhibition of reactive oxygen species (ROS) (Gilgun-Sherki et al., 2004; Miller et al., 2010a). ROS is a cause of damage to cellular structures such as proteins, nucleic acids (e.g., DNA) and lipids and is implicated in neuronal damage resulting in cellular necrosis and subsequent pathogenesis of MS (Gilgun-Sherki et al., 2004; Miller et al., 2010a).

Dangers, contraindications and adverse event reporting for cryotherapy

Although low risk, adverse reactions to the application of local cryotherapy are reported (Cipollaro, 1992; Cuthill and Cuthill, 2006; O'Toole and Rayatt, 1999; Selfe et al., 2007), these include reductions in muscle function, nerve damage and scarring of the skin. Contraindications due

Box 7.3 **Contraindications to cryotherapy**

- Acute cardiovascular disorders
- Acute respiratory disorders
- Any mental disorders which may affect cooperation of the exposure protocol
- Cachexia
- Claustrophobia
- Cold intolerance
- Cryoglobulinaemia
- Hypothermia
- Hypothyroidism
- Local blood flow disorders
- Purulent or gangrenous cutaneous lesions
- Raynaud's syndrome
- Sympathetic neuropathies

Lombardi, G., Ziemann, E., Banfi, G., 2017. Whole-body cryotherapy in athletes: from therapy to stimulation. An updated review of the literature. Frontiers in Physiology 8 (258), 1–16.

to physiological changes caused by more extensive cooling, such as WBC as a medical treatment are noted and clinicians should follow current guidelines (Box 7.3). Clinicians should be aware of contraindications prior to cryotherapy application and should carefully monitor patients for any adverse reactions during the application of cryotherapy.

Only one study to date has reported on adverse reactions during WBC exposure (Selfe et al., 2014). Selfe et al. (2014) investigated the effects of WBC in a group of elite rugby league players and reported a mild superficial skin burn in one Samoan player with a known intolerance to cold. This player had failed to disclose this information prior to WBC exposure despite careful screening. This superficial burn resulted in minor blistering and erythema bilaterally over the player's anterior thigh. Although able to train and play competitively following this adverse reaction, it emphasizes the importance of careful screening of athletes or patients prior to applying any form of cryotherapy.

References

Abaïdia, A.E., Lambin, J., Delecroix, B., Leduc, C., McCall, A., Nédélec, M., et al., 2017. Recovery from exercise-induced muscle damage: cold-water immersion versus whole-body cryotherapy. International Journal of Sports Physiology and Performance 12 (3), 402–409.

Alexander, J., Selfe, J., Oliver, B., Mee, D., Carter, A., Scott, M., et al., 2016. An exploratory study into the effects of a 20 minute crushed ice application on knee joint position sense during a small knee bend. Physical Therapy Sport 18, 21–26.

Alexander, J., Richards, J., Attah, O., Cheema, S., Snook, J., Wisdell, C., et al., 2018. Delayed effects of a 20-min crushed ice application on knee joint position sense assessed by a functional task during a re-warming period. Gait & Posture 62, 173–178.

Alexander, J., Selfe, J., Oliver, B., Mee, D., Carter, A., Scott, M., et al., 2016. The effects of a 20 minute crushed ice application on knee joint position sense during a small knee bend. Physical Therapy Sport 18, 21–26.

Algafly, A., George, K., 2007. The effect of cryotherapy on nerve conduction velocity, pain threshold and pain tolerance. British Journal of Sports Medicine 41 (6), 365–369.

Allan, R., Mawhinney, C., 2017. Is the ice bath finally melting? Cold water immersion is no greater than active recovery upon local and systemic inflammatory cellular stress in humans. The Journal of Physiology 595 (6), 1857–1858.

Ammer, K., 2012. Temperature of the human knee – a review. Thermology International 22 (4), 137–151.

Anderson, M., Hall, S., 1995. *Sports Injury Management*. Lippincott Williams and Wilkins, Baltimore, MD.

Banfi, G., Lombardi, G., Columbini, A., Melegati, G., 2010. Whole-body cryotherapy in athletes. Sports Medicine 40 (6), 509–517.

Banfi, G., Melegati, G., Barassi, A., Dogliotti, G., d'Egril, G., Dugue, B., Corsi Romanelli, M., 2009. Effects of whole-body cryotherapy on serum mediators of inflammation and serum muscle enzymes in athletes. Journal of Thermal Biology 34 (2), 55–59.

Baranov, A., Malyseva, T., 2006. Thermophysical processes of cryotherapy. In: Podbielska, H., Strek, W., Bialy, D. (Eds.), Whole-Body Cryotherapy. Acta of Biomedical Engineering. Kriotechnika Medyczna Sp., Warsaw, pp. 27–33.

Bettoni, L., Bonomi, F., Zani, V., Manisco, L., Indelicato, A., Lanteri, P., et al., 2013. Effects of 15 consecutive cryotherapy sessions on the clinical output of fibromyalgia patients. Clinical Rheumatology 32 (9), 1337–1345.

Bleakley, C., Costello, J.T., Glasgow, P.D., 2012a. Should athletes return to sport after applying ice. A systematic review of the effect of local cooling on functional performance. Sports Medicine 42 (1), 69–87.

Bleakley, C., McDonough, S., MacAuley, D., 2006. Cryotherapy for acute ankle sprains: a randomised controlled study of two different icing protocols. British Journal of Sports Medicine 40, 700–705.

Bleakley, C., McDonough, S., Gardner, E., Baxter, G.D., Hopkins, J.T., Davison, G.W., 2012b. Cold-water immersion (cryotherapy) for preventing and treating muscle soreness after exercise. Cochrane Database of Systematic Reviews (2), CD008262.

Bleakley, C., McDonough, S., MacAuley, D., 2004. The use of ice in the treatment of acute soft-tissue injury: a systematic review of randomized controlled trials. American Journal of Sports Medicine 32 (1), 251–261.

Bleakley, C.M., Costello, J.T., 2013. Do thermal agents affect range of movement and mechanical properties in soft tissues? A systematic review. Archives of Physical Medicine and Rehabilitation 94 (1), 149–163.

Bleakley, C.M., Glasgow, P.D., Philips, N., Hanna, L., Callaghan, M.J., Davison, G.W., et al., 2011. Management of Acute Soft Tissue Injury Using Protection Rest Ice Compression and Elevation: Recommendations from the Association of Chartered Physiotherapists in Sports Medicine (ACPSM). ACPSM, London.

Bleakley, C.M., Hopkins, J.T., 2010. Is it possible to achieve optimal levels of tissue cooling in cryotherapy? Physical Therapy Reviews 15 (4), 344–351.

Bleakley, C.M., O'Connor, S., Tully, M.A., Rocke, L.G., Macauley, D.C., McDonough, S.M., 2007. The PRICE study (Protection Rest Ice Compression Elevation): design of a randomised controlled trial comparing standard versus cryokinetic ice applications in the management of acute ankle sprain [IS-RCTN13903946]. BMC Musculoskeletal Disorders 8, 125.

Bleakley, C., Bieuzen, F., Davison, G.W., Costello, J.T., 2014. Whole-body cryotherapy: empirical evidence and theoretical perspectives. Journal of Sports Medicine 5, 25–36.

Bleakley, C.M., Glasgow, P., MacAuley, D.C., 2012c. PRICE needs updating should we call the POLICE? British Journal of Sports Medicine 46 (4), 220–221.

Bugaj, R., 1975. The cooling, analgesic, and rewarming effects of ice massage on localized skin. Physical Therapy 55 (1), 11–1.

Burgh, U., Ekblom, B., 1979. Influence of muscle temperature on maximal muscle strength and power output in human skeletal muscles. Acta Physiologica Scandinavica 107 (1), 33–37.

Cameron, M., 1999. Physical Agents in Rehabilitation. From Research to Practice. W.B. Saunders Company, Philadelphia, PA.

Chatap, G., De Sousa, A., Giraud, K., Vincent, J.P., 2007. Pain in the elderly: prospective study of hyperbaric CO_2 cryotherapy (neurocryostimulation). Joint Bone Spine 74 (6), 617–621.

Cipollaro, V.A., 1992. Cryogenic injury due to local application of a reusable cold compress. Cutis 50 (2), 111–112.

Costello, J.T., Algar, L.A., Donnelly, A.E., 2012a. Effects of whole-body cryotherapy (−110°C) on proprioception and indices of muscle damage. Scandinavian Journal of Medicine & Science in Sports 22 (2), 190–198.

Costello, J.T., Culligan, K., Selfe, J., Donnelly, A.E., 2012b. Muscle, skin and core temperature after −110°C cold air and 8°C water treatment. PLoS One 7 (11):e48190.

Costello, J.T., Donnelly, A.E., Karki, A., Selfe, J., 2014. Effects of whole body cryotherapy and cold water immersion on knee skin temperature. International Journal of Sports Medicine 35 (1), 35–40.

Costello, J., Donnelly, A.E., 2011. Effects of cold water immersion on knee joint position sense in healthy volunteers. Journal of Sports Science 29 (5), 449–456.

Costello, J.T., Donnelly, A.E., 2010. Cryotherapy and joint position sense in healthy participants: a systematic review. Journal of Athletic Training 45 (3), 306–316.

Costello, J.T., Baker, P.R.A., Minett, G.M., Bieuzen, F., Stewart, I.B., Bleakley, C., 2015. Whole-Body cryotherapy (extreme cold air exposure) for preventing and treating muscle soreness after exercise in adults (Review). Cochrane Database of Systematic Reviews (9), CD010789.

Costello, J.T., McInerney, C., Bleakley, C., Selfe, J., Donnelly, A.E., 2012c. The use of thermal imaging in assessing skin temperature following cryotherapy: a review. Journal of Thermal Biology 37 (2), 103–110.

Crystal, N.J., Townson, D.H., Cook, S.B., LaRoche, D.P., 2013. Effect of cryotherapy on muscle recovery and inflammation following a bout of damaging exercise. European Journal of Applied Physiology 113 (10), 2577–2586.

Cuthill, J.A., Cuthill, G.S., 2006. Partial-thickness burn to the leg following application of a cold pack: case report and results of a questionnaire survey of Scottish physiotherapists in private practice. Physiotherapy 92 (1), 61–65.

Cuttell, S., Hammond, L., Langdon, D., Costello, J., 2017. Individualising the exposure of −110°C whole body cryotherapy: the effects of sex and body composition. Journal of Thermal Biology 65, 41–47.

De Nardi, M., Pizzigalli, L., Benis, R., Caffaro, F., Cremasco, M., Micheletti, M., 2017. Acute effects of partial-body cryotherapy on isometric strength: maximum handgrip strength evaluation. Journal of Strength and Conditioning Research 31 (12), 3497–3502.

Demoulin, C., Vanderthommen, M., 2012. Cryotherapy in rheumatic diseases. Joint Bone Spine 79 (2), 117–118.

Dewhurst, S., Macaluso, A., Gizzi, L., Felici, F., Forina, D., De Vito, G., 2010. Effects of altered muscle temperature on neuromuscular properties in young and older women. European Journal of Applied Physiology 108 (3), 451–458.

Dover, G., Powers, M.E., 2004. Cryotherapy does not impair shoulder joint position sense. Archives of Physical Medicine and Rehabilitation 85, 1241–1246.

Dykstra, J.H., Hill, H.M., Miller, M.G., Cheatham, C.C., Michael, T.J., Baker, R.J., 2009. Comparisons of cubed ice, crushed ice, and wetted ice on intramuscular and surface temperature changes. Journal of Athletic Training 44 (2), 136–141.

Erande, R., Dey, M., Richards, J., Selfe, J., 2016. An investigation of the relationship between thermal imaging and digital thermometer testing at the knee. Physiotherapy Practice and Research 37 (1), 41–47.

FDA, 2016. Whole Body Cryotherapy (WBC): a 'Cool' trend that lacks evidence, poses risks. Available at: https://www.fda.gov/ForConsumers/ConsumerUpdates/ucm508739.htm.

FDA, 2017. https://www.accessdata.fda.gov/scripts/cdrh/cfdocs/cfRL/rl.cfm

Ferreira-Junior, J.B., Bottaro, M., Loenneke, J.P., Vieira, A., Vieira, C., Bemben, M.G., 2014. Could whole-body cryotherapy (below −100°C) improve muscle recovery from muscle damage? Frontiers in Physiology 5, 247.

Ferretti, G., 1992. Cold and muscle performance. International Journal of Sports Medicine 13 (Suppl. 1), S185–S187.

Fonda, B., Sarabon, N., 2013. Effects of whole-body cryotherapy on recovery after hamstring damaging exercise: a crossover study. Scandinavian Journal of Medicine and Science in Sports 23 (5), 270–278.

Fu, M., Weng, W., Chen, W., Luo, N., 2016. Review on modelling heat transfer and thermoregulatory responses in the human body. Journal of Thermal Biology 62, 189–200.

Fullam, K., Caulfield, B., Coughlan, G.F., McGroarty, M., Delahunt, E., 2015. Dynamic postural-stability deficits after cryotherapy to the ankle joint. Journal of Athletic Training 50 (9), 893–904.

Furmanek, M.P., Slomka, K., Juras, G., 2014. The effects of cryotherapy on proprioception system. Biomed Research International 2014, 696397.

Galliera, E., Dogliotti, D., Melegati, G., Corsi Romanelli, M.M., Cabitza, P., Banfi, G., 2012. Bone remodelling biomarkers after whole-body cryotherapy (WBC) in elite rugby players. Injury 44 (8), 1117–1121.

Gilgun-Sherki, Y., Melamed, E., Offen, D., 2004. The role of oxidative stress in the pathogenesis of multiple sclerosis. The need for the effective antioxidant therapy. Journal of Neurology 251 (3), 261–268.

Gonzalez, C., 2015. What's the difference between conduction, convection, and radiation? machine design. Available at: http://machinedesign.com/whats-difference-between/what-s-difference-between-conduction-convection-and-radiation.

Grasso, D., Lanteri, P., Di Bernardo, C., Mauri, C., Porcelli, S., Colombini, A., et al., 2014. Salivary steroid hormones response to whole-body cryotherapy in elite rugby players. Journal of Biological Regulators and Homeostatic Agents 28 (2), 291–300.

Green, J.H., 1981. An Introduction to Human Physiology, Forth ed, Oxford University Press, Oxford.

Grob, K.R., Kuster, M.S., Higgins, S.A., Lloyd, D.G., Yata, H., 2002. Lack of correlation between different measurements of proprioception in the knee. The Journal of Bone and Joint Surgery British 84 (4), 614–618.

Guillot, X., Tordi, N., Mourot, L., Demougeot, C., Dugue, B., Prati, C., et al., 2014. Cryotherapy in inflammatory rheumatic diseases: a systematic review. Expert Review of Clinical Immunology 10 (2), 281–294.

Hammond, L.E., Cuttell, S., Nunley, P., Meyler, J., 2014. Anthropometric characteristics and sex influence magnitude of skin cooling following exposure to whole body cryotherapy. Biomed Research International 2014, 628724.

Hardaker, N., Moss, A., Richards, J., Jarvis, S., McEwan, I., Selfe, J., 2007. The relationship between skin surface temperatures measured via non-contact thermal imaging and intra-muscular temperature of the rectus femoris muscle. Thermology International 17 (1), 45–50.

Hardy, M., Woodall, W., 1998. Therapeutic effects of heat, cold and stretch and connective tissue. Journal of Hand Therapy 11 (2), 148–156.

Hawkins, J.R., 2016. Is the clinical use of ice still relevant? Experimental Physiology 101, 789-789.

Hawkins, S.W., Hawkins, J.R., 2016. Clinical applications of cryotherapy among sports physical therapists. International Journal of Sports Physical Therapy 11 (1), 141–148.

Herrera, E., Sandoval, M.C., Camargo, D.M., Salvini, T.F., 2010. Motor and sensory nerve conduction are affected differently via ice pack, ice massage and cold water immersion. Physical Therapy 90 (4), 581–591.

Hildebrandt, C., Raschner, C., Ammer, K., 2010. An overview of recent application of medical infrared thermography in sports medicine in Austria. Sensors 10 (5), 4700–4715.

Hohenauer, E., Taeymans, J., Baeyens, J.P., Clarys, P., Clijsen, R., 2015. The effect of post-exercise cryotherapy on recovery characteristics: a systematic review and meta-analysis. PLoS One 10 (9):e0139028.

Holmes, M., Willoughby, D.S., 2016. The effectiveness of whole body cryotherapy compared to cold water immersion: implications for sports and exercise recovery. International Journal of Kinesiology and Sports Science 4 (4), 32–39.

Hopper, D., Whittington, D., Davies, J., 1997. Does ice immersion influence ankle joint position sense? Physiotherapy Research International 2 (4), 223–236.

Hornery, D.J., Papalia, S., Mujika, I., Hann, A., 2005. Physiological and performance of half-time cooling. Journal of Science and Medicine in Sport 8 (1), 15–25.

Jutte, L.S., Merrick, M.A., Ingersoll, C.D., Edwards, J.E., 2001. The relationship between intramuscular temperature, skin temperature, and adipose thickness during cryotherapy and rewarming. Archives of Physical Medicine and Rehabilitation 82 (6), 845–850.

Jutte, L.S., Merrick, M.A., Ingersoll, C.D., Edwards, J.E., 2001. The relationship between intramuscular temperature, skin temperature, and adipose thickness during cryotherapy and rewarming. Archives of Physical Medicine and Rehabilitation 82 (6), 845–850.

Kaynak, H., Altun, M., Tok, S., 2019. Effect of force sense to active joint position sense and relationships between active joint position sense, force sense, jumping and muscle strength. Journal of Motor Behavior 1–10.

Kelman, G.R., 1980. Physiology: a Clinical Approach, third ed, Churchill Livingstone, Edinburgh.

Kennet, J., Hardaker, N., Hobbs, S., Selfe, J., 2007. A comparison of four cryotherapeutic modalities on skin temperature reduction in the healthy ankle. Journal of Athletic Training 42 (3), 343–348.

Kępińska, M., Bednarek, J., Szygua, Z., Teleglow, A., Dabrowski, Z., 2013. A comparison of the efficacy of three different cryotherapy treatments used in the athletic recovery of sports people – literature review. Medicina Sportiva 17 (3), 142–146.

Knight, K.L., 1995. Cryotherapy in Sport Injury Management. Human Kinetics, Champaign, IL.

Knight, K.L., Brucker, J.B., Stoneman, P.D., Rubley, M.D., 2000. Muscle injury management with cryotherapy. Athletic Therapy Today 5 (4), 26–30.

Kruger, M., de Marees, M., Dittmar, K., Sperlich, B., Mester, J., 2015. Whole-body cryotherapy's enhancement of acute recovery of running performance in well-trained athletes. International Journal of Sports Physiology and Performance 10 (5), 605–612.

Lange, U., Uhlemann, C., Muller-Ladner, U., 2008. [Serial whole-body cryotherapy in the criostream for inflammatory rheumatic diseases. A pilot study]. Med Klin 103 (6), 383–388.

LaRiviere, J., Osternig, L.R., 1994. The effect of ice immersion on joint position sense. Journal of Sport Rehabilitation 3 (1), 58–67.

LaVelle, B.E., Snyder, M., 1985. Differential conduction of cold though barriers. Journal of Advanced Nursing 10 (1), 55–61.

Lephart, S.M., Pincivero, D.M., Giraldo, J.L., Fu, F.H., 1997. The role of proprioception in the management and rehabilitation of athletic injuries. The American Journal of Sports Medicine 25, 130–137.

Lombardi, G., Ziemann, E., Banfi, G., 2017. Whole-body cryotherapy in athletes: from therapy to stimulation. an updated review of the literature. Frontiers in Physiology 8 (258), 1–16.

Louis, J., Schaal, K., Bieuzen, F., Le Meur, Y., Filliard, J.R., Volondat, M., et al., 2015. Head exposure to cold during whole body cryostimulation: Influence on thermal response and autonomic modulation. PLoS One 10 (4), 1–18.

Lubkowska, A., Banfi, G., Doidgowska, B., Melzi d'Eril, V.G., Guczak, J., Barassi, A., 2010. Changes in lipid profile in response to three different protocols of whole-body cryostimulation treatments. Cryobiology 61 (1), 22–26.

Lubkowska, A., Szygula, Z., Chlubek, D., Banfi, G., 2011. The effect of prolonged whole body cryostimulation treatment with different amounts of sessions on chosen pro- and anti-inflammatory cytokines levels in healthy men. Scandinavian Journal of Clinical and Laboratory Investigation 71 (5), 419–425.

Lubkowska, A., Szygula, Z., Klimek, A.J., Torii, M., 2010. Do sessions of cryostimulation have influence on white blood cell count, level of IL6 and total oxidative and antioxidative status in healthy men? European Journal of Applied Physiology 109 (1), 67–72.

MacAuley, D.C., 2001. Ice therapy: how good is the evidence? International Journal of Sports Medicine 22 (5), 379–384.

Markovic, G., Fonda, B., Nejc, Š., 2014. Does whole-body cryotherapy affect the recovery process after hamstring damaging exercise: A crossover study. British Journal of Sports Medicine 48 (7), 633.

McMaster, W.C., Liddle, S., 1980. Cryotherapy influence on post-traumatic limb edema. Clinical Orthopaedics and Related Research 150, 283–287.

Meeusen, R., Lievens, P., 1986. The use of cryotherapy in sports injuries. Journal of Sports Medicine 3 (6), 398–414.

Merrick, M., 2007. Physiological basis of physical agents. In: Magee, D.J., Zachazewski, J.E., Quillen, W.S. (Eds.), Scientific Foundations and Principles of Practice in Musculoskeletal Rehabilitation. Saunders, St Louis, MO.

Merrick, M., Jutte, L., Smith, M., 2003. Cold modalities with different thermodynamic properties produce different surface and intramuscular temperatures. Journal of Athletic Training 38 (1), 28–33.

Merrick, M., Knight, K., Ingersoll, C., Potteiger, J., 1993. The effects of ice and compression wraps on intramuscular temperatures at various depths. Journal of Athletic Training 28 (3), 236–245.

Merrick, M.A., 2002. Secondary injury after musculoskeletal trauma: a review and update. Journal of Athletic Training 37 (2), 209–217.

Miller, E., Mrowicka, M., Malinowska, K., Mrowicki, J., Saluk-Juszczak, J., Kędziora, J., 2010a. Effects of whole-body cryotherapy on a total antioxidative status and activities of antioxidative enzymes in blood of depressive multiple sclerosis patients. World Journal of Biological Psychiatry 12 (3), 223–227.

Miller, E., Mrowicka, M., Malinowska, K., Saluk-Juszczak, J., Kędziora, J., 2010c. Effects of whole body cryotherapy on oxidative stress in multiple sclerosis patients. Journal of Thermal Biology 35 (8), 406–410.

Miller, E., Mrowicka, M., Malinowska, K., Zołyński, K., Kędziora, J., 2010b. Effects of the whole-body cryotherapy on a total antioxidative status and activities of some antioxidative enzymes in blood of patients with multiple sclerosis. Journal of Medical Investigation 57 (1-2), 168–173.

Miller, E., Markiewicz, L., Saluk, J., Majsterek, I., 2012. Effect of short-term cryostimulation on antioxidative status and its clinical application in humans. European Journal of Applied Physiology 112 (5), 1645–1652.

Moreira, D.G., Costello, J.T., Brito, C.J., Adamczyk, J.G., Ammer, K., Bach, A.J.E., et al., 2017. Thermographic imaging in sports and exercise medicine: A Delphi study and consensus statement on the measurement of human skin temperature. Journal of Thermal Biology 69, 155–162.

Myrer, J.W., Myrer, K.A., Meason, G.J., Fellingham, G.W., Evers, S.L., 2001. Muscle temperature is affected by overlying adipose when cryotherapy is administered. Journal of Athletic Training 36 (1), 32–36.

O'Toole, G., Rayatt, S., 1999. Frostbite at the gym: a case report of an ice pack burn. British Journal of Sports Medicine 33 (4), 278–279.

Oksa, J., Rintamaki, H., Rissanen, S., Rytky, S., Tolonen, U., Kami, P., 2000. Stretch and H-Reflexes of the lower leg during whole body cooling and local warming. Aviation Space and Environmental Medicine 71 (2), 156–161.

Oosterveld, F.G., Rasker, J.J., 1994. Treating arthritis with locally applied heat or cold. Seminars in Arthritis and Rheumatism 24 (2), 82–90.

Otte, J.W., Merrick, M.A., Ingersoll, C.D., Cordova, M.L., 2002. Subcutaneous adipose tissue thickness alters cooling time during cryotherapy. Archives of Physical Medicine and Rehabilitation 83 (11), 1501–1505.

Palmieri-Smith, R., Leanard-Frye, J., Garrison, C., Welman, A., Ingersoll, C., 2007. Peripheral joint cooling increases spinal reflex excitability and serum norepinephrine. International Journal of Neuroscience 117 (2), 229–242.

Pathak, H.,M., 2014. Effect of cryotherapy on the intrinsic muscle strength of the hand. Indian Journal of Physiotherapy and Occupational Therapy 8 (4), 202–206.

Peake, J.M., Roberts, L.A., Figueiredo, V.C., Egner, I., Krog, S., Aas, S.N., et al., 2017. The effects of cold water immersion and active recovery on inflammation and cell stress responses in human skeletal muscle after resistance exercise. Journal of Physiotherapy 595 (3), 695–711.

Point, M., Gulhem, G., Hug, F., Nordez, A., Frey, A., Lacourpaille, L., 2017. Cryotherapy induces an increase in muscle stiffness. Scandinavian Journal of Medicine and Science in Sports 28 (1), 260–266.

Pointon, M., Duffield, R., Cannon, J., Marino, F.E., 2012. Cold water immersion recovery following intermittent-sprint exercise in the heat. European Journal of Applied Physiology 112, 2483–2494.

Poppendieck, W., Faude, O., Wegmann, M., Meyer, T., 2013. Cooling and performance recovery of trained athletes: a meta-analytical review. International Journal of Sports Physiology and Performance 8 (3), 227–242.

Pournot, H., Bieuzen, F., Louis, J., Fillard, J.R., Barbiche, E., Hausswirth, C., 2011. Time-course of changes in inflammatory response after whole-body cryotherapy multi exposures following severe exercise. PLoS One 6 (7), 227–248.

Rabelo, P., Botelho, K., Oliveria, F., 2016. Grip strength after forearm cooling in healthy subjects. Fisioterapia em Movimento 29 (4), 685–692.

Ranatunga, K.W., Sharpe, B., Turnbull, B., 1987. Contractions of human skeletal muscle at different temperatures. Jounal of Physiology (London) 390, 383–395.

Ring, Ammer, K., 2000. The technique of infrared imaging in medicine. Thermology International 10 (1), 7–14.

Roberts, L.A., Noska, K., Coombes, J.S., Peake, J.M., 2014. Cold water immersion enhances recovery of submaximal muscle function after resistance exercise. American Journal of Physiology. Regulatory, Integrative and Comparative Physiology 307 (8), R998–R1008.

Russell, M., Birch, J., Love, T., Cook, C.J., Bracken, R.M., Taylor, T., et al., 2017. The effects of a single whole-body cryotherapy exposure on physiological, performance, and perceptual responses of professional academy soccer players after repeated sprint exercise. Journal of Strength and Conditioning Research 31 (2), 415–421.

Rutkove, S.B., 2001. Effects of temperature on neuromuscular electrophysiology. Muscle Nerve 24, 867–882.

Rymaszewska, J., Ramse, D., Chladzinska-Kiejna, S., 2007. Whole-body cryotherapy as an adjunct treatment of depressive and anxiety disorders. Archive Immunologia et Therapiae Experimentalis 56 (1), 63–68.

Sanya, A., Bello, A., 1999. Effects of cold application on isometric strength and endurance of quadriceps femoris muscle. African Journal of Medicine and Medical Sciences 28, 195–198.

Sawka, M., Wegner, C., 1988. Physiological responses to acute-exercise heat stress. In: Pandolf, K.B., Gonzalez, R.R., Sawka, M.N. (Eds.), Human Performance Physiology and Environmental Medicine at Terrestrial Extremes. Benchmark Press, Indianapolis, IN.

Schaal, K., Le Meur, Y., Louis, J., Filliard, J.R., Hellanrd, P., Casazza, G., Hausswirth, C., 2015. Whole-body cryostimulation limits overreaching in elite synchronised swimmers. Medicine and Science in Sports and Exercise 47 (7), 1416–1425.

Selfe, J., Hardaker, N., Whittaker, J., Hayes, C., 2007. Thermal imaging of an ice burn over the patella following clinically relevant cryotherapy application during a clinical research study. Physical Therapy in Sport 8 (3), 153–158.

Selfe, J., Hardaker, N., Thewlis, D., Karki, A., 2006. An accurate and reliable method of thermal data analysis in thermal imaging of the anterior knee for use in cryotherapy research. Archives of Physical Medicine and Rehabilitation 87 (12), 1630–1635.

Selfe, J., Alexander, J., Costello, J., May, K., Garratt, N., Atkins, S., et al., 2014. The effect of three different (−135°C) whole body cryotherapy exposure durations on elite rugby league players. PLoS One (9), 1–8 1.

Selfe, J., Hardaker, N., Whittaker, J., Hayes, C., 2009. An investigation into the effect on skin surface temperature of three cryotherapy modalities. Thermology International 19 (4), 121–126.

Sieroń, A., Stanek, A., Cieślar, G., Pasek, J., 2007. Cryorehabilitation – Role of cryotherapy in the contemporary rehabilitation. Fizjoterapia 15 (2), 3–8.

Smith, M., 2005. A review of the initial management of soft tissue sports injuries. Journal of Orthopaedic Nursing 9 (2), 103–107.

Song, M., Sun, X., Tian, X., Zhang, X., Shi, T., Sun, R., et al., 2016. Compressive cryotherapy versus cryotherapy alone in patients undergoing knee surgery: a meta-analysis. Springerplus 5 (1), 1074.

Stanek, A., Cieslar, G., Strzelczyk, J., Kasperczyk, S., Sieron-Stoltny, K., Wiczkowski, A., et al., 2010. Influence of cryogenic temperatures on inflammatory markers in patients with ankylosing spondylitis. Polish Journal of Environmental Studies 19 (1), 167–175.

Stephens, J.M., Halson, S., Miller, J., Slater, G.J., Askew, C.D., 2017. Cold-water immersion for athletic recovery: one size does not fit all. International Journal of Sports Physiology and Performance 12 (1), 2–9.

Sürenkök, Ö., Aytar, A., Tüzün, E.H., Akman, M.N., 2008. Cryotherapy impairs knee joint position sense and balance. Isokinetics and Exercise Science 16 (1), 69–73.

Sutkowy, P., Augustunska, B., Wozniak, A., Rakowski, A., 2014. Physical exercise combined with whole-body cryotherapy in evaluating the level of lipid peroxidation products and other oxidant stress indicators in kayakers. Oxidative Medicine and Cellular Longevity 2014, 402631.

Szczepańska-Gierachaa, J., Borsuka, P., Pawika, M., Rymaszewskaa, J., 2014. Mental state and quality of life after 10 session whole-body cryotherapy. Psychology, Health & Medicine 19 (1), 40–46.

Thain, P., Bleakley, C., Mitchell, A.C., 2015. Muscle reaction time during a simulated lateral ankle sprain after wet-ice application or cold-water immersion. Journal of Athletic Training 50 (7), 697–703.

Thornley, L., Ledford, E., Jacks, D., 2003. Local tissue temperature effects on peak torque and muscular endurance during isometric knee extension. European Journal of Applied Physiology 90 (5–6), 588–594.

Tomchuk, D., Rubley, M.D., Holcomb, W.R., Guadagnoli, M., Tarno, J.M., 2010. The magnitude of tissue cooling during cryotherapy with varied types of compression. Journal of Athletic Training 45 (3), 230–237.

Topp, C., Hesselholt, P., Trier, MR., Nielsen, PV., 2003. Influence of geometry of thermal manikins on room airflow. Proceedings of the 7th International Conference on Healthy Buildings 2003, vol. 2. Singapore, pp. 339–344.

Torres, R., Silva, F., Pedrosa, V., Ferreira, J., Lopes, A., 2017. The acute effect of cryotherapy on muscle strength and shoulder proprioception. Journal of Sports Rehabilitation 26 (6), 497–506.

Twist, C., Waldron, M., Highton, J., Burt, D., Daniels, M., 2012. Neuromuscular, biochemical and perceptual post-match fatigue in professional rugby league forwards and backs. Journal of Sports Science 30 (4), 359–367.

Uchio, Y., Ochi, M., Fujihara, A., Adachi, N., Iwasa, J., Sakai, Y., 2003. Cryotherapy influences joint laxity and position sense of the healthy knee joint. Archives of Physical Medicine and Rehabilitation 84 (1), 131–135.

Vincent, M., Tipton, M., 1988. The effect of cold immersion and hand protection on grip strength. Aviation, Space and Environmental Medicine 59 (8), 738–741.

Wassinger, C.A., Myers, J.B., Gatti, J.M., Conley, K.M., Lephart, S.M., 2007. Proprioception and throwing accuracy in the dominant shoulder after cryotherapy. Journal of Athletic Training 42 (1), 84–89.

Watsford, M.L., Murphey, A.J., McLachlan, K.A., 2010. A prospective study of the relationship between lower body stiffness and hamstring injury in professional Australian rules footballers. American Journal of Sports Medicine 38 (10), 2058–2064.

Watson, P., Watson, I., Batt, R., 1980. Total body water volumes for adult males and females estimated from simple anthropometric measurements. The American Journal of Clinical Nutrition 33 (1), 27–39.

White, G.E., Wells, G.D., 2013. Cold-water immersion and other forms of cryotherapy: physiological changes potentially affecting recovery from high-intensity exercise. Extreme Physiology and Medicine 2 (1), 26.

Wozniak, A., Mila-Kierzenkowska, C., Szpinda, M., Chwalbinska-Moneta, J., Augustynska, B., Jurecka, A., 2013. Whole-body cryostimulation and oxidative stress in rowers: the preliminary results. Archives of Medicine & Science 9 (2), 303–308.

Wozniak, A., Wozniak, B., Drewa, G., Mila-Kierzenkowska, C., Rokowski, A., 2007. The effect of whole-body cryostimulation on lysosomal enzyme activity in kayakers during training. European Journal of Applied Physiology 100 (2), 137–142.

Yamauchi, T., Kim, S., Nogami, S., Kwano, A.D., 1981a. Extreme cold treatment (−150°C) on the whole body in rheumatoid arthritis. Reviews in Rheumatology 48 (Suppl.), 1054.

Yamauchi, T., Nogami, S., Miura, K., 1981b. Various applications of the extreme cryotherapy and strenuous exercise program. Physiotherapy Rehabilitation 5, 35–39.

Young, A., 1988. Human adaptation to cold. In: Pandolf, K.B., Gonzalez, R.R., Sawka, M.N. (Eds.), Human Performance Physiology and Environmental Medicine at Terrestrial Extremes. Benchmark Press, Indianapolis, IN.

Zalewski, P., Bitner, A., Slomko, J., Szrajda, J., Klawe, J.J., Tafil-Klawe, M., et al., 2014. Whole-body cryostimulation increases parasympathetic outflow and decreases core body temperature. Journal of Thermal Biology 45, 75–80.

Ziemann, E., Olek, R.A., Grzywacz, T., Kaczor, J.J., Antosiewicz, J., Skrobot, W., et al., 2014. Whole-body cryostimulation as an effective way of reducing exercise-induced inflammation and blood cholesterol in young men. European Cytokine Network 25 (1), 14–23.

Ziemann, E., Olek, R.A., Kujach, S., Grzywacz, T., Antosiewicz, J., Garrsztka, T., et al., 2012. Five-day whole-body cryostimulation, blood inflammatory markers, and performance in high-ranking professional tennis players. Journal of Athletic Training 47 (6), 664–672.

Chapter | 8 |

Physiology of sporting and athletic recovery

Tony Tompos

Introduction

It has been suggested that the most researched fields of athletic performance are currently focused primarily on the improvements available through various modes of exercise training, whilst the physiology of recovery in athletic performance has been underresearched despite the possibility that many professional athletes spend similar, if not more time, in recovery than in active training (Hausswirth and Mujika, 2013). The aim of this chapter is to provide the reader with evidence-based approaches to the recovery period and how these may be practically utilized within their field of work.

Within the fields of professional sports, many methods of recovery have been proposed and are currently used in daily practice including, but not limited to, cold water immersion, contrast bathing, massage and physiotherapy, cross-training, electrostimulation, nutrition and hydration strategies, modification of training, training periodization, stretching, compression garments, whole-body cryotherapy, laser, sauna and other thermal applications (Howatson et al., 2016). The evidence for and applications of some of these modalities will be discussed with the aim of giving the reader clear and concise takeaway messages to apply to their sports-specific setting.

Members of the sports science multidisciplinary team (MDT) all have a responsibility to ensure that each athlete under their care does not reach an overtrained state which may lead to significant losses in training and competition time. It is probable that MDTs that plan realistic opportunities for recovery in between active training schedules are likely to be rewarded with athletes of superior capabilities and with less risk of injury (Hausswirth and Mujika, 2013).

A discussion and appraisal of training periodization as a subject is not within the scope of this chapter; instead it will focus and consolidate the current evidence on recovery adjuncts and provide recommendations for practice based upon the current literature.

Functional foods

The utilization of functional foods, with supposed antioxidant capacity, has received much attention recently given that supplements such as Montmorency tart cherry concentrate has been found to aid recovery in cycling (Bell et al., 2014), running (Howatson et al., 2010), strength training (Bowtell et al., 2011) and prolonged, intermittent exercise (Bell et al., 2016). It has also been suggested that the beneficial effects of Montmorency tart cherry concentrate are due to its high levels of polyphenolic compounds, including flavonoids and anthocyanins, possessing antioxidant and antiinflammatory properties (Bowtell et al., 2011).

Further research has found that cherries and raspberries have an antiinflammatory effect similar to that of Ibuprofen and Naproxen due to high activity levels of cyclooxygenase (COX) inhibitors (Seeram et al., 2001).

Hyldahl et al. (2014) postulated that muscle damage following repeated sprint activity may be due to muscle membrane damage, sarcomere disorganization and inflammation. It has also been suggested that following intense exercise there are rapid perturbations in the nervous, endocrine, immune and musculoskeletal systems, with an increased formation of reactive oxygen species (ROS) (Bogdanis et al., 2013). The generation of ROS following intense exercise is a likely consequence of inflammatory-mediated repair processes, which may exacerbate existing muscle damage. It is possible that the endogenous antioxidant system is unable to cope with the excessive demands placed upon it during intense exercise. This leads to the possibility that supplements that control oxidative stress, such as antioxidant functional foods, may help accelerate muscle recovery following intense exercise (Clifford et al., 2016). Legal, noninvasive strategies that can impact upon exercise-induced oxidative stress and inflammation may therefore be of benefit to the professional athlete (Cockburn and Bell, 2017).

Bell et al. (2016) in a recent study showed that participants who ingested Montmorency tart cherry concentrate pre- and postexercise over a 7-day period had significant improvements in recovery markers compared to those in the placebo group. Subjects who ingested the tart cherry concentrate had significantly less decrements in performance during countermovement jump (CMJ) (6%), 20-m sprint (4%), quadriceps isometric strength (17%) and agility (3%) at 72 hours posttesting.

Additional research has supported the use of Montmorency tart cherry concentrate supplements on improving the total sleep time and sleep efficiency in a randomized controlled trial (RCT). Subjects who ingested tart cherry juice over a 7-day period had significantly improved sleep in terms of efficiency and duration. The authors postulated that this was due to higher exogenous melatonin levels found during testing (Howatson et al., 2012).

Short-term ingestion of powdered Montmorency tart cherries has also been found to benefit subjects when completing heavy resistance exercise. In a more recent RCT it was found that by supplementing 480 mg/day for 10 days, the Montmorency tart cherries appeared to attenuate muscle soreness, strength decrement during recovery and also markers of muscle catabolism (serum cortisol) (Levers et al., 2015). An earlier study also found that by supplementing long-distance runners with tart cherry juice twice daily for 7 days leading up to a long-distance relay race, subjects reported a significantly smaller increase in pain postrace compared to subjects who ingested a placebo drink (Kuehl et al., 2010).

Beetroot juice has also been the subject of recent attention, in part due to its supposed antioxidant effects and nitrate content. Beetroot juice is also a beneficial source of polyphenols and provides betalains which give the vegetable its red/violet colour. Betalains are water-soluble phytochemicals; they have been found to have antiinflammatory and antioxidant properties and may attenuate ROS-mediated injury (Clifford et al., 2016). The phytonutrient compounds contained in beetroot juice have been shown to scavenge ROS, which may limit cellular injury (El Gamal, 2014). Additionally, Jadert et al. (2012) propose that there may be an indirect antioxidant effect due to the high nitrate content in beetroots suppressing the main producers of ROS, leukocytes.

Research studies into the use of beetroot juice as a recovery aid are fewer in number than those on tart cherry concentrate. However, a recent study suggests that acute beetroot supplementation may attenuate muscle soreness and decrements in CMJ performance following a bout of

plyometric exercise when the juice is ingested immediately, 24 hours and 48 hours after exercise. Although performance was more quickly recovered in CMJ (relative to baseline) and pressure pain threshold was reduced compared to the placebo group, there was no difference between the groups for measurements of the inflammatory markers creatine kinase (CK), interleukin-6, interleukin-8 and tumour necrosis factor-α (Clifford et al., 2015).

The same research group also performed a study on muscle function following repeated sprint exercises, where the subjects consumed beetroot juice for the 3 days following those exercises and compared these to a matching group ingesting a placebo drink. Compared to the placebo group, those who ingested the beetroot juice showed improvements on the CMJ (7.6% less decrement) and reactive strength index (13.8% less decrement) (Clifford et al., 2016).

In summary, there are promising results from research into the benefits of beetroot juice and Montmorency tart cherry concentrate following pre- and postexercise supplementation on differing aspects of athletic recovery. These include decreased delayed onset muscle soreness (DOMS); attenuating losses of power, speed and agility; improved sleep patterns; and decreased pain following long-distance running. It would be interesting to see if other high-antioxidant polyphenol-rich foods such as pomegranate, grape, blackberry or blueberry had similar effects on recovery markers following pre- and postexercise ingestion.

Compression garments

Exercise-induced muscle damage (EIMD) is a frequent consequence of training and competition with the amount of damage dependent upon exercise type, duration and intensity (Tee et al., 2007). Strategies enabling the reduction of EIMD are therefore of importance to the elite athlete aiming to optimally recover between sessions.

It has been proposed that the wearing of compression garments postexercise may have a physiological benefit due to the creation of an external pressure gradient and enhanced blood flow; this may reduce any swelling and also enhance the removal of waste products, such as CK which is considered to be an indirect marker of muscle damage (Baird et al., 2012), lactate and interleukin-6 (Davies et al., 2009).

Because of this, compression garments have recently received much attention, with researchers focusing on the impact these garments may have on DOMS, CK levels, recovery of maximal strength, blood lactate, muscle damage and other inflammatory responses. Some results have shown positive benefits. A recent study has suggested that DOMS and recovery of maximal isometric strength were significantly improved in subjects wearing compression sleeves that provided compression of 5–10 mmHg over the biceps immediately following a bout of eccentric bicep exercises (Kim et al., 2017). Although there was an improvement in DOMS and maximal isometric strength, there was no significant improvement in CK activity or tumour necrosis factor-α (TNF-α), suggesting that the inflammatory response is not associated with the reduction of DOMS (Kim et al., 2017). It is important to note that this study was conducted on a small number (n = 16) of untrained students who were not blind to which group they were in; therefore there may have been a psychological effect with their perceived recovery.

Similar results were found in a comparison study of different whole-body compression garments, in which cricket players performed a series of sprint and upper limb throwing exercises (Duffield and Portus, 2007). The results showed that the majority of physiological markers, including blood lactate, pH, body mass, O_2 saturation and O_2 partial pressure were no different whether a compression garment was worn or not. Interestingly, however, this study did find a reduction in absolute CK values when wearing compression garments compared to the control, and also a reduction in the rating of perceived muscle soreness for both upper and lower limbs (Duffield and Portus, 2007).

This decrease in CK levels has been noted in other studies (Gill et al., 2006; Kraemer et al., 2001) with both groups of authors suggesting these may be due to the compression provided in reducing swelling and therefore limiting the inflammatory response to muscle damage caused by exercise.

In a recent study Goto et al. (2017) assessed the efficacy of the potential benefits of compression garments on recovery of athletic performance within a 24-hour period, as many athletes are required to conduct strenuous exercise twice a day with less than 12 hours of rest separating these bouts of exercise. Following two bouts of exercise (focusing on strength, power and repeated sprints), it was found that physiological muscle damage markers of serum myoglobin, CK, leptin and plasma were no different between the two groups (whole-body compression garment vs. normal garment without compression). There was also no difference in muscular strength observed between the groups. However, a significant difference was observed for subjective muscle soreness, with improvement shown in the compression garment group compared to the control group. Given that muscle damage and inflammatory markers peak at 24–48 hours after exercise (Fatouros et al., 2010) but blood measurements were taken prior to this period, a lack of blinding, and the lack of pressure level measurement applied to participants, results of this study should be interpreted with caution.

Marqués-Jiménez et al. (2017) compared the use of three different types of compression garment in semi-professional soccer players: compression stockings, shorts and full-leg tights. Measurements of DOMS, EIMD biomarkers and swelling were collected prematch and 24, 48 and 72 hours postmatch. With similarities to other studies mentioned, all three compression garments attenuated EIMD biomarkers in a positive, but nonsignificant, manner when compared to not wearing a compression garment, although full-leg compression tights showed the greatest improvement. The authors suggest that this was possibly due to a greater venous return, thus improving the removal of myofibrillar proteins and other waste products. Swelling and DOMS were also attenuated postmatch when wearing compression garments. This suggests that during periods of high training loads and volumes, such as preseason, compression garments may offer a positive, if not significant, benefit to soccer players postmatch.

Cold water immersion

Cold water immersion (CWI) has emerged as one of the most popular recovery interventions for athletes and sports medicine teams to employ in an effort to improve the rate of athletic recovery (Bleakley and Davison, 2010). It has been suggested that the mechanisms underpinning the benefits of CWI are related to temperature, pressure-induced changes in blood flow and reduced muscle temperature, leading to a decrease in postexercise inflammation and subsequent DOMS (Leeder et al., 2012). It has also been proposed that CWI ameliorates DOMS via localized cooling, hydrostatic pressures and redirection of blood flow (Ihsan et al., 2016). For example, postexercise oedema within the muscle impedes oxygen delivery to the muscles as compression of local capillaries is increased resulting in an increased distance between capillaries and muscle fibres for oxygen exchange. Cold-induced vasoconstriction and hydrostatic changes increase central blood volume by increasing the central venous pressure, thus facilitating movement of fluids from the intracellular and interstitial spaces to the intravascular compartments.

This fluid movement therefore encourages and facilitates the clearance of cellular debris via an intracellular–extracellular osmotic gradient (Ihsan et al., 2016). CWI may thus improve DOMS by reducing oedema via cold-induced vasoconstriction, which facilitates the clearance of peripheral fluid and inflammation attenuating DOMS and decrements in muscle function (Ihsan et al., 2016).

CWI has been found to provide improvement in DOMS (Ingram et al., 2009; Jakeman et al., 2009; Vaile et al., 2008), decreased CK levels (Goodall, 2008; Vaile, 2008) and improved rate of recovery for muscle power (Eston 1999; Vaile, 2008). Despite the increasing body of evidence to support CWI as a recovery tool, there remains some resistance to its use due to a lack of clear guidelines on time immersed, depth of immersion and temperature, which may place the athlete at risk of enduring extreme temperatures for longer than required (Bleakley and Davison, 2010). A systematic review of the literature related to CWI found that studies used water temperatures of 5–15°C for either continuous or intermittent sets of between 5 and 24 min (Bleakley et al., 2012).

In an effort to clarify which temperatures and immersion times may be of most benefit to athletes, one study has assessed the efficacy of five different CWI protocols in 50 students (1 min 38°C/1 min 10°C × 3; 1 min CWI in 10°C followed by no immersion for 1 min × 3; 10 min CWI in 10°C; 10 min CWI in 6°C; or control (seated rest)). All four CWI protocols had a beneficial effect on DOMS compared to the control group. However, there was no significant statistical difference between these four groups. Nevertheless, there was a positive trend for 10 min of immersion in 6°C water, demonstrating the greatest results for DOMS at 96 hours postexercise (Glasgow et al., 2014). A systematic review found similar results in that CWI postexercise across a range of 14 studies provided favourable results for DOMS at 24, 48, 72 and 96 hours postexercise (Bleakley et al., 2012).

A systematic review found that across a range of studies reporting a significant result favouring CWI over passive interventions, the mean temperature for alleviating subjective symptoms of DOMS was 10°C, and the suggested mean immersion time was 13 min (Hohenauer et al., 2015). A similar review also found comparable results when investigating CWI versus passive therapies. Results indicated that CWI with a water temperature of 11–15°C with an immersion time of 11–15 min provided the best results for DOMS (Machado et al., 2016).

An earlier study by Leeder et al. (2012) also found that CWI alleviated symptoms of DOMS at 24, 48, 72 and 96 hours postexercise, significantly decreased levels of CK, and also showed improved recovery of muscle power at 24, 48 and 72 hours postexercise, but not muscular strength. The results of this study showed that CWI reduced the perception of DOMS by an average of 16% and that it appears to be more effective as an analgesic following high-intensity exercise rather than eccentric-biased exercises.

Given these meta-analyses and systematic reviews, it may be reasonable to suggest that CWI can be of benefit to athletes looking to decrease DOMS and reduce the loss of power in between training and competition. However, understanding the mechanisms by which CWI benefits athletes is of critical importance to the sports medical professional to ensure that the periodization of recovery is intertwined with longer term goals for training-induced adaptation (Ihsan et al., 2016).

Contrast bathing

Contrast water therapy (CWT) is another recovery strategy that has become a commonplace modality available to high-performance sports athletes. It has the purported benefit of decreasing DOMS via a 'pumping action' created by vasoconstriction and vasodilation following immersions in cold and hot water respectively (Vaile et al., 2007). In addition, it has been suggested that CWT may aid recovery by reducing muscle spasm, inflammation and improving range of motion (Biuzen et al., 2013). Commonly practiced methods include ratios of warm baths to cold at 3:1 or 4:1, respectively, ending on cold treatment to encourage sufficient vasoconstriction (Cochrane, 2004). However, these strategies have been challenged, with the suggestion that 1 min of cold exposure is not sufficient to decrease muscle temperature following warm water immersion, thereby nullifying any physiological effects (Higgins and Kaminski, 1998).

There is currently a marked lack of research in the area of CWT in comparison to other recovery approaches. In an attempt to establish the effects of CWT on recovery following exercise, a study compared passive recovery (15 min seated), to a contrast bathing protocol of 60 s immersion in cold water (8–10°C) followed by immersion in hot water (40–42°C) for 120 s. Compared to the passive recovery group, the CWT group demonstrated a significantly smaller loss of isometric and dynamic force-generating capacity (assessed via isometric squat and jump squat), significantly smaller increase in thigh volume (swelling), a trend towards lower levels of pain (perceived soreness), and also a trend towards lower levels of CK concentration at 48 and 72 hours (Vaile et al., 2007).

In a systematic review and meta-analysis comparing CWT to other recovery techniques following exercise, muscle soreness was significantly lower in CWT groups compared to passive recovery in all 13 studies analysed within the review, at all follow up times (<6, 24, 48, 72, >96 hours). Muscle strength (six studies) and muscle power (nine studies) were also significantly improved in the CWT compared to passive recovery groups when compared to baseline scores. The authors suggest that, due to the majority of studies ending their CWT protocol with cold water immersion, this may have had an analgesic effect by decreasing the nerve conduction velocity and excitability, and reduced neural (nociceptive) transmission. Another theory that has been postulated is that, following cold water immersion, there is activation of thermal nociceptors which causes a change in sympathetic nerve activity; this reduces arterial blood flow causing a reduction in microvascular blood flow surrounding the damaged site, reducing oedema and inflammatory events. However, the main finding of this systematic review and meta-analysis is that when compared to other recovery methods, including CWI, compression and active recovery, there was little difference found between the groups, with all giving superior outcomes on recovery compared to passive recovery (Bieuzen et al., 2013).

Whole-body cryotherapy

Whole-body cryotherapy (WBC) has now also become a popular treatment method and has increasingly been used as a recovery tool for athletes. Within an environmentally controlled room, athletes enter a vestibule chamber at −60°C for approximately 30 s for body adaptation prior to entering the cryochamber where they are exposed to extremely cold, dry air (usually between −100°C and −140°C) for between 2 and 5 min wearing minimal clothing and an air mask to protect from cold-related injury (Bleakley et al., 2014).

WBC was initially intended for use in the clinical setting to aid patients with conditions such as multiple sclerosis and rheumatoid arthritis. However, more recently athletes have started to use WBC in an attempt to gain a competitive advantage through improved recovery (Costello et al., 2015). WBC is often used immediately after or soon after (within 24 hours) intensive exercise, with the treatment often being repeated the same day or over several days (Costello et al., 2012).

WBC as a recovery tool following intensive exercise has been found to decrease CK levels (Banfi et al., 2009), improve psychological recovery including perception of tiredness and pain in runners (Hausswirth et al., 2011) and decrease inflammatory markers and enhance muscular recovery (Pournot et al., 2011). It has been suggested that the significantly cold temperatures elicited during WBC compared to CWI may lead athletes to believe that recovery is enhanced, contributing to some or all of the observed effects. The physiological benefits of WBC have been hypothesized to be related to vasoconstriction, thus limiting oedema and inflammation, causing an analgesic effect due to the cold air, which may limit muscle soreness following exercise (Cockburn and Bell, 2017).

In a recent review of the literature (Lombardi et al., 2017) the authors observed significantly enhanced psychological recovery in runners following a simulated trail run, relating to perceptions of pain and tiredness after the first session of WBC (Hausswirth et al., 2011). Within the review, it was also noted that CK levels were reduced by as much as 40% in rugby players following five sessions on alternate days of WBC when compared to without WBC (Banfi et al., 2009). Similar results were observed in kayakers, with a 34% decrease in CK levels following 3 times

daily WBC sessions during a 10-day training cycle (Wozniak et al., 2007). CK levels, interleukin 6 (60%) and tumour necrosis factor (63%) were also found to have decreased levels in professional tennis players following 5 days of twice daily WBC sessions in a cryogenic chamber during a moderate-intensity training schedule when compared to training without WBC (Ziemann et al., 2012); stroke effectiveness and performance recovery also improved in the WBC group.

WBC was also found to have a beneficial impact on athletes' sleep duration and limiting sleep latency in synchronized swimmers, when the athletes were randomly assigned to either WBC or non-WBC supported recovery following training sessions (Schaal et al., 2015). The authors of this systematic review suggested that WBC improves acute recovery via beneficial effects on inflammation, enhanced oxygenation and reduced cardiovascular strain caused by peripheral vasoconstriction (Lombardi et al., 2017).

In a review of current evidence on WBC, the researchers found that there was evidence to support the notion that WBC could improve subjective outcome measures of perceived recovery and muscle soreness whilst also having an analgesic effect if skin cooling was sufficient enough (<13°C) (Bleakley et al., 2014). A key objective for the review by Bleakley et al. (2014) was to determine the magnitude of tissue temperature reductions associated with WBC compared to other, traditional methods of cooling. It may be suggested that due to the significantly colder temperatures associated with WBC, that this method of cryotherapy may be superior to crushed ice application or CWI. However, due to the poor thermal conductivity of air and water, ice application is more efficient at extracting heat energy from the body (Bleakley et al., 2014). Despite this, a potential advantage may be that WBC is able to cool larger surface areas of the body simultaneously.

A systematic review in 2015 studied the effects of WBC on muscle soreness postexercise. The authors found a reduction in muscle soreness of between 7% and 20% among the studies analysed, whilst four studies found significantly reduced soreness at 1, 24, 48 and 72 hours after exercise when compared to rest or no WBC (Costello et al., 2015). Due to the lack of high-quality RCTs in this area, the high risk of bias within the included studies, the lack of evidence on adverse events and the lack of studies on females or elite athletes, the authors suggest that there is little or no evidence that informs on the relevant effects of WBC versus other interventions such as CWI (Costello et al., 2015). Until further research is available, athletes should be aware that less expensive modes of cryotherapy, such as CWI or ice pack application, appear to offer comparable physiological and clinical benefits to WBC (Bleakley et al., 2014).

Sleep

Sleep is an essential component of health and well-being and there is accumulating evidence suggesting that improved sleep quality and duration in athletes is correlated with improved performance, competitive success and a reduced risk of both injury and illness (Watson, 2017). Sleep is therefore considered to be the main method of recovery in athletes. Persistent poor sleep in athletes is associated with a range of adverse health outcomes (Biggins et al., 2018). The management of an athlete's sleep is especially important during intense training and competition periods, with athletes often reporting sleep as their most important recovery strategy (Halson, 2008). Unfortunately though, it has been reported that elite athletes often experience inadequate sleep compared to nonathletes (Simpson et al., 2017). This is further supported by a study on Olympic Games athletes 3 months prior to the 2016 Olympics that found that as many as 49% of the athletes presented with poor sleep quality as measured by the Pittsburgh Sleep Quality Index (Drew et al., 2018).

In an attempt to clarify the importance of sleep in athletes as a recovery tool postcompetition, a study was performed on amateur rugby league players whereby the participants were randomized to a sleep-deprivation group (0 hours sleep), or control (8 hours sleep) following a competitive rugby league match. The results indicated that for the sleep-deprived group there was a decrease in neuromuscular recovery (mean and peak countermovement jump distance); biochemical recovery (increased CK and C-reactive protein levels); and cognitive function (slowed recovery of reaction-time responses for colour–word cognitive tasks) (Skein et al., 2013).

A similar study found sleep deprivation to have a significantly detrimental effect on the physiological recovery process, producing elevated minute ventilation and oxygen uptake during the recovery period (McMurray and Brown, 1984). Further research has suggested that significant reductions in sleep quantity and quality are associated with increased fatigue and decreased exercise capacity in elite synchronized swimmers (Schaal et al., 2015). Sleep loss has also been associated with impaired muscle protein accumulation, decreased mood and vigour, overtraining syndrome, higher rates of upper respiratory tract infections and it may also hinder the learning of new skills (Fullagar et al., 2015).

A reduction in sleep duration and quality has been reported in both individual and team athletes, especially at times of congested competition, during short- and long-haul travel and when training and playing at night (Fullagar et al., 2015). A recent study assessed objective sleep quantity and calculated the association with perceived training load in elite athletes; although results indicated healthy sleep durations, there was elevated wake after sleep onset (amount of time spent awake after initially falling asleep) suggesting the need for sleep optimization (Knufinke et al., 2017). Similar results have been found in academy soccer players during intensive training periods where young subjects did not meet national sleep guidelines of 8–10 hours for 14- to 17-year-olds, further suggesting a need for sleep education and interventions (Fowler et al., 2017). A decreased total sleep time has also been correlated with decreased performance in elite female gymnasts when assessing sleep as a recovery tool in 26 female gymnasts (Dumortier et al., 2018).

Sleep education has been proposed as one method of improving sleep in patients with insomnia (Stepanski et al., 2003). O'Donnell and Driller (2017) initiated a study utilizing sleep education as an intervention in elite-level netballers. Using a single group pre–post design whereby athletes received a sleep hygiene education presentation in the middle of a 2-week testing period where participants were educated on the maintenance of regular bedtime and wake time, ensuring a quiet, cool bedroom, avoidance of stimulants prior to sleep, avoidance of light-emitting technology and relaxation strategies prior to sleep. Results indicated that the sleep hygiene education presentation resulted in a significant improvement in total sleep time and wake variance. Results also indicated positive trends, although not significantly, to the improvements in total time in bed, sleep efficiency and sleep latency.

Sleep hygiene education has also been shown to have a significant beneficial effect on sleep quantity in highly trained tennis players (Duffield et al., 2014).

Another method put forward to improve recovery was restorative napping when in a sleep-depleted state. Subjects in a sleep-depleted state (<4 hours sleep the previous night) napped or rested for 30 min postlunch and were compared with the control group who did not. Napping was associated with significant improvements in alertness, sleepiness and short-term memory, with positive improvements in 20-m sprint times when compared to the non-napping control group (Waterhouse et al., 2007). It has also been suggested that napping midafternoon, between 1 p.m. and 3 p.m., may be the most optimal time due to a spike in circadian rhythm producing an increased urge and need to sleep if in a sleep-depleted state (Littlehales, 2016).

Much shorter periods of sleep, as little as 6 min, have also been suggested to improve cognitive performance (Lahl et al., 2008), whilst 10-min naps produced the most immediate results for subjective sleepiness, fatigue, vigour and cognitive performance when compared to other nap durations (Brooks and Lack, 2006).

Although sleep is often reported to be of critical importance to recovery, it is currently an underresearched aspect, with limited studies assessing its efficacy on athletic recovery. The limited research that exists does suggest that athletes often have reductions in sleep quality and duration following periods of fixture congestion, evening games and training and during periods of excess travel. Interventions that may improve the recovery of athletes include sleep hygiene education, focusing on improving athletes' pre-sleep routine, and afternoon napping when an athlete is sleep deprived.

References

Baird, M., Graham, S., Baker, J., Bickerstaff, G., 2012. Creatine kinase- and exercise-related muscle damage implications for muscle performance and recovery. Journal of Nutrition and Metabolism 2012, 1–13.

Banfi, G., Melegati, G., Barassi, A., Dogliotti, G., Melzi d'Eril, G., Dugué, B., et al., 2009. Effects of whole-body cryotherapy on serum mediators of inflammation and serum muscle enzymes in athletes. Journal of Thermal Biology 34 (2), 55–59.

Bell, P., Stevenson, E., Davison, G., Howatson, G., 2016. The effects of montmorency tart cherry concentrate supplementation on recovery following prolonged, intermittent exercise. Nutrients 8 (8), 441.

Bell, P., Walshe, I., Davison, G., Stevenson, E., Howatson, G., 2014. Montmorency cherries reduce the oxidative stress and inflammatory responses to repeated days high-intensity stochastic cycling. Nutrients 6 (2), 829–843.

Bieuzen, F., Bleakley, C., Costello, J., 2013. Contrast water therapy and exercise induced muscle damage: a systematic review and meta-analysis. PLoS ONE 8 (4), e62356.

Biggins, M., Cahalan, R., Comyns, T., Purtill, H., O'Sullivan, K., 2018. Poor sleep is related to lower general health, increased stress and increased confusion in elite Gaelic athletes. The Physician and Sportsmedicine 46 (1), 14–20.

Bleakley, C., Davison, G., 2010. What is the biochemical and physiological rationale for using cold-water immersion in sports recovery? A systematic review. British Journal of Sports Medicine 44 (3), 179–187.

Bleakley, C., Bieuzen, F., Davison, G., Costello, J., 2014. Whole-body cryotherapy: empirical evidence and theoretical perspectives. Open Access Journal of Sports Medicine 5, 25–36.

Bleakley, C., McDonough, S., Gardner, E., Baxter, G., Hopkins, J., Davison, G., 2012. Cold-water immersion (cryotherapy) for preventing and treating muscle soreness after exercise. Cochrane Database of Systematic Reviews 2012 (2), CD008262.

Bogdanis, G.C., Stavrinou, P., Fatouros, I.G., Philippou, A., Chatzinikolaou, A., Draganidis, D., et al., 2013. Short-term high-intensity interval exercise training attenuates oxidative stress responses and improves antioxidant status in healthy humans. Food and Chemical Toxicology 61, 171–177.

Bowtell, J., Sumners, D., Dyer, A., Fox, P., Mileva, K., 2011. Montmorency cherry juice reduces muscle damage caused by intensive strength exercise. Medicine and Science in Sports and Exercise 43 (8), 1544–1551.

Brooks, A., Lack, L., 2006. A Brief afternoon nap following nocturnal sleep restriction: which nap duration is most recuperative? Sleep 29 (6), 831–840.

Clifford, T., Bell, O., West, D., Howatson, G., Stevenson, E., 2015. The effects of beetroot juice supplementation on indices of muscle damage following eccentric exercise. European Journal of Applied Physiology 116 (2), 353–362.

Clifford, T., Berntzen, B., Davison, G., West, D., Howatson, G., Stevenson, E., 2016. Effects of beetroot juice on recovery of muscle function and performance between bouts of repeated sprint exercise. Nutrients 8 (8), 506.

Cochrane, D., 2004. Alternating hot and cold-water immersion for athlete recovery: a review. Physical Therapy in Sport 5 (1), 26–32.

Cockburn, E., Bell, P., 2017. Strategies to enhance athlete recovery. In: Turner, A., Comfort, P. (Eds.), Advanced Strength and Conditioning – An Evidence Based Approach, first st ed. Routledge, Oxon, p. 168.

Costello, J.T., Baker, P.R.A., Minett, G.M., Bieuzen, F., Stewart, I.B., Bleakley, C., 2015. Whole-body cryotherapy (extreme cold air exposure) for preventing and treating muscle soreness after exercise in adults. Cochrane Database of Systematic Reviews. Issue 9. Art. No.: CD010789.

Costello, J., Culligan, K., Selfe, J., Donnelly, A., 2012. Muscle, skin and core temperature after −110°C cold air and 8°C water treatment. PLoS ONE 7 (11), e48190.

Davies, V., Thompson, K., Cooper, S., 2009. The effects of compression garments on recovery. Journal of Strength and Conditioning Research 23 (6), 1786–1794.

Drew, M., Vlahovich, N., Hughes, D., Appaneal, R., Burke, L., Lundy, B., et al., 2018. Prevalence of illness, poor mental health and sleep quality and low energy availability prior to the 2016 Summer Olympic Games. British Journal of Sports Medicine 52 (1), 47–53.

Duffield, R., Portus, M., 2007. Comparison of three types of full-body compression garments on throwing and repeat-sprint performance in cricket players. British Journal of Sports Medicine 41, 409–414.

Duffield, R., Murphy, A., Kellett, A., Reid, M., 2014. Recovery from repeated on-court tennis sessions: combining cold-water immersion, compression, and sleep interventions. International Journal of Sports Physiology and Performance 9 (2), 273–282.

Dumortier, J., Mariman, A. Boone, J., Delesie, L., Tobback, E., Vogelaers, D., Bourgois, J.G., 2018. Sleep, training load and performance in elite female gymnasts. European Journal of Sport Science.18(2),151–161.

El Gamal, A., AL Said, M., Raish, M., Al-Sohaibani, M., Al-Massarani, S., Ahmad, A., et al., 2014. Beetroot (Beta vulgaris L.) Extract ameliorates gentamicin-induced nephrotoxicity associated oxidative stress, inflammation, and apoptosis in rodent model. Mediators of Inflammation 2014, 983952.

Eston, R., Peters, D., 1999. Effects of cold water immersion on the symptoms of exercise induced muscle damage. Journal Sports Sciences 17 (3), 231–238.

Fatouros, I.G., Chatzinikolaou, A., Douroudos, I.I., Nikolaidis, M.G., Kyparos, A., Margonis, K., et al., 2010. Time-course of changes in oxidative stress and antioxidant status responses following a soccer game. The Journal of Strength and Conditioning Research 24 (12), 3278–3286.

Fowler, P., Paul, D., Tomazoli, G., Farooq, A., Akenhead, R., Taylor, L., 2017. Evidence of sub-optimal sleep in adolescent Middle Eastern academy soccer players which is exacerbated by sleep intermission proximal to dawn. European Journal of Sport Science 17 (9), 1110–1118.

Fullagar, H., Duffield, R., Skorski, S., Coutts, A., Julian, R., Meyer, T., 2015. Sleep and recovery in team sport: current sleep-related issues facing professional team-sport athletes. International Journal of Sports Physiology and Performance 10 (8), 950–957.

Gill, N., Beavan, C., Cook, c., 2006. Effectiveness of post-match recovery strategies in rugby players. British Journal of Sports Medicine 40 (3), 260–263.

Glasgow, P., Ferris, R., Bleakley, C., 2014. Cold water immersion in the management of delayed-onset muscle soreness: Is dose important? A randomised controlled trial. Physical Therapy in Sport 15 (4), 228–233.

Goodall, S., Howatson, G., 2008. The effects of multiple cold-water immersions on indices of muscle damage. Journal of Sports Science and Medicine 7, 235–241.

Goto, K., Mizuno, S., Mori, A., 2017. Efficacy of wearing compression garments during post-exercise period after two repeated bouts of strenuous exercise: a randomized crossover design in healthy, active males. Sports Medicine - Open 3 (1), 25.

Halson, S.L., 2008. Nutrition, sleep and recovery. European Journal Sports Science 8 (2), 119–126.

Hausswirth, C., Mujika, I., 2013. Recovery for Performance in Sport. The National Institute of Sport for Expertise and Performance (INSEP), Leeds, UK, Human Kinetics p. xi.

Hausswirth, C., Louis, J., Bieuzen, F., Pournot, H., Fournier, J., Filliard, J., et al., 2011. Effects of whole-body cryotherapy vs. far-infrared vs. passive modalities on recovery from exercise-induced muscle damage in highly trained runners. PLoS One 6 (12), e27749.

Higgins, D., Kaminski, T.W., 1998. Contrast therapy does not cause fluctuations in human gastrocnemius. Journal of Athletic Training 33 (4), 336–340.

Hohenauer, E., Taeymans, J., Baeyens, J., Clarys, P., Clijsen, R., 2015. The effect of post-exercise cryotherapy on recovery characterstics: a systematic review and meta-analysis. PLoS One 10 (9), e0139028.

Howatson, G., Bells, P.G., Tallent, J., Middleton, B., McHugh, M.P., Ellis, J., 2012. Effect of tart cherry juice (Prunus cerasus) on melatonin levels and enhanced sleep quality. European Journal of Nutrition. 51 (8), 909–916.

Howatson, G., Leeder, J., van Someren, K., 2016. The BASES Expert Statement on Athletic Recovery Strategies. British Association of Sport and Exercise Sciences (BASES), Leeds, UK. Available at: https://www.bases.org.uk/imgs/tses_expert_statement_spread_recovery_strategies947.pdf.

Howatson, G., McHugh, M.P., Hill, J.A., Brouner, J., Jewell, A.P., Van Someren, K.A., et al., 2010. Influence of tart cherry juice on indices of recovery following marathon running. Scandinavian Journal of Medicine and Science in Sports 20 (6), 843–852.

Hyldahl, R.D., Hubal, M.J., 2014. Lengthening our perspective: morphological, cellular, and molecular responses to eccentric exercise. Muscle and Nerve Journal 49 (2), 155–170.

Ihsan, M., Watson, G., Abiss, C.R., 2016. What are the physiological mechanisms for post exercise cold water immersion in the recovery from prolonged endurance and intermittent exercise? Sports Medicine 46 (8), 1095–1109.

Ingram, J., Dawson, B., Goodman, C., Wallman, K., Beilby, J., 2009. Effect of water immersion methods on post-exercise recovery from simulated team sport exercise. Journal of Science and Medicine in Sport 12 (3), 417–421.

Jadert, C., Petersson, J., Massena, S., Ahl, D., Grapensparr, L., Holm, L., et al., 2012. Decreased leukocyte recruitment by inorganic nitrate and nitrite in microvascular inflammation and NSAID-induced intestinal injury. Free Radical Biology and Medicine 52 (3), 683–692.

Jakeman, J.R., Macrae, R., Eston, R., 2009. A single 10-min bout of cold-water immersion therapy after strenuous plyometric exercise has no beneficial effect on recovery from the symptoms of exercise-induced muscle damage. Ergonomics 52 (4), 456–460.

Kim, J., Kim, J., Lee, J., 2017. Effect of compression garments on delayed-onset muscle soreness and blood inflammatory markers after eccentric exercise: a randomized controlled trial. Journal of Exercise Rehabilitation 13 (5), 541–545.

Knufinke, M., Nieuwenhuys, A., Geurts, S., Møst, E., Maase, K., Moen, M., et al., 2017. Train hard, sleep well? perceived training load, sleep quantity and sleep stage distribution in elite level athletes. Journal of Science and Medicine in Sport.

Kraemer, W.J., Bush, J.A., Wickham, R.B., Denegar, C.R., Gómez, A.L., Gotshalk, L.A., et al., 2001. Influence of compression therapy on symptoms following soft tissue injury from maximal eccentric exercise. Journal of Orthopaedic Sports Physical Therapy 31 (6), 282–290.

Kuehl, K., Perrier, E., 2010. Efficacy of tart cherry juice in reducing muscle pain during running. Journey of The International Society of Sports Nutrition 7, 17.

Lahl, O., Wispel, C., Willigens, B., Pietrowsky, R., 2008. An ultra-short episode of sleep is sufficient to promote declarative memory performance. Journal of Sleep Research 17 (1), 3–10.

Leeder, J., Gissane, C., van Someren, K., Gregson, W., Howatson, G., 2012. Cold water immersion and recovery from strenuous exercise: a meta-analysis. British Journal of Sports Medicine 46 (4), 233–240.

Levers, K., Dalton, R., Galvan, E., Goodenough, C., O'Connor, A., Simbo, S., Barringer, N., Mertens-Talcott, S.U., Rasmussen, C., Greenwood, M., Riechman, S., Crouse, S., Kreider, R.B., 2015. Effects of powdered Montmorency tart cherry supplementation on an acute bout of intense lower body strength exercise in resistance trained males. Journal of the International Society of Sports Nutrition. 12, 41.

Littlehales, N., 2016. Sleep, first ed. Penguin Random House, London, UK, p. 60.

Lombardi, G., Ziemann, E., Banfi, G., 2017. Whole-body cryotherapy in athletes: from therapy to stimulation. an updated review of the literature. Frontiers in Physiology 8, 258.

Machado, A.F., Ferreira, P.H., Micheletti, J.K., De Almeida, A.C., Lemes, I.R., Vanderlei, F.M., et al., 2016. Can water temperature and immersion time influence the effect of cold water immersion on muscle soreness? a systematic review and meta-analysis. Sports Medicine 46 (4), 503–514.

Marqués-Jiménez, D., Calleja-González, J., Arratibel-Imaz, I., Delextrat, A., Uriarte, F., Terrados, N., 2017. Influence of different types of compression garments on exercise-induced muscle damage markers after a soccer match. Research in Sports Medicine 26 (1), 27–42.

McMurray, R.G., Brown, C.F., 1984. The effect of sleep loss on high intensity exercise and recovery. Aviation, Space and Environmental Medicine 55 (11), 1031–1035.

O'Donnell, S., Driller, M.W., 2017. Sleep-hygiene education improves sleep indices in elite female athletes. International Journal of Exercise Science 10 (4), 522–530.

Pournot, H., Bieuzen, F., Louis, J., Mounier, R., Fillard, J.R., Barbiche, E., et al., 2011. Time-course of changes in inflammatory response after whole-body cryotherapy multi exposures following severe exercise. PLos One 6, e22748.

Schaal, K., Le Meur, Y., Louis, J., Filliard, J., Hellard, P., Casazza, G., et al., 2015. Whole-body cryostimulation limits overreaching in elite synchronized swimmers. Medicine and Science in Sports and Exercise 47 (7), 1416–1425.

Seeram, N.P., Momin, R.A., Nair, M.G., Bourquin, L.D., 2001. Cyclooxygenase inhibitory and antioxidant cyaniding glycosides in cherries and berries. Phytomedicine 8 (5), 362–369.

Simpson, N.S., Gibbs, E.L., Matheson, G.O., 2017. Optimizing sleep to maximize performance: implications and recommendations for elite athletes. Scandinavian Journal of Medicine and Science in Sports 27 (3), 266–274.

Skein, M., Duffield, R., Minett, G., Snape, A., Murphy, A., 2013. The effect of overnight sleep deprivation after competitive rugby league matches on post-match physiological and perceptual recovery. International Journal of Sports Physiology and Performance 8 (5), 556–564.

Stepanski, E., Wyatt, J., 2003. Use of sleep hygiene in the treatment of insomnia. Sleep Medicine Reviews 7 (3), 215–225.

Tee, J.C., Bosch, A.N., Lambert, M.I., 2007. Metabolic consequences of exercise-induced muscle thrombosis: a randomized cross-over trial. Journal of Thrombosis and Haemostasis 1, 494–499.

Vaile, J.M., Gill, N.D., Blazevich, A.J., 2007. The effect of contrast water therapy on symptoms of delayed onset muscle soreness. Journal of Strength and Conditioning Research 21 (3), 697–702.

Vaile, J., Halson, S., Gill, N., Dawson, B., 2008. Effect of hydrotherapy on recovery from fatigue. International Journal of Sports Medicine 29 (7), 539–544.

Waterhouse, J., Atkinson, G., Edwards, B., Reilly, T., 2007. The role of a short post-lunch nap in improving cognitive, motor, and sprint performance in participants with partial sleep deprivation. Journal of Sports Science 25 (14), 1557–1566.

Watson, A.M., 2017. Sleep and athletic performance. Current Sports Medicine Reports 16 (6), 413–418.

Wozniak, A., Wozniakn, B., Drewa, G., Mila-Kierzenkowska, C. Rakowski, A., 2007. The effect of whole-body cryostimulation on lysosomal enzyme activity in kayakers during training. European Journal of Applied Physiology. 100 (2), 137–142.

Ziemann, E., Olek, R.A., Kujach, S., Grzywacz, T., Antosiewicz, J., Garsztka, T., et al., 2012. Five-day whole-body cryostimulation, blood inflammatory markers, and performance in high-ranking professional tennis players. Journal of Athletic Training 47 (6), 664–672.

Chapter | **9** |

Making sense of pain in sports physiotherapy: applying the Pain and Movement Reasoning Model

Des O'Shaughnessy and Lester E. Jones

Introduction

Clinical management of sports injury and rehabilitation incorporates an understanding of pain science (Hainline et al., 2017a; 2017b). The complexity of pain experiences in training, competition and all stages of recovery is relevant to clinicians working in the sporting arena. As in all fields of musculoskeletal care, a working understanding of the mechanisms of pain is important, so that athletes at all levels receive care that is personalized and evidence based. It is now recognized that the central nervous system (CNS) is always involved in how pain is perceived. This is reflected in clinical studies of athletes that show that although athletes' threshold to recognizing pain is similar to population norms, their ability to tolerate it is different (Hainline et al., 2017b). Matching the relevant rehabilitation principles to the individual requires an understanding of how seemingly similar presentations can arise from different physiological mechanisms. It also demands a knowledge of how assessment processes may discern these various mechanisms, as well as a sound reasoning process that facilitates tailoring of care. For example, delayed recovery may be due to ongoing inflammatory processes, altered biomechanics or the lack of confidence the athlete has in the process. A clinical reasoning strategy that can work across more than one domain is considered important.

Reframing the relationship between pain and tissue damage

Although there is sufficient evidence to suggest that pain in not a good indicator of tissue health, for most people the attribution of pain to a damaged structure is automatic. This is especially the case when tissue damage brings visible inflammation. Therefore it is easy to develop the belief that it is solely tissue disruption that is responsible for the perception of pain. It is widely acknowledged that the main purpose of pain is to drive safety behaviour in the injured or at risk athlete. However the relationship between pain and the state of tissue health is arguably incidental to this. In recent years there has been growing acceptance that the nerve signals that come from the tissues in response to tissue stress or injury are not pain signals. Instead they should simply be considered as messages to the CNS processors that there is potential danger (Catley et al., 2019).

Experienced rehabilitation practitioners have recognized that seemingly similar injuries can impact on different sportspeople in different ways and can even vary for the same person, depending on how an individual is performing or depending on the pressure they may be experiencing. Therefore, a more robust view of pain is that it is part of the body's protection system (Janig et al., 2006). Pain occurs when appraisal of the internal environment, together with memories, context, attention, mood and self-confidence brings conscious awareness to an individual that a body area is vulnerable (Baliki and Apkarian, 2015).

This means that pain is like other internal states of awareness such as feeling anxious, cold, hungry or thirsty, where information is filtered according to what is deemed important to react to at that time (Legrain et al., 2011; Wallwork et al., 2016). These states are perceptions and are experienced when reasonable information suggests that the body is in jeopardy. Importantly, the feeling of thirst to increase water intake is based on more than just blood volume levels. Pain is similar in that it is not solely reliant on a single source of input (i.e., nociception) to determine level of intensity, or even the quality, of pain felt. This reinforces the need to reframe pain as part of a collection of protective responses.

Where loads on tissue may place tissue at risk of injury, it makes sense for a body protection system to produce pain in order to alter behaviour and so protect the tissue under stress. When injury occurs, sensitizing inflammatory processes subsequent to tissue damage enhance this perception of vulnerability, and pain again facilitates tissue protection. These nociceptive mechanisms indicate a threat to safety and coordinate with other processes so the athlete might protect him/herself – including through appropriate responsive motor patterns, behaviours, psychological strategies and autonomic, immune and endocrine function (Baliki and Apkarian, 2015; Cortelli et al., 2013; Legrain et al., 2011; Melzack, 2005; Sullivan and Vowles, 2017).

Reframing the relationship between pain and movement

The protective processing of engaging movement physiology is complex, and contemporary theoretical models explain how the processing of pain and motor outputs occurs concurrently, rather than sequentially as is usually thought (Melzack, 2005; Wallwork et al., 2016). There is a simultaneous, continual and unconscious appraisal of both nociceptive activity and associated motor behaviours working to minimize any threats to tissue health (Baliki and Apkarian, 2015; Hodges, 2011; Sullivan and Vowles, 2017). Responses associated with pain can include alterations to muscle activity, such as accelerating motion so a body part is removed from an environmental danger, bringing cocontraction to internally splint a body segment, inhibiting activity to distance the body from a hazard, vocalizing a call for help or making a facial expression to elicit support to manage the threat (Hodges and Smeets, 2015). Accordingly, from a neurological perspective, pain is considered to be a sensorimotor experience (Sullivan and Vowles, 2017).

Sensitization postinjury occurs in the periphery and within the CNS and facilitates greater vigilance of the internal and external environments (Arendt-Nielsen et al., 2018; Pelletier et al., 2015a). This amplified processing of potentially threatening stimuli more easily engages the appropriate protective outputs, including changes in motor patterning and glial-enhanced nociception (Grace et al., 2014; Meulders et al., 2011; Nijs et al., 2014b; Schabrun et al., 2015a). A person's adaptations in movement are individualized to her or his perception of pain, her or his body, available motor strategies and experiences, as well as the goal task (Falla and Hodges, 2017; Hodges, 2011). When these adjustments outlast a period of tissue threat, there are subsequent long-term changes in neurological processing of sensory information, in motor coordination and in

activity in the relevant higher centres involved (Baliki et al., 2011; Moseley and Flor, 2012; Vrana et al., 2015; Zusman, 2008a). Such central processing of peripheral inputs allows modulation in both directions; either more sensitivity or, at times, more inhibition.

Central processing to produce pain

Neuroscience has identified that pain exists when thalamic and somatosensory pathways are stimulated, but it is also dependent on activity in multiple emotional and thought processing centres including the insula, the cingulate cortex, the limbic system and the prefrontal cortex, as well as areas dedicated to motor outputs (Apkarian et al., 2011; Bushnell et al., 2013). This neurological complexity of pain is accompanied by the modulation activity of glial cells within the CNS, which links to the body's immune system, and endogenous substances such as endorphins, oxytocin and the stress hormones (Grace et al., 2014; Jones, 2017). Consequently, a pain experience is a neuroimmunoendocrine event.

With such a complex interaction of motor, salience, emotional, cognitive and immunological processes, it is not surprising that pain experiences can vary so greatly (Apkarian et al., 2011; Baliki and Apkarian, 2015). As a result, the same stimulus can be perceived very differently, athletes can continue to move despite nociceptive drive occurring (e.g., on the sporting field) and pain can be reported in the absence of nociception (e.g., phantom limb pain).

Pain and Movement Reasoning Model

Assessment supported by comprehensive clinical reasoning is required to capture this sophisticated physiology. A mechanism-based approach that considers all contributors to the pain experience allows the key influences to be identified and addressed in treatment (Falla and Hodges, 2017; Hush et al., 2013; Nijs et al., 2014b; Smart et al., 2010; Stanos et al., 2016; Wijma et al., 2016). This requires assessment expertise and also a strategy that incorporates all relevant information gathered in the clinical interaction. The authors have developed the *pain and movement reasoning model* to facilitate clinical reasoning where multiple mechanisms may be implicated in pain states (Fig. 9.1) (Jones and O'Shaughnessy, 2014). It is thought there are three potentially coexisting categories of pain mechanisms that require appraisal and assimilation into a management plan. This includes (1) the state of the central neuroimmunological matrix, (2) discretely local issues and (3) a grouping labelled as 'regional factors'. Being aware of the potential for overlap of these three categories, clinicians are guided to match their

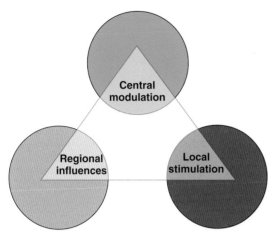

Fig. 9.1 Categories of the Pain and Movement Reasoning Model. (The Pain and Movement Reasoning Model by Des O'Shaughnessy and Lester Jones is licenced under a Creative Commons Attribution-NonCommercial-Share Alike 4.0 International (CC BY-NC-SA 4.0) License.)

treatment to what they judge to be the predominant component in a person's presentation. For clinicians supporting sportspeople working to optimize motor performance, it is important to acknowledge that physiological mechanisms of altered movement can be captured in a similar way – central, regional and local influences.

Local stimulation

Nociception leads to transmission of signals that reach the CNS, and these arise from activity related to biomechanical deformation and chemical stimulation.

The triggering of high-threshold mechanical nociceptors can occur with compression of tissues, via an external force, or when movement is constrained either by the translational movement at a joint or with traction of tissues, e.g., when structures are extended close to ranges where loads will exceed tissue integrity (Smart et al., 2010). This may sometimes occur under the threshold of the perception of pain (Baliki and Apkarian, 2015). At a significant level of aggravation, pain will most likely occur, arising from, for example, a shoulder dislocation or a quadriceps contusion.

When any tissue is damaged, inflammation is produced as the body works to heal itself. Fortunately, the chemicals involved in this inflammatory soup, such as various cytokines, are also pronociceptive (Smart et al., 2012a). This supports protective behaviour such as guarding and reducing tissue loads that facilitate the healing of tissue.

There is evidence that chemical nociceptors are also sensitive to an excess of adenosine triphosphate (ATP) associated with muscle spasm and pH imbalances arising from ischaemia (McGill et al., 2000; Mense, 2008; Rio et al.,

2014). These additional local biochemical changes can occur through activation of muscles in prolonged static or protective postures or as a result of strong and persistent muscle spasm in response to injury or pain.

In addition, inflammation sensitizes mechanical nociceptors, which then are able to send danger signals with low levels of tissue pressure. Therefore, even small movements can be painful, promoting protective behaviours with minimal disturbance (Jones and O'Shaughnessy, 2014). As tissue healing progresses through the stages, with the diminution of pronociceptive chemicals, the pain experience usually resolves accordingly.

Clinical note

The features that suggest local stimulation factors are predominant include the presence of insult to tissue and the demonstration of a clear mechanical pattern that matches the clinical rationale of nociception in a target tissue (Fig. 9.2) (Smart et al., 2012a). Improvement occurs with expected or observed healing processes and in response to care that emphasizes a local cause, e.g., protection of movement, mechanical-focused therapy, use of nonsteroidal anti-inflammatory drug (NSAID) medication or surgery. For pain to be considered as principally arising from local mechanisms, the contributions from other factors (i.e., regional influences or central modulation) are determined as less significant (Nijs et al., 2014b; Smart et al., 2012a). The presence of a predominantly nociceptive contribution to pain does not mean that only a single structure is at fault. In the majority of low back pain presentations there is no identifiable pathoanatomic cause (Müller-Schwefe et al., 2017). For cases where the pain is chiefly due to local stimulation, it is believed that the most appropriate rehabilitation should focus on alleviating any inflammation present and prescribing exercises that address loading anomalies or reduce excessive muscle activation to normalize blood flow and reestablish tissue oxygen levels (Falla and Hodges, 2017; McGill et al., 2000).

Regional influences

This category recognizes that pain can arise remote to the actual location of pathology or dysfunction. Three subcategories of mechanisms are considered as 'regional influences': kinetic chain, neuropathodynamics and CNS convergence. The relationship between pain and movement and the need to consider mechanisms of pain and movement in parallel is arguably best displayed in this category.

Kinetic chain

Athletes will move in quite individual ways and their chosen activity will require a range of postures and movement variance across multiple body segments. Where pain is attributed

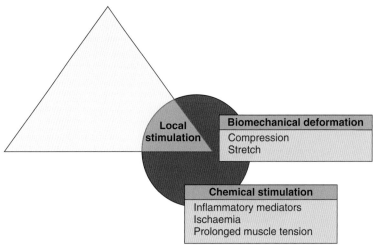

Fig. 9.2 Local stimulation subcategories. (The Pain and Movement Reasoning Model by Des O'Shaughnessy and Lester Jones is licenced under a Creative Commons Attribution-NonCommercial-Share Alike 4.0 International (CC BY-NC-SA 4.0) License.)

to the motion of the kinetic chain, the assumption is that the forces at one region are triggering altered stress patterns and local stimulation of nociceptors at the place of symptoms. A clinical example might be an athlete experiencing altered joint stress patterns and knee pain; the clinician must determine whether there are also changes in calf length, gluteal forces or ankle proprioceptive ability. The chain may extend further to include the spine and thoracolumbar fascia, which in turn has linkages to multiple muscles as well as related visceral fascial tissue (Standring, 2015). It seems appropriate that the impact of mechanical force modifications caused by equipment, bracing and other support devices are also considered within this subcategory.

Pathoneurodynamics

A second subcategory of regional influences is the presence of changes in sensitivity of the peripheral neural tissue or the mobility of the surrounding connective tissue along the entire nerve (Schmid et al., 2013; 2018). Peripheral neuropathy, i.e., disease or damage to nerve tissue, would fit here. Most commonly for musculoskeletal practitioners, this involves nerve compression or entrapment and the pathophysiological ramifications, also described as *pathoneurodynamic* changes (Jones and O'Shaughnessy, 2014). This can often involve more than a simple biomechanical effect, such as nerve movement or restriction, and can occur when part of the connective tissue adjacent to the nerve bed loses its mobility and Schwann cells degenerate at the point of strain. This in turn leads to an inflammatory response to promote healing, again with the release of pronociceptive chemicals (Schmid et al., 2013; 2018; Smart et al., 2012b; Zusman, 2008b; 2009). Action potentials are created bidirectionally in the nerve. Orthodromically (i.e., distal to proximal) these

reach second-order neurones in the dorsal horn that conduct signals to higher centres. Antidromically (i.e., proximal to distal) the change in potential reaches the site of the receptor and causes a release of chemicals. These in turn are able to restimulate action potentials as well as create a neurogenic inflammatory response, so that an element of swelling may occur at a site distal to the original lesion.

This is a good example of regional influences, where a tissue stress or injury leads to an attribution of pain at a remote site. Indeed, pain can become quite widespread, with responses in spinal cord, cortical and glia processes within days of the initial peripheral processes (Arendt-Nielsen et al., 2018; Baliki and Apkarian, 2015; Grace et al., 2014; Nijs et al., 2017a; Schmid et al., 2013; 2018; Zusman, 2008b). Motor patterning can also be affected as these events can alter the contractile ability of the adjacent muscle (Hodges, 2011).

These presentations are most easily identified when pain follows structures along a nerve bed and with the presence of positive neurodynamic tests (Smart et al., 2012b). Other potential clues include where there is a collection of pain, paraesthesia, proprioceptive and power changes; where the pain is described as having a burning quality; or when there is a connection, potentially only vague, between symptoms in different parts of the body (Smart et al., 2010). Neurological screening assesses changes to lower motor neuron reflexes, power, sensation or movement of the nerve beds. These essentially test the whole nervous system, so if there are CNS changes, the ability to discern dysfunction in the peripheral nervous system specifically is reduced. It is also difficult to discriminate whether a limitation is at the level of the peripheral nerve and/or the plexus and/or nerve root (Nee and Butler, 2006; Schmid et al., 2013; 2018). Similarly, determining the nerve root level responsible is difficult due to the degree of

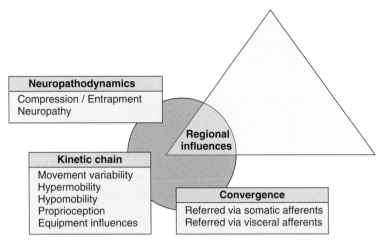

Fig. 9.3 Central modulation subcategories. (The Pain and Movement Reasoning Model by Des O'Shaughnessy and Lester Jones is licenced under a Creative Commons Attribution-NonCommercial-Share Alike 4.0 International (CC BY-NC-SA 4.0) License.)

anatomical variation between individuals and the high level of crossover between levels, which becomes magnified in the presence of compression neuropathies (Anderberg et al., 2006; Schmid et al., 2013; 2018; Smart et al., 2012b). Neurodynamic examination involves stretching tissue at the site of perceived pain initially, and then moving a distant body part to see if symptoms are altered (Nee and Butler, 2006). This assessment routine is not perfect, as cases of entrapment neuropathies can still be missed if looking only for neurological signs as confirmation (Baselgia et al., 2017).

Musculoskeletal clinicians will regularly see such cases as: carpal tunnel-like presentations when the wrist is under load, being resolved through addressing interfaces in the cervicothoracic spine and along the median nerve bed; hamstring symptoms occurring due to sciatic nerve bed compression arising at the lumbar spine or at piriformis; and superior tibiofibular joint management improving movement of lower leg nerves and as a result addressing foot and ankle dysfunction.

CNS convergence

Comprehensive musculoskeletal care also considers the role of distant peripheral nerve signals converging within the CNS (Graven-Nielsen and Arendt-Nielsen, 2010). This crosswiring mechanism improves the body's resilience to avoid reliance on one solitary path for afferent information. Again, this process can limit the ability of practitioners to pinpoint the exact structures at fault. A common example is nonspecific low back pain with accompanying leg symptoms, where referral patterns can be similar for adjacent tissue such as facet joints, paraspinal muscles, periosteum or sacroiliac structures (LaPlante et al., 2012; Schwarzer et al., 1994). Locating the predominant source of symptoms is further complicated when referral areas for structures increases in the presence

of dysfunctions, such as whiplash-associated disorders or arthropathies (Graven-Nielsen and Arendt-Nielsen, 2010).

To add further complexity, convergence mechanisms are not always somatosomatic; viscerosomatic referral may also occur. The latter is a pain mechanism that enables the identification of pathologies of viscera (Giamberardino et al., 2010). Visceral mesenteric structures are reported to be the source of referred pain, and manual therapy that targets viscera can improve low back pain outcomes, presumably either via convergence processes or structural connectivity (Gebhart and Bielefeldt, 2016; McSweeney et al., 2012; Tozzi, et al., 2012).

Clinical note

The features that suggest regional influences are predominant in a case include movement limitations linked to the painful site by kinetic chain, sensitivity or reduced mobility in relevant neural structures and evidence of pathology or stress in tissues with convergent innervation (Fig. 9.3). Establishing the extent and the location of regional limitations in a clinical presentation requires the comprehensive assessment of potentially implicated structures. For example, a jumping athlete with lateral thigh symptoms could be managed with consideration of local structures such as iliotibial band (ITB) tension. However, investigation of broader influences (i.e., remote to the site of pain) may include gluteal imbalance; mobility of the sciatic nerve with a bias towards the common peroneal nerve; piriformis tension; and referral from the lumbar spine. It would not be an uncommon presentation to have all of these involved, and a deductive reasoning process may be more appropriate where a valid and relevant objective measure is assessed for pre- and posttreatment changes with various techniques. Addressing these remote structures sequentially with targeted assessment and observing for the alteration of symptoms determines which structures are likely to be associated in the reported dysfunction.

Central modulation

This category includes mechanisms that might sensitize or inhibit the body's protection system. Central components, predominantly involving the CNS, play a critical role both in pain processing and motor patterning.

Predisposing factors

Pain levels and movement patterning may be significantly affected by the preexisting state of central systems prior to a loading event on the musculoskeletal system. The central modulation can be influenced by the plasticity of the nervous system, as well as of the immune and endocrine systems. Systems can become pro- or antiinflammatory and nerve responsiveness can be primed or dampened, which then influences the degree to which an individual might be considered pain vulnerable (Flor et al., 2001; Generaal et al., 2016; Grace et al., 2014).

The term 'central sensitization' is increasingly used to describe any amplification of nociception by CNS mechanisms (spinal cord or cortical), and is increasingly understood to be influenced by immune and endocrine mechanisms. It has been reported to be a significant factor in a variety of pain conditions including tendinopathies, ligamentous injury, arthropathies, low back pain, elbow dysfunction, pelvic pain disorder and fibromyalgia (Arendt-Nielsen et al., 2018; Kapreli et al., 2009; Murphy et al., 2012; Needle et al., 2017; Pelletier et al., 2015a; Plinsinga et al., 2015; Rio et al., 2014; Sluka and Clauw, 2016; Wolfe et al., 2016). Importantly, central sensitizing processes can occur in the acute phase of an injury and so the term should not solely be used to describe presentations of chronic or persistent pain. The new term 'nociplastic' has recently been introduced to describe this type of influence on pain. However, note that the International Association for the Study of Pain (IASP) definition of *nociplastic pain* is one of exclusion (i.e., no identified nociceptive or neuropathic contributions), which is not reflective of clinical presentations where pain can be attributed to multiple mechanisms (Aydede and Shriver, 2018).

People will be predisposed to experience pain to differing degrees dependent on their prior physical, psychological and social health baselines. It follows that sensitivity to pain is an expression of global sensitivity to the body's various signals for maintaining equilibrium in response to internal and external threats to physiology (Arendt-Nielsen et al., 2018; Yunus, 2015). Pain is only one warning system amongst others such as signals to rest and sleep, to renew energy levels, to avoid stimuli that may damage sense organs such as the

eyes, to empty the bowel of waste product, to keep upright balance, to reduce blood flow to the periphery in order to maintain core temperature, or to deal with social environmental risks (Gracely and Schweinhardt, 2015). Rather than seeing persistent pain as a frequent comorbidity alongside other functional sensitivity syndromes (i.e., chronic fatigue syndrome, photophobia, irritable bowel, benign paroxysmal positional vertigo, Raynaud's phenomenon or posttraumatic stress disorder), persistent pain and these syndromes are seen as a collection of amplified responses to unconscious homeostatic processes, driven by a sensitized CNS (Gracely and Schweinhardt, 2015; Maixner et al., 2016).

Measurement scales for determining a person's susceptibility to heightened responses to stimuli include assessing not only sensitivity to painful experiences but also to feelings of fatigue, previous pain experiences, mood changes, a history of trauma, other physical symptoms and concentration abilities (Scerbo et al., 2018; Wolfe et al., 2016). Analyses of the prevalence of these syndromes in populations reveal that rather than these syndromes being present or not in a binary fashion, it appears that all people are on a continuum and experience a constellation of symptoms to varying degrees (Wolfe et al., 2013). This goes some way to explaining how people considered to be healthy demonstrate a breadth of reported pain levels in experiments. It seems that the extent of central sensitization or inhibition prior to a painful experience affects subsequent pain levels and functional outcomes after a pain event or surgery (Clark et al., 2017; Coghill et al., 2003). This is the case even for those who do not have any sensitization syndrome diagnosis (Brummett et al., 2013; 2015)

The health of an individual also affects their susceptibility to pain via three different expressions of the immune system: (1) The presence of autoimmune diseases can elevate pain sensitivity; (2) there is an increase in sensitivity in the presence of raised immune activity such as fighting an infection; and (3) there appears to be a relationship between amplified sensitivity syndrome symptoms and recent major immunological challenge such as post-glandular fever (Jones, 2017; Klein et al., 2012; Phillips and Clauw, 2013).

Recent research is bringing to light the complex physiology that underlies this immune–nervous systems interaction, and a major focus is on the interface provided by the glial system. Glia are considered to be the specialized protective cells for the CNS, which respond not only to potential infections but also other states of duress such as current and past stresses or sleep deprivation (Grace et al., 2014; Loggia et al., 2015; Nijs et al., 2017b). When the CNS is confronted by such challenges, glia become activated to address this threatened state, releasing mediating chemicals that promote neuroinflammation and by doing so, increase pain sensitivity (Grace et al., 2014; Nijs et al., 2017b). This process has also been suggested as one of those responsible for the development of opioid-induced hyperalgesia, where use of opiate medication leads to a heightened sensitivity of the CNS (Grace et al., 2014). Importantly, these cells, after responding to a perceived risk, do not reduce their activity levels to the prethreat levels, so that pain sensitivity will remain slightly elevated (Grace et al., 2014; Nicotra et al., 2012). This stimulus–incomplete decline cycle may be repeated over time and therefore when immunological–neurological threats are faced over multiple occasions, the end result is a pain system that has become more responsive to movement of musculoskeletal structures. This is a likely mechanism for the impact of traumas on central sensitivity scores, muscle fatigue and pain (Burke et al., 2017; Generaal et al., 2016; Keller-Ross et al., 2014; Sueki et al., 2014; Tsur et al., 2017).

Also important in body protection is the endocrine system. Both elevated and reduced levels of the stress hormone cortisol are associated with pain conditions. In addition, stress-buffering substances such as oxytocin and endorphins alter pain perception (Chapman et al., 2008; Hannibal and Bishop, 2014; Wippert et al., 2017). Respiratory system dysfunction alters the ability of the diaphragm to achieve both breathing and spinal control functions (Hodges et al., 2001), as well as affecting tissue oxygenation levels in concert with the cardiovascular system. The health of the intestinal system has recently gained attention in understanding pain states, through what has been labelled the gut–brain axis, predominantly driven by the vagus nerve (Farmer et al., 2014; Moloney et al., 2014).

Inherited characteristics are believed to play a role in both an individual's baseline motor performance skills and pain sensitivity, and the expression of genes, influenced by external and internal events, is gaining much attention in the research area known as epigenetics (Denk and McMahon, 2012; Huijnen et al., 2015). Researchers are exploring the mechanisms that lead to individual pain phenotypes, in particular how the interaction between genetics and the environment can alter characteristics such as pain sensitivity, including through the neuroimmune and neuroendocrine mechanisms described here.

Together a person's past experiences, immune status, the environment, genetics and overall health, sets an individual amplification level of centrally mediated sensitivity. These predisposing factors dictate how and to what degree stimuli, including those related to movement and the musculoskeletal system, are interpreted (Phillips and Clauw, 2013; Yunus, 2015).

Activity-dependent plasticity

Another major influence on how movement and pain are encoded within the CNS is the role of learned activity patterns. This can be described as activity-dependent plasticity as the learning is dependent on the activity in neurons and

nerve pathways. Persistent patterns of activation reinforce the responsiveness of neurons and associated immune and endocrine function, leading to strengthened neural connections and enhanced transmission. Sports rehabilitation is encouraged to utilize this knowledge for recovery from sports injuries (Wallwork et al., 2016).

There is recognition that changes in the spinal cord and higher centres (i.e. structural, chemical and connectivity) have a bearing on pain perception which relates to the duration of a pain condition (Apkarian et al., 2011; Arendt-Nielsen et al., 2018; Baliki et al., 2011; Coppieters et al., 2016; Kuner and Flor, 2017; Pelletier et al., 2015a; Pomares et al., 2017). In particular, the transition from an acute to a persistent pain state involves increased involvement of the emotional processing centres and less involvement of the somatosensory cortical centres (Baliki and Apkarian, 2015; Hashmi et al., 2013; Vachon-Presseau et al., 2016). Most importantly, these changes are mirrored by additional alterations in the motor cortex, again reinforcing the intimacy of the pain and movement relationship (Hodges and Smeets, 2015; Moseley and Flor, 2012; Pelletier et al., 2015a; Vrana et al., 2015). This includes increased activity for those with ongoing pain when anticipating pain or simply when imagining movements, without peripheral nociceptive signalling (Tucker et al., 2012; Zusman, 2008a). Perhaps unsurprisingly, these transformations in higher centres involved in both pain processing and motor performance have been found to correlate with pain intensity levels across a broad scope of conditions (Boudreau et al., 2010; Meeus et al., 2012; Pelletier et al., 2015a; Schabrun et al., 2015b; 2017; Stanton et al., 2012; Te et al., 2017; Tsao et al., 2011; Ung et al., 2012).

Processing of acute pain brings both motor patterning alterations, to find the most appropriate muscle activation, and sensitizing mechanisms, which together minimize risk and promote healing (Boudreau et al., 2010; Hodges, 2011; Nijs et al., 2014a; Sullivan and Vowles, 2017; van Dieën et al., 2017). When this activation persists, new biomechanical learnings occur which can vary from a subtle redistribution of load, to new movement patterning in order to complete an action, through to avoidant behaviours (Hodges and Smeets, 2015). With healing, generally, there is a separation of the need to minimize pain from these learned motor strategies (Zusman, 2012). However, if the sense of vulnerability remains high, with repetition it can lead to a learning both of what biomechanics are threatening and what are appropriate avoidant behaviours (den Hollander et al., 2010; Hodges and Smeets, 2015; Madden et al., 2015; Nijs et al., 2017a; van Dieën et al., 2017; Zusman, 2008a). If unchallenged, this can eventually lead to alterations to the number and variety of available movement patterns at a person's disposal, and an expansion of avoidant behaviours across a broader suite of movements (Meulders et al., 2011; Vlaeyen et al., 2016; Wallwork et al., 2016).

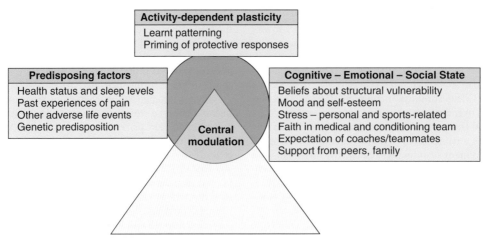

Fig. 9.4 The spectrum of factors that influence pain and movement and the effect of central neuroimmunological changes include an individual's past experiences, health status, beliefs and emotions. (The Pain and Movement Reasoning Model by Des O'Shaughnessy and Lester Jones is licenced under a Creative Commons Attribution-NonCommercial-Share Alike 4.0 International (CC BY-NC-SA 4.0) License.)

Fear avoidance/protection models have evolved to view these learnings not as pathological but rather as a normal response associated with a heightened sense of damage, vigilance and an emphasis of removing pain as a primary focus (Bunzli et al., 2015; Crombez et al., 2012; Wideman et al., 2013). These attitudes may have been gained from various well-meaning sources such as teammates, coaches, family or a variety of health professionals. When subtle mechanical input is believed to be a representation of current or future tissue vulnerability, this encourages someone to move differently and avoid those actions that activate pain and are perceived to cause damage. As the CNS becomes more responsive to afferent information and accentuates the threat value of such information, neuroplasticity facilitates this sensitized patterning to become initially acquired, then embedded, eventually automated and then transferred to other similar movements or neighbouring structures. This overapplied protection leads to pain being experienced more readily, perceived in previously nonpainful structures, and provoked by a greater range of movements and postures.

Cognitive–emotive–social state

The learning of altered neural patterns, whether it be a fine motor skill or adapting to minimize pain levels, will depend on time, but also a person's psychosocial state. Activation of cognitive and emotional centres is implicated in the resistance of the athlete's presenting condition to treatment (Bushnell et al., 2013; Malfliet et al., 2017; Nijs et al., 2014a). This crosses a variety of domains where pain and accompanying functional levels relate not only to fear, but also memories of similar pain events or previously unsuccessful care; tendency to catastrophize; resilience; degree of emotional

insight; sense of injustice; acceptance; guilt; coping strategies; social anxiety; self-efficacy; social support; depression; current stresses to do with performance or potential selection; or other occupational, family or personal stresses (Bunzli et al., 2015; Gatchel et al., 2007; Hasenbring et al., 2012; Linton and Shaw, 2011; Lumley et al., 2011; Quartana et al., 2009; Serbic and Pincus, 2017; Sullivan et al., 2012; Wippert et al., 2017; Wurm et al., 2016). Such factors influence a spectrum of scenarios including experimental situations involving pain-free participants, someone recovering from a painful event and where pain is ongoing.

Similarly, motor performance has also been found to rely on psychosocial factors and provides the basis for sports psychology to play a role in maximizing motor performance (Benedetti, 2013; Pelletier et al., 2015b; Swinkels-Meewisse et al., 2006). A system of 'yellow flags' has been developed to help identify psychological risk factors that have the potential to slow recovery if left unaddressed during rehabilitation (Nicholas et al., 2011).

Clinical note

It has been highlighted that no matter what stage of healing the athlete presents, central factors are always involved to some degree (Hainline et al., 2017a). Musculoskeletal practice that identifies the complex interactions and influences that lead to pain and movement will be best placed to address the central neuroimmunological changes associated with an individual's past experiences, health status, beliefs and emotions at all stages of presentation to a clinic (Fig. 9.4) (Wallwork et al., 2016; Wijma et al., 2016). This will assist practitioners to recognize the various factors which can lead to pain being experienced and expressed in a myriad of ways and sensitivities. Taking a biopsychosocial approach including fostering a therapeutic partnership with the athlete can influence CNS, immune and endocrine outputs (Benedetti, 2013; Diener et al., 2016; Nijs et al., 2014a; O'Keeffe et al., 2016). For example, for people accessing care for an acute episode of low back pain, building trust and the delivery of reassuring information about the resilience of the spine and normal results for imaging, all facilitate an improvement in long-term outcomes (Frederiksen et al., 2017; Hasenbring and Pincus, 2015).

The assessment of central contributing factors is an emerging area. Questionnaires that help to identify levels of self-efficacy, fear, catastrophizing, depression, anxiety and stress can be used as part of the clinical judgement, but translating and relating this to the pain experience is difficult. One might expect that someone who scores highly on these scales would have higher central sensitization contributing to pain but it is unlikely that there is a clear-cut relationship. The validity of sensory testing strategies assessing for tactile acuity, including two-point discrimination, and cold hyperalgesia are being explored (Harvie et al., 2017; Hübscher et al., 2014; Moss et al., 2016).

A greater awareness of the impact of central modulating factors allows for a reinterpretation of exercise programmes. Rather than attributing outcomes solely to biomechanical efficiencies, coordination and cardiovascular output, it becomes important to maximize the benefits of targeting central influences. Further, it allows for exercise prescribers to develop a person's self-assurance in their ability to achieve desired movement patterning, or perform an activity without triggering painful responses (Wallwork et al., 2016). Although the load may vary greatly depending on whether the intention is to improve confidence in a highly acquired skilled movement or to be more able at achieving everyday activities, the principles of graded progression are the same (Moseley, 2003). In the presence of persistent pain, the encouragement to exercise in order to facilitate endorphin release is now seen as an inappropriate goal as the normal opioid-induced hypoalgesic response is suppressed (Brellenthin et al., 2016). Similarly, the prime focus for functional activity gains is no longer considered to be targeting deconditioning, but is seen as reversing the sensorimotor cautiousness and physiological vigilance related to a heightened sense of structural vulnerability (Hodges and Smeets, 2015; Sullivan and Vowles, 2017; Vlaeyen et al., 2016; Wideman et al., 2013).

Such nonpharmacological care requires the clinician and athlete to work at skilfully adapting the body's protection systems to be less reactive. This includes reinforcing that pain is a personalized perception and experience, and altering beliefs about the levels of safety that are appropriate (Louw et al., 2016). Experiential learning integrates cognitive behavioural techniques with the principles of graded exposure, where the baseline of threat levels attached to

movements is gradually progressed (Blickenstaff and Pearson, 2016; Louw et al., 2016; Moseley, 2003; Nijs et al., 2017a; Pelletier et al., 2015a; Sullivan and Vowles, 2017).

Tailoring of expectations is essential based on the degree of catastrophizing thoughts and fearful beliefs, as well as exploring how to move without the learned fear response activating centres of the pain matrix (Blickenstaff and Pearson, 2016; Huijnen et al., 2015; Moseley, 2003; Nijs et al., 2015; Wijma et al., 2016; Zusman, 2008a). Priming appropriate neuroplastic mechanisms of recovery may need to start in the absence of movement when healing processes or sensitivity to movement preclude normal loading. This can be achieved using graded motor imagery, before advancing to mirrored movements or by maximizing visual feedback (Daffada et al., 2015; Guillot and Collet, 2008; Moseley and Flor, 2012; Wallwork et al., 2016). Activities can be progressed by increasing repetition or the duration of time spent on a task, even in the presence of pain, although the rate of increase often needs to be very low. Progression can also be achieved by challenging the system to cope with changes in musculoskeletal load, the physical or social environment, the cognitive–emotional demands and confidence levels, or by introducing movement where pain is provoked (Moseley, 2003; Nijs et al., 2015; O'Sullivan et al., 2015; Pelletier et al., 2015b; Sullivan and Vowles, 2017).

Implications for integrated sports rehabilitation

An applied knowledge of pain physiology is important in achieving best outcomes for the injured athlete. Effective clinical reasoning requires consideration of all potential mechanisms that impact on performance. Pain can be seen to be a signal to change, and this may occur in response to biomechanical issues or training regimes. In addition, now it is defined as a perception of threat, and the judgement that something needs addressing can be sensitized by other regional musculoskeletal factors or modulated by a myriad of personal stresses, related to the sport or other pressures, beliefs, memories and expectations.

Management approaches founded on central sensitization principles and psychosocial foci have brought functional improvements in outcomes for people, with accompanying changes in higher centres within the pain matrix (Boudreau et al., 2010; Kregel et al., 2017; Nijs et al., 2017a; Pelletier et al., 2015b; Richmond et al., 2015; Seminowicz et al., 2013; Shpaner et al., 2014; Snodgrass et al., 2014; Veehof et al., 2016; Vowles et al., 2017; Wälti et al., 2015) Addressing these central mechanisms and targeting individual fears should occur through all stages of rehabilitation including in early stages (Boudreau et al., 2010;

Pelletier et al., 2015b; Wallwork et al., 2016). It is recognized that this requires specialized skills, experience and time. When such care is required it may be appropriate to refer sportspeople to multidisciplinary pain clinics, even at an early stage in rehabilitation. In Australia, referral to recognized *pain* physiotherapists provides another avenue for enhancing recovery where pain is predominantly centrally modulated. Being aware of the central modulation of pain and the referral options that are available may be important first steps in improving pain management in sport.

Pursuing professional development activities to enhance knowledge and skills in pain management is encouraged although it is important that the impact on clinical practice is more than just an addition to a biomedical paradigm.

Summary

Acknowledging that multiple dysfunctions are at play, the Pain and Movement Reasoning Model is designed to assist clinicians in scrutinizing all the possible contributors and enables priorities for intervention to be established. This ensures the sports clinician directs management to the most significant factor. Importantly if someone does present with high psychometric scores suggesting central factors at play, it cannot be assumed that other mechanisms are excluded. Equally, when someone presents with frank tissue damage, the potential for central modulating influences may be relevant, particularly relating to self-identity (Hainline et al., 2017a). The description of pain as either acute or chronic pain heightens the risk of this reasoning error. All pain is complex and likely to be provoked by the multiple concurrent mechanisms that have been discussed above.

Through providing musculoskeletal care that takes into account the various elements involved in the multifactorial experience of pain and movement, more sustainable outcomes for athletes, and others accessing care, becomes possible.

References

Anderberg, L., Annertz, M., Rydholm, U., Brandt, L., Säveland, H., 2006. Selective diagnostic nerve root block for the evaluation of radicular pain in the multilevel degenerated cervical spine. European Spine Journal 15 (6), 794–801.

Apkarian, A.V., Hashmi, J.A., Baliki, M.N., 2011. Pain and the brain: specificity and plasticity of the brain in clinical chronic pain. Pain 152 (3, Suppl. 1), S49–S64.

Arendt–Nielsen, L., Morlion, B., Perrot, S., Dahan, A., Dickenson, A., Kress, H., et al., 2018. Assessment and manifestation of central sensitisation across different chronic pain conditions. European Journal of Pain 22 (2), 216–241.

Aydede, M., Shriver, A., 2018. Recently introduced definition of 'nociplastic pain' by the international association for the study of pain needs better formulation. Pain 159 (6), 1176–1177.

Baliki, M.N., Apkarian, A.V., 2015. Nociception, pain, negative moods, and behavior selection. Neuron 87 (3), 474–491.

Baliki, M.N., Schnitzer, T.J., Bauer, W.R., Apkarian, A.V., 2011. Brain morphological signatures for chronic pain. PloS ONE 6 (10), e26010.

Baselgia, L.T., Bennett, D.L., Silbiger, R.M., Schmid, A.B., 2017. Negative neurodynamic tests do not exclude neural dysfunction in patients with entrapment neuropathies. Archives of Physical Medicine and Rehabilitation 98 (3), 480–486.

Benedetti, F., 2013. Placebo and the new physiology of the doctor-patient relationship. Physiological Reviews 93 (3), 1207–1246.

Blickenstaff, C., Pearson, N., 2016. Reconciling movement and exercise with pain neuroscience education: a case for consistent education. Physiotherapy Theory and Practice 32 (5), 396–407.

Boudreau, S.A., Farina, D., Falla, D., 2010. The role of motor learning and neuroplasticity in designing rehabilitation approaches for musculoskeletal pain disorders. Manual Therapy 15 (5), 410–414.

Brellenthin, A.G., Crombie, K.M., Cook, D.B., Sehgal, N., Koltyn, K.F., 2016. Psychosocial influences on exercise-induced hypoalgesia. Pain Medicine 18 (3), 538–550.

Brummett, C.M., Janda, A.M., Schueller, C.M., Tsodikov, A., Morris, M., Williams, D.A., et al., 2013. Survey criteria for fibromyalgia independently predict increased postoperative opioid consumption after lower-extremity joint arthroplastya prospective, observational cohort study. The Journal of the American Society of Anesthesiologists 119 (6), 1434–1443.

Brummett, C.M., Urquhart, A.G., Hassett, A.I., Tsodikov, A., Hallstrom, B.R., Wood, N.I., et al., 2015. Characteristics of fibromyalgia independently predict poorer long–term analgesic outcomes following total knee and hip arthroplasty. Arthritis & Rheumatology 67 (5), 1386–1394.

Bunzli, S., Smith, A., Schütze, R., O'Sullivan, P., 2015. Beliefs underlying pain-related fear and how they evolve: a qualitative investigation in people with chronic back pain and high pain-related fear. BMJ Open 5 (10), e008847.

Burke, N.N., Finn, D.P., McGuire, B.E., Roche, M., 2017. Psychological stress in early life as a predisposing factor for the development of chronic pain: clinical and preclinical evidence and neurobiological mechanisms. Journal of Neuroscience Research 95 (6), 1257–1270.

Bushnell, M.C., Čeko, M., Low, L.A., 2013. Cognitive and emotional control of pain and its disruption in chronic pain. Nature Reviews Neuroscience 14 (7), 502–511.

Catley, M.J., Moseley, G.L., Jones, M.A., 2019. Understanding pain in order to treat patients in pain. In: Jones, M.A., Rivett, D.A. (Eds.), Clinical Reasoning in Musculoskeletal Practice, second ed. Elsevier Health Sciences, Oxford, p. 32.

Chapman, C.R., Tuckett, R.P., Song, C.W., 2008. Pain and stress in a systems perspective: reciprocal neural, endocrine, and immune interactions. The Journal of Pain 9 (2), 122–145.

Clark, J., Nijs, J., Yeowell, G., Goodwin, P., 2017. What are the predictors of altered central pain modulation in chronic musculoskeletal pain populations? A systematic review. Pain Physician 20 (6), 487–500.

Coghill, R.C., McHaffie, J.G., Yen, Y.-F., 2003. Neural correlates of interindividual differences in the subjective experience of pain. Proceedings of the National Academy of Sciences 100 (14), 8538–8542.

Coppieters, I., Meeus, M., Kregel, J., Caeyenberghs, K., De Pauw, R., Goubert, D., et al., 2016. Relations between brain alterations and clinical pain measures in chronic musculoskeletal pain: a systematic review. The Journal of Pain 17 (9), 949–962.

Cortelli, P., Giannini, G., Favoni, V., Cevoli, S., Pierangeli, G., 2013. Nociception and autonomic nervous system. Neurological Sciences 34 (1), 41–46.

Crombez, G., Eccleston, C., Van Damme, S., Vlaeyen, J.W., Karoly, P., 2012. Fear-avoidance model of chronic pain: the next generation. The Clinical Journal of Pain 28 (6), 475–483.

Daffada, P., Walsh, N., McCabe, C., Palmer, S., 2015. The impact of cortical remapping interventions on pain and disability in chronic low back pain: a systematic review. Physiotherapy 101 (1), 25–33.

den Hollander, M., De Jong, J.R., Volders, S., Goossens, M.E., Smeets, R.J., Vlaeyen, J.W., 2010. Fear reduction in patients with chronic pain: a learning theory perspective. Expert Review of Neurotherapeutics 10 (11), 1733–1745.

Denk, F., McMahon, S.B., 2012. Chronic pain: emerging evidence for the involvement of epigenetics. Neuron 73 (3), 435–444.

Diener, I., Kargela, M., Louw, A., 2016. Listening is therapy: patient interviewing from a pain science perspective. Physiotherapy Theory and Practice 32 (5), 356–367.

Falla, D., Hodges, P.W., 2017. Individualized exercise interventions for spinal pain. Exercise and Sport Sciences Reviews 45 (2), 105–115.

Farmer, A.D., Randall, H.A., Aziz, Q., 2014. It's a gut feeling: how the gut microbiota affects the state of mind. The Journal of Physiology 592 (14), 2981–2988.

Flor, H., Denke, C., Schaefer, M., Grusser, S., 2001. Effect of sensory discrimination training on cortical reorganisation and phantom limb pain. Lancet 357 (9270), 1763–1764.

Frederiksen, P., Indahl, A., Andersen, L.L., Burton, K., Hertzum-Larsen, R., Bendix, T., 2017. Can group-based reassuring information alter low back pain behavior? A cluster-randomized controlled trial. PloS One 12 (3), e0172003.

Gatchel, R.J., Peng, Y.B., Peters, M.L., Fuchs, P.N., Turk, D.C., 2007. The biopsychosocial approach to chronic pain: scientific advances and future directions. Psychological Bulletin 133 (4), 581.

Gebhart, G., Bielefeldt, K., 2016. Physiology of visceral pain. Comprehensive Physiology 6 (4), 1609–1633.

Generaal, E., Vogelzangs, N., Macfarlane, G.J., Geenen, R., Smit, J.H., de Geus, E.J., et al., 2016. Biological stress systems, adverse life events and the onset of chronic multisite musculoskeletal pain: a 6-year cohort study. Annals of the Rheumatic Diseases 75 (5), 847–854.

Giamberardino, M.A., Affaitati, G., Costantini, R., 2010. Visceral referred pain. Journal of Musculoskeletal Pain 18 (4), 403–410.

Grace, P.M., Hutchinson, M.R., Maier, S.F., Watkins, L.R., 2014. Pathological pain and the neuroimmune interface. Nature Reviews Immunology 14 (4), 217–231.

Gracely, R.H., Schweinhardt, P., 2015. Programmed symptoms: disparate effects united by purpose. Current Rheumatology Reviews 11 (2), 116–130.

Graven-Nielsen, T., Arendt-Nielsen, L., 2010. Assessment of mechanisms in localized and widespread musculoskeletal pain. Nature Reviews Rheumatology 6 (10), 599–606.

Guillot, A., Collet, C., 2008. Construction of the motor imagery integrative model in sport: a review and theoretical investigation of motor imagery use. International Review of Sport and Exercise Psychology 1 (1), 31–44.

Hainline, B., Derman, W., Vernec, A., Budgett, R., Deie, M., Dvořák, J., et al., 2017a. International olympic committee consensus statement on pain management in elite athletes. British Journal of Sports Medicine 51 (17), 1245–1258.

Hainline, B., Turner, J.A., Caneiro, J., Stewart, M., Moseley, G.L., 2017b. Pain in elite athletes –neurophysiological, biomechanical and psychosocial considerations: a narrative review. British Journal of Sports Medicine 51 (17), 1259–1264.

Hannibal, K.E., Bishop, M.D., 2014. Chronic stress, cortisol dysfunction, and pain: a psychoneuroendocrine rationale for stress management in pain rehabilitation. Physical Therapy 94 (12), 1816–1825.

Harvie, D.S., Kelly, J., Buckman, H., Chan, J., Sutherland, G., Catley, M., et al., 2017. Tactile acuity testing at the neck: a comparison of methods. Musculoskeletal Science and Practice 32, 23–30.

Hasenbring, M.I., Hallner, D., Klasen, B., Streitlein-Böhme, I., Willburger, R., Rusche, H., 2012. Pain-related avoidance versus endurance in primary care patients with subacute back pain: psychological characteristics and outcome at a 6-month follow-up. Pain 153 (1), 211–217.

Hasenbring, M.I., Pincus, T., 2015. Effective reassurance in primary care of low back pain: what messages from clinicians are most beneficial at early stages? The Clinical Journal of Pain 31 (2), 133–136.

Hashmi, J.A., Baliki, M.N., Huang, L., Baria, A.T., Torbey, S., Hermann, K.M., et al., 2013. Shape shifting pain: chronification of back pain shifts brain representation from nociceptive to emotional circuits. Brain 136 (9), 2751–2768.

Hodges, P.W., Heijnen, I., Gandevia, S.C., 2001. Postural activity of the diaphragm is reduced in humans when respiratory demand increases. The Journal of Physiology 537 (3), 999–1008.

Hodges, P.W., Smeets, R.J., 2015. Interaction between pain, movement, and physical activity: short-term benefits, long-term consequences, and targets for treatment. The Clinical Journal of Pain 31 (2), 97–107.

Hodges, P.W., 2011. Pain and motor control: from the laboratory to rehabilitation. Journal of Electromyography and Kinesiology 21 (2), 220–228.

Hübscher, M., Moloney, N., Rebbeck, T., Traeger, A., Refshauge, K.M., 2014. Contributions of mood, pain catastrophizing, and cold hyperalgesia in acute and chronic low back pain: a comparison with pain-free controls. The Clinical Journal of Pain 30 (10), 886–893.

Huijnen, I.P., Rusu, A.C., Scholich, S., Meloto, C.B., Diatchenko, L., 2015. Subgrouping of low back pain patients for targeting treatments: evidence from genetic, psychological, and activity-related behavioral approaches. The Clinical Journal of Pain 31 (2), 123–132.

Hush, J.M., Stanton, T.R., Siddall, P., Marcuzzi, A., Attal, N., 2013. Untangling nociceptive, neuropathic and neuroplastic mechanisms underlying the biological domain of back pain. Pain 3 (3), 223–236.

Janig, W., Chapman, C., Green, P., 2006. Pain and body protection: sensory, autonomic, neuroendocrine and behavioural mechanisms in control of inflammation and hyperalgesia. In: Flor, H., Kaslo, E., Dostrovsky, J.O. (Eds.), Proceedings of the 11th World Congress on Pain. IASP Press, Seattle.

Jones, L.E., 2017. Stress, pain and recovery: neuro-immune-endocrine interactions and clinical practice. In: Porter, S. (Ed.), Psychologically Informed Physiotherapy: Embedding Psychosocial Perspectives Within Clinical Management. Elsevier, Edinburgh, pp. 78–106.

Jones, L.E., O'Shaughnessy, D.F., 2014. The Pain and Movement Reasoning Model: introduction to a simple tool for integrated pain assessment. Manual Therapy 19 (3), 270–276.

Kapreli, E., Athanasopoulos, S., Gliatis, J., Papathanasiou, M., Peeters, R., Strimpakos, N., et al., 2009. Anterior cruciate ligament deficiency causes brain plasticity: a functional MRI study. The American Journal of Sports Medicine 37 (12), 2419–2426.

Keller-Ross, M.L., Schlinder-Delap, B., Doyel, R., Larson, G., Hunter, S.K., 2014. Muscle fatigability and control of force in men with posttraumatic stress disorder. Medicine and Science in Sports and Exercise 46 (7), 1302–1313.

Klein, C.J., Lennon, V.A., Aston, P.A., McKeon, A., Pittock, S.J., 2012. Chronic pain as a manifestation of potassium channel-complex autoimmunity. Neurology 79 (11), 1136–1144.

Kregel, J., Coppieters, I., De Pauw, R., Malfliet, A., Danneels, L., Nijs, J., et al., 2017. Does conservative treatment change the brain in patients with chronic musculoskeletal pain? A systematic review. Pain Physician 20 (3), 139–154.

Kuner, R., Flor, H., 2017. Structural plasticity and reorganisation in chronic pain. Nature Reviews Neuroscience 18 (1), 20–30.

LaPlante, B.L., Ketchum, J.M., Saullo, T.R., DePalma, M.J., 2012. Multivariable analysis of the relationship between pain referral patterns and the source of chronic low back pain. Pain Physician 15, 171–178.

Legrain, V., Iannetti, G.D., Plaghki, L., Mouraux, A., 2011. The pain matrix reloaded: a salience detection system for the body. Progress in Neurobiology 93 (1), 111–124.

Linton, S.J., Shaw, W.S., 2011. Impact of psychological factors in the experience of pain. Physical Therapy 91 (5), 700–711.

Loggia, M.L., Chonde, D.B., Akeju, O., Arabasz, G., Catana, C., Edwards, R.R., et al., 2015. Evidence for brain glial activation in chronic pain patients. Brain 138 (3), 604–615.

Louw, A., Zimney, K., Puentedura, E.J., Diener, I., 2016. The efficacy of pain neuroscience education on musculoskeletal pain: a systematic review of the literature. Physiotherapy Theory and Practice 32 (5), 332–355.

Lumley, M.A., Cohen, J.L., Borszcz, G.S., Cano, A., Radcliffe, A.M., Porter, L.S., et al., 2011. Pain and emotion: a biopsychosocial review of recent research. Journal of Clinical Psychology 67 (9), 942–968.

Madden, V.J., Harvie, D.S., Parker, R., Jensen, K.B., Vlaeyen, J.W., Moseley, G.L., et al., 2015. Can pain or hyperalgesia be a classically conditioned response in humans? A systematic review and meta-analysis. Pain Medicine 17 (6), 1094–1111.

Maixner, W., Fillingim, R.B., Williams, D.A., Smith, S.B., Slade, G.D., 2016. Overlapping chronic pain conditions: implications for diagnosis and classification. The Journal of Pain 17 (9), T93–T107.

Malfliet, A., Coppieters, I., Van Wilgen, P., Kregel, J., De Pauw, R., Dolphens, M., et al., 2017. Brain changes associated with cognitive and emotional factors in chronic pain: a systematic review. European Journal of Pain 21 (5), 769–786.

McGill, S.M., Hughson, R.L., Parks, K., 2000. Lumbar erector spinae oxygenation during prolonged contractions: implications for prolonged work. Ergonomics 43 (4), 486–493.

McSweeney, T.P., Thomson, O.P., Johnston, R., 2012. The immediate effects of sigmoid colon manipulation on pressure pain thresholds in the lumbar spine. Journal of Bodywork and Movement Therapies 16 (4), 416–423.

Meeus M., Vervisch S., De Clerck, L.S., Moorkens G., Hans G., Nijs J., editors., 2012. Central sensitization in patients with rheumatoid arthritis: a systematic literature review. Seminars in Arthritis and Rheumatism 41 (4), 556-567.

Melzack, R., 2005. Evolution of the neuromatrix theory of pain. The Prithvi Raj lecture: presented at the third world congress of world institute of pain, barcelona 2004. Pain Practice 5 (2), 85–94.

Mense, S., 2008. Muscle pain: mechanisms and clinical significance. Deutsches Ärzteblatt International 105 (12), 214.

Meulders, A., Vansteenwegen, D., Vlaeyen, J.W., 2011. The acquisition of fear of movement-related pain and associative learning: a novel pain-relevant human fear conditioning paradigm. Pain 152 (11), 2460–2469.

Moloney, R.D., Desbonnet, L., Clarke, G., Dinan, T.G., Cryan, J.F., 2014. The microbiome: stress, health and disease. Mammalian Genome 25 (1-2), 49–74.

Moseley, G., 2003. A pain neuromatrix approach to patients with chronic pain. Manual Therapy 8 (3), 130–140.

Moseley, G.L., Flor, H., 2012. Targeting cortical representations in the treatment of chronic pain: a review. Neurorehabilitation and Neural Repair 26 (6), 646–652.

Moss, P., Knight, E., Wright, A., 2016. Subjects with knee osteoarthritis exhibit widespread hyperalgesia to pressure and cold. PloS One 11 (1), e0147526.

Müller-Schwefe, G., Morlion, B., Ahlbeck, K., Alon, E., Coaccioli, S., Coluzzi, F., et al., 2017. Treatment for chronic low back pain: the focus should change to multimodal management that reflects the underlying pain mechanisms. Current Medical Research and Opinion 33 (7), 1199–1210.

Murphy, S.L., Phillips, K., Williams, D.A., Clauw, D.J., 2012. The role of the central nervous system in osteoarthritis pain and implications for rehabilitation. Current Rheumatology Reports 14 (6), 576–582.

Nee, R.J., Butler, D., 2006. Management of peripheral neuropathic pain: integrating neurobiology, neurodynamics, and clinical evidence. Physical Therapy in Sport 7 (1), 36–49.

Needle, A.R., Lepley, A.S., Grooms, D.R., 2017. Central nervous system adaptation after ligamentous injury: a summary of theories, evidence, and clinical interpretation. Sports Medicine 47 (7), 1271–1288.

Nicholas, M.K., Linton, S.J., Watson, P.J., Main, C.J., 'Decade of the flags' working group, 2011. Early identification and management of psychological risk factors ('yellow flags') in patients with low back pain: a reappraisal. Physical Therapy 91 (5), 737–753.

Nicotra, L., Loram, L.C., Watkins, L.R., Hutchinson, M.R., 2012. Toll-like receptors in chronic pain. Experimental Neurology 234 (2), 316–329.

Nijs, J., Clark, J., Malfliet, A., Ickmans, K., Voogt, L., Don, S., et al., 2017a. In the spine or in the brain? Recent advances in pain neuroscience applied in the intervention for low back pain. Clinical and Experimental Rheumatology 35 (5), 108–115.

Nijs, J., Girbés, E.L., Lundberg, M., Malfliet, A., Sterling, M., 2015. Exercise therapy for chronic musculoskeletal pain: innovation by altering pain memories. Manual Therapy 20 (1), 216–220.

Nijs, J., Loggia, M.L., Polli, A., Moens, M., Huysmans, E., Goudman, L., et al., 2017b. Sleep disturbances and severe stress as glial activators: key targets for treating central sensitization in chronic pain patients? Expert Opinion on Therapeutic Targets 21 (8), 817–826.

Nijs, J., Meeus, M., Cagnie, B., Roussel, N.A., Dolphens, M., Van Oosterwijck, J., et al., 2014a. A modern neuroscience approach to chronic spinal pain: combining pain neuroscience education with cognition-targeted motor control training. Physical Therapy 94 (5), 730–738.

Nijs, J., Torres-Cueco, R., van Wilgen, P., Lluch Girbés, E., Struyf, F., Roussel, N., et al., 2014b. Applying modern pain neuroscience in clinical practice: criteria for the classification of central sensitization pain. Pain Physician 17 (5), 447–457.

O'Keeffe, M., Cullinane, P., Hurley, J., Leahy, I., Bunzli, S., O'Sullivan, P.B., et al., 2016. What influences patient–therapist interactions in musculoskeletal physical therapy? Qualitative systematic review and meta-synthesis. Physical Therapy 96 (5), 609–622.

O'Sullivan, K., Dankaerts, W., O'Sullivan, L., O'Sullivan, P.B., 2015. Cognitive functional therapy for disabling nonspecific chronic low back pain: multiple case-cohort study. Physical Therapy 95 (11), 1478–1488.

Pelletier, R., Higgins, J., Bourbonnais, D., 2015a. Addressing neuroplastic changes in distributed areas of the nervous system associated with chronic musculoskeletal disorders. Physical Therapy 95 (11), 1582–1591.

Pelletier, R., Higgins, J., Bourbonnais, D., 2015b. Is neuroplasticity in the central nervous system the missing link to our understanding of chronic musculoskeletal disorders? BMC Musculoskeletal Disorders 16 (1), 25.

Phillips, K., Clauw, D.J., 2013. Central pain mechanisms in the rheumatic diseases: future directions. Arthritis & Rheumatology 65 (2), 291–302.

Plinsinga, M.L., Brink, M.S., Vicenzino, B., Van Wilgen, C.P., 2015. Evidence of nervous system sensitization in commonly presenting and persistent painful tendinopathies: a systematic review. Journal of Orthopaedic & Sports Physical Therapy 45 (11), 864–875.

Pomares, F.B., Funck, T., Feier, N.A., Roy, S., Daigle-Martel, A., Ceko, M., et al., 2017. Histological underpinnings of grey matter changes in fibromyalgia investigated using multimodal brain imaging. Journal of Neuroscience 37 (5), 1090–1101.

Quartana, P.J., Campbell, C.M., Edwards, R.R., 2009. Pain catastrophizing: a critical review. Expert Review of Neurotherapeutics 9 (5), 745–758.

Richmond, H., Hall, A.M., Copsey, B., Hansen, Z., Williamson, E., Hoxey-Thomas, N., et al., 2015. The effectiveness of cognitive behavioural treatment for non-specific low back pain: a systematic review and meta-analysis. PloS One 10 (8), e0134192.

Rio, E., Moseley, L., Purdam, C., Samiric, T., Kidgell, D., Pearce, A.J., et al., 2014. The pain of tendinopathy: physiological or pathophysiological? Sports Medicine 44 (1), 9–23.

Scerbo, T., Colasurdo, J., Dunn, S., Unger, J., Nijs, J., Cook, C., 2018. Measurement properties of the central sensitization inventory: a systematic review. Pain Practice 18 (4), 544–554.

Schabrun, S.M., Christensen, S.W., Mrachacz-Kersting, N., Graven-Nielsen, T., 2015a. Motor cortex reorganization and impaired function in the transition to sustained muscle pain. Cerebral Cortex 26 (5), 1878–1890.

Schabrun, S.M., Elgueta-Cancino, E.L., Hodges, P.W., 2017. Smudging of the motor cortex is related to the severity of low back pain. Spine 42 (15), 1172–1178.

Schabrun, S.M., Hodges, P.W., Vicenzino, B., Jones, E., Chipchase, L.S., 2015b. Novel adaptations in motor cortical maps: the relationship to persistent elbow pain. Medicine and Science in Sports and Exercise 47 (4), 681–690.

Schmid, A.B., Hailey, L., Tampin, B., 2018. Entrapment neuropathies: challenging common beliefs with novel evidence. Journal of Orthopaedic & Sports Physical Therapy 48 (2), 58–62.

Schmid, A.B., Nee, R.J., Coppieters, M.W., 2013. Reappraising entrapment neuropathies – mechanisms, diagnosis and management. Manual Therapy 18 (6), 449–457.

Schwarzer, A.C., Aprill, C.N., Derby, R., Fortin, J., Kine, G., Bogduk, N., 1994. The relative contributions of the disc and zygapophyseal joint in chronic low back pain. Spine 19 (7), 801–806.

Seminowicz, D.A., Shpaner, M., Keaser, M.L., Krauthamer, G.M., Mantegna, J., Dumas, J.A., et al., 2013. Cognitive-behavioral therapy increases prefrontal cortex gray matter in patients with chronic pain. The Journal of Pain 14 (12), 1573–1584.

Serbic D., Pincus T., 2017. The relationship between pain, disability, guilt and acceptance in low back pain: a mediation analysis. Journal of Behavioral Medicine 40 (4), 651–658. 119.

Sturgeon J.A., Zautra, A.J., 2013. Psychological resilience, pain catastrophizing, and positive emotions: perspectives on comprehensive modeling of individual pain adaptation. Current Pain and Headache Reports 17 (3), 317.

Shpaner, M., Kelly, C., Lieberman, G., Perelman, H., Davis, M., Keefe, F.J., et al., 2014. Unlearning chronic pain: a randomized controlled trial to investigate changes in intrinsic brain connectivity following cognitive behavioral therapy. NeuroImage: Clinical 5, 365–376.

Sluka, K.A., Clauw, D.J., 2016. Neurobiology of fibromyalgia and chronic widespread pain. Neuroscience 338, 114–129.

Smart, K.M., Blake, C., Staines, A., Doody, C., 2010. Clinical indicators of 'nociceptive', 'peripheral neuropathic' and 'central' mechanisms of musculoskeletal pain. A Delphi survey of expert clinicians. Manual Therapy 15 (1), 80–87.

Smart, K.M., Blake, C., Staines, A., Thacker, M., Doody, C., 2012a. Mechanisms-based classifications of musculoskeletal pain: part 3 of 3: symptoms and signs of nociceptive pain in patients with low back (±leg) pain. Manual Therapy 17 (4), 352–357.

Smart, K.M., Blake, C., Staines, A., Thacker, M., Doody, C., 2012b. Mechanisms-based classifications of musculoskeletal pain: part 2 of 3: symptoms and signs of peripheral neuropathic pain in patients with low back (±leg) pain. Manual Therapy 17 (4), 345–351.

Snodgrass, S.J., Heneghan, N.R., Tsao, H., Stanwell, P.T., Rivett, D.A., Van Vliet, P.M., 2014. Recognising neuroplasticity in musculoskeletal rehabilitation: a basis for greater collaboration between musculoskeletal and neurological physiotherapists Manual Therapy 19 (6), 614–617.

Standring, S., 2015. Gray's Anatomy: The Anatomical Basis of Clinical Practice, forty-first ed. Elsevier Health Sciences, Oxford.

Stanos, S., Brodsky, M., Argoff, C., Clauw, D.J., D'Arcy, Y., Donevan, S., et al., 2016. Rethinking chronic pain in a primary care setting. Postgraduate Medicine 128 (5), 502–515.

Stanton, T.R., Lin, C.-W.C., Smeets, R.J., Taylor, D., Law, R., Moseley, G.L., 2012. Spatially defined disruption of motor imagery performance in people with osteoarthritis. Rheumatology 51 (8), 1455–1464.

Sueki, D., Dunleavy, K., Puentedura, E., Spielholz, N., Cheng, M., 2014. The role of associative learning and fear in the development of chronic pain—a comparison of chronic pain and post-traumatic stress disorder. Physical Therapy Reviews 19 (5), 352–366.

Sullivan, M.D., Vowles, K.E., 2017. Patient action: as means and end for chronic pain care. Pain 158 (8), 1405–1407.

Sullivan, M.J., Scott, W., Trost, Z., 2012. Perceived injustice: a risk factor for problematic pain outcomes. The Clinical Journal of Pain 28 (6), 484–488.

Swinkels-Meewisse, I.E., Roelofs, J., Oostendorp, R.A., Verbeek, A.L., Vlaeyen, J.W., 2006. Acute low back pain: pain-related fear and pain catastrophizing influence physical performance and perceived disability. Pain 120 (1), 36–43.

Te, M., Baptista, A.F., Chipchase, L.S., Schabrun, S.M., 2017. Primary motor cortex organization is altered in persistent patellofemoral pain. Pain Medicine 18 (11), 2224–2234.

Tozzi, P., Bongiorno, D., Vitturini, C., 2012. Low back pain and kidney mobility: local osteopathic fascial manipulation decreases pain perception and improves renal mobility. Journal of Bodywork and Movement Therapies 16 (3), 381–391.

Tsao, H., Danneels, L.A., Hodges, P.W., 2011. ISSLS prize winner: smudging the motor brain in young adults with recurrent low back pain. Spine 36 (21), 1721–1727.

Tsur, N., Defrin, R., Ginzburg, K., 2017. Posttraumatic stress disorder, orientation to pain, and pain perception in ex-prisoners of war who underwent torture. Psychosomatic Medicine 79 (6), 655–663.

Tucker, K., Larsson, A.-K., Oknelid, S., Hodges, P., 2012. Similar alteration of motor unit recruitment strategies during the anticipation and experience of pain. Pain 153 (3), 636–643.

Ung, H., Brown, J.E., Johnson, K.A., Younger, J., Hush, J., Mackey, S., 2012. Multivariate classification of structural MRI data detects chronic low back pain. Cerebral Cortex 24 (4), 1037–1044.

Vachon-Presseau, E., Tétreault, P., Petre, B., Huang, L., Berger, S.E., Torbey, S., et al., 2016. Corticolimbic anatomical characteristics predetermine risk for chronic pain. Brain 139 (7), 1958–1970.

van Dieën, J.H., Flor, H., Hodges, P.W., 2017. Low-back pain patients learn to adapt motor behavior with adverse secondary consequences. Exercise and Sport Sciences Reviews 45 (4), 223–229.

Veehof, M., Trompetter, H., Bohlmeijer, E.T., Schreurs, K.M.G., 2016. Acceptance- and mindfulness-based interventions for the treatment of chronic pain: a meta-analytic review. Cognitive Behaviour Therapy 45 (1), 5–31.

Vlaeyen, J.W., Morley, S., Crombez, G., 2016. The experimental analysis of the interruptive, interfering, and identity-distorting effects of chronic pain. Behaviour Research and Therapy 86, 23–34.

Vowles, K.E., Witkiewitz, K., Levell, J., Sowden, G., Ashworth, J., 2017. Are reductions in pain intensity and pain-related distress necessary? An analysis of within-treatment change trajectories in relation to improved functioning following interdisciplinary acceptance and commitment therapy for adults with chronic pain. Journal of Consulting and Clinical Psychology 85 (2), 87.

Vrana, A., Hotz-Boendermaker, S., Stämpfli, P., Hänggi, J., Seifritz, E., Humphreys, B.K., et al., 2015. Differential neural processing during motor imagery of daily activities in chronic low back pain patients. PloS One 10 (11), e0142391.

Wallwork, S.B., Bellan, V., Catley, M.J., Moseley, G.L., 2016. Neural representations and the cortical body matrix: implications for sports medicine and future directions. British Journal of Sports Medicine 50, 990–996.

Wälti, P., Kool, J., Luomajoki, H., 2015. Short-term effect on pain and function of neurophysiological education and sensorimotor retraining compared to usual physiotherapy in patients with chronic or recurrent nonspecific low back pain, a pilot randomized controlled trial. BMC Musculoskeletal Disorders 16 (1), 83.

Wideman, T.H., Asmundson, G.G., Smeets, R.J.M., Zautra, A.J., Simmonds, M.J., Sullivan, M.J., et al., 2013. Re-thinking the fear avoidance model: toward a multi-dimensional framework of pain-related disability. Pain 154 (11), 2262–2265.

Wijma, A.J., van Wilgen, C.P., Meeus, M., Nijs, J., 2016. Clinical biopsychosocial physiotherapy assessment of patients with chronic pain: the first step in pain neuroscience education. Physiotherapy Theory and Practice 32 (5), 368–384.

Wippert, P.-M., Fliesser, M., Krause, M., 2017. Risk and protective factors in the clinical rehabilitation of chronic back pain. Journal of Pain Research 10, 1569–1579.

Wolfe, F., Brähler, E., Hinz, A., Häuser, W., 2013. Fibromyalgia prevalence, somatic symptom reporting, and the dimensionality of polysymptomatic distress: results from a survey of the general population. Arthritis Care & Research 65 (5), 777–785.

Wolfe, F., Clauw, D.J., Fitzcharles, M.-A., Goldenberg, D.L., Häuser, W., Katz, R.L., et al., 2016. Revisions to the 2010/2011 fibromyalgia diagnostic criteria. Seminars in Arthritis and Rheumatism 46 (3), 319–329.

Wurm, M., Edlund, S., Tillfors, M., Boersma, K., 2016. Characteristics and consequences of the co-occurrence between social anxiety and pain-related fear in chronic pain patients receiving multimodal pain rehabilitation treatment. Scandinavian Journal of Pain 12, 45–52.

Yunus, M.B., 2015. Editorial review (Thematic issue: an update on central sensitivity syndromes and the issues of nosology and psychobiology). Current Rheumatology Reviews 11 (2), 70–85.

Zusman, M., 2012. A review of the proposal that innocuous proprioceptive input may maintain movement-evoked joint pain. Physical Therapy Reviews 17 (5), 346–349.

Zusman, M., 2008a. Associative memory for movement-evoked chronic back pain and its extinction with musculoskeletal physiotherapy. Physical Therapy Reviews 13 (1), 57–68.

Zusman, M., 2008b. Mechanisms of peripheral neuropathic pain: implications for musculoskeletal physiotherapy. Physical Therapy Reviews 13 (5), 313–323.

Zusman, M., 2009. Pain science and mobilization of painful compressive neuropathies. Physical Therapy Reviews 14 (4), 285–289.

Chapter | **10** |

The physiology of manual therapy

Christopher J. McCarthy, Elaine Lonnemann, Jackie Hindle, Ruth MacDonald and Ioannis Paneris

Introduction

Manual therapy (MT) is considered to be a therapeutic intervention method involving the skilled application of movement to the body. This commonly takes the form of movement that is applied to the recipient rather than movement generated by the recipient and thus is termed passive movement (Maitland, 1986; Vicenzino et al., 2007). However, forms of guided active movement and isometric muscle contractions (Day and Nitz, 2012; Sharman et al., 2006; Smith and Fryer, 2008) are also considered to fall under the umbrella term of manual therapy. Manual therapy is intended to have any or all of the following effects: improve tissue extensibility; increase range of motion; mobilize or manipulate soft tissues and joints; induce relaxation; change muscle function; stabilize the joint complex; modulate pain; reduce soft tissue swelling, inflammation or movement restriction (IFOMPT Standards, 2016). There are numerous texts describing joint mobilizations (Maitland, 1986; McCarthy, 2010; Vicenzino et al., 2007), muscle techniques (Smith and Fryer, 2008) and nerve techniques (Shacklock, 2005). The application of contact to the body with the intention of guiding or evoking motion will influence skin, fascia, neural, vascular, lymphatic, myogenic and arthrogenic tissue and thus such labels are a little artificial.

Manual therapy can also be subcategorized based on the parameters of the movement produced. Nonlocalized, light pressure, large amplitude, stroking movement could be considered to characterize 'soft-tissue massage' (Lindgren et al., 2010) whilst small-amplitude, high-velocity movement would be considered to be typical of 'manipulative thrust' techniques (Evans, 2010; McCarthy et al., 2015). Whilst there are differences in the methods whereby one might introduce movement to the body, there appear to be some common responses to applied touch and movement that can offer therapeutic benefits to those experiencing pain. Certainly the consideration of MT (as a component of a multimodal package of care) is recommended in the majority of international guidelines for the management of low back pain and sciatica, and its use is considered to be cost effective (Chou et al. 2007; NICE, 2016).

Effects on pain

The mechanical stimulus of applied movement generates a series of neurophysiological responses from multiple systems including the peripheral nervous system, the spinal cord and supraspinal structures (Bialosky et al., 2009; Lascurain-Aguirrebena et al., 2016; Pickar, 2002). In addition to the neurophysiological effects, some biomechanical effects have been noted. These include short-term to permanent change in connective tissue length and stiffness (Bialosky et al., 2009; Martinez-Segura et al., 2006; 2012). The simple act of applying touch to the skin can have beneficial effects on the perception of pain (Mancini et al., 2015). Brief applications of light-touch, small-amplitude, low-pressure motion can evoke sufficient afferent stimulation to reduce dorsal horn sensitization and amplification resulting in a reduction in temporal summation phenomenon, an observable index of dorsal horn 'wind-up' (Mancini et al., 2015). Similar central nervous system (CNS) inhibitory mediation is also observed after high-velocity, small-amplitude stimulation (spinal manipulation) (Bishop et al., 2011). In addition, large-amplitude, light-pressure 'stroking' touch of the skin, stimulating C-tactile skin receptors, has been shown to reduce pain. This is linked with responses in the orbitofrontal cortex associated with pleasure, suggesting an inhibition of pain at a supraspinal level being produced in the context of a pleasant touch sensation (Leknes and Tracey, 2008; Liljencrantz and Olausson, 2014). The 'hands on effects' communication and feedback, personal attention and examination are part of the clinical management process of a manual therapist. These factors may produce a placebo effect which must be considered in the plausible mechanisms for improvement.

There is a considerable body of evidence describing the influence of afferent stimulation from various types of MT on the mediation of CNS-orchestrated inhibitory pain mechanisms (Bialosky et al., 2009; Bishop et al., 2011; Coronado et al., 2012; Skyba et al., 2003; Vicenzino et al., 1999; Wright, 1999; Wright and Sluka, 2001; Yeo and Wright, 2011). The precise type of afferent stimulation does not seem to be critical, with similar responses being reported with mobilization techniques (slow, non-localized, large-amplitude, low-pressure movements) and manipulative thrust techniques (localized, fast, high-pressure, small-amplitude movements) (Bishop et al., 2015; Moulson and Watson, 2006). A fast-acting, short-term sympathetoexcitatory response to MT has been well documented (Zusman, 2012), with this 'fight or flight' mechanism providing reductions in perception of nociceptive afferent information local to the region of application and, to a lesser extent, systemically (Hegedus et al., 2011; Voogt et al., 2015).

There is some evidence to suggest that the application of deep-pressure touch and movement sufficient to stimulate high-threshold mechanoreceptors and local nociceptors can evoke diffuse noxious inhibitory control (DNIC) cortical shifts (Granot et al., 2008; Kunz et al., 2006; Peters et al., 1992; Ram et al., 2008; Staud et al., 2003). The diversion of cortical attention from pathologic pain to a non-threatening, 'less-significant' nociceptive stimulus (similar to that observed with the insertion of acupuncture needles) can reduce painful states (Staud et al., 2003). In addition, functional magnetic resonance imaging evidence has shown that the perception of nonthreatening discomfort can be interpreted in the pain neuromatrix (Moseley, 2003) as pleasure, resulting in a systemic hypoalgesia (Leknes and Tracey, 2008).

The relief of pain following the application of MT can be interpreted by the brain as a reward, particularly so if it is unexpected or greater than expected (Bissonette and Roesch, 2016; Leknes et al., 2011; 2013; Morita et al., 2013; Navratilova and Porreca, 2014; Wise, 2005). Unexpected reward sensations result in phasic release of the neurotransmitter dopamine which, in addition to contributing to systemic hypoalgesia, will facilitate motivation to seek that reward sensation again (Navratilova and Porreca, 2014). Thus, motivation to repeat movement can be facilitated and a process of graded exposure to movement undertaken (Jones et al., 2002). A gradual upgrading of movement will lead to neurophysiological adaptations facilitating habituation to the nociceptive stimulus, resulting in a gradual reduction in pain (Zusman, 2004).

The influence MT has on the neuroendocrine system is not clear and is relatively underresearched. The initial mechanical stimulus affects the peripheral nervous system and may cause a reduction in inflammatory mediators such as cytokines (Kovanur Sampath et al., 2015; Teodorczyk-Injeyan et al., 2006; 2010). Alterations in levels of neuropeptides and nerve growth factor have also been noted (Bialosky et al., 2018). The peripheral nervous system response to the mechanical stimulus not only affects the spinal cord but portions of the brain that modulate pain such as the anterior cingular cortex, periaqueductal grey and rostral ventromedial medulla. These areas affect the autonomic nervous system and cause changes in skin temperature and conduction, cortisol levels and heart rate (Coronado and Bialosky, 2017). They also stimulate an endocrine response producing β-endorphins and endogenous opioids. In addition, the pain-modulating areas of the brain create placebo effects and psychological changes in pain catastrophizing, kinesiophobia and fear (Coronado and Bialosky, 2017).

There is some suggestion that spinal manipulation may result in small increases in endogenous opioid levels (Vernon, 1989; Vernon et al., 1986) and small reductions in inflammatory cytokines (Kovanur Sampath et al., 2015; Teodorczyk-Injeyan et al., 2006; 2010). However further work is needed to establish if these findings will have any clinical relevance to lumbar spine pain. Thus, the evidence would suggest that introducing touch and passive/active movement can influence perceptions of pain through a series of complex interactions of the peripheral nervous system, central nervous system and neuroendocrine system.

Mechanical effects

There is a growing body of evidence indicating that the mechanical interactions between the cells and their extracellular matrix (ECM) have a significant effect on the cells' development and function that is as important as the biochemical signalling (Ingber, 2010; Swanson, 2013). This notion gives MT, as well as other mechanical therapies (such as electrotherapy) and exercise, another basis for influencing tissue healing and improving function. Tissues and cells translate mechanical loads into biochemical processes that switch on and off cellular functions such as inflammation, cellular proliferation and migration, stem cell differentiation and maturation, and tissue remodelling and repair; this process is termed 'mechanotransduction' (Chaitow, 2013; Dunn and Olmedo, 2016). Chalkias and Xanthos (2013) state, 'Mechanotransduction describes the molecular mechanisms by which cells respond to mechanical changes in their physical environment. It reflects the process whereby mechanical forces are converted into biochemical or electrical signals that are able to promote structural and functional remodelling in cells and tissues.'

The role of mechanical loading and exercise has been long recognized in enhancing the structural properties and morphology of bone whilst vigorous exercise can reduce the rate of bone loss associated with osteoporosis. Mechanical stimulation can also accelerate bone healing. The addition of rhythmical compression to immobilized fractures accelerated callus formation, improved the quality of the new-formed bone tissue (Challis et al., 2006; Henstock et al., 2014) and improved muscle power and joint range of motion postimmobilization (Challis et al., 2007). In joint cartilage, mechanical stimulation in the form of low-grade cyclic compression has been shown to supress the production of proinflammatory regulators and antagonize inflammatory and matrix catabolic processes *in vitro* (Leong et al., 2011). Further, studies have shown that compressive and tensile stresses produce changes in the cell shape that augment the accumulation of newly synthesized proteoglycans, increase the production of matrix molecules and type II collagen, induce cell proliferation and increase the synthesis of the lubricant glycoprotein lubricin (Jaumard et al., 2011).

Mechanical loading affects connective tissue in a number of ways. Tension induces cytoskeletal and morphological remodelling of the fibroblast, allowing for the connective tissue to relax and achieve lower levels of resting tension in a short period of time (Langevin et al., 2011). Cells also respond in a similar manner to cyclic loads which, if applied for a longer period of time, may lead to reduction of the stress further towards the preloaded values (Humphrey et al., 2014). Mechanical loading has also positive effects on ECM turnover as it increases the cellular production of ECM structural constituents and accelerates the removal of old ECM (Chiquet et al., 2003; Humphrey et al., 2014; Jaumard et al., 2011). However, ECM compliance (Abbott et al., 2013) and fibroblast cytoskeleton pre-stress (Chiquet et al., 2003) are prerequisites for the above responses of the fibroblasts. In tendons, stretching and cyclic loading was found to increase the proliferation of tendon fibroblasts and gene expression of type I collagen, whilst low-grade cyclic stretching produced an antiinflammatory effect on the tendon and increased proliferation of tendon stem cells (TSC), TSCs' collagen production and TSC differentiation into tenocytes (Wang et al., 2012).

Mechanical stimulation can produce adverse effects that seem to be dependent on the magnitude of the stimulation. Whilst a 4% cyclical stretching appears to have an antiinflammatory effect on the tendon by reducing the gene expression of proinflammatory cytokines, increasing the stretch to 8% promotes the expression of these cytokines (Wang et al., 2012). Further, a large mechanical stretch leads to differentiation of TSC into nontenocytes such as adipocytes, chondrocytes and osteocytes (Wang et al., 2012). The rate of application of the mechanical load to tissues seems also to be of importance. Acute increases in strain and stress can lead to failure of the mechanism of cellular tension homeostasis and can result in continuing ECM stiffening and fibrosis (Humphrey et al., 2014).

Effects on motor control

In addition to reductions in pain, the reported effects of MT include improvements in range of motion, reductions in resistance to passive movement (spinal stiffness) and alterations in paraspinal muscle activity (Edgecombe et al., 2015; Pickar, 2002). However, this body of evidence is surprisingly small, and at times contradictory. Interestingly, there is evidence to suggest that the effect MT on stiffness may not be uniform throughout the spine, with regional differences in reductions in stiffness being observed in animal models (Edgecombe, et al., 2015). There is debate regarding the mediation of motor activity following spinal manipulation, with evidence to support both short-term facilitation and attenuation of spinal reflex loops and paraspinal muscle activity (DeVocht et al., 2005; Keller and Colloca, 2000).

How manual therapy influences the learning of motor control is an important area for development. There are a number of theories of motor learning suggesting that manual therapy has a role in influencing the input, interpretation and biopsychosocial integrations necessary for controlled movement. One such theory is the 'optimizing performance through intrinsic motivation and attention for learning' (OPTIMAL) theory of motor learning (Fig. 10.1). This builds on the premise that motor learning cannot be understood without considering the motivational (e.g., social-cognitive and affective) and attentional influences on behaviour (Wulf and Lewthwaite, 2016), and it offers a useful framework for the optimization of motor performance in relation to the use of movement 'therapy'. This is done by adapting the therapeutic alliance in manner that addresses the sociocognitive and affective (biopsychosocial) profile of the patient to allow:

- therapeutic conditions that enhance expectancies of effect
- patient choice in therapeutic movement, thereby increasing their sense of autonomy
- promoting an external focus of attention to movement retraining, by directing concentration to a relevant and appropriate external goal.

In doing so, motor relearning and concomitant reductions in disability can be optimized (see Fig. 10.1).

These strategies incorporate positive and social comparative feedback on performance, selective attention (external focus on the therapy and not the pain) and learner autonomy and self-efficacy. In the context of manual therapy, this includes realistic functional goal setting in conjunction with the patient, graded quota-based rehabilitation and positive reinforcement of active participation and positive

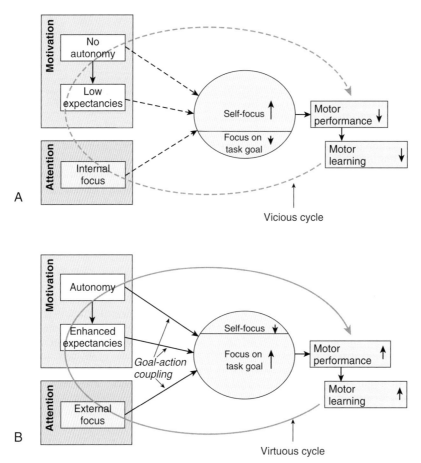

Fig. 10.1 Optimizing performance through intrinsic motivation and attention for learning (OPTIMAL) theory of motor learning. Conditions that fail to enhance patient expectancies, support their need for autonomy and promote an internal focus of attention result in a vicious cycle of nonoptimal learning (A); in contrast, conditions that enhance expectancies, provide autonomy support and promote an external focus result in a virtuous cycle of enhanced motor learning (B).

pain behaviours (Bunzli et al., 2011). Within classical conditioning, pairing manual therapy with a positive experience can have a marked impact on an individual's response and can be integrated to further intrinsic motivation and behavioural change (Fordyce et al., 1968).

Conclusion

Whilst there is confidence that MT is an effective modality in the relief of pain and reduction in disability, its specific biomedical, psychological and social influences and interactions are still to be fully understood. Manual therapy is a complex intervention and will require further mixed methodology research to fully appreciate its role within the biopsychosocial management of pain and disability. The effective utilization of MT requires the synthesis of patient and therapist factors, which include personal and condition-specific patient characteristics, and also the cultural biases, beliefs, and experiences of both the patient and therapist (Coronado and Bialosky, 2017). Additionally, it is important to use methods to integrate adjunct interventions such as psychosocial motor learning strategies, pain education, and exercise that enhances the effectiveness of manual therapy in reducing pain and disability (Coronado and Bialosky, 2017) (Fig. 10.2). The clinical reasoning for the use of manual therapy requires an appreciation of the influence of touch and movement on the psychological, biomechanical and neurophysiological profile of the patient. An understanding of the personal biopsychosocial interaction of these mechanisms enables effective and efficient integration of manual therapy with other rehabilitation approaches in the management of musculoskeletal dysfunction.

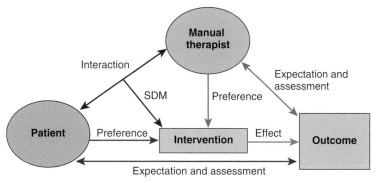

Fig. 10.2 A comprehensive approach to manual physical therapy effectiveness. This approach takes into account interaction between patient, therapist and intervention factors. Examples of these factors include preferences, expectations, outcome assessment, and shared decision making *(SDM)*. From Coronado R.A., Bialosky, J.E., 2017. Manual physical therapy for chronic pain: the complex whole is greater than the sum of its parts. Journal of Manual & Manipulative Therapy 25, 115–117.

References

Abbott, R.D., Koptiuch, C., Iatridis, J.C., Howe, A.K., Badger, G.J., Langevin, H.M., 2013. Stress and matrix-responsive cytoskeletal remodeling in fibroblasts. Journal of Cellular Physiology 228, 50–57.

Bialosky, J.E., Beneciuk, J.M., Bishop, M.D., Coronado, R.A., Penza, C.W., Simon, C.B., et al., 2018. Unraveling the mechanisms of manual therapy: modeling an approach. The Journal of Orthopaedic and Sports Physical Therapy 48, 8–18.

Bialosky, J.E., Bishop, M.D., Price, D.D., Robinson, M.E., George, S.Z., 2009. The mechanisms of manual therapy in the treatment of musculoskeletal pain: a comprehensive model. Manual Therapy 14, 531–538.

Bishop, M.D., Beneciuk, J.M., George, S.Z., 2011. Immediate reduction in temporal sensory summation after thoracic spinal manipulation. Spine Journal 11, 440–446.

Bishop, M.D., Torres-Cueco, R., Gay, C.W., Lluch-Girbes, E., Beneciuk, J.M., Bialosky, J.E., 2015. What effect can manual therapy have on a patient's pain experience? Pain Management 5, 455–464.

Bissonette, G.B., Roesch, M.R., 2016. Neurophysiology of reward-guided behavior: correlates related to predictions, value, motivation, errors, attention, and action. Current Topics in Behavioral Neurosciences 27, 199–230.

Bunzli, E., Gillham, D., Esterman, A., 2011. Physiothrapy-provided operant conditioning in the management of low back pain: a systematic review. Physiotherapy Research International 16 (1), 4–19.

Chaitow, L., 2013. Understanding mechanotransduction and biotensegrity from an adaptation perspective. Journal of Bodywork and Movement Therapies 17, 141–142.

Chalkias, A., Xanthos, T., 2013. Mechanotransduction and cardiac arrest during marathon running. American Journal of Medicine 126 (3), e23.

Challis, M.J., Gaston, P., Wilson, K., Jull, G.A., Crawford, R., 2006. Cyclic pneumatic soft-tissue compression accelerates the union of distal radial osteotomies in an ovine model. Journal of Bone and Joint Surgery British 88, 411–415.

Challis, M.J., Jull, G.J., Stanton, W.R., Welsh, M.K., 2007. Cyclic pneumatic soft-tissue compression enhances recovery following fracture of the distal radius: a randomised controlled trial. Australian Journal of Physiotherapy 53, 247–252.

Chiquet, M., Renedo, A.S., Huber, F., Flück, M., 2003. How do fibroblasts translate mechanical signals into changes in extra-cellular matrix production? Matrix Biology 22, 73–80.

Chou, R., Qaseem, A., Snow, V., et al. 2007. Diagnosis and treatment of low back pain: a joint clinical practice guideline from the American College of Physicians and the American Pain Society [published correction appears in Annals of Internal Medicine. 2008 Feb 5;148(3):247–8. Annals of Internal Medicine. 147 (7), 478–491.

Coronado, R.A., Bialosky, J.E., 2017. Manual physical therapy for chronic pain: the complex whole is greater than the sum of its parts. Journal of Manual & Manipulative Therapy 25, 115–117.

Coronado, R.A., Gay, C.W., Bialosky, J.E., Carnaby, G.D., Bishop, M.D., George, S.Z., 2012. Changes in pain sensitivity following spinal manipulation: a systematic review and meta-analysis. Journal of Electromyography & Kinesiology 22, 752–767.

Day, J.M., Nitz, A.J., 2012. The effect of muscle energy techniques on disability and pain scores in individuals with low back pain. Journal of Sport Rehabilitation 21, 194–198.

DeVocht, J.W., Pickar, J.G., Wilder, D.G., 2005. Spinal manipulation alters electromyographic activity of paraspinal muscles: a descriptive study. Journal of Manipulative and Physiological Therapeutics 28, 465–471.

Dunn, S.L., Olmedo, M.L., 2016. Mechanotransduction: relevance to physical therapist practice – understanding our ability to affect genetic expression through mechanical forces. Physical Therapy 96, 712–721.

Edgecombe, T.L., Kawchuk, G.N., Long, C.R., Pickar, J.G., 2015. The effect of application site of spinal manipulative therapy (SMT) on spinal stiffness. Spine Journal 15, 1332–1338.

Evans, D.W., 2010. Why do spinal manipulation techniques take the form they do? towards a general model of spinal manipulation. Manual Therapy 15, 212–219.

Fordyce, W.E., Fowler, R., Delateur, B., 1968. An application of behaviour modification technique to a problem of chronic pain. Behaviour Research and Therapy 6 (1), 105–107.

Granot, M., Weissman-Fogel, I., Crispel, Y., Pud, D., Granovsky, Y., Sprecher, E., et al., 2008. Determinants of endogenous analgesia magnitude in a diffuse noxious inhibitory control (DNIC) paradigm: do conditioning stimulus painfulness, gender and personality variables matter? Pain 136, 142–149.

Hegedus, E.J., Goode, A., Butler, R.J., Slaven, E., 2011. The neurophysiological effects of a single session of spinal joint mobilization: does the effect last? The Journal of Manual & Manipulative Therapy 19, 143–151.

Henstock, J.R., Rotherham, M., Rashidi, H., Shakesheff, K.M., El Haj, A.J., 2014. Remotely activated mechanotransduction via magnetic nanoparticles promotes mineralization synergistically with bone morphogenetic protein 2: applications for injectable cell therapy. Stem Cells Translational Medicine 3, 1363–1374.

Humphrey, J.D., Dufresne, E.R., Schwartz, M.A., 2014. Mechanotransduction and extracellular matrix homeostasis. Nature Reviews Molecular Cell Biology 15 (12), 802–812.

IFOMPT Standards, 2016. Educational Standards In Orthopaedic Manipulative Therapy. International Federation of Orthopaedic Manipulative Physical Therapists, Auckland, New Zealand. Available at: https://www.ifompt.org/site/ifompt/IFOMPT %20Standards%20Document%20definitive%202016.pdf.

Ingber, D.E., 2010. From cellular mechanotransduction to biologically inspired engineering: 2009 Pritzker Award Lecture, BMES annual meeting October 10, 2009. Journal of Biomechanical Engineering 38 (3), 1148–1161.

Jaumard, N.V., Welch, W.C., Winkelstein, B.A., 2011. Spinal facet joint biomechanics and mechanotransduction in normal, injury and degenerative conditions. Journal of Biomechanical Engineering 133 (7), 071010.

Jones, M., Edwards, I., Gifford, L., 2002. Conceptual models for implementing biopsychosocial theory in clinical practice. Manual Therapy 7 (1), 2–9.

Keller, T.S., Colloca, C.J., 2000. Mechanical force spinal manipulation increases trunk muscle strength assessed by electromyography: a comparative clinical trial. Journal of Manipulative and Physiological Therapeutics 23, 585–595.

Kovanur Sampath, K., Mani, R., Cotter, J.D., Tumilty, S., 2015. Measureable changes in the neuro-endocrinal mechanism following spinal manipulation. Medical Hypotheses 85, 819–824.

Kunz, M., Scholl, K.E., Schu, U., Lautenbacher, S., 2006. GABAergic modulation of diffuse noxious inhibitory controls (DNIC): a test by use of lorazepam. Experimental Brain Research 175, 363–371.

Langevin, H.M., Bouffard, N.A., Fox, J.R., Palmer, B.M., Wu, J., Iatridis, J.C., et al., 2011. Fibroblast cytoskeletal remodeling contributes to connective tissue tension. Journal of Cellular Physiology 226, 1166–1175.

Lascurain-Aguirrebena, I., Newham, D., Critchley, D.J., 2016. Mechanism of action of spinal mobilizations: a systematic review. Spine (Phila Pa 1976) 41, 159–172.

Leknes, S., Berna, C., Lee, M.C., Snyder, G.D., Biele, G., Tracey, I., 2013. The importance of context: when relative relief renders pain pleasant. Pain 154, 402–410.

Leknes, S., Lee, M., Berna, C., Andersson, J., Tracey, I., 2011. Relief as a reward: hedonic and neural responses to safety from pain. PLoS One 6, e17870.

Leknes, S., Tracey, I., 2008. A common neurobiology for pain and pleasure. Nature Reviews Neuroscience 9, 314–320.

Leong, D.J., Hardin, J.A., Cobelli, N.J., Sun, H.B., 2011. Mechanotransduction and cartilage integrity. Annals of the New York Academy of Sciences 1240, 32–37.

Liljencrantz, J., Olausson, H., 2014. Tactile C fibers and their contributions to pleasant sensations and to tactile allodynia. Frontiers in Behavioral Neuroscience 8, 37.

Lindgren, L., Rundgren, S., Winsö, O., Lehtipalo, S., Wiklund, U., Karlsson, M., et al., 2010. Physiological responses to touch massage in healthy volunteers. Autonomic Neuroscience 158, 105–110.

Maitland, G.D., 1986. Vertebral Manipulation, fifth ed. Butterworth-Heinemann, Oxford.

Mancini, F., Beaumont, A.L., Hu, L., Haggard, P., Iannetti, G.D., 2015. Touch inhibits subcortical and cortical nociceptive responses. Pain 156, 1936–1944.

Martinez-Segura, R., De-la-Llave-Rincon, A.I., Ortega-Santiago, R., Cleland, J.A., Fernandez-de-Las-Penas, C., 2012. Immediate changes in widespread pressure pain sensitivity, neck pain, and cervical range of motion after cervical or thoracic thrust manipulation in patients with bilateral chronic mechanical neck pain: a randomized clinical trial. Journal of Orthopaedic & Sports Physical Therapy 42, 806–814.

Martinez-Segura, R., Fernandez-de-las-Penas, C., Ruiz-Saez, M., Lopez-Jimenez, C., Rodriguez-Blanco, C., 2006. Immediate effects on neck pain and active range of motion after a single cervical high-velocity low-amplitude manipulation in subjects presenting with mechanical neck pain: a randomized controlled trial. Journal of Manipulative and Physiological Therapeutics 29, 511–517.

McCarthy, C.J., Bialoski, J., Rivett, D., 2015. Spinal manipulation. In: Jull, G., Moore, A., Falla, D., Lewis, J., McCarthy, C., Sterling, M. (Eds.), Grieve's Modern Musculoskeletal Physiotherapy, fourth ed. Elsevier, Oxford.

McCarthy, C.J., 2010. Combined Movement Theory: Rational Mobilization and Manipulation of the Vertebral Column. Elsevier Health Sciences, Oxford.

Morita, K., Morishima, M., Sakai, K., Kawaguchi, Y., 2013. Dopaminergic control of motivation and reinforcement learning: a closed-circuit account for reward-oriented behavior. Journal of Neuroscience 33, 8866–8890.

Moseley, G.L., 2003. A pain neuromatrix approach to patients with chronic pain. Manual Therapy 8, 130–140.

Moulson, A., Watson, T., 2006. A preliminary investigation into the relationship between cervical snags and sympathetic nervous system activity in the upper limbs of an asymptomatic population. Manual Therapy 11, 214–224.

Navratilova, E., Porreca, F., 2014. Reward and motivation in pain and pain relief. Nature Neuroscience 17, 1304–1312.

NICE, 2016. Low Back Pain and Sciatica in Over 16s: Assessment and Management. NICE Guideline, No. 59. National Institute for Health and Care Excellence, London.

Peters, M.L., Schmidt, A.J., Van den Hout, M.A., Koopmans, R., Sluijter, M.E., 1992. Chronic back pain, acute postoperative pain and the activation of diffuse noxious inhibitory controls (DNIC). Pain 50, 177–187.

Pickar, J.G., 2002. Neurophysiological effects of spinal manipulation. Spine Journal 2, 357–371.

Ram, K.C., Eisenberg, E., Haddad, M., Pud, D., 2008. Oral opioid use alters DNIC but not cold pain perception in patients with chronic pain – new perspective of opioid-induced hyperalgesia. Pain 139, 431–438.

Shacklock, M., 2005. Improving application of neurodynamic (neural tension) testing and treatments: a message to researchers and clinicians. Manual Therapy 10, 175–179.

Sharman, M.J., Cresswell, A.G., Riek, S., 2006. Proprioceptive neuromuscular facilitation stretching: mechanisms and clinical implications. Sports Medicine 36, 929–939.

Skyba, D.A., Radhakrishnan, R., Rohlwing, J.J., Wright, A., Sluka, K.A., 2003. Joint manipulation reduces hyperalgesia by activation of monoamine receptors but not opioid or GABA receptors in the spinal cord. Pain 106, 159–168.

Smith, M., Fryer, G., 2008. A comparison of two muscle energy techniques for increasing flexibility of the hamstring muscle group. Journal of Bodywork and Movement Therapies 12, 312–317.

Staud, R., Robinson, M.E., Vierck Jr., C.J., Price, D.D., 2003. Diffuse noxious inhibitory controls (DNIC) attenuate temporal summation of second pain in normal males but not in normal females or fibromyalgia patients. Pain 101, 167–174.

Swanson 2nd., R. L., 2013. Biotensegrity: a unifying theory of biological architecture with applications to osteopathic practice, education, and research – a review and analysis. Journal of the American Osteopathic Association 113 (1), 34–52.

Teodorczyk-Injeyan, J.A., Injeyan, H.S., Ruegg, R., 2006. Spinal manipulative therapy reduces inflammatory cytokines but not substance p production in normal subjects. Journal of Manipulative and Physiological Therapeutics 29, 14–21.

Teodorczyk-Injeyan, J.A., McGregor, M., Ruegg, R., Injeyan, H.S., 2010. Interleukin 2-regulated in vitro antibody production following a single spinal manipulative treatment in normal subjects. Chiropractic & Osteopathy 18, 26.

Vernon, H., 1989. Exploring the effect of a spinal manipulation on plasma beta-endorphin levels in normal men. Spine (Phila Pa 1976) 14, 1272–1273.

Vernon, H.T., Dhami, M.S., Howley, T.P., Annett, R., 1986. Spinal manipulation and beta-endorphin: a controlled study of the effect of a spinal manipulation on plasma beta-endorphin levels in normal males. Journal of Manipulative and Physiological Therapeutics 9, 115–123.

Vicenzino, B., Cartwright, T., Collins, D., Wright, A., 1999. An investigation of stress and pain perception during manual therapy in asymptomatic subjects. European Journal of Pain 3, 13–18.

Vicenzino, B., Paungmali, A., Teys, P., 2007. Mulligan's mobilization-with-movement, positional faults and pain relief: current concepts from a critical review of literature. Manual Therapy 12, 98–108.

Voogt, L., de Vries, J., Meeus, M., Struyf, F., Meuffels, D., Nijs, J., 2015. Analgesic effects of manual therapy in patients with musculoskeletal pain: a systematic review. Manual Therapy 20, 250–256.

Wang, J.H., Guo, Q., Li, B., 2012. Tendon biomechanics and mechanobiology – a minireview of basic concepts and recent advancements. Journal of Hand Therapy 25, 133–140; Quiz 141.

Wise, R.A., 2005. Forebrain substrates of reward and motivation. Journal of Comparative Neurology 493, 115–121.

Wright, A., Sluka, K.A., 2001. Nonpharmacological treatments for musculoskeletal pain. Clinical Journal of Pain 17, 33–46.

Wright, A., 1999. Recent concepts in the neurophysiology of pain. Manual Therapy 4, 196–202.

Wulf, G., Lewthwaite, R., 2016. Optimizing performance through intrinsic motivation and attention for learning: The OPTIMAL theory of motor learning. Psychonomic Bulletin & Review 23, 1382–1414.

Yeo, H.K., Wright, A., 2011. Hypoalgesic effect of a passive accessory mobilisation technique in patients with lateral ankle pain. Manual Therapy 16, 373–377.

Zusman, M., 2012. A note to the musculoskeletal physiotherapist. Journal of Back and Musculoskeletal Rehabilitation 25, 103–107.

Zusman, M., 2004. Mechanisms of musculoskeletal physiotherapy. Physical Therapy Reviews 9 (1), 39–49.

Chapter | 11 |

The physiology of acupuncture analgesia

Jonathan Hobbs

Introduction

The early research into the physiological mechanisms of acupuncture analgesia (AA) began towards the end of the 1960s (Zhao, 2008). Over recent decades, numbers of those seeking acupuncture as a treatment modality has grown steadily. Analysis of the National Health Interview Survey (NHIS) from 2002 and 2007 demonstrated that acupuncture usage had increased from 0.4% of population in 1990 to 1.01% in 1998 within the United States. From 2002, the figure increased from 1.1% to 1.4% in 2007 (Barnes et al., 2004; 2009; Eisenberg et al., 1998). These figures demonstrate a modest yet persistent increase in overall usage which equates to an estimate of over 14 million individuals in the United States regularly utilizing acupuncture by 2007 (Burke et al., 2006). Data from the 2007 survey suggests that the majority of those individuals sought acupuncture for the treatment of pain, which included musculoskeletal pain, headaches and fibromyalgia (Barnes et al., 2009).

Although there is a documented growth in the usage of acupuncture, there continues to be considerable debate as to its value, the nature of its proposed mechanisms and relevance to clinical application (Colquhoun and Novella, 2013). There is some evidence to suggest that expectation and belief affect the experience of pain and its management and that these components exist within the placebo response of analgesia (Richardson and Vincent, 1986; Wager et al., 2004). The early work of Price et al. (1984) highlighted these aspects and acknowledged that psychological factors exist within acupuncture analgesia, but acupuncture's analgesic properties have a neurophysiological underpinning (Zhao, 2008). A recent systematic review and meta-analysis of trials for acupuncture for nonspecific low back pain concluded that both sham and placebo acupuncture were more efficacious than routine care or waiting list (Xiang et al., 2017). The existence of a tactile component,

which can create a physiological response similar to verum acupuncture, can cause issues when attempting to evaluate and understand the various components of acupuncture treatment (Makary et al., 2018). These findings may bring into question the use of sham or placebo acupuncture as interventions in research trials where they are compared with verum acupuncture. Early evaluation of placebo and acupuncture effect in the treatment of chronic pain suggested that acupuncture could be effective in 50–80% of patients. These are significant suggestions when compared to morphine, which was found to help 30% of those evaluated (Lewith and Machin, 1983; Richardson and Vincent, 1986).

Application and mechanisms

During acupuncture and dry needling (DN), a narrow-gauge filiform needle, which will typically range between 0.16 and 0.35 mm in diameter, is inserted into the body to stimulate both proposed local and systemic effects. Whilst some seek to differentiate the processes and techniques of acupuncture and DN, suggesting fundamental differences in ideology, both approaches can be considered to share significant components including the needle itself and the crossover between classical acupuncture points and DN sites. Dorscher (2006) has suggested a significant anatomical correlation of over 93% between myofascial trigger points and classical acupuncture points. Approaches such as Western medical acupuncture (WMA) may take the application of technique from traditional Chinese acupuncture (TCA) and seek to underpin the practice with physiological explanation and mechanistic theory whilst casting aside esoteric concepts such as *yin* and *yang* and *qi*.

Both traditional acupuncture and DN utilize the concept of specific locations for needling and set techniques of needle insertion and manipulation to create a stimulus and subsequent response from the patient. Inserting a filiform needle into skeletal muscle tissue has been shown to stimulate A delta (Aδ) or group III small-diameter myelinated primary afferents in the skin and muscle (Pomeranz, 1987). These fibres are responsible for the initial pinprick sensation of needling. Early studies in primates demonstrated that the stimulation of Aδ fibres had significant effects on pain inhibition via the spinothalamic tract (Chung et al., 1984). Following insertion, the needles are manipulated either by rotation or repeated penetration into the underlying muscle fibres, creating localized trauma and strong mechanical stimulation. The level of manipulation dictates stimulus level (Zhao, 2008). The numbness, heaviness and distension experienced during the mechanical stimulus of needling of deeper tissues is thought to be attributed to the stimulation of a combination of A beta (Aβ) and Aδ fibres (Zhang et al., 2012). The trauma caused by needle penetration and manipulation also triggers an inflammatory response stimulating the release of a variety of proinflammatory mediators. These include serotonin, bradykinin, histamine, adenosine triphosphate (ATP), prostaglandin E2 and calcitonin gene-related peptide (CGRP) that can excite local nociceptors (Boucher et al., 2000; Meyer et al., 2006).

During acupuncture needling, C fibres that are responsible for aching pain are also stimulated (Pomeranz, 1987). C unmyelinated fibres have a slower conduction and are responsible for a dull, more burning, aching, throbbing pain and are usually felt after the initial sharp stimulus of needle insertion (Wilkinson, 2001). C fibres are thought to contribute to the overall analgesic effect generated by acupuncture and the associated phenomenon of *de qi* as they give rise to a feeling of heaviness and soreness (Wang et al., 1985; 1989). Wang et al. (1990) concluded however that C fibre activation was not necessary for AA, after the chemical denervation of C fibres did not subsequently negatively affect AA.

Since the seminal work of Pomeranz and Chiu (1976), numerous studies have shown that acupuncture analgesia in both humans and animals can be reversed or abolished by naloxone, the opioid receptor antagonist. This process suggests that acupuncture's mechanism is opioidergic. The endogenous opioid group that influence acupuncture analgesia consist of Leu-enkephalin, Met-enkephalin, β-endorphin and dynorphins. For a considerable time there has been evidence to demonstrate an involvement of a number of monoamines, including noradrenaline, serotonin (5HT), dopamine and substance P (Han and Terenius, 1982). It has also been shown that when a nerve is blocked by local anaesthesia, acupuncture is ineffective in the region innervated by that nerve. The suggestion follows that acupuncture's effect is being transmitted via neural pathways (Stux et al., 2003; Stux and Hammerschlag, 2001). Seminal work by Chiang and colleagues (1973)

demonstrated that needling of the midbelly of the first dorsal interosseous muscle (meridian point: Large Intestine 4) increased the pain threshold in study participants. Following the administration of procaine to the cutaneous branches of the radial nerve there was no alteration in threshold response. Administering the same application of procaine to the deeper muscular branches of the ulnar and median nerve, however, countered the analgesia effect suggesting that is was in fact derived from the afferent innervation from the muscles.

Langevin et al. (2001a; 2002) demonstrated that the manipulation of the needle via rotation leads to the needle-grasp sensation associated with acupuncture and a subsequent mechanical coupling of the needle and its surrounding connective tissue. This phenomenon is considered to transmit signals to the adjacent connective tissue cells via mechanotransduction and support acupuncture's proposed therapeutic effects (Langevin et al., 2001b). Evidence suggests that significantly greater C fibre stimulus is elicited in superficial and deep mechanoreceptors through rotation than is achieved with thrusting, flicking or scraping the needle (Zhang et al., 2012). Zhang et al. (2008) concluded that mast cells had a significant role in the analgesic mechanism of acupuncture, as analgesia was lessened following chemically mediated mast cell destruction.

Acupuncture analgesia

The mechanical manipulation of the needle within the target tissue triggers a response in small-diameter myelinated afferent Aδ fibres (Fig. 11.1). On reaching the spinal cord these first-order Aδ neurons synapse mainly in the superficial dorsal horn (laminae I and V) of the spinal cord with cells of the anterolateral tract (ALT). The Aδ fibres also send short branches to intermediate endorphinergic cells of the substantia gelatinosa within the same spinal segment (Sugiura et al., 1986). The ALT proceeds cephalad to communicate with the midbrain and the pituitary hypothalamic complex (PHTC). The synapsing of Aδ fibres within the spinal cord stimulates a release of the endorphins enkephalin and dynorphin. Although β-endorphin is also considered to play a role in acupuncture analgesia, it is not involved in the spinal cord–mediated response. The release of spinal cord endorphins generates a presynaptic inhibitory effect within the local segmental region, limiting transmission of the pain signals initiated from C fibres to the spinothalamic tract (STT) (Stux and Hammerschlag, 2001).

The ALT ascends to and communicates with the midbrain and stimulates cells within the periaquaductal grey (PAG). Numerous studies highlight the role of the PAG in the management of pain, with Wang et al. (1990) demonstrating that lesions of the PAG abolish AA in the pain

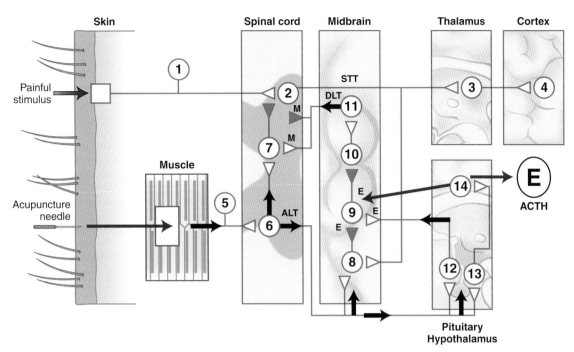

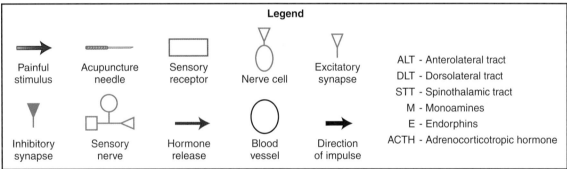

Fig. 11.1 **The mechanism of acupuncture analgesia.** *Pain*: A painful stimulus of small afferent Aδ and C nerve fibres (*1*) synapse in the dorsal horn of the spinal cord (*2*) before ascending the spinothalamic tract (STT) to the thalamus (*3*) and terminating in the cortex (*4*) where pain can be perceived at a conscious level. *Needling*: Needling the muscle stimulates Aδ fibres (*5*) which synapse in the spinal cord (*6*) and stimulate cell (*7*) where enkephalin is released causing presynaptic inhibition of cell (*1*). Cell (*6*) also synapses with the anterolateral tract (ALT) to the midbrain and stimulates cells (*8*) and (*9*) in the periaquaductal grey (PAG) which release β-endorphin to excite cell (*10*) (raphe nucleus) and cell (*11*), triggering impulses along the dorsolateral tract (DLT) to release monoamines (M) onto the cells (*2*) and (*7*) in the spinal cord. Cell (*1*) is presynaptically inhibited by M (serotonin) via cell (*7*), whilst cell (*2*) is postsynaptically inhibited by M (noradrenaline). ALT stimulus at cells (*12*) and (*13*) within the pituitary hypothalamic complex releases ACTH and β-endorphin into the circulation in equal measures. ACTH modulates the antiinflammatory response. The stimulation of cell (*8*) by cell (*2*) via the STT also causes analgesia through the mechanism of diffuse noxious inhibitory control (DNIC), where one noxious stimulus may inhibit another.

model in rats. Stimuli descending from the arcuate nucleus of the hypothalamus generate the release of β-endorphin. The limbic system, considered to be influential in the perception of pain due to its role in emotion, also delivers stimulus to the PAG. The modulation of activity in the limbic and subcortical structures has previously been demonstrated in a variety of studies examining the effects of point specificity via functional magnetic resonance imaging scanning (Li et al., 2000; Wu et al., 1999; Yan et al., 2005).

There also occurs the excitation of cells within the raphe nucleus in the medulla oblongata. These trigger impulses along the dorsolateral tract (DLT), which initiate the release of the monoamines serotonin and noradrenaline. The release of monoamines within the spinal cord supports further analgesic mechanisms. In one descending mechanism, noradrenaline acts to inhibit the postsynaptic membrane of the transmission cell within the STT, limiting propagation of nociceptive input from C fibres (Pomeranz, 1987; Stux and Hammerschlag, 2001; Zhao, 2008). This system acts diffusely throughout the spinal cord. Within the other descending inhibitory system, serotonin supports presynaptic inhibition further by exciting segmental intermediate cells and reinforcing the release of Met-enkephalin. Either or both of the two monoamines released can support the suppression of nociceptive transmission (Stux and Hammerschlag, 2001). Further ascending stimulus that is carried via the ALT reaches cells within the PHTC and triggers the release of adrenocorticotropic hormone (ACTH) and β-endorphin into the circulation in equal measure. ACTH influences the adrenal cortex and modulates cortisol production, which is considered to influence inflammatory responses within the body (Stux and Hammerschlag, 2001).

Layering effect

When acupuncture is performed in a region close to the site of pain or tender points within the local soft tissues, both the local inflammatory response and segmental circuits operating within the same spinal cord segment are utilized as the primary analgesic mechanisms (Baeumler et al., 2015). Local needling at points of myofascial pain occurs both within the practice of acupuncture and DN, with a significant crossover in the target areas for insertion (Dorsher, 2006). Within DN, trigger points are tender points located within the local soft tissues that are used to relieve the symptoms of myofascial pain (Cagnie et al., 2013). A systematic review conducted by Wong et al. (2014) concluded that local tender points are beneficial for short-term pain relief in the management of chronic myofascial pain.

Acupuncture, both TCA and WMA, may also employ needles placed in distal points some distance away from the painful region, either within the same dermatome or myotome or completely heterosegmental in location (White et al., 2018). DN focuses on the local myofascial target tissue and does not generally seek to utilize distally initiated stimuli. The addition of distal needling may contribute to a more profound activation of stimulus to the supraspinal regions of the central nervous system. By combining the documented benefits of the segmental

and local effects of needling with that of distal needling, it is proposed that the overall effect of acupuncture may be enhanced (Bradnam, 2007a; 2007b). This concept of a layering effect is considered to create the potential for widespread analgesia throughout the body (Stux and Hammerschlag, 2001). Therefore, local segmental needling usually gives more intensive analgesia than distal nonsegmental needling because it uses all three centres. Distal points are less likely to fall within the same segment, although this does occur in some cases. A study conducted by Srbely et al. (2010) demonstrated that by needling an area of myofascial pain defined as a trigger point there was a short-term antinociceptive response in an adjacent muscle. They concluded that there was a segmental mechanism of analgesia in effect. The work of Baeumler and colleagues (2015) also supports the conclusion that pain threshold changes with electroacupuncture (EA) are mediated via segmental inhibition at segmental level within the spinal cord. Another study examining needling for myofascial pain demonstrated that distant myofascial trigger points could reduce the irritability of painful areas in more proximal muscles within the same myotome via the proposed mechanism of segmental spinal cord inhibition (Hsieh et al., 2014).

A study examining neuropathic pain in a spinal nerve–ligated rat model demonstrated with the use of naloxone that the opioid system was involved in the acupuncture-reduced hypersensitivity. Acupuncture also displayed a similar efficacy to gabapentin in the same model and there was no subsequent increase in tolerance with continued treatment, suggesting its positive potential role in the treatment of neuropathic pain (Cidral-Filho et al., 2011). The heterosegmental effect of needling is brought about by a neurohormonal mechanism involving the release of β-endorphin and the two descending neuronal mechanisms which are serotonergic and adrenergic. There is also considered to be some involvement of diffuse noxious inhibitory control (DNIC) in the overall analgesic effect where one pain may inhibit another (Filshie and White, 1998).

Inflammation and healing

In a number of studies in rats it was demonstrated that manual acupuncture can increase local muscle blood flow via the release of nitric oxide, CGRP, adenosine diphosphate (ADP) and ATP (Nagaoka et al., 2016; Shinbara et al., 2013; 2015; 2017). Shinbara et al. (2017) concluded that adenosine may also have influence on acupuncture's analgesic effect by assisting with the removal of algesic substances. It has been suggested that due to its role in the increase of local muscle blood flow, acupuncture may also have a role to play in tissue healing (White et al., 2018). In studies examining acupuncture's role in inflammation, it was demonstrated that electroacupuncture (EA) enhanced corticotrophin-releasing hormone and ACTH levels in rats via stimulation of the hypothalamic-pituitary-adrenal axis (Li et al., 2008). A previous study had also shown that the experimental blocking of corticosterone receptors resulted in a measurable loss of the antiinflammatory effects of EA (Li et al., 2007). A more recent study by Yang et al. (2017) demonstrated that EA significantly reduced chronic mechanical and thermal hyperalgesia in the chronic inflammatory pain model in mice when compared to sham EA. This provides some level of evidence to support the clinical application of EA in the treatment of chronic inflammatory pain.

Summary

With breakthroughs in investigative research and deeper understanding of neurophysiology, there continues to be new evidence highlighting the underlying mechanisms of acupuncture and the potential benefits from its clinical application. Some of the more established mechanisms of acupuncture analgesia have been touched upon in this chapter but acupuncture's physiological effects are proposed to be much broader. Outside of the spectrum of myofascial pain, evidence exists for the use of acupuncture in the treatment of a range of problems including nausea, headaches, migraines and overactive bladder, to name but a few (Carlsson et al., 2000; Linde et al., 2016a; 2016b; Wang et al., 2012). With further research still, a more profound knowledge of mechanisms and application surely awaits.

References

Baeumler, P.I., Fleckensteina, J.B., Benedikta, F., Badera, J., Irnicha, D., 2015. Acupuncture-induced changes of pressure pain threshold are mediated by segmental inhibition – A randomized controlled trial. Pain 156 (11), 2245–2255.

Barnes, P.M., Bloom, B., Nahin, R.L., 2009. Complementary and alternative medicine use among adults and children: United States, 2007. National Health Statistics Reports (12), 1–23.

Barnes, P.M., Powell-Griner, E., McFann, K., Nahin, R.L., 2004. Complementary and alternative medicine use among adults: United States, 2002. Advance Data (343), 1–19.

Boucher, T.J., Okuse, K., Bennett, D.L., Munson, J.B., Wood, J.N., McMahon, S.B., 2000. Potent analgesic effects of GDNF in neuropathic pain states. Science 290, 124–127.

Bradnam, L., 2007a. A proposed clinical reasoning model for western acupuncture. Journal of the Acupuncture Association of Chartered Physiotherapists 21–30.

Bradnam, L., 2007b. A physiological underpinning for treatment progression of western acupuncture. Journal of the Acupuncture Association of Chartered Physiotherapists 25–33 Autumn.

Burke, D., Upchurch, M., Dye, C., Chyu, L., 2006. Acupuncture use in the United States: findings from the national health interview survey. Journal of Alternative and Complementary Medicine 12 (7), 639–648.

Cagnie, B., Dewitte, V., Barbe, T., Timmermans, F., Delrue, N., Meeus, M., 2013. Physiologic effects of dry needling. Current Pain and Headache Reports 17, 348.

Carlsson, C.P.O., Axemo, P., Bodin, A., Carstensen, H., Ehrenroth, B., Madegård-Lind, I., et al., 2000. Manual acupuncture reduces hyperemesis gravidarum: a placebo-controlled, randomized, single-blind, crossover study. Journal of Pain and Symptom Management 20 (4), 273–279.

Chiang, C.Y., Chang, C.T., Chu, H.C., Yang, L.F., 1973. Peripheral afferent pathway for acupuncture analgesia. Scientia Sinica - Series B 16, 210–217.

Chung, J.M., Willis, W.D., Lee, K.H., 1984. Factors influencing peripheral nerve stimulation produced inhibition of primate spinothalamic tract cells. Pain 19, 227–293.

Cidral-Filho, F.J., da Silva, M.D., Moré, A.O., Córdova, M.M., Werner, M.F., Santos, A.R., 2011. Manual acupuncture inhibits mechanical hypersensitivity induced by spinal nerve ligation in rats. Neuroscience 193, 370–376.

Colquhoun, D., Novella, S.P., 2013. Acupuncture is theatrical placebo. Anesthesia & Analgesia 116 (6), 1360–1363.

Dorsher, P.T., 2006. Trigger points and acupuncture points: anatomic and clinical correlations. Medical Acupuncture 17, 21–24.

Eisenberg, D.M., Davis, R.B., Ettner, S.L., 1998. Trends in alternative medicine use in the United States, 1990–1997: results of a follow-up national survey. Journal of the American Medical Association 280 (18), 1569–1575.

Filshie, J., White, 1998. Medical Acupuncture – a Western Scientific Approach. Churchill Livingstone, Edinburgh.

Han, J.S., Terenius, L., 1982. Neurochemical basis of acupuncture analgesia. Annual Review of Pharmacology and Toxicology 22, 193–220.

Hsieh, Y.L., Yang, C.C., Liu, S.Y., Chou, L.W., Hong, C.Z., 2014. Remote dose-dependent effects of dry needling at distant myofascial trigger spots of rabbit skeletal muscles on reduction of substance p levels of proximal muscle and spinal cords. Biomedical Research International 2014, 982121.

Langevin, H.M., Churchill, D.L., Cipolla, M.J., 2001a. Mechanical signalling through connective tissue: a mechanism for the therapeutic effect of acupuncture. FASEB Journal 15, 2275–2282.

Langevin, H.M., Churchill, D.L., Fox, J.R., Badger, G.J., Garra, B.S., Krag, M.H., 2001b. Biomechanical response to acupuncture needling in humans. Journal of Applied Physiology 91, 2471–2478.

Langevin, H.M., Churchill, D.L., Wu, J., Badger, G.J., Yandow, J.A., Fox, J.R., et al., 2002. Evidence of connective tissue involvement in acupuncture. FASEB Journal 16, 872–874.

Lewith, G.T., Machin, D., 1983. On the evaluation of the clinical effects of acupuncture. Pain 16, 111–127.

Li, A., Lao, L., Wang, Y., Xin, J., Ren, K., 2008. Electroacupuncture activates corticotrophin-releasing hormone-containing neurons in the paraventricular nucleus of the hypothalamus to alleviate edema in a rat model of inflammation. BMC Complementary and Alternative Medicine 8, 20.

Li, A., Zhang, R.X., Wang, Y., Zhang, H., Ren, K., 2007. Corticosterone mediates electroacupuncture-produced anti-edema in a rat model of inflammation. BMC Complementary and Alternative Medicine 7, 27.

Li, W.C., Hung, D.L., Kalnin, A., Holodny, A., Komisaruk, B., 2000. Brain activation of acupuncture induced analgesia. Neuroimage 11, S701.

Linde, K., Allais, G., Brinkhaus, B., Fei, Y., Mehring, M., Shin, B.C., et al., 2016a. Acupuncture for the prevention of tension-type headache. Cochrane Database of Systematic Reviews 4, CD007587.

Linde, K., Allais, G., Brinkhaus, B., Fei, Y., Mehring, M., Vertosick, E.A., et al., 2016b. Acupuncture for the prevention of episodic migraine. Cochrane Database of Systematic Reviews 2016 (6), CD001218 2016.

Makary, M.M., Lee, J., Lee, E., Eun, S., Kim, J., Jahng, G.H., et al., 2018. Phantom acupuncture induces placebo credibility and vicarious sensations: a parallel fMRI study of low back pain patients. Scientific Reports 8 (1), 930.

Meyer, R.A., Ringkamp, M., Campbell, J.N., Raja, S.N., 2006. Peripheral mechanisms of cutaneous nociception. In: McMahon, S.B., Koltzenburg, M. (Eds.), Wall and Melzack's Textbook of Pain, fifth ed. Elsevier/Churchill Livingstone, Edinburgh, pp. 3–34.

Nagaoka, S., Shinbara, H., Okubo, M., Kawita, T., Hino, K., Sumiya, E., 2016. Contributions of ADP and ATP to the increase in skeletal muscle blood flow after manual acupuncture stimulation in rats. Acupuncture in Medicine 2016 34 (3), 229–234.

Pomeranz, B., 1987. Scientific basis of acupuncture. In: Stux, G., Pomeranz, B. (Eds.), Acupuncture Textbook and Atlas. Springer-Verlag; 1987, Heidelberg, pp. 1–18.

Pomeranz, B., Chiu, D., 1976. Naloxone blocks acupuncture analgesia and causes hyperalgesia: endorphin is implicated. Life Sciences 19 (11), 1757–1762.

Price, D.D., Rafii, A., Watkins, L.R., Buckingham, B., 1984. A psychophysical analysis of acupuncture analgesia. Pain 19 (1), 27–42.

Richardson, H., Vincent, C.A., 1986. Acupuncture for the treatment of pain: a review of evaluative research. Pain 24, 15–40.

Shinbara, H., Nagaoka, S., Izutani, Y., Okubo, M., Kimura, K, Mizunuma, K., Sumiya, E., (2017) Contributions of adenosine to the increase in muscle blood flow caused by manual acupuncture in rats. Acupuncture in Medicine 35 (4), 284–288.

Shinbara, H., Okubo, M., Kimura, K., Mizunuma, K., Sumiya, E., 2013. Participation of calcitonin gene related peptide released via axon reflex in the local increase in muscle blood flow following manual acupuncture. Acupuncture in Medicine 31 (1), 81–87.

Shinbara, H., Okubo, M., Kimura, K, Mizunuma, K., Sumiya, E., 2015. Contributions of nitric oxide and prostaglandins to the local increase in muscle blood flow following manual

acupuncture in rats. Acupuncture in Medicine 33 (1), 65–71.

Srbely, J.Z., Dickey, J.P., Lee, D., Lowerison, M., 2010. Dry needle stimulation of myofascial trigger points evokes segmental anti-nociceptive effects. Journal of Rehabilitation Medicine 42, 463–468.

Stux, G., Berman, B., Pomeranz, B., 2003. Basics of Acupuncture, fifth ed. Springer, Berlin.

Stux, G., Hammerschlag, R. (Eds.), 2001. Clinical Acupuncture: Scientific Basis. Springer, Berlin.

Sugiura, Y., Lee, C.L., Perl, E.R., 1986. Central projection of identified, unmyelinated (C) afferent fibers innervating mammalian skin. Science 234, 358–361.

Wager, T.D., Riling, J.K., Smith, E.E., Sokolik, A., Casey, K.L., Davidson, R.J., et al., 2004. Placebo-induced changes in FMRI in the anticipation and experience of pain. Science 303, 1162–1167.

Wang, H., Tanaka, Y., Kawauchi, A., Miki, T., Kayama, Y., Koyama, Y., 2012. Acupuncture of the sacral vertebrae suppresses bladder activity and bladder activity-related neurons in the brainstem micturition center. Neuroscience Research 72 (1), 43–49.

Wang, K.M., Liu, J., 1989. Needling sensation receptor of an acupoint supplied by the median nerve studies of their electrophysiological characteristics. The American Journal of Chinese Medicine 17 (3–4), 145–156.

Wang, K.M., Yao, S.M., Xian, Y.L., Hou, Z.L., 1985. A study on the receptive field of acupoints and the relationship between characteristics of needling sensation and groups of afferent fibres. Scientia Sinica Series B 28 (9), 963–971.

Wang, Q., Mao, L., Han, J.S., 1990. The arcuate nucleus of hypothalamus mediates low but not high frequency electroacupuncture in rats. Brain Research 513, 60–66.

White, A., Cummings, M., Filshie, J., 2018. An Introduction to Western Medical Acupuncture, second ed. Churchill Livingstone/Elsevier, Edinburgh.

Wilkinson, P.R., 2001. Neurophysiology of pain. Part 1: mechanisms of pain in the peripheral nervous system. CPD Anaesthesia 3 (3), 103–108.

Wong Lit Wan, D., Wang, Y., Xue, C.C., Wang, L.P., Liang, F.R., Zheng, Z., 2015. Local and distant acupuncture points stimulation for chronic musculoskeletal pain: A systematic review on the comparative effects. European Journal of Pain 19 (9), 1232–1247.

Wu, M.T., Hsieh, J.C., Xiong, J., Yang, C.F., Pan, H.B., Chen, Y.C., et al., 1999. Central nervous pathway for acupuncture stimulation: localization of processing with functional MR imaging of the brain—preliminary experience. Radiology 212, 133–141.

Xiang, Y., He, J.Y., Li, R., 2017. Appropriateness of sham or placebo acupuncture for randomised controlled trials of acupuncture for nonspecific low back pain: a systematic review and meta-analysis. Journal of Pain Research 11, 83–94.

Yan, B., Li, K., Xu, J.X., Wang, W., Li, K., Liu, H., et al., 2005. Acupoint specific fMRI patterns in human brain. Neuroscience Letters 383, 236–240.

Yang, J., Hsieh, C.L., Lin, Y.W., 2017. Role of transient receptor potential vanilloid 1 in electroacupuncture analgesia on chronic inflammatory pain in mice. BioMed Research International 2017, 5068347.

Zhang, D., Ding, G., Shen, X., Yao, W., Zhang, Z., Zhang, Y., et al., 2008. Role of mast cells in acupuncture effect: a pilot study. Explore 4 (3), 170–177.

Zhang, Z.J., Wang, X.M., McAlonan, G.M., 2012. Neural acupuncture unit: a new concept for interpreting effects and mechanisms of acupuncture. Evidence-Based Complementary and Alternative Medicine 2012, 429412.

Zhao, Z.Q., 2008. Neural mechanism underlying acupuncture analgesia. Progress in Neurobiology 85, 355–375.

Chapter | **12** |

Physiological determinants of endurance performance: maximal oxygen uptake ($\dot{V}O_{2max}$)

Testing, training and practical application

Paul Sindall

Introduction

The ability to endure is an essential characteristic underpinning optimal outcomes in a variety of forms of organized sport. Furthermore, a fundamental requirement for cardiorespiratory and muscular endurance underpins optimal performance and function in everyday life. A number of physiological factors determine endurance performance, most notably oxygen availability (Weltman et al., 1978), altitude (Wehrlin and Hallén, 2006), economy [oxygen uptake ($\dot{V}O_2$) at a given work-rate] (Saunders et al., 2004), mechanical efficiency (Kyröläinen et al., 1995), muscle fibre type (Taylor and Bachman, 1999), mitochondrial number and size (Meinild Lundby et al., 2018), blood lactate transition thresholds (Yoshida et al., 1987), energy stores (Bjorntorp, 1991), hydration (Goulet, 2012), tactics (Hanley, 2015) and mental resilience (Crust and Clough, 2005). However, maximal oxygen uptake ($\dot{V}O_{2max}$) is generally accepted as the most important determinant. As $\dot{V}O_{2max}$ is defined as the maximal volume of oxygen the body can uptake and utilize at sea-level during high-intensity, dynamic exercise, it represents an individual's peak capacity for aerobic metabolism (Kavcic et al., 2012; Tran, 2018). Whilst 'maximal oxygen uptake' is the preferred description of $\dot{V}O_{2max}$, various terms are used interchangeably to describe the same phenomenon, depending on the setting and population group(s) involved:

- peak/maximal/maximum aerobic capacity
- peak/maximal/maximum oxygen consumption
- maximal aerobic power
- aerobic fitness
- functional capacity

- cardiorespiratory endurance, capacity and/or fitness
- cardiovascular endurance, capacity and/or fitness.

This chapter outlines the most common methods by which $\dot{V}O_{2max}$ can be measured and thereafter used to offer guidance on exercise training intensities for optimization of health and performance outcomes. As a considerable volume of high-quality information is available on the assessment of $\dot{V}O_{2max}$ and oxygen uptake kinetics during exercise, here we offer an overview of commonly available test options, so that practitioners can apply these with relative ease, in a way that is appropriate to the testing context and implicated population group(s). Example data are also presented in the form of a case study to outline the process of exercise training prescription to prompt increases in $\dot{V}O_{2max}$ and enhance associated physiological markers.

Central vs. peripheral considerations

The Fick equation states that in any physiological state, whether resting or under exertion, $\dot{V}O_{2max}$ is a product of cardiac output (Q) multiplied by arteriovenous oxygen difference (a-vO_{2diff}). As Q is a product of heart rate (HR) multiplied by left ventricular stroke volume (= end diastolic volume – end systolic volume), $\dot{V}O_{2max}$ is determined, in part, by *central factors*, namely transport of O_2 from ambient air into the lungs, diffusion into the arterial blood supply and subsequent translocation to the periphery via systemic circulatory mechanisms. In contrast, a-vO_{2diff} is related to cellular and molecular processes within skeletal muscle whereby O_2 is diffused into the mitochondria from arterial blood to enable regeneration of ATP and promote aerobic energy production. Therefore, $\dot{V}O_{2max}$ is also determined by *peripheral factors*. So, if $\dot{V}O_{2max}$ is a product of $Q \times \text{a-vO}_{2diff}$, $\dot{V}O_{2max}$ is quite simply the collective product of maximal Q (oxygen supply) and maximal a-vO$_{2diff}$ (oxygen extraction).

However, the question of which factor(s) limits $\dot{V}O_{2max}$ is not as simple and remains a controversial topic lacking clarity (Noakes, 2008). The traditional view that central factors predominate in the realization of peak physiological effort (Bassett and Howley, 1997; 2000) has been questioned; some argue that the characteristics of muscle and its oxidative potential act as the primary determinant (Noakes, 1998; 2008; Sloth et al., 2013).

$\dot{V}O_{2max}$ and its association with optimal sports performance

Stakeholders within the world of elite sport require information on peak endurance capacity for talent identification (Burgess and Naughton, 2010), to establish baseline fitness at specific points within the competitive calendar and to fine tune performance for competition (Ishak et al., 2016) with a view to ensuring a physiological 'edge' over competitors. A high $\dot{V}O_{2max}$ offers a distinct advantage for competition in individual sports such as long-distance running (Sjödin and Svedenhag, 1985) and tennis (Kovacs, 2006), and team sports such as basketball (Metaxas et al., 2009), football (soccer) (Metaxas et al., 2009), field-hockey (Reilly and Borrie, 1992), ice-hockey (Cox et al., 1995; Ransdell et al., 2013), netball (Bell et al., 1994), rugby league (Brewer and Davis, 1995; Gabbett et al., 2013) and rugby union (Duthie et al., 2003; Vaz et al., 2016). Elite athletes typically have $\dot{V}O_{2max}$ values 50–100% above those observed in active people (Joyner and Coyle, 2008). Therefore, athletic populations can essentially sustain double the work rate of their less-trained counterparts. In terms of performance, this confers a significant advantage as participants are able to sustain aerobic activity for a longer duration and/or a higher proportion of a competitive athletic event.

Whilst it is prudent to note that $\dot{V}O_{2max}$ is not the only implicated physiological factor in deciding performance outcomes (Coyle, 1995; Sjödin and Svedenhag, 1985), it is closely correlated with performance times in triathletes (Butts et al., 1991) and in endurance-trained runners (Freeman, 1990; Hagan et al., 1981; 1987). Further indicators of performance in endurance-based sports have been proposed. For example, running velocity at $\dot{V}O_{2max}$ (Hill and Rowell, 1996) has been deemed useful due to its ability to effectively combine $\dot{V}O_{2max}$ and economy into a single factor (Billat and Koralsztein, 1996). More recently, the concept of critical power has been mooted (Jones et al., 2010), referring to the point at which physiological responses

cannot be stabilized with an increase in exercise intensity. Whilst this has been challenged, mainly due to its application of potentially inappropriate terminology (Winter, 2011), there remains potential for the application of critical power for optimization of athletic training programmes (Poole et al., 2016).

In a more holistic sense, sport should be considered a vehicle for physical activity and is a viable activity option for those who have a requirement for, and interest in, a more competitive physical activity environment. For example, positive changes in $\dot{V}O_{2max}$ have been reported for recreational football (Milanović et al., 2015a; 2015b), with considerable potential for health-enhancing effects (Bangsbo et al., 2015; Eime et al., 2015b). Fitness levels are typically lower in middle-aged people (Lindgren et al., 2016) and young girls (Bohr et al., 2013) with a low socioeconomic status (SES). However, there is some evidence that participation in team sports is greater for people with a low SES, and those living in remote areas (Eime et al., 2015a). Nevertheless, facility provision (Eime et al., 2017) and accessibility (Karusisi et al., 2013) are considerable barriers to participation.

$\dot{V}O_{2max}$ and its association with optimal health

A negative correlation is associated with $\dot{V}O_{2max}$ and age due to chronic decreases in cardiac output and a decline in skeletal muscle oxidative capacity prompting decreases in peripheral tissue oxygen utilization (Betik and Hepple, 2008). This natural decline in $\dot{V}O_{2max}$ is expected with increasing age in both males and females (0.45 and 0.30 mL·kg·min^{-1} per year respectively) from the age of 25 years onwards (Stamford, 1988). However and in addition, the prevalence of sedentary behaviour and obesity in adolescents (Carnethon et al., 2005; Pate et al., 2006), adults (Carnethon et al., 2005; Wang et al., 2010), and those with intellectual (Oppewal et al., 2013) or physical impairments and/or disabilities (van den Berg-Emons et al., 2008), has exacerbated and unnecessarily accelerated the decline in $\dot{V}O_{2max}$ at a population level. Activity level for both males and females decreases with increasing age (MacAuley et al., 1998). This has placed considerable burden on healthcare systems around the world as $\dot{V}O_{2max}$ is accepted to be the strongest single predictor of all-cause and, specifically, cardiovascular mortality (Keteyian et al., 2008; Myers et al., 2002). Consequently, there has never been a more opportune time for examination and critique of testing and training methodologies for respective identification and enhancement of aerobic capacity.

Considerable attention has been paid in the scientific literature to associations made between $\dot{V}O_{2max}$ and optimal health. An elevated $\dot{V}O_{2max}$ offers a protective health effect, with reduced incidence of all-cause mortality and coronary heart disease in those with a high $\dot{V}O_{2max}$ (Kodama et al., 2009). In contrast, a low $\dot{V}O_{2max}$ has been strongly linked with premature death (Lee et al., 2010). The study of Harvard University alumni focused attention on the characteristics of physical activity for optimal health gains, with a reduction in mortality and stroke rates associated with chronic vigorous activity (Lee and Paffenbarger, 1998; 2000; Lee et al., 1995). Great gains in fitness and function can be made with a commitment to exercise, with considerable crossover into individual health status and quality of life. In terms of life expectancy, increases in $\dot{V}O_{2max}$ are profound, with an increase as small as 3.5 mL·kg·min^{-1} (~1 MET) associated with large (10 to 25%) increases in survival rate (Kaminsky et al., 2013). Therefore, $\dot{V}O_{2max}$ should not solely be considered a preserve of the athletic world. Furthermore, $\dot{V}O_{2max}$ should be used as a tool by practitioners working with general populations (i.e., unfit, deconditioned, apparently healthy sedentary) to inform health-related exercise prescription, lifestyle guidance and health-based education.

Physiological assessment of $\dot{V}O_{2max}$

Laboratory-based approaches

Assessment of $\dot{V}O_{2max}$ is conventionally done in climate-controlled laboratory conditions where a direct analysis of expired air is undertaken during progressive exercise. When collected, $\dot{V}O_{2max}$ is expressed in either absolute (L·min^{-1}) or relative (mL·kg·min^{-1}) units, with the latter allowing for comparison between individuals of differing body mass. A traditional approach involving manual collection of expired air using Douglas bags (Fig. 12.1A) followed by analysis of oxygen and carbon dioxide concentrations using respective paramagnetic and infrared analysers is still adopted in some testing settings. However, modern analysers enable measurement of breath-by-breath pulmonary gas exchange (Fig. 12.1B) and are therefore more commonly used to assess physiological cost during incremental testing for research and applied physiological consultancy.

Metabolic carts are easily calibrated (Macfarlane, 2001), allow rapid turn-around times to enable more prompt data reporting and feedback (Macfarlane, 2001), and offer valid and reliable data in comparison to manual methods (Lee et al., 2011; Nieman et al., 2007). Reference values for $\dot{V}O_{2max}$ are provided with relative ease and accuracy (Macfarlane, 2001), with test output used to inform training prescription (see Fig. 12.1), to act as a baseline to assess chronic training responses or to detect irregularities and diagnose specific health conditions. However, such testing requires expensive equipment, is time consuming and requires trained personnel for data collection and subsequent interpretation (Abut and Akay, 2015). Also, identification of peak physiological variables requires a maximal exertion on behalf of the participant. Attainment of peak performance is a complex process which requires application of physiological test-termination criteria and is affected by age (Huggett et al., 2005) and influenced by psychobiological factors (Midgley et al., 2017), most notably motivation and commitment to perform a maximal effort (Moffatt et al., 1994).

Considerations in selection of exercise test modality

As exercise modality influences determination of $\dot{V}O_{2max}$ (Keren et al., 1980; Millet et al., 2009) and subsequent training priorities (Sousa et al., 2015), careful consideration should be given to this aspect prior to testing. Treadmill

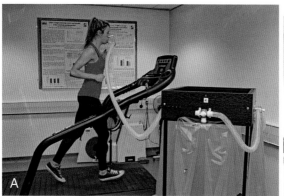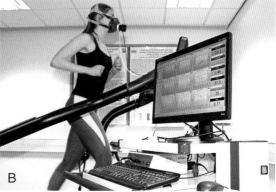

Fig. 12.1 Collection of expired air samples in a controlled laboratory environment using Douglas bags (A) and an online, breath-by-breath analyser (B).

testing is the most commonly used modality as upright locomotion is a familiar movement that involves activation of all major muscle groups (McConnell, 1988; Weiglein et al., 2011). This modality is therefore associated with the highest observed values in studies comparing modes (Keren et al., 1980), with runners (Caputo and Denadai, 2004; Millet et al., 2009), triathletes (Caputo and Denadai, 2004) and untrained populations (Caputo and Denadai, 2004) obtaining higher values using a motorized treadmill versus a static cycle. Highly trained runners should therefore be tested, where possible, using this modality.

Whilst road cycling is a complex motor task involving pedalling, braking and steering, the action of cycling is a relatively low-skill, easy-to-learn task as it involves an innate voluntary motor rhythm (Hansen, 2015). Use of a static upright cycle ergometer, which requires no such responses to external stimuli, represents an ideal testing option for low-skill or low-fit groups. Cycling protocols are a popular option for those with limitations or impairments as these groups can be tested easily (Beltz et al., 2016), although lower values for $\dot{V}O_{2max}$ are likely to be reported due to sole recruitment of the lower limb musculature (Loftin et al., 2004; McKay and Bannister, 1976).

Trained cyclists will require a more specific testing setup. Use of a turbo trainer enables a customized setup, whereby the rider is tested on his/her own cycle. This facilitates a more specific and valid data collection with no trade-off in mechanical efficiency versus a treadmill-based cycle assessment (Arkesteijn et al., 2013). However, in situations where repeat testing is required (e.g., pre- to posttraining intervention), it may be preferable to use a cycle ergometer, as the protocol, power output and rider configuration can more easily be exactly replicated from test to test. Trained cyclists achieve higher peak outcomes on a static cycle ergometer than a treadmill (Caputo and Denadai, 2004; Ricci and Léger, 1983), but even though constrained by a smaller amount of active muscle mass, highly conditioned cyclists can achieve a similar $\dot{V}O_{2max}$ to runners using this modality (Millet et al., 2009). This is due to the considerable peripheral adaptations prompted by repeated strain on the lower limb musculature (Atkinson et al., 2003).

Arm-trained athletes (e.g., rowers, swimmers, cross-country skiers) can achieve an upper body $\dot{V}O_{2max}$ which surpasses their equivalent performance in a lower body test (Secher and Volianitis, 2006) and therefore arm-crank ergometry is the preferred modality for these populations, along with those who are unable to cycle (Orr et al., 2013). Subtle differences in the movement characteristics can also influence test performance. For example, the $\dot{V}O_{2max}$ of elite hand-cyclists is 10% lower during an asynchronous arm-crank ergometer when compared with their more familiar synchronous pattern on the same ergometer (Goosey-Tolfrey and Sindall, 2007). Therefore, determination of $\dot{V}O_{2max}$ is both highly

mode-specific (Millet et al., 2009) and task-dependent (Smirmaul et al., 2013), and careful thought should be given to mode selection based on situational (i.e., resources, facilities) and individual (i.e., sport, position) considerations and constraints prior to testing. Pedal cadence is also a factor which is known to influence economy (Hansen and Smith, 2009), thereby influencing internal physiological load. An individual's preferred, 'freely-chosen' cadence tends to be higher than their most economical pedal frequency (Marsh and Martin, 1997; Vercruyssen and Brisswalter, 2010). Therefore, lack of cadence standardization potentially introduces bias in test-to-test scenarios. Less-trained, noncyclists may subconsciously choose lower pedal rates to minimize aerobic demand (Marsh and Martin, 1997). In contrast, the freely chosen cadence of well-trained cyclists is closer to energetically optimal pedal rates (Brisswalter et al., 2000). Therefore, the decision to fix or allow freely chosen cadence should be made prior to implementation of cycle-based exercise testing and be informed by training status.

Considerations in test protocol selection and design

To ensure an accurate determination of $\dot{V}O_{2max}$, and that appropriate recommendations are made regarding training, test protocol must be carefully considered (Riboli et al., 2017). Test durations approximating 7 to 12 min are considered optimal (Astorino et al., 2004; McConnell, 1988; Poole and Jones, 2012; Yoon et al., 2007). Whilst this represents an appropriate general target, it is useful to note that the steeper $\Delta \dot{V}O_2/\Delta$ work-rate slope in shorter protocols may be challenging for low-fit individuals, with premature fatigue potentially confounding outcomes (Beltz et al., 2016). Therefore, selection should always be dictated by the testing scenario and the individual to be tested. For example, a competitive athlete will require a comparatively greater stimulus (e.g., speed and gradient in a treadmill running test) to elicit a maximal effort than a counterpart with low fitness or a functional impairment. Fig. 12.2 offers a comparison of commonly used treadmill testing protocols, whereby increments are fixed. Included are two examples of testing protocols used within the author's laboratory for assessment of elite professional football players and boxers. These can easily be applied in a controlled setting and show how speed and gradient can be manipulated to prompt ultimate progression to maximal exertion. In both cases, gradient is fixed at 1% to best represent the energetic cost of outdoor running (Jones and Doust, 1996).

Athletic protocols, such as those shown in Fig. 12.2, may appear tentative. However, their application may provide a simpler, quicker and more effective means to ascertain peak physiological attributes than more established protocols (Hamlin et al., 2012). An alternative approach is

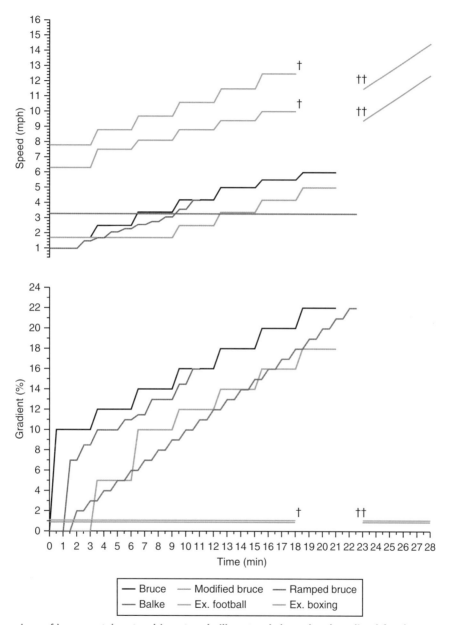

Fig. 12.2 Comparison of incremental motor-driven treadmill protocols (speed and gradient) for the assessment of oxygen uptake during exercise Common (Bruce, modified Bruce, ramped Bruce and Balke) are presented against two example protocols used with professional football players and boxers. *†*, End of submaximal graded testing followed by a 5-min recovery period prior to *††*, start of peak testing to exhaustion.

for individuals to self-select pace, with duration specified and ratings of perceived exertion (RPE) (Borg, 1982) used as an anchor to empower self-selection of target pace/intensity. Such an approach compares favourably to traditional ramp-incremental protocols for quantification of $\dot{V}O_{2max}$ (Chidnok et al., 2013; Straub et al., 2014) and offers a simple, reliable means to administer graded exercise testing (Beltz et al., 2016).

Identification of peak physiological exertion during laboratory-based exercise testing

$\dot{V}O_{2max}$ increases linearly with work rate. Therefore, observation of a $\dot{V}O_{2max}$ plateau with increasing work rate is generally accepted as the prime method for defining peak capacity (Howley et al., 1995). Indeed, the absence of an increase in $\dot{V}O_{2max}$ with further increases in workload during incremental exercise was the means by which $\dot{V}O_{2max}$ was first defined in the seminal works of Hill and Lupton (1923). However, a plateau is not seen in all individuals. In a study involving 804 participants aged 20 to 85 years, a plateau was observed in only 43% (Edvardsen et al., 2014). In these cases, the term $\dot{V}O_{2peak}$ is advocated in preference to $\dot{V}O_{2max}$ and secondary criteria such as blood lactate (BLa^-), maximal HR, respiratory exchange ratio (RER) and RPE are used to coinform identification of peak physiological effort (Duncan et al., 1997; Howley et al., 1995).

Proposed secondary criteria to support test termination and identification of $\dot{V}O_{2max}$:

- $BLa^- \geq 8.0$ mmol·L^{-1}
- maximal HR $\geq$ (220 – age)
- RER $\geq$ 1.15
- RPE $\geq$ 19

It should be noted however that these parameters are often achieved at intensities below $\dot{V}O_{2max}$ (Edvardsen et al., 2014; Schaun, 2017) and there is considerable variation in how these criteria are applied, both in the literature and in practice (Howley et al., 1995). For example, the practice is to accept two criteria to represent end-test termination point, although this is not always the case. Also, volitional exhaustion is highly variable and intrinsically generated. Consequently, a further, more rigorous option is to administer a posttest verification stage (Poole and Jones, 2017) whereby one additional supramaximal exercise bout is undertaken (~110% final workload) posttest to verify end-stage $\dot{V}O_{2max}$. Whilst some evidence suggests that similar values for $\dot{V}O_{2max}$ are obtained during conventional and supramaximal testing (Hawkins et al., 2007), others state that this approach increases the accuracy of $\dot{V}O_{2max}$ measurements in athletic and apparently healthy populations (Midgley and Carroll, 2009; Mier et al., 2012). Nevertheless, tolerance to supramaximal effort in less-able groups (i.e., children, obese people and the elderly) could be questioned (Midgley and Carroll, 2009). Therefore, where verification is applied it should be population specific and further work should be completed to refine and standardize protocols for this purpose (Schaun, 2017).

Field-based approaches

The advantages of testing $\dot{V}O_{2max}$ in a controlled laboratory setting are well documented (Beltz et al., 2016). Conditions can be easily replicated from test to test, offering an ideal means to monitor training programme effectiveness and for research purposes, where the need to limit confounding factors is of prime concern (McConnell, 1988; Skelly et al., 2012). However, a mechanistic approach to physiological testing is not always appropriate, nor feasible.

Due to the highly specialized and unique characteristics of specific sporting tasks, laboratory testing is not always the most attractive option for coaches who are more focused on the specific movement demands and physiological traits underpinning athletic performance in a given sporting domain. Coupled with the fact that direct testing is often impractical (Lindberg et al., 2014) and invasive (Nakagaichi et al., 2001), issues such as cost and the requirement for trained personnel may present a challenge to accessing facilities (Barbieri et al., 2017). Novel field tests involving assessment in a more natural, 'simulated' sporting environment have become increasingly popular in recent years, with acceptable accuracy and reliability proven for a range of popular sports including, but not limited to, indoor track cycling (González-Haro et al., 2007; Karsten et al., 2014), football (Castagna et al., 2014; Da Silva et al., 2011; Teixeira et al., 2014), futsal (Barbieri et al., 2017), karate (Tabben et al., 2014), rugby union (Moore and Murphy, 2003), tennis (Fernandez, 2005) and a range of wheelchair sports (Goosey-Tolfrey and Leicht, 2013), e.g., sitting volleyball (Marszalek et al., 2015).

Similarly positive observations have been noted for a range of highly specific aerobic field tests in a health context, with good reproducibility and repeatability reported for the 6-min walk test in patients with chronic obstructive pulmonary disease (COPD) (Fotheringham et al., 2015; Jenkins and Čečins, 2011; Poulain et al., 2003), and in an occupational setting for firefighters (Lindberg et al., 2013; 2014; Michaelides et al., 2011) and the military (Hauschild et al., 2017; Weiglein et al., 2011). Such testing approaches have considerable value in terms of ecological validity and should therefore not be overlooked (Goosey-Tolfrey and Leicht, 2013). Indeed, in some cases, field testing may offer a more effective means to assess actual performance (Rylands et al., 2015; Wells et al., 2012) and more effectively simulate the demands of any given sport (Fernandez, 2005). This argument has to be counterbalanced as submaximal tests can underestimate (Bennett et al., 2016a; Fitchett, 1985; Hartung et al., 1993; Jamnick et al., 2016) or overestimate (Bennett et al., 2016b) observed $\dot{V}O_{2max}$ and are reliant on appropriate monitoring during exercise (Caputo and Denadai, 2004). Also, field testing has not been proven effective for all subgroups of the population, with questionable outcomes in some children and those with intellectual disabilities (Wouters et al., 2017). Therefore caution must be observed when interpreting outcomes from testing, particularly those that relate to validity.

Chronic disease, physical impairments and sedentary lifestyles are all associated with a reduction in function. Hence, when such groups embark on an exercise regime, the testing modality must be appropriate and low risk. In health-based or recreational leisure settings, specialist testing equipment is unlikely to be available. Also, testing involving a maximal effort may be contraindicated for individuals with exertional intolerance. In these cases, prediction of $\dot{V}O_{2max}$ using submaximal testing offers a low-cost, low-risk, low-supervision option (Sartor et al., 2013). In summary, careful consideration should be given to the context within which testing is completed, i.e., sporting, clinical, leisure facility, community (Sartor et al., 2013); the purpose of testing (West et al., 2015); specific movement or activity requirements/restrictions; available equipment; the number of participants; and any temporal constraints. For ease of reference, a range of popular testing options and their characteristics are summarized in Table 12.1.

Walking tests

Walking is a familiar and easily accessible mode of activity for a large cross-section of the population and is therefore a highly applicable modality for exercise testing, encompassing a wide spectrum of individuals. Testing can be completed indoors or outside, with similar values obtained (Brooks et al., 2003). A simple Rockport walking test is ideal for those with low fitness due to its low-risk attributes (Kline et al., 1987). Participants walk at a self-selected pace for 1 mile, with weight, age, gender, walk time and HR entered into a regression equation to determine $\dot{V}O_{2max}$. Validity has been confirmed with acceptable agreement with a laboratory-based treadmill testing protocol (Weiglein et al., 2011) and both test duration and data processing times compare favourably to other, more time- and labour-intensive methods (see Table 12.1). Some tests can also be customized to suit the participant. For example, the Fox walking test allows the individual to self-select test distance, with speed and gradient entered into the regression equation for determination of $\dot{V}O_{2max}$ (Nordgren et al., 2014). As test outcomes are reliable on a test-to-test basis (Verberkt et al., 2012), individuals can effectively take ownership of the fitness-testing process, tracking changes in $\dot{V}O_{2max}$ over time. Where time constraints are an issue, very short tests (~3 min) can be administered with ease and with acceptable relation to reference measures (Cao et al., 2013).

Running tests

Due to the large amount of muscle mass recruited during running, this mode of exercise arguably offers the best indication of aerobic power, especially in trained runners who replicate this motion in training and performance (McConnell, 1988). The multistage fitness test is a viable and valid option for testing adults involved in running-based sports (Léger, 1982) and for children (20-m variant) (Artero et al., 2011; Batista et al., 2017; Castro-Piñero et al., 2010), with acceptable test-to-test reliability against reference measures (Léger, 1982; Metsios et al., 2008). The initial work rate is low (light jog), progressing to running and ultimately, maximal exertion. As increments of speed are fixed, unskilled or deconditioned individuals may find testing overly challenging and demotivating if participating with more capable counterparts. A square version (i.e., linear motion with 4 × 90-degree turns vs. standard linear motion with 2 × 180-degree turns) of the same test can be applied where prediction of $\dot{V}O_{2max}$ is important (Flouris et al., 2009; Metsios et al., 2008) or revised algorithms can be applied to the traditional test to increase accuracy (Flouris et al., 2005).

The manner in which running field tests are applied is also an important consideration. Offering performance feedback during both linear and square 20-m shuttle tests reduces the limits of agreement and coefficient of variation, thereby yielding more accurate outcomes (Metsios et al., 2006). Alternatively, the 1.5-mile endurance test allows individuals to self-select pace, opting to walk, jog or run. This type of testing is ideal for assessment of large groups with varying fitness levels or when laboratory based assessment is not an available option (Mayorga-Vega et al., 2016). $\dot{V}O_{2max}$ is accurately predicted ($R = 0.86$, $SEE = 3.4$ mL·kg·min^{-1}) using test duration, with marginal improvements if HR is also factored into the model ($R = 0.90$, $SEE = 2.9$ mL·kg·min^{-1}) (Larsen et al., 2002). The yo-yo test is a popular choice for team sports, most notably football where its application enables effective training programme formation, providing useful data to monitor player progress in exercise capacity (Krustrup et al., 2003; Metaxas et al., 2005). Furthermore, the level 2 variant is sensitive to player position and level of competition (i.e., international elite vs. moderate elite) (Krustrup et al., 2006), which is useful given that elite endurance athletes typically have a higher $\dot{V}O_{2max}$ than non-elite athletes (Lorenz et al., 2013; Metaxas et al., 2009).

Step tests

If correctly and properly executed, step testing can provide reliable data which does not deviate significantly from reference measures for $\dot{V}O_{2max}$ (Keren et al., 1980). Technique must be standardized and, most importantly for

Table 12.1 Summary of laboratory and commonly used field-based tests for quantification of $\dot{V}O_{2max}$

	TEST				TEST DETAILS
Type	Name(s)	Method	Mode	Exertion required	Equipment
Gas analysis		Direct	Cycle, treadmill, ergometer (i.e., rower, arm-crank, wheelchair)	100% (maximal)	a) Douglas bags, dry gas mete mouthpiece/mask, HR monitor, RPE scale b) Metabolic cart, mouthpiece/mask, HR monitor, RPE scale
Running	Cooper's run	Indirect	Overground running	100% (maximal)	Running track,[c] measuring tape
	Multistage shuttle	Indirect	Overground running	100% (maximal)	Sports hall or equivalent space (flat and nonslip[d]), cones, 20-m measuring tape, specific reporting sheets, audio track with system for playback
	Yo-yo	Indirect	Overground running	100% (maximal)	Sports hall or equivalent space (flat and nonslip[d]), cones, 20-m measuring tape, specific reporting sheets, audio track with system for playback
	1.5-mile endurance	Indirect	Overground walking, jogging or running	Freely chosen	Stopwatch, weighing scales, running track,[c] HR monitors,[c] flat surface.
Walk testing	Rockport; Fox	Indirect	Overground walking	Low but variable (walking pace)	Smooth and level surface,[d] marked track,[c] stopwatch, weighing scales, HR monitors[c]
Step	McArdle, Chester	Indirect	Stepping	<85% HR max	Step boxes, HR monitors, RPE scales, dedicated scoring/reporting sheet
Cycle ergometer testing	Astrand-Rhyming, YMCA, Ekblom-Bak	Indirect	Static cycle	Low (submaximal)	Static cycle, HR monitors,[c] RPE scale, BP monitor[c]
Prediction		Nonexercise	None	None	Calculator, weighing scales, specific physical activity scoring sales

Test times are based on assessment of one individual and are approximate.
[a]Protocol dependent.
[b]Variable analysis duration (i.e., shorter time if investigator uses built-in reporting tools, longer if calculations are made and reported by hand).
[c]Desirable (not essential).
[d]Essential.
BP, Blood pressure; *HR*, heart rate; *RPE*, ratings of perceived exertion.

Scope	Setting	TIME			Overall total
		Calibration and Setup	Test implementation	Data processing, analysis, feedback	
Limited to one individual and access to/availability of specialist equipment/ personnel	Controlled laboratory environment	~20 min	12 to 20 min[a]	10 to 90 min[b]	~40 to 130 min
Limited by available space only	Outside	Negligible	12 min	8 min	~20 min
Limited by available equipment and space	Inside/outside	~10 min	22 min (maximum)	5 min	~20 to 40 min
Limited by available equipment and space	Inside/outside	~10 min	Level 1: 6 to 20 min	5 min	25 to 40 min
Limited by available space only	Inside/outside	Negligible	Level 2: 2 to 10 min	5 min	<40 min
Limited by available space only	Inside/outside	Negligible	<20 min	5 min	<30 min
Limited by available equipment and space	Inside/outside	Negligible	<20 min	10 min	<35 min
Limited by available space only	Inside	Negligible	~30 min	10 min	~40 min
Unlimited	Anywhere	None	None	5 min	~5 min

inexperienced exercisers, a prior familiarization test must be completed to ensure optimal outcomes. Under these conditions, step tests provide ecologically valid and suitably robust outcomes (Bennett et al., 2016). The Chester step test (CST) is a good example of an easy-to-administer stepping field test. A minimum of two submaximal HRs are collected, regressed against $\dot{V}O_{2max}$ and extrapolated to age-predicted maximum HR. As maximal HR coincides with maximal $\dot{V}O_{2max}$, this enables estimation of $\dot{V}O_{2max}$. Face validity has been confirmed (Sykes and Roberts, 2004). However, due to underestimation of laboratory-based reference values and a lack of linearity in HR and $\dot{V}O_{2max}$ responses during progressive, incremental work (Buckley et al., 2004), the accuracy of CST in identifying true $\dot{V}O_{2max}$ is questionable. However, as test-to-test reliability is acceptable (intertest bias and 95% limits of agreement (LoA): −0.8 and 3.7 mL·kg·min^{-1}, respectively) (Buckley et al., 2004), CST has considerable applicability for testing scenarios where the aim is to monitor temporal alterations in performance or health prompted by training (Bennett et al., 2016). Moreover, as large numbers can be accommodated in single testing bouts, full teams/squads can be assessed simultaneously. Where time pressures are an issue, shorter tests have been validated such as the single-stage, 5-min continuous step test, which reports excellent association with reference measures (Keren et al., 1980). This has application for practitioners setting exercise programmes in recreational leisure settings, who do not have recourse to high-tech facilities or equipment, and have a finite time for induction of new clients.

Submaximal cycling tests

Cycle tests have been used with good effect for prediction of peak performance in trained individuals (Lamberts et al., 2011) and to inform training prescription in such groups (Lamberts, 2014). The Astrand-Ryhming test (Astrand and Ryhming, 1954) has been considered an appropriate submaximal test for estimation of peak capacity for many years, with preferentially low error levels and high validity observed in comparison to other methods (Grant et al., 1999). Also, the YMCA cycle test is a long-established method and a popular option in recreational and clinical settings for testing general populations due to its relative ease of application and low-risk attributes (Garatachea et al., 2007). Blood pressure, HR and RPE are monitored towards the end of a series of 3-min steady-state exercise stages. In contrast, the Ekblom-Bak test (Björkman et al., 2016; Ekblom-Bak et al., 2012) includes one fixed and one individually chosen submaximal workload. This test confers similar advantages to more established tests, and compares favourably with observed $\dot{V}O_{2max}$ ($R = 0.91$, SEE = 0.302 L·min^{-1}). Indeed, it outperforms the Astrand-Ryhming test (Björkman et al., 2016; Ekblom-Bak et al., 2012). The availability of newly validated submaximal cycle tests emphasizes the importance of appropriate critique of the literature when deciding on test type, as opposed to a default position whereby a test is selected as it has been used for many years. The consensus, however, is that whichever cycle tests is applied, it should be minimally invasive and of a short duration (Capostagno et al., 2016).

Nonexercise prediction equations

Quantification of $\dot{V}O_{2max}$ without exercise confers considerable advantages where testing resources and/or equipment is restricted or medical conditions preclude exertion; a vast array of equations are validated within the literature. Most often, regression equations rely on basic quantitative measures such as percentage body fat (Robert McComb et al., 2006) and/or self-reported estimations of function and/or physical activity levels (Bradshaw et al., 2005; Malek et al., 2004; Schembre and Riebe, 2011). As a consequence they are particularly easy to administer and can be used with acceptable levels of accuracy. The caveat, however, is that in order to ensure validity, application must only be made to the population group(s) stated (Evans et al., 2015). Some example equations are listed below in order of strength of association between regression equation and reference values for $\dot{V}O_{2max}$ (R) (Box 12.1).

Exercise training prescription

$\dot{V}O_{2max}$ is highly responsive to exercise training at all ages, even in later life (Chodzko-Zajko et al., 2009; Stamford, 1988), with increased cardiac output, blood volume and both capillary and mitochondrial density realized through regular aerobic activity (Costill et al., 1976). Therefore, sport and exercise scientists working across the entire spectrum of physical conditioning levels (i.e., deconditioned, apparently healthy but inactive, chronic disease, recreational exercisers, athletic populations) dedicate considerable time and attention to the design, delivery and review of bespoke plans to promote positive alterations in $\dot{V}O_{2max}$.

Collection of HR and RPE alongside measurement of $\dot{V}O_{2max}$ during laboratory-based testing enables a training prescription to be defined and translated into practice. Such variables are easily monitored during training and match-play conditions, thereby enabling an understanding of internal physiological load and facilitating a training environment which is conducive to required adaptation(s). This is of prime importance given that some investigators have identified insufficiencies in the physiological load experienced by players during training (Eniseler, 2005; Fulton et al., 2010). Whilst RPE has considerable practical value in a sport performance context (Lambert and Borresen, 2010) it it is not commonly used for exercise prescription in athletes. However, it can be administered to good effect with general populations who intend to develop cardiorespiratory and muscular fitness (Garnacho-Castaño et al., 2018) and can act as a useful adjunct measure to enhance the accuracy of indirect determinations of $\dot{V}O_{2max}$ (Davies et al., 2008).

Note that in a sporting context, cardiorespiratory endurance is only one aspect of performance. Where programmes are designed for enhancement of this aspect, other important attributes as defined by the sport, i.e., all-out speed, speed–endurance (Iaia and Bangsbo, 2010), muscular strength and power (Suchomel et al., 2016), agility (Sheppard and Young, 2006), motor skill (Annett, 1994), balance (Hrysomallis, 2011; Zemková, 2014), coordination (Lech et al., 2011), should also be periodized into an athlete's plan. Whilst such attributes are outside the scope of this chapter, they require due consideration by practicing sport and exercise scientists.

Dose–response relationships and $\dot{V}O_{2max}$

Training load can be simplified and summarized by its characteristics in terms of physiological stress (dose) and resultant outcomes (response) (Lambert and Borresen, 2010). In general terms, a greater weekly volume of physical activity will equate to a greater improvement in cardiorespiratory fitness (Oja, 2001). Consequently, an inverse linear dose–response relation is said to exist between physical activity volume and all-cause mortality (Lee and Skerrett, 2001). However, the dose for realizing positive alterations in $\dot{V}O_{2max}$ is not likely to be consistent across all populations. A greater magnitude of benefit is experienced over time for less active persons when compared to highly active counterparts (Haskell, 1994). Hence, novice, deconditioned

---

Box 12.1 Nonexercise prediction equations

Healthy adults aged 18 to 65 years

$$\dot{V}O_{2max} \sim 40 \pm 10 \text{ mL kg min}^{-1}$$

$(R = 0.93, SEE = 3.5 \text{ mL kg min}^{-1})$:

$$\dot{V}O_{2max} = 48.0730 + (6.1779 \times S) -$$
$$(0.2463 \times A) - (0.6186 \times BMI) +$$
$$(0.7115 \times PFA) + (0.6709 \times PA\text{-}R)$$

where S = sex (female = 0, male = 1); A = age (years); BMI = body mass index (kg·m²); PFA = perceived functional ability; $PA\text{-}R$ = physical activity rating (Bradshaw et al., 2005). Procedures for determination of PFA (George, 1996) and PA-R (Jackson et al., 1990) have previously been defined and offer a quick and easy means to quantify function and activity levels.

Trained females aged 38 ± 10 years (range unavailable)

$$\dot{V}O_{2max} \sim 43 \pm 7 \text{ mL kg min}^{-1}$$

$\left(R = 0.83, SEE = 259 \text{ mL min}^{-1}\right)$:

$$\dot{V}O_{2max} = (18.528 \times W) + (11.993 \times H) -$$
$$(17.197 \times A) + (23.522 \times D) + (62.118 \times I)$$
$$+ (278.262 \times Y) - 1375.878$$

where W = weight (kg); H = height (cm); A = age (years); D = training duration (h·wk⁻¹); I = training intensity using the Borg 6–20 scale; Y = years of training (Malek et al., 2004).

Trained males aged 40 ± 12 years (range unavailable)

$$\dot{V}O_{2max} \sim 53 \pm 9 \text{ mL kg min}^{-1}$$

$\left(R = 0.82, SEE = 382 \text{ mL min}^{-1}\right)$:

$$\dot{V}O_{2max} = (27.387 \times W) + (26.634 \times H) -$$
$$(27.572 \times A) + (26.161 \times D) + (114.904 \times I)$$
$$+ (506.752 \times Y) - 4609.791$$

where W = weight (kg); H = height (cm); A = age (years); D = training duration (h·wk⁻¹); I = training intensity using the Borg 6–20 scale; Y = years of training (Malek et al., 2005).

Healthy adults aged 46 ± 13 years (range unavailable)

$$\dot{V}O_{2max} \sim 34 \pm 12 \text{ mL kg min}^{-1}$$

$\left(R = 0.79, SEE = 7.2 \text{ mL kg min}^{-1}\right)$:

$$\dot{V}O_{2max} = 79.9 - (0.39 \times A) -$$
$$(13.7 \times S) + (0.127 \times W)$$

where A = age (years); S = sex (female = 1, male = 0); W = weight (lb) (Myers et al., 2017).

Healthy adults aged 18 to 25 years

$$\dot{V}O_{2max} \sim 42 \pm 7 \text{ mL kg min}^{-1}$$

$\left(R = 0.65, SEE = 5.5 \text{ mL kg min}^{-1}\right)$:

$$\dot{V}O_{2max} = 47.749 - (6.493 \times S) + (0.140 \times VA)$$

where S = sex (female = 2, male = 1); VA = vigorous activity (Schembre and Riebe, 2011).
Calculation of VA is straightforward using outcomes from application of the International Physical Activity Questionnaire – Short Form (IPAQ-SF) (Craig et al., 2003) (VA (MET min·wk⁻¹) = 8.0 METs × VA min per day × VA days per week).

---

exercisers will experience greater improvements over a shorter time than more well-conditioned populations, who typically have a higher $\dot{V}O_{2max}$ (Rankovic et al., 2010). In a mixed sample of 20- to 60-year-old apparently healthy individuals, low-intensity moderate- and high-duration (<200 and >200 min per week, respectively) walking exercise groups displayed a greater $\dot{V}O_{2max}$ than those who did no exercise (Gim and Choi, 2016). Furthermore, aerobic training at 63–73% of HR reserve for 40–50 min, 3 to 4 days per week is effective in optimizing cardiorespiratory benefits in apparently healthy but sedentary older adults (Huang et al., 2016). Therefore, positive adaptations can be seen with relatively low levels of physical activity in low-fit groups. This is encouraging given that such individuals struggle to maintain commitment to exercise programmes (Dishman, 2001), with a considerable percentage (~50%) giving up after 6 months (Robison and Rogers, 1994). However, such doses are likely to be insufficient for athletic gains, or even perhaps a recreational exerciser who is training for an event such as a marathon or triathlon.

Factors confounding and limiting chronic alterations in $\dot{V}O_{2max}$

Whilst clear evidence exists to support the trainability of $\dot{V}O_{2max}$, sport and exercise scientists should not automatically expect exponential increases in exercise capacity with chronic training. With respect to exercise programming, considerable interindividual variability exists in training responses (Williams et al., 2017). Beyond the exercise programme, many factors will influence an individual's predisposition for an elevation in $\dot{V}O_{2max}$. Factors such as age (Legaz Arrese et al., 2005), injury, disuse and detraining (Neufer, 1989; Petibois and Déléris, 2003), player position (Duthie et al., 2003; Ransdell et al., 2013) and sporting modality (Metaxas et al., 2009) will influence peak capacity. Also, highly trained athletes will eventually reach a genetic 'ceiling' for $\dot{V}O_{2max}$ (Sjödin and Svedenhag, 1985). Moreover, genes responsible for muscular subsystem encoding, electrolyte balance, lipid metabolism, oxidative phosphorylation and oxygen delivery combine to build a unique individual profile characterized by inherent systemic variability in motor performance (Bray et al., 2009; Williams et al., 2017). This individually unique signature will be one of the major factors defining performance potential and limiting performance gains. This reason, coupled with the fact that improvements in submaximal physiological variables (e.g., ventilatory threshold) can be seen without changes in $\dot{V}O_{2max}$ (Millet et al., 2009) emphasize the importance of avoiding a sole reliance on maximal capacity. Hence, submaximal physiological markers of performance, most notably BLa^- transition thresholds, $\dot{V}O_{2max}$ at submaximal workloads and mechanical efficiency, should also be

examined to ensure a thorough and accurate picture of performance or functional potential is obtained.

Exercise prescription for promoting increases in $\dot{V}O_{2max}$

Traditional approaches to training have favoured high-volume, continuous endurance exercise involving rhythmic, large muscle–group activity for elevation of $\dot{V}O_{2max}$. However, such activities are time consuming and do not naturally align with complex sport-specific demands, which often require intermittent, rather than continuous, exertion. A more modern approach is to administer high-intensity interval training (HIIT), whereby bouts of high-intensity work are interspersed with periods of active recovery. This approach to training has become popular due to its considerable time efficiency (Burgomaster et al., 2008; Gibala et al., 2006; Gist et al., 2014) and positive impact on skeletal muscle physiology (Burgomaster et al., 2008; Cochran et al., 2014; Gibala et al., 2006; Little et al., 2010; Sjödin and Svedenhag, 1985). Specifically, increases in muscle oxidative capacity (Burgomaster et al., 2008; Gibala et al., 2006), muscle buffering capacity (Gibala et al., 2006), glycogen content (Gibala et al., 2006; Little et al., 2010), muscle glycogenolytic enzyme activity (Kubukeli et al., 2002) and sarcolemmal lactate transport capacity (Kubukeli et al., 2002) are observed after high-intensity training. Indeed, physiological adaptations are consistent with those observed during a continuous endurance regime, yet the volume of training is considerably lower (~90 %) (Gibala et al., 2006), with large increases in $\dot{V}O_{2max}$ (~10%) expected over short time periods using this approach (Munoz et al., 2015; Støren et al., 2012). Therefore, from a practical perspective, high-intensity training strategies should be considered equally effective as traditional continuous, steady-state endurance training (Burgomaster et al., 2008; Gibala et al., 2006; Gist et al., 2014; Macpherson et al., 2011; Milanović et al., 2015c; Sloth et al., 2013), with clear applicability for elite athletes (Iaia and Bangsbo, 2010; Ní Chéilleachair et al., 2017), active (nonathletic) (Weston et al., 2014) and sedentary (Weston et al., 2014) individuals.

Manipulation of intensity, duration and work-to-rest ratio enables the sport and exercise scientist to optimize high-intensity training strategies for enhancement of $\dot{V}O_{2max}$, with sprint training being a desirable option. Durations between 10 and 30 s are effective in elevating $\dot{V}O_{2max}$ (Hazell et al., 2010; McKie et al., 2018) and effects can be realized in relatively short timeframes (3 to 4 weeks) (Astorino et al., 2013; McKie et al., 2018; Rønnestad et al., 2014). Indeed, short-duration sprints (~5 s), completed over more repetitions may represent an ideal strategy due to higher perceived enjoyment over longer sprint strategies (Islam et al., 2017; Townsend et al., 2017).

Case study

The following example illustrates how collection of physiological measures, specifically $\dot{V}O_{2max}$ can be used to individualize and optimize training prescription.

Participant profile and testing protocol

Characteristics	56-year-old apparently healthy male
	Trained, recreational cyclist
	Daily long, slow distance road cycling ($\geq$ 60-min sessions)
Weight	79.0 kg
Height	176 cm
Test protocol	All testing completed using a static cycle (Lode BV, the Netherlands) configured by the participant to the desired position
	Graded exercise test involving eight, 3-min submaximal stages (30–240 W, 30-W increments); 10-min active recovery
	Peak exercise test to exhaustion (0–345 W, 15-W increments applied every 30 s)
Measures	HR, $\dot{V}O_{2max}$ and respiratory parameters ($\dot{V}O_{2max}$, VE, RER) monitored continuously using an online metabolic cart. RPE at the end of each submaximal stage and immediately after peak testing

Determination of $\dot{V}O_{2max}$

Primary criteria were met for determination of peak physiological exertion with a $\dot{V}O_{2max}$ plateau observed. Hence there was no requirement for a verification stage nor consideration of secondary criteria. However, in this case these are listed for reference:

$\dot{V}O_{2max}$ (absolute)	3.84 L·min^{-1}
$\dot{V}O_{2max}$ (relative)	49.0 mL·kg·min^{-1}
BLa$^-_{peak}$	7.49 mmol·L^{-1}
HR$_{peak}$	169 b·min^{-1} (~103% of age-predicted maximum)
RER$_{peak}$	1.25
RPE$_{peak}$	Overall RPE of 20 (RPE 6 to 20 scale: Borg, 1982)

Comparisons to normative data

Once identified, $\dot{V}O_{2max}$ should be contrasted to normative data to facilitate athlete feedback. In this case, a functional classification of superior was defined (>45.3 mL·kg·min^{-1}) using accepted normative data for general populations (Heyward and Gibson, 2014). However, as the majority of classification systems relate to associations between $\dot{V}O_{2max}$ and cardiovascular health status (Duncan et al., 2005; Heyward and Gibson, 2014; Sanders and Duncan, 2006),

they have limited application for athletic populations who display a significantly higher $\dot{V}O_{2max}$ (Rankovic et al., 2010). Useful normative data exits for a number of sports, including male football players (Helgerud et al., 2011; Hoff, 2005; Tønnessen et al., 2013; Ziogas et al., 2011), female football players (Haugen et al., 2014), rugby sevens (Higham et al., 2013), rugby league (Brewer and Davis, 1995) and trained runners (Barnes and Kilding, 2015). In addition, physiological data is available for some sports to enable comparison to standards at specific phases of the competitive cycle (Miller et al., 2011). However, normative data is not available for all discrete sporting disciplines or to enable sex-specific profiling in all cases. Where data collected from athletes competing within the same sport are available, a more specific comparison can, and should, be made according to player position, league and/or discipline.

Using the HR and $\dot{V}O_{2max}$ relationship to inform training prescription

Physiological measures obtained during testing can be used to identify target training intensities to optimize chronic effects. One of the most commonly applied approaches for this purpose is to undertake basic linear regression of HR and $\dot{V}O_{2max}$ (Fig. 12.3). At any given percentage of $\dot{V}O_{2max}$ a target HR or RPE can be provided, dependent upon which variable is plotted on the y axis. In this case, as the client had access to a HR monitor, training zones were offered to match.

Blood lactate responses and training prescription

Due to limitations of scope, this chapter has not considered the significance of blood lactate transition thresholds in detail, yet their relative role in demarcating important physiological phenomena is not to be underestimated. Collection of BLa$^-$ data during graded exercise testing offers a valid and reliable alternative to ventilatory thresholds identified using respiratory measures (Pallarés et al., 2016). Therefore, testing can be highly useful in defining the exercise training prescription. A curvilinear speed (or work-rate) lactate profile (Fig. 12.4) is generated by collecting a small blood sample from the earlobe or fingertip, with measures obtained towards the end of each submaximal, steady-state stage (3- or 4-min stage duration with a 1-min rest interval is ideal).

Visual inspection of these data allows for determination of lactate threshold (LT$_1$) where an elevation in BLa$^-$ from rest is first observed (<1.0 mmol·L^{-1}), and lactate turnpoint (LT$_2$), where lactate production and clearance are no longer in equilibrium during exercise (see Fig. 12.4). Following identification of LT$_1$ and LT$_2$, three training zones can easily be defined (Faude et al., 2009) and these have been applied to this case study (Fig. 12.5).

Continued

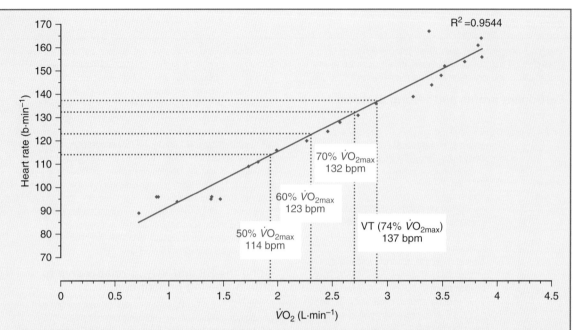

Fig. 12.3 Simple linear regression of heart rate (HR) and $\dot{V}O_{2max}$ during laboratory-based graded exercise testing *Red dotted line* indicates process for extrapolation of HR (*y*) from $\dot{V}O_{2max}$ (*x*) using fixed percentages. *Blue dotted line* indicates ventilatory threshold (VT) as defined by separate analysis of respiratory responses to incremental work to exhaustion. *bpm*, Beats per minute.

Prior to attainment of LT_1, lactate production is negligible and therefore, physiological load is at its lowest. For this case study example, this equates to a HR of 113 b·min⁻¹ (see Fig. 12.4) and a relative exercise intensity, work rate and RPE of 50% $\dot{V}O_{2max}$, 120 W, and 10, respectively (Table 12.2). Therefore, exercise at or below this intensity should be advocated for warm-up sessions and bouts of active recovery interspersed between high-intensity intervals. Past LT_1, but below LT_2, lactate begins to rise. However, increases are aligned to changes in exercise intensity and a physiological equilibrium remains (i.e., work rate increases = lactate increases; work rate stays constant = lactate stays constant). With respect to the case example, HRs of 114 to 137 b·min⁻¹ (51–74% $\dot{V}O_{2max}$; 125–210 W; RPE of 11–12) should therefore be advised for long, slow distance training (see Fig. 12.5), with likely chronic adaptations being: increased capillary density and arterial compliance, decreased resting and submaximal HRs, increased Q and left ventricular ejection fraction (Clausen, 1977).

In exercise conditions where O_2 is no longer available in sufficient quantities, large amounts of lactate begin to accumulate through predominant reliance upon anaerobic systems. For this case study, this can be seen at work rates beyond LT_2, where BLa⁻ levels rise disproportionately over time, with rate of production exceeding clearance (see Fig. 12.4). Whilst this point has been described as the 'anaerobic threshold', and used to demarcate progression from aerobic to anaerobic metabolism (Wasserman, 1986), use of this

terminology can be misleading as energy systems and their relative contribution to overall net physiological output are not mutually exclusive. Nevertheless, the physiological events that occur around this point are generally accepted to be representative of transition from moderate to vigorous internal physiological load; therefore this point is highly significant. Ability to sustain a high factional component of $\dot{V}O_{2max}$ for an extended duration delays metabolic acidosis (Ghosh, 2004) and thus, the anaerobic threshold is highly correlated to distance running performance. Exceeding this threshold is typified by excessive plasma carbon dioxide and hydrogen ion concentrations, produced as a consequence of increased metabolic activity within muscle, causing a reduction in blood pH. This stimulates an immediate increase in minute ventilation (V_E), as clearing excess CO_2 produced by buffering of hydrogen ions, becomes a priority for avoidance of metabolic acidosis. Therefore, analysis of respiratory gases (i.e., V_E, $\dot{V}O_2$, $\dot{V}CO_2$) and, specifically, changes in linearity in these relationships support threshold identification; hence, the term 'ventilatory threshold' (VT) may be more appropriate. In this case study, VT was determined to occur at 74% $\dot{V}O_{2max}$ (137 b·min⁻¹). Cross-checking the BLa⁻ data (see Fig. 12.4) reveals that LT_2 occurred at the same point (136 b·min⁻¹) during graded testing. Furthermore, BLa⁻ concentration prior to the break in linearity observed during and prior to maximal lactate steady state was ~4.0 mmol·L⁻¹ (see Fig. 12.4), which is generally accepted to represent the onset of blood lactate

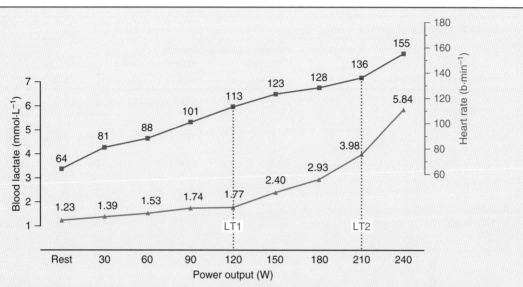

Fig. 12.4 **Blood lactate and heart rate response to incremental exercise during a graded exercise test on a static cycle ergometer** *Red dotted lines* indicate lactate threshold (LT_1) and turnpoint (LT_2), respectively, as defined by visual inspection of the lactate curve.

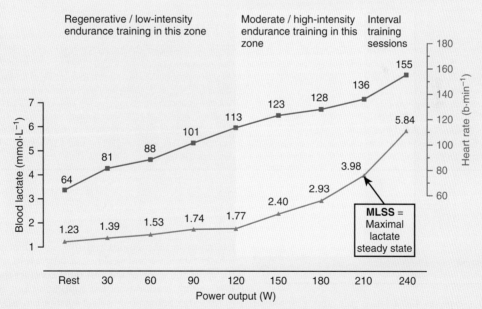

Fig. 12.5 **Heart rate training zones as defined by blood lactate transition thresholds identified during incremental work** (Adapted from Faude, O., Kindermann, W., Meyer, T., 2009. Lactate threshold concepts: how valid are they? Sports Medicine, 39 (6), 469–490.)

Continued

Table 12.2 Summary of exercise training prescription based on percentage of $\dot{V}O_{2max}$

Training type	Notes	Target training intensity % $\dot{V}O_{2max}$	Power output Watts	HR b·min⁻¹	$\dot{V}O_{2max}$ mL·kg·min⁻¹	RPE
Warm up/cool down	Less than LT₁	<50%	<120	≤113	24–29	10
Endurance – level 1	Cycling with lactate accumulation – easy	50–60%	125–160	114–123	24–29	11
Endurance – level 2	Cycling with lactate accumulation – moderate	60–74%	161–210	124–137	29–34	12
Anaerobic threshold (LT₂)	Transfer to anaerobic work – train up to this level	74%	210–225	137	34	13
Intervals	High-intensity interval training (HIIT) – work at this level interspersed with active recovery (<50%)	>74%	225–345	137–169	34–49	≥13
Peak capacity	Maximal effort	100%	345	169	49	20

HR, Heart rate; *LT1*, lactate threshold; *LT2*, lactate turnpoint; *RPE*, ratings of perceived exertion.

accumulation (OBLA) across individuals. Collectively, these data reinforce the premise that anaerobic processes become dominant at 137 b·min⁻¹ and that 210 W is representative of critical power.

As LT₂ occurs at a higher percentage of $\dot{V}O_{2max}$ in elite athletes than active, non-elite equivalents (Joyner and Coyle, 2008), it is generally accepted that elevation of LT₂/VT translates directly into improved performance in endurance-based sports. Elevation is achieved through threshold training,

at, or slightly above, the anaerobic threshold (Ghosh, 2004). Such an intensity has the added effect of increasing $\dot{V}O_{2max}$, as stated previously. The intermittent nature of interval training, particularly using very high intensities, but low volume, is important to maximize skeletal muscle adaptations (Cochran et al., 2014), thereby enhancing $\dot{V}O_{2max}$. Therefore, the client should incorporate high-intensity intervals into his training plan, elevating HR beyond 137 b·min⁻¹, ideally towards the top end of the range (169 b·min⁻¹).

Summary

This chapter explores the relative role and purpose of $\dot{V}O_{2max}$ as the primary physiological determinant of endurance capacity. A number of methods exist for quantification of this parameter, with a variety of field- and laboratory-based methods available, each characterized by inherent strengths and weaknesses. Where tests are applied, the sport and exercise scientist must consider the population, setting, feasibility of test application and availability of resources. Subsequently, data must be carefully analysed and interpreted to ensure that appropriate training targets and modes can be determined and optimized for health or performance gains.

References

Abut, F., Akay, M.F., 2015. Machine learning and statistical methods for the prediction of maximal oxygen uptake: recent advances. Medical Devices (Auckland) 8, 369–379.

Annett, J., 1994. The learning of motor skills: sports science and ergonomics perspectives. Ergonomics 37 (1), 5–16.

Arkesteijn, M., Hopker, J., Jobson, S.A., Passfield, L., 2013. The effect of turbo trainer cycling on pedalling technique and cycling efficiency. International Journal of Sports Medicine 34 (6), 520–525.

Artero, E.G., España-Romero, V., Castro-Piñero, J., Ortega, F.B., Suni, J., Castillo-Garzon, M.J., et al., 2011. Reliability of field-based fitness tests in youth. International Journal of Sports Medicine 32 (3), 159–169.

Astorino, T., Rietschel, J.C., Tam, P.A., Taylor, K., Johnson, S.M., Freedman, T.P., et al., 2004. Reinvestigation of optimal duration of $\dot{V}O_{2max}$ testing. Journal of Exercise Physiology 7 (6), 1–8.

Astorino, T.A., Schubert, M.M., Palumbo, E., Stirling, D., McMillan, D.W., Cooper, C., et al., 2013. Magnitude and time course of changes in maximal oxygen uptake in response to distinct regimens of chronic interval training in sedentary women. European Journal of Applied Physiology 113 (9), 2361–2369.

Astrand, P.O., Ryhming, I., 1954. A nomogram for calculation of aerobic capacity (physical fitness) from pulse rate during submaximal work. Journal of Applied Physiology 7, 218–221.

Atkinson, G., Davison, R., Jeukendrup, A., Passfield, L., 2003. Science and cycling: current knowledge and future directions for research. Journal of Sports Science 21 (9), 767–787.

Bangsbo, J., Hansen, P.R., Dvorak, J., Krustrup, P., 2015. Recreational football for disease prevention and treatment in untrained men: a narrative review examining cardiovascular health, lipid profile, body composition, muscle strength and functional capacity. British Journal of Sports Medicine 49 (9), 568–576.

Barbieri, R., Barbieri, F., Milioni, F., Dos-Santos, J., Soares, M., Zagatto, A., et al., 2017. Reliability and validity of a new specific field test of aerobic capacity with the ball for futsal players. International Journal of Sports Medicine 38 (3), 233–240.

Barnes, K.R., Kilding, A.E., 2015. Running economy: measurement, norms, and determining factors. Sports Medicine Open 1, 8.

Bassett, D.R., Howley, E.T., 1997. Maximal oxygen uptake: "classical" versus "contemporary" viewpoints. Medicine and Science in Sports and Exercise 29 (5), 591–603.

Bassett, D.R., Howley, E.T., 2000. Limiting factors for maximum oxygen uptake and determinants of endurance performance. Medicine and Science in Sports and Exercise 32 (1), 70–84.

Batista, M.B., Romanzini, C.L.P., Castro-Piñero, J., Vaz Ronque, E.R., 2017. Validity of field tests to estimate cardiorespiratory fitness in children and adolescents: a systematic review. Revista Paulista de Pediatria 35 (2), 222–233.

Bell, W., Cooper, S.M., Cobner, D., Longville, J., 1994. Physiological changes arising from a training programme in under-21 international netball players. Ergonomics 37 (1), 149–157.

Beltz, N.M., Gibson, A.L., Janot, J.M., Kravitz, L., Mermier, C.M., Dalleck, L.C., et al., 2016. Graded exercise testing protocols for the determination of $\dot{V}O_{2max}$: historical perspectives, progress, and future considerations. Journal of Sports Medicine. https://doi.org/10.1155/2016/3968393.

Bennett, H., Davison, K., Parfitt, G., Eston, R., 2016a. Validity of a perceptually-regulated step test protocol for assessing cardiorespiratory fitness in healthy adults. European Journal of Applied Physiology 116 (11-12), 2337–2344.

Bennett, H., Parfitt, G., Davison, K., Eston, R., 2016b. Validity of submaximal step tests to estimate maximal oxygen uptake in healthy adults. Sports Medicine 46 (5), 737–750.

Betik, A.C., Hepple, R.T., 2008. Determinants of $\dot{V}O_{2max}$ decline with aging: an integrated perspective. Applied Physiology, Nutrition and Metabolism 33 (1), 130–140.

Billat, L.V., Koralsztein, J.P., 1996. Significance of the velocity at $\dot{V}O_{2max}$ and time to exhaustion at this velocity. Sports Medicine 22 (2), 90–108.

Björkman, F., Ekblom-Bak, E., Ekblom, O., Ekblom, B., 2016. Validity of the revised Ekblom Bak cycle ergometer test in adults. European Journal of Applied Physiology 116, 1627–1638.

Bjorntorp, P., 1991. Importance of fat as a support nutrient for energy: metabolism of athletes. Journal of Sports Science 9 (7), 1–6.

Bohr, A.D., Brown, D.D., Laurson, K.R., Smith, P.J., Bass, R.W., 2013. Relationship between socioeconomic status and physical fitness in junior high school students. Journal of School Health 83 (8), 542–547.

Borg, G.A., 1982. Psychophysical bases of perceived exertion. Medicine and Science in Sports and Exercise 14, 377–381.

Bradshaw, D.I., George, J.D., Hyde, A., LaMonte, M.J., Vehrs, P.R., Hager, R.L., et al., 2005. An accurate $\dot{V}O_{2max}$ nonexercise regression model for 18–65-year-old adults. Research Quarterly for Exercise and Sport 76 (4), 426–432.

Bray, M.S., Hagberg, J.M., Pérusse, L., Rankinen, T., Roth, S.M., Wolfarth, B., et al., 2009. The human gene map for performance and health-related fitness phenotypes: the 2006–2007 update. Medicine and Science in Sports and Exercise 41 (1), 35–73.

Brewer, J., Davis, J., 1995. Applied physiology of rugby league. Sports Medicine 20 (3), 129–135.

Brisswalter, J., Hausswirth, C., Smith, D., Vercruyssen, F., Vallier, J.M., 2000. Energetically optimal cadence vs. freely-chosen cadence during cycling: effect of exercise duration. International Journal of Sports Medicine 21 (1), 60–64.

Brooks, D., Solway, S., Weinacht, K., Wang, D., Thomas, S., 2003. Comparison between an indoor and an outdoor 6-minute walk test among individuals with chronic obstructive pulmonary disease. Archives of Physical Medicine and Rehabilitation 84 (6), 873–876.

Buckley, J.P., Sim, J., Eston, R.G., Hession, R., Fox, R., 2004. Reliability and validity of measures taken during the Chester step test to predict aerobic power and to prescribe aerobic exercise. British Journal of Sports Medicine 38, 197–205.

Burgess, D.J., Naughton, G.A., 2010. Talent development in adolescent team sports: a review. International Journal of Sports Physiology and Performance 5 (1), 103–116.

Burgomaster, K.A., Howarth, K.R., Phillips, S.M., Rakobowchuk, M., Macdonald, M.J., McGee, S.L., et al., 2008. Similar metabolic adaptations during exercise after low volume sprint interval and traditional endurance training in humans. Journal of Physiology 586 (1), 151–160.

Butts, N.K., Henry, B.A., Mclean, D., 1991. Correlations between $\dot{V}O_{2max}$ and performance times of recreational triathletes. Journal of Sports Medicine and Physical Fitness 31 (3), 339–344.

Cao, Z.B., Miyatake, N., Aoyama, T., Higuchi, M., Tabata, I., 2013. Prediction of maximal oxygen uptake from a 3-minute walk based on gender, age, and body composition. Journal of Physical Activity and Health 10 (2), 280–287.

Capostagno, B., Lambert, M.I., Lamberts, R.P., 2016. Systematic review of submaximal cycle tests to predict, monitor and optimize cycling performance. International Journal of Sports Physiology and Performance 11 (6), 707–714.

Caputo, F., Denadai, B.S., 2004. Effects of aerobic endurance training status and specificity on oxygen uptake kinetics during maximal exercise. European Journal of Applied Physiology 93 (1-2), 87–95.

Carnethon, M.R., Gulati, M., Greenland, P., 2005. Prevalence and cardiovascular disease correlates of low cardiorespiratory fitness in adolescents and adults. The Journal of the American Medical Association 294 (23), 2981–2988.

Castagna, C., Iellamo, F., Impellizzeri, F.M., Manzi, V., 2014. Validity and reliability of the 45-15 test for aerobic fitness in young soccer players. International Journal of Sports Physiology and Performance 9 (3), 525–531.

Castro-Piñero, J., Artero, E.G., España-Romero, V., Ortega, F.B., Sjöström, M., Suni, J., et al., 2010. Criterion-related validity of field-based fitness tests in youth: a systematic review. British Journal of Sports Medicine 44 (13), 934–943.

Chidnok, W., Dimenna, F.J., Bailey, S.J., Burnley, M., Wilkerson, D.P., Vanhatalo, A., et al., 2013. $\dot{V}O_{2max}$ is not altered by self-pacing during incremental exercise. European Journal of Applied Physiology 113 (2), 529–539.

Chodzko-Zajko, W.J., Proctor, D.N., Fiatarone Singh, M.A., Minson, C.T., Nigg, C.R., Salem, G.J., et al., 2009. American College of Sports Medicine position stand. Exercise and physical activity for older adults. Medicine and Science in Sports and Exercise 41 (7), 1510–1530.

Clausen, J.P., 1977. Effect of physical training on cardiovascular adjustments to exercise in man. Physiological Reviews 57 (4), 779–815.

Cochran, A.J., Percival, M.E., Tricarico, S., Little, J.P., Cermak, N., Gillen, J.B., et al., 2014. Intermittent and continuous high-intensity exercise training induce similar acute but different chronic muscle adaptations. Experimental Physiology 99 (5), 782–791.

Costill, D., Fink, W.J., Pollock, M.L., 1976. Muscle fiber composition and enzyme activities of elite distance runners. Medicine and Science in Sports and Exercise 8, 96–100.

Cox, M.H., Miles, D.S., Verde, T.J., Rhodes, E.C., 1995. Applied physiology of ice hockey. Sports Medicine 19 (3), 184–201.

Coyle, E.F., 1995. Integration of the physiological factors determining endurance performance ability. Exercise and Sports Science Reviews 23, 25–63.

Craig, C.L., Marshall, A.L., Sjostrom, M., Bauman, A., Booth, M.L., Ainsworth, B.E., et al., 2003. International Physical Activity Questionnaire: 12-country reliability and validity. Medicine and Science in Sports and Exercise 35, 1381–1395.

Crust, L., Clough, P.J., 2005. Relationship between mental toughness and physical endurance. Perception and Motor Skills 100 (1), 192–194.

Da Silva, J.F., Guglielmo, L.G., Carminatti, L.J., De Oliveira, F.R., Dittrich, N., Paton, C.D., et al., 2011. Validity and reliability of a new field test (Carminatti's test) for soccer players compared with laboratory-based measures. Journal of Sports Science 29 (15), 1621–1628.

Davies, R.C., Rowlands, A.V., Eston, R.G., 2008. The prediction of maximal oxygen uptake from submaximal ratings of perceived exertion elicited during the multistage fitness test. British Journal of Sports Medicine 42 (12), 1006–1010.

Dishman, R.K., 2001. The problem exercise adherence: fighting sloth in nations with market economics. Quest 53, 279–294.

Duncan, G.E., Howley, E.T., Johnson, B.N., 1997. Applicability of $\dot{V}O_{2max}$ criteria: discontinuous versus continuous protocols. Medicine and Science in Sports and Exercise 29 (2), 273–278.

Duncan, G.E., Li, S.M., Zhou, X.H., 2005. Cardiovascular fitness among U.S. adults: NHANES 1999–2000 and 2001–2002. Medicine and Science in Sports and Exercise 37 (8), 1324–1328.

Duthie, G.1, Pyne, D., Hooper, S., 2003. Applied physiology and game analysis of rugby union. Journal of Sports Medicine 33 (13), 973–991.

Edvardsen, E., Hem, E., Anderssen, S.A., 2014. End criteria for reaching maximal oxygen uptake must be strict and adjusted to sex and age: a cross-sectional study. PLoS One 9 (1), e85276.

Eime, R.M., Charity, M.J., Harvey, J.T., Payne, W.R., 2015a. Participation in sport and physical activity: associations with socio-economic status and geographical remoteness. BMC Public Health 15, 434.

Eime, R.M., Harvey, J., Charity, M.J., Casey, M., Westerbeek, H., Payne, W.R., et al., 2017. The relationship of sport participation to provision of sports facilities and socioeconomic status: a geographical analysis. Australian and New Zealand Journal of Public Health 41 (3), 248–255.

Eime, R.M., Harvey, J.T., Charity, M.J., Casey, M.M., van Uffelen, J.G.Z., Payne, W.R., et al., 2015b. The contribution of sport participation to overall health enhancing physical activity levels in Australia: a population-based study. BMC Public Health 15, 806.

Ekblom-Bak, E., Björkman, F., Hellenius, M.L., Ekblom, B., 2012. A new submaximal cycle ergometer test for prediction of $\dot{V}O_{2max}$. Scandinavian Journal of Medicine and Science in Sports 24 (2), 319–326.

Eniseler, N., 2005. Heart rate and blood lactate concentrations as predictors of physiological load on elite soccer players during various soccer training activities. Journal of Strength and Conditioning Research 19 (4), 799–804.

Evans, H.J.L., Ferrar, K.E., Smith, A.E., Parfitta, G., Eston, R.G., 2015. A systematic review of methods to predict maximal oxygen uptake from submaximal, open circuit spirometry in healthy adults. Journal of Science and Medicine in Sport 18, 183–188.

Faude, O., Kindermann, W., Meyer, T., 2009. Lactate threshold concepts: how valid are they? Sports Medicine 39 (6), 469–490.

Fernandez, J., 2005. Specific field tests for tennis players. Medicine and Science in Tennis 10, 22–23.

Fitchett, M.A., 1985. Predictability of $\dot{V}O_{2max}$ from submaximal cycle ergometer and bench stepping tests. British Journal of Sports Medicine 19, 85–88.

Flouris, A.D., Metsios, G.S., Koutedakis, Y., 2005. Enhancing the efficacy of the 20 m multistage shuttle run test. British Journal of Sports Medicine 39 (3), 166–170.

Flouris, A.D., Metsios, G.S., Famisis, K., Geladas, N., Koutedakis, Y., 2009. Prediction of $\dot{V}O_{2max}$ from a new field test based on portable indirect calorimetry. Journal of Science and Medicine in Sport 13 (1), 70–73.

Fotheringham, I., Meakin, G., Punekar, Y.S., Riley, J.H., Cockle, S.M., Singh, S.J., et al., 2015. Comparison of laboratory- and field-based exercise tests for COPD: a systematic review. International Journal of Chronic Obstructive Pulmonary Disease 10, 625–643.

Freeman, W., Williams, C., Nute, M.G., 1990. Endurance running performance in athletes with asthma. Journal of Sports Science 8 (2), 103–117.

Fulton, S.K., Pyne, D.B., Hopkins, W.G., Burkett, B., 2010. Training characteristics of paralympic swimmers. Journal of Strength and Conditioning Research 24 (2), 471–478.

Gabbett, T.J., Stein, J.G., Kemp, J.G., Lorenzen, C., 2013. Relationship between tests of physical qualities and physical match performance in elite rugby league players. Journal of Strength and Conditioning Research 27 (6), 1539–1545.

Garatachea, N., Cavalcanti, E., García-López, D., González-Gallego, J., de Paz, J.A., 2007. Estimation of energy expenditure in healthy adults from the YMCA submaximal cycle ergometer test. Evaluation and the Health Professions 30 (2), 138–149.

Garnacho-Castaño, M.V., Domínguez, R., Muñoz González, A., Feliu-Ruano, R., Serra-Payá, N., Maté-Muñoz, J.L., et al., 2018. Exercise prescription using the Borg rating of perceived exertion to improve fitness. International Journal of Sports Medicine 39 (2), 115–123.

George, J.D., 1996. Alternative approach to maximal exercise testing and V̇O₂max prediction in college students. Research Quarterly for Exercise and Sport 67 (4), 452–457.

Ghosh, A.K., 2004. Anaerobic threshold: its concept and role in endurance sport. Malaysian Journal of Medical Sciences 11 (1), 24–36.

Gibala, M.J., Little, J.P., van Essen, M., Wilkin, G.P., Burgomaster, K.A., Safdar, A., et al., 2006. Short-term sprint interval versus traditional endurance training: similar initial adaptations in human skeletal muscle and exercise performance. Journal of Physiology 575 (3), 901–911.

Gim, M.N., Choi, J.H., 2016. The effects of weekly exercise time on V̇O₂max and resting metabolic rate in normal adults. Journal of Physical Therapy Science 28 (4), 1359–1363.

Gist, N.H., Fedewa, M.V., Dishman, R.K., Cureton, K.J., 2014. Sprint interval training effects on aerobic capacity: a systematic review and meta-analysis. Sport Medicine 44 (2), 269–279.

González-Haro, C., Galilea, P.A., Drobnic, F., Escanero, J.F., 2007. Validation of a field test to determine the maximal aerobic power in triathletes and endurance cyclists. British Journal of Sports Medicine 41 (3), 174–179.

Goosey-Tolfrey, V.L., Leicht, C.A., 2013. Field-based physiological testing of wheelchair athletes. Sports Medicine 43 (2), 77–91.

Goosey-Tolfrey, V.L., Sindall, P., 2007. The effects of arm crank strategy on physiological responses and mechanical efficiency during submaximal exercise. Journal of Sports Science 25 (4), 453–460.

Goulet, E.D., 2012. Dehydration and endurance performance in competitive athletes. Nutrition Reviews 70 (2), S132–S136.

Grant, J.A., Joseph, A.M., Campagna, P.D., 1999. The prediction of V̇O₂max: a comparison of 7 indirect tests of aerobic power. Journal of Strength and Conditioning Research 13 (4), 346–352.

Hagan, R.D., Smith, M.G., Gettman, L.R., 1981. Marathon performance in relation to maximal aerobic power and training indices. Medicine and Science in Sports and Exercise 13 (3), 185–189.

Hagan, R.D., Upton, S.J., Duncan, J.J., Gettman, L.R., 1987. Marathon performance in relation to maximal aerobic power and training indices in female distance runners. British Journal of Sports Medicine 21 (1), 3–7.

Hamlin, M.J., Draper, N., Blackwell, G., Shearman, J.P., Kimber, N.E., 2012. Determination of maximal oxygen uptake using the Bruce or a novel athlete-led protocol in a mixed population. Journal of Human Kinetics 31, 97–104.

Hanley, B., 2015. Pacing profiles and pack running at the IAAF World Half Marathon Championships. Journal of Sports Science 33 (11), 1189–1195.

Hansen, E.A., 2015. On voluntary rhythmic leg movement behaviour and control during pedalling. Acta Physiologica 214 (702), 1–18.

Hansen, E.A., Smith, G., 2009. Factors affecting cadence choice during submaximal cycling and cadence influence on performance. International Journal of Sports Physiology and Performance 4 (1), 3–17.

Hartung, G.H., Krock, L.P., Crandall, C.G., Bisson, R.U., Myhre, L.G., 1993. Prediction of maximal oxygen uptake from submaximal exercise testing in aerobically fit and non-fit men. Aviation Space and Environmental Medicine 64 (8), 735–740.

Haskell, W.L., 1994. Health consequences of physical activity: understanding and challenges regarding dose-response. Medicine and Science in Sports and Exercise 26, 649–660.

Haugen, T.A., Tønnessen, E., Hem, E., Leirstein, S., Seiler, S., 2014. V̇O₂max characteristics of elite female soccer players, 1989-2007. International Journal of Sports Physiology and Performance 9 (3), 515–521.

Hauschild, V.D., DeGroot, D.W., Hall, S.M., Grier, T.L., Deaver, K.D., Hauret, K.G., et al., 2017. Fitness tests and occupational tasks of military interest: a systematic review of correlations. Occupational and Environmental Medicine 74 (2), 144–153.

Hawkins, M.N., Raven, P.B., Snell, P.G., Stray-Gundersen, J., Levine, B.D., 2007. Maximal oxygen uptake as a parametric measure of cardiorespiratory capacity. Medicine and Science in Sports and Exercise 39 (1), 103–107.

Hazell, T.J., Macpherson, R.E., Gravelle, B.M., Lemon, P.W., 2010. 10 or 30-s sprint interval training bouts enhance both aerobic and anaerobic performance. European Journal of Applied Physiology 110 (1), 153–160.

Helgerud, J., Rodas, G., Kemi, O.J., Hoff, J., 2011. Strength and endurance in elite football players. International Journal of Sports Medicine 32 (9), 677–682.

Heyward, V.H., Gibson, A.L., 2014. Advanced Fitness Assessment and Exercise Prescription, seventh ed. Human Kinetics, Champaign, IL.

Higham, D.G., Pyne, D.B., Anson, J.M., Eddy, A., 2013. Physiological, anthropometric, and performance characteristics of rugby sevens players. International Journal of Sports Physiology and Performance 8 (1), 19–27.

Hill, A.V., Lupton, H., 1923. Muscular exercise, lactic acid, and the supply and utilization of oxygen. QJM. An International Journal of Medicine 16 (62), 135–171.

Hill, D.W., Rowell, A.L., 1996. Running velocity at V̇O₂max. Medicine and Science in Sports and Exercise 28 (1), 114–119.

Hoff, J., 2005. Training and testing physical capacities for elite soccer players. Journal of Sports Science 23 (6), 573–582.

Howley, E.T., Bassett Jr., D.R., Welch, H.G., 1995. Criteria for maximal oxygen uptake: review and commentary. Medicine and Science in Sports and Exercise 27 (9), 1292–1301.

Hrysomallis, C., 2011. Balance ability and athletic performance. Journal of Sports Medicine 41 (3), 221–232.

Huang, G., Wang, R., Chen, P., Huang, S.C., Donnelly, J.E., Mehlferber, J.P., et al., 2016. Dose-response relationship of cardiorespiratory fitness adaptation to controlled endurance training in sedentary older adults. European Journal of Preventative Cardiology 23 (5), 518–529.

Huggett, D.L., Connelly, D.M., Overend, T.J., 2005. Maximal aerobic capacity testing of older adults: a critical review. Journal of Gerontology 60A (1), 57–66.

Iaia, F.M., Bangsbo, J., 2010. Speed endurance training is a powerful stimulus for physiological adaptations and performance improvements of athletes. Scandinavian Journal of Medicine and Science in Sports 20 (S2), 11–23.

Ishak, A., Hashim, H.A., Krasilshchikov, O., 2016. The effects of modified exponential tapering technique on perceived exertion, heart rate, time trial performance, $\dot{V}O_{2max}$ and power output among highly trained junior cyclists. Journal of Sports Medicine and Physical Fitness 56 (9), 961–967.

Islam, H., Townsend, L.K., Hazell, T.J., 2017. Modified sprint interval training protocols. Part I: physiological responses. Applied Physiology, Nutrition and Metabolism 42 (4), 339–346.

Jackson, A.S., Blair, S.N., Maher, M.T., Wier, L.T., Ross, R.M., Stuteville, J.E., et al., 1990. Prediction of functional aerobic capacity without exercise testing. Medicine and Science in Sports and Exercise 22, 863–870.

Jamnick, N.A., By, S., Pettitt, C.D., Pettitt, R.W., 2016. Comparison of the YMCA and a custom submaximal exercise test for determining $\dot{V}O_{2max}$. Medicine and Science in Sports and Exercise 48 (2), 254–259.

Jenkins, S., Čečins, N., 2011. Six-minute walk test: observed adverse events and oxygen desaturation in a large cohort of patients with chronic lung disease. International Medicine Journal 41 (5), 416–422.

Jones, A.M., Doust, J.H., 1996. A 1% treadmill grade most accurately reflects the energetic cost of outdoor running. Journal of Sports Science 14 (4), 321–327.

Jones, A.M., Vanhatalo, A., Burnley, M., Morton, R.H., Poole, D.C., 2010. Critical power: implications for determination of $\dot{V}O_{2max}$ and exercise tolerance. Medicine and Science in Sports and Exercise 42 (10), 1876–1890.

Joyner, M.J., Coyle, E.F., 2008. Endurance exercise performance: the physiology of champions. Journal of Physiology 586 (1), 35–44.

Kaminsky, L.A., Arena, R., Beckie, T.M., Brubaker, P.H., Church, T.S., Forman, D.E., et al., 2013. The importance of cardiorespiratory fitness in the United States: the need for a national registry: a policy statement from the American Heart Association. Circulation 127, 652–662.

Karsten, B., Jobson, S.A., Hopker, J., Jimenez, A., Beedie, C., 2014. High agreement between laboratory and field estimates of critical power in cycling. International Journal of Sports Medicine 35 (4), 298–303.

Karusisi, N., Thomas, F., Méline, J., Chaix, B., 2013. Spatial accessibility to specific sport facilities and corresponding sport practice: the RECORD Study. International Journal of Behavioural Nutrition and Physical Activity 20, 10–48.

Kavcic, I., Milic, R., Jourkesh, M., Ostojic, S.M., Ozkol, M.Z., 2012. Comparative study of measured and predicted $\dot{V}O_{2max}$ during a multi-stage fitness test with junior soccer players. Kinesiology 44 (1), 18–23.

Keren, G., Magazanik, A., Epstein, Y., 1980. A comparison of various methods for the determination of $\dot{V}O_{2max}$. European Journal of Applied Physiology and Occupational Physiology 45 (2-3), 117–124.

Keteyian, S.J., Brawner, C.A., Savage, P.D., Ehrman, J.K., Schairer, J., Divine, G., et al., 2008. Peak aerobic capacity predicts prognosis in patients with coronary heart disease. American Heart Journal 156, 292–300.

Kline, G.M., Porcari, J.P., Hintermeister, R., Freedson, P.S., Ward, A., McCarron, R.F., et al., 1987. Estimation of $\dot{V}O_{2max}$ from a one mile track walk, gender, age and body weight. Medicine and Science in Sports and Exercise 19, 253–259.

Kodama, S., Saito, K., Tanaka, S., Maki, M., Yachi, Y., Asumi, M., et al., 2009. Cardiorespiratory fitness as a quantitative predictor of all-cause mortality and cardiovascular events in healthy men and women. The Journal of the American Medical Association 301, 2024–2035.

Kovacs, M.S., 2006. Applied physiology of tennis performance. British Journal of Sports Medicine 40 (5), 381–386.

Krustrup, P., Mohr, M., Amstrup, T., Rysgaard, T., Johansen, J., Steensberg, A., et al., 2003. The Yo-Yo intermittent recovery test: physiological response, reliability, and validity. Medicine and Science in Sports and Exercise 35 (4), 697–705.

Krustrup, P., Mohr, M., Nybo, L., Jensen, J.M., Nielsen, J.J., Bangsbo, J., et al., 2006. The Yo-Yo IR2 test: physiological response, reliability, and application to elite soccer. 48. Medicine and Science in Sports and Exercise 38 (9), 1666–1673.

Kubukeli, Z.N., Noakes, T.D., Dennis, S.C., 2002. Training techniques to improve endurance exercise performances. Sports Medicine 32 (8), 489–509.

Kyröläinen, H., Komi, P.V., Belli, A., 1995. Mechanical efficiency in athletes during running. Scandinavian Journal of Medicine and Science in Sports 5 (4), 200–208.

Lambert, M.I., Borresen, J., 2010. Measuring training load in sports. International Journal of Sports Physiology and Performance 5 (3), 406–411.

Lamberts, R.P., 2014. Predicting cycling performance in trained to elite male and female cyclists. 223. International Journal of Sports Physiology and Performance 9 (4), 610–614.

Lamberts, R.P., Swart, J., Noakes, T.D., Lambert, M.I., 2011. A novel submaximal cycle test to monitor fatigue and predict cycling performance. British Journal of Sports Medicine 45 (10), 797–804.

Larsen, G.E., George, J.D., Alexander, J.L., Fellingham, G.W., Aldana, S.G., Parcell, A.C., et al., 2002. Prediction of maximum oxygen consumption from walking, jogging, or running. Research Quarterly for Exercise and Sport 73 (1), 66–72.

Lech, G., Jaworski, J., Lyakh, V., Krawczyk, R., 2011. Effect of the level of coordinated motor abilities on performance in junior judokas. Journal of Human Kinetics 30, 153–160.

Lee, D., Artero, E.G., Sui, X., Blair, S.N., 2010. Mortality trends in the general population: the importance of cardiorespiratory fitness. Psychopharmacology 24 (4), 27–35.

Lee, I.M., Paffenbarger Jr., R.S., 1998. Physical activity and stroke incidence: the Harvard Alumni Health Study. Stroke 29 (10), 2049–2054.

Lee, I.M., Paffenbarger Jr., R.S., 2000. Associations of light, moderate, and vigorous intensity physical activity with longevity. The Harvard Alumni Health Study. American Journal of Epidemiology 151 (3), 293–299.

Lee, I.M., Skerrett, P.J., 2001. Physical activity and all-cause mortality: what is the dose–response relation? Medicine and Science in Sports and Exercise 33 (S6), 459–471.

Lee, I.M., Hsieh, C.C., Paffenbarger Jr., R.S., 1995. Exercise intensity and longevity in men. The Harvard Alumni Health Study. The Journal of the American Medical Association 273 (15), 1179–1184.

Lee, J.M., Bassett Jr., D.R., Thompson, D.L., Fitzhugh, E.C., 2011. Validation of the Cosmed Fitmate for prediction of maximal oxygen consumption. Journal of Strength and Conditioning Research 25 (9), 2573–2579.

Legaz Arrese, A., Serrano Ostáriz, E., Casajús Mallén, J.A., Munguía Izquierdo, D., 2005. The changes in running performance and maximal oxygen uptake after long-term training in elite athletes. Journal of Sports Medicine and Physical Fitness 45 (4), 435–440.

Léger, L.A., 1982. A maximal multistage 20-m shuttle run test to predict $\dot{V}O_{2max}$. European Journal of Applied Physiology and Occupational Physiology 49 (1), 1–12.

Lindberg, A.S., Oksa, J., Malm, C., 2014. Laboratory or field tests for evaluating firefighters' work capacity? PLoS One 9 (3), e91215.

Lindberg, A.S., Oksa, J., Gavhed, D., Malm, C., 2013. Field tests for evaluating the aerobic work capacity of firefighters. PLoS One 8 (7), e68047.

Lindgren, M., Börjesson, M., Ekblom, Ö., Bergström, G., Lappas, G., Rosengrena, A., et al., 2016. Physical activity pattern, cardiorespiratory fitness, and socioeconomic status in the SCAPIS pilot trial: a cross-sectional study. Preventative Medicine Reports 4, 44–49.

Little, J.P., Safdar, A., Wilkin, G.P., Tarnopolsky, M.A., Gibala, M.J., 2010. A practical model of low-volume high-intensity interval training induces mitochondrial biogenesis in human skeletal muscle: potential mechanisms. Journal of Physiology 588 (6), 1011–1022.

Loftin, M., Sothern, M., Warren, B., Udall, J., 2004. Comparison of $\dot{V}O_{2max}$ during treadmill and cycle ergometry in severely overweight youth. Journal of Sports Science and Medicine 3 (4), 554–560.

Lorenz, D.S., Reiman, M.P., Lehecka, B.J., Naylor, A., 2013. What performance characteristics determine elite versus nonelite athletes in the same sport? Sports Health 5 (6), 542–547.

MacAuley, D., McCrum, E.E., Stott, G., Evans, A.E., Gamble, R.P., McRoberts, B., et al., 1998. Levels of physical activity, physical fitness and their relationship in the Northern Ireland Health and Activity Survey. International Journal of Sports Medicine 19 (7), 503–511.

Macfarlane, D.J., 2001. Automated metabolic gas analysis systems: a review. Journal of Sports Medicine 31 (12), 841–861.

Macpherson, R.E., Hazell, T.J., Olver, T.D., Paterson, D.H., Lemon, P.W., 2011. Run sprint interval training improves aerobic performance but not maximal cardiac output. Medicine and Science in Sports and Exercise 43 (1), 115–122.

Malek, M.H., Housh, T.J., Berger, D.E., Coburn, J.W., Beck, T.W., 2005. A new non-exercise-based $\dot{V}O_{2max}$ prediction equation for aerobically trained men. Journal of Strength and Conditioning Research 19 (3), 559–565.

Malek, M.H., Housh, T.J., Berger, D.E., Coburn, J.W., Beck, T.W., 2004. A new nonexercise-based $\dot{V}O_{2max}$ equation for aerobically trained females. Medicine and Science in Sports and Exercise 36 (10), 1804–1810.

Marsh, A.P., Martin, P.E., 1997. Effect of cycling experience, aerobic power, and power output on preferred and most economical cycling cadences. Medicine and Science in Sports and Exercise 29 (9), 1225–1232.

Marszalek, J., Molik, B., Gomez, M.A., Skučas, K., Lencse-Mucha, J., Rekowski, W., et al., 2015. Relationships between anaerobic performance, field tests and game performance of sitting volleyball players. Journal of Human Kinetics 48, 25–32.

Mayorga-Vega, D., Bocanegra-Parrilla, R., Ornelas, M., Viciana, J., 2016. Criterion-related validity of the distance- and time-based walk/run field tests for estimating cardiorespiratory fitness: a systematic review and meta-analysis. PLoS One 11 (3), e0151671.

McConnell, T.R., 1988. Practical considerations in the testing of $\dot{V}O_{2max}$ in runners. Journal of Sports Medicine 5 (1), 57–68.

McKay, G.A., Bannister, E.W., 1976. A comparison of maximum oxygen uptake determination by bicycle ergometry at various pedaling frequencies and by treadmill running at various speeds. European Journal of Applied Physiology 35, 191–200.

McKie, G.L., Islam, H., Townsend, L.K., Robertson-Wilson, J., Eys, M., Hazell, T.J., et al., 2018. Modified sprint interval training protocols: physiological and psychological responses to four weeks of training. Applied Physiology, Nutrition and Metabolism 43 (6), 595–601.

Meinild Lundby, A.K., Jacobs, R.A., Gehrig, S., de Leur, J., Hauser, M., Bonne, T.C., et al., 2018. Exercise training increases skeletal muscle mitochondrial volume density by enlargement of existing mitochondria and not de novo biogenesis. Acta Physiologica 222 (1), e12976.

Metaxas, T., Koutlianos, N., Sendelides, T., Mandrouka, A., 2009. Preseason physiological profile of soccer and basketball players in different divisions. 182. Journal of Strength and Conditioning Research 23 (6), 1704–1713.

Metaxas, T.I., Koutlianos, N.A., Kouidi, E.J., Deligiannis, A.P., 2005. Comparative study of field and laboratory tests for the evaluation of aerobic capacity in soccer players. Journal of Strength and Conditioning Research 19 (1), 79–84.

Metsios, G.S., Flouris, A.D., Koutedakis, Y., Nevill, A., 2008. Criterion-related validity and test-retest reliability of the 20-m square shuttle test. Journal of Science and Medicine in Sport 2008 11 (2), 214–217.

Metsios, G.S., Flouris, A.D., Koutedakis, Y., Theodorakis, Y., 2006. The effect of performance feedback on cardiorespiratory fitness field tests. Journal of Science and Medicine in Sport 9 (3), 263–266.

Michaelides, M.A., Parpa, K.M., Henry, L.J., Thompson, G.B., Brown, B.S., 2011. Assessment of physical fitness aspects and their relationship to firefighters' job abilities. Journal of Strength and Conditioning Research 25 (4), 956–965.

Midgley, A.W., Carroll, S., 2009. Emergence of the verification phase procedure for confirming 'true' $\dot{V}O_{2max}$. Scandinavian Journal of Medicine and Science in Sports 19 (3), 313–322.

Midgley, A.W., Earle, K., McNaughton, L.R., Siegler, J.C., Clough, P., Earle, F., et al., 2017. Exercise tolerance during $\dot{V}O_{2max}$ testing is a multifactorial psychobiological phenomenon. Research in Sports Medicine 25 (4), 480–494.

Mier, C.M., Alexander, R.P., Mageean, A.L., 2012. Achievement of $\dot{V}O_{2max}$ criteria during a continuous graded exercise test and a verification stage performed by college athletes. Journal of Strength and Conditioning Research 26 (10), 2648–2654.

Milanović, Z., Pantelić, S., Čović, N., Sporiš, G., Krustrup, P., 2015a. Is recreational soccer effective for improving $\dot{V}O_{2max}$? A systematic review and meta-analysis. Journal of Sports Medicine 45 (9), 1339–1353.

Milanović, Z., Pantelić, S., Sporiš, G., Mohr, M., Krustrup, P., 2015b. Health-related physical fitness in healthy untrained men: effects on $\dot{V}O_{2max}$, jump performance and flexibility of soccer and moderate-intensity continuous running. PLoS One 10 (8), e0135319.

Milanović, Z., Sporiš, G., Weston, M., 2015c. Effectiveness of high-intensity interval training (HIT) and continuous endurance training for $\dot{V}O_{2max}$ improvements: a systematic review and meta-analysis of controlled trials. Journal of Sports Medicine 45 (10), 1469–1481.

Miller, D.K., Kieffer, H.S., Kemp, H.E., Torres, S.E., 2011. Off-season physiological profiles of elite National Collegiate Athletic Association Division III male soccer players. Journal of Strength and Conditioning Research 25 (6), 1508–1513.

Millet, G.P., Vleck, V.E., Bentley, D.J., 2009. Physiological differences between cycling and running: lessons from triathletes. Journal of Sports Medicine 39 (3), 179–206.

Moffatt, R.J., Chitwood, L.F., Biggerstaff, K.D., 1994. The influence of verbal encouragement during assessment of maximal oxygen uptake. Journal of Sports Medicine and Physical Fitness 34 (1), 45–49.

Moore, A., Murphy, A., 2003. Development of an anaerobic capacity test for field sport athletes. Journal of Science and Medicine in Sport 6 (3), 275–284.

Munoz, I., Seiler, S., Alcocer, A., Carr, N., Esteve-Lanao, J., 2015. Specific intensity for peaking: is race pace the best option? Asian Journal of Sports Medicine 6 (3), e24900.

Myers, J., Kaminsky, L.A., Lima, R., Christle, J.W., Ashley, E., Arena, R., et al., 2017. A reference equation for normal standards for $\dot{V}O_{2max}$: analysis from the Fitness Registry and the Importance of Exercise National Database (FRIEND Registry). Progress in Cardiovascular Diseases 60 (1), 21–29.

Myers, J., Prakash, M., Froelicher, V., Do, D., Partington, S., Atwood, J.E., et al., 2002. Exercise capacity and mortality among men referred for exercise testing. New England Journal of Medicine 346, 793–801.

Nakagaichi, M., Lee, M.S., Tanaka, K., 2001. Accuracy of two simple methods for the assessment of health-related physical fitness. Perception and Motor Skills 92 (1), 37–49.

Neufer, P.D., 1989. The effect of detraining and reduced training on the physiological adaptations to aerobic exercise training. Journal of Sports Medicine 8 (5), 302–320.

Ní Chéilleachair, N.J., Harrison, A.J., Warrington, G.D., 2017. HIIT enhances endurance performance and aerobic characteristics more than high-volume training in trained rowers. Journal of Sports Science 35 (11), 1052–1058.

Nieman, D.C., Lasasso, H., Austin, M.D., Pearce, S., McInnis, T., Unick, J., et al., 2007. Validation of Cosmed's FitMate in measuring exercise metabolism. Research in Sports Medicine 15 (1), 67–75.

Noakes, T.D., 1998. Maximal oxygen uptake: "classical" versus "contemporary" viewpoints: a rebuttal. Medicine and Science in Sports and Exercise 30 (9), 1381–1398.

Noakes, T.D., 2008. How did A V Hill understand the $\dot{V}O_{2max}$ and the "plateau phenomenon"? Still no clarity? British Journal of Sports Medicine 42 (7), 574–580.

Nordgren, B., Fridén, C., Jansson, E., Österlund, T., Wilhelmus, J.G., Opava, C.H., et al., 2014. Criterion validation of two submaximal aerobic fitness tests, the self-monitoring Fox-walk test and the Åstrand cycle test in people with rheumatoid arthritis. BMC Musculoskeletal Disorders 15, 305.

Oja, P., 2001. Dose response between total volume of physical activity and health and fitness. Medicine and Science in Sports and Exercise 33 (S6), 428–437.

Oppewal, A., Hilgenkamp, T.I., van Wijck, R., Evenhuis, H.M., 2013. Cardiorespiratory fitness in individuals with intellectual disabilities: a review. Research in Developmental Disabilities 34 (10), 3301–3316.

Orr, J.L., Williamson, P., Anderson, W., Ross, R., McCafferty, S., Fettes, P., et al., 2013. Cardiopulmonary exercise testing: arm crank vs cycle ergometry. Anasthesia 68 (5), 497–501.

Pallarés, J.G., Morán-Navarro, R., Ortega, J.F., Fernández-Elías, V.E., Mora-Rodriguez, R., 2016. Validity and reliability of ventilatory and blood lactate thresholds in well-trained cyclists. PLoS One 11 (9), e0163389.

Pate, R.R., Wang, C.Y., Dowda, M., Farrell, S.W., O'Neill, J.R., 2006. Cardiorespiratory fitness levels among US youth 12 to 19 years of age: findings from the 1999–2002 National Health and Nutrition Examination Survey. Archives of Paediatric and Adolescent Medicine 160 (10), 1005–1012.

Petibois, C., Déléris, G., 2003. Effects of short- and long-term detraining on the metabolic response to endurance exercise. International Journal of Sports Medicine 24 (5), 320–325.

Poole, D.C., Jones, A.M., 2012. Oxygen uptake kinetics. Comprehensive Physiology 2, 933–996.

Poole, D.C., Jones, A.M., 2017. Measurement of the maximum oxygen uptake $\dot{V}O_{2max}$: is no longer acceptable. Journal of Applied Physiology 122 (4), 997–1002.

Poole, D.C., Burnley, M., Vanhatalo, A., Rossiter, H.B., Jones, A.M., 2016. Critical power: an important fatigue threshold in exercise physiology. Medicine and Science in Sports and Exercise 48 (11), 2320–2334.

Poulain, M., Durand, F., Palomba, B., Ceugniet, F., Desplan, J., Varray, A., et al., 2003. 6-Minute walk testing is more sensitive than maximal incremental cycle testing for detecting oxygen desaturation in patients with COPD. Chest 123 (5), 1401–1407.

Rankovic, G., Mutavdzic, V., Toskic, D., Preljevic, A., Kocic, M., Nedin Rankovic, G., et al., 2010. Aerobic capacity as an indicator in different kinds of sports. Bosnian Journal of Basic Medical Science 10 (1), 44–48.

Ransdell, L.B., Murray, T.M., Gao, Y., 2013. Off-ice fitness of elite female ice hockey players by team success, age, and player position. Journal of Strength and Conditioning Research 27 (4), 875–884.

Reilly, T., Borrie, A., 1992. Physiology applied to field hockey. Journal of Sports Medicine 14 (1), 10–26.

Riboli, A., Cè, E., Rampichini, S., Venturelli, M., Alberti, G., Limonta, E., et al., 2017. Comparison between continuous and discontinuous incremental treadmill test to assess velocity at $\dot{V}O_{2max}$. Journal of Sports Medicine and Physical Fitness 57 (9), 1119–1125.

Ricci, J., Léger, L.A., 1983. $\dot{V}O_{2max}$ of cyclists from treadmill, bicycle ergometer and velodrome tests. European Journal of Applied Physiology and Occupational Physiology 50 (2), 283–289.

Robert McComb, J.J., Roh, D., Williams, J.S., 2006. Explanatory variance in maximal oxygen uptake. Journal of Sports Science and Medicine 5 (2), 296–303.

Robison, J.I., Rogers, M.A., 1994. Adherence to exercise programmes. Recommendations. Sports Medicine 17 (1), 39–52.

Rønnestad, B.R., Hansen, J., Ellefsen, S., 2014. Block periodization of high-intensity aerobic intervals provides superior training effects in trained cyclists. Scandinavian Journal of Medicine and Science in Sports 24 (1), 34–42.

Rylands, L.P., Roberts, S.J., Hurst, H.T., 2015. Variability in laboratory vs. field testing of peak power, torque, and time of peak power production among elite bicycle motocross cyclists. Journal of Strength and Conditioning Research 29 (9), 2635–2640.

Sanders, L.F., Duncan, G.E., 2006. Population-based reference standards for cardiovascular fitness among U.S. adults: NHANES 1999–2000 and 2001–2002. Medicine and Science in Sports and Exercise 38 (4), 701–707.

Sartor, F., Vernillo, G., de Morree, H.M., Bonomi, A.G., La Torre, A., Kubis, H.P., et al., 2013. Estimation of maximal oxygen uptake via submaximal exercise testing in sports, clinical, and home settings. Journal of Sports Medicine 43 (9), 865–873.

Saunders, P.U., Pyne, D.B., Telford, R.D., Hawley, J.A., 2004. Factors affecting running economy in trained distance runners. Journal of Sports Medicine 34 (7), 465–485.

Schaun, G.Z., 2017. The maximal oxygen uptake verification phase: a light at the end of the tunnel? Sports Medicine – Open 3 (1), 44.

Schembre, S.M., Riebe, D.A., 2011. Non-exercise estimation of $\dot{V}O_{2max}$ using the International Physical Activity Questionnaire. Measurement in Physical Education and Exercise Science 15 (3), 168–181.

Secher, N.H., Volianitis, S., 2006. Are the arms and legs in competition for cardiac output? Medicine and Science in Sports and Exercise 38 (10), 1797–1803.

Sheppard, J.M., Young, W.B., 2006. Agility literature review: classifications, training and testing. Journal of Sports Science 24 (9), 919–932.

Sjödin, B., Svedenhag, J., 1985. Applied physiology of marathon running. Journal of Sports Medicine 2 (2), 83–99.

Skelly, A.C., Dettori, J.R., Brodt, E.D., 2012. Assessing bias: the importance of considering confounding. Evidence Based Spine Care Journal 3 (1), 9–12.

Sloth, M., Sloth, D., Overgaard, K., Dalgas, U., 2013. Effects of sprint interval training on $\dot{V}O_{2max}$ and aerobic exercise performance: a systematic review and meta-analysis. Scandinavian Journal of Medicine and Science in Sports 23 (6), 341–352.

Smirmaul, B.P.C., Bertucci, D.R., Teixeira, I.P., 2013. Is the $\dot{V}O_{2max}$ that we measure really maximal? Frontiers in Physiology 4, 203.

Sousa, A., Rodríguez, F.A., Machado, L., Vilas-Boas, J.P., Fernandes, R.J., 2015. Exercise modality effect on oxygen uptake off-transient kinetics at maximal oxygen uptake intensity. Experimental Physiology 100 (6), 719–729.

Stamford, B.A., 1988. Exercise and the elderly. Exercise and Sports Science Reviews 16, 341–379.

Støren, Ø., Bratland-Sanda, S., Haave, M., Helgerud, J., 2012. Improved $\dot{V}O_{2max}$ and time trial performance with more high aerobic intensity interval training and reduced training volume: a case study on an elite national cyclist. Journal of Strength and Conditioning Research 26 (10), 2705–2711.

Straub, A.M., Midgley, A.W., Zavorsky, G.S., Hillman, A.R., 2014. Ramp-incremented and RPE-clamped test protocols elicit similar $\dot{V}O_{2max}$ values in trained cyclists. European Journal of Applied Physiology 114 (8), 1581–1590.

Suchomel, T.J., Nimphius, S., Stone, M.H., 2016. The importance of muscular strength in athletic performance. Journal of Sports Medicine 46 (10), 1419–1449.

Sykes, K., Roberts, A., 2004. The Chester step test: a simple yet effective tool for the prediction of aerobic capacity. Physiotherapy 90, 183–188.

Tabben, M., Coquart, J., Chaabène, H., Franchini, E., Chamari, K., Tourny, C., et al., 2014. Validity and reliability of new karate-specific aerobic test for karatekas. International Journal of Sports Physiology and Performance 9 (6), 953–958.

Taylor, A.W., Bachman, L., 1999. The effects of endurance training on muscle fibre types and enzyme activities. Canadian Journal of Applied Physiology 24 (1), 41–53.

Teixeira, A.S., da Silva, J.F., Carminatti, L.J., Dittrich, N., Castagna, C., Guglielmo, L.G., et al., 2014. Reliability and validity of the Carminatti's test for aerobic fitness in youth soccer players. Journal of Strength and Conditioning Research 28 (11), 3264–3273.

Tønnessen, E., Hem, E., Leirstein, S., Haugen, T., Seiler, S., 2013. Maximal aerobic power characteristics of male professional soccer players, 1989–2012. International Journal of Sports Physiology and Performance 8 (3), 323–329.

Townsend, L.K., Islam, H., Dunn, E., Eys, M., Robertson-Wilson, J., Hazell, T.J., et al., 2017. Modified sprint interval training protocols. Part II: psychological responses. Applied Physiology, Nutrition and Metabolism 42 (4), 347–353.

Tran, D., 2018. Cardiopulmonary exercise testing. Methods in Molecular Biology 67 (1735), 285–295.

van den Berg-Emons, R.J., Bussmann, J.B., Haisma, J.A., Sluis, T.A., van der Woude, L.H., Bergen, M.P., et al., 2008. A prospective study on physical activity levels after spinal cord injury during inpatient rehabilitation and the year after discharge. Archives of Physical Medicine and Rehabilitation 89, 2094–2101.

Vaz, L., Vasilica, I., Carreras, D., Kraak, W., Nakamura, F.Y., 2016. Physical fitness profiles of elite under-19 rugby union players. Journal of Sports Medicine and Physical Fitness 56 (4), 415–421.

Verberkt, C.A., Fridén, C., Grooten, W.J., Opava, C.H., 2012. Reliability of the Fox-walk test in patients with rheumatoid arthritis. Disability and Rehabilitation 34 (23), 2001–2006.

Vercruyssen, F., Brisswalter, J., 2010. Which factors determine the freely chosen cadence during submaximal cycling? Journal of Science and Medicine in Sport 13 (2), 225–231.

Wang, C.Y., Haskell, W.L., Farrell, S.W., Lamonte, M.J., Blair, S.N., Curtin, L.R., et al., 2010. Cardiorespiratory fitness levels among US adults 20–49 years of age: findings from the 1999–2004 National Health and Nutrition Examination Survey. American Journal of Epidemiology 171 (4), 426–435.

Wasserman, K., 1986. The anaerobic threshold: definition, physiological significance and identification. Advances in Cardiology 35, 1–23.

Wehrlin, J.P., Hallén, J., 2006. Linear decrease in $\dot{V}O_{2max}$ and performance with increasing altitude in endurance athletes. European Journal of Applied Physiology 96 (4), 404–412.

Weiglein, L., Herrick, J., Kirk, S., Kirk, E.P., 2011. The 1-mile walk test is a valid predictor of $\dot{V}O_{2max}$ and is a reliable alternative fitness test to the 1.5-mile run in U.S. Air Force males. Military Medicine 176 (6), 669–673.

Wells, C.M., Edwards, A.M., Winter, E.M., Fysh, M.L., Drust, B., 2012. Sport-specific fitness testing differentiates professional from amateur soccer players where $\dot{V}O_{2max}$ and $\dot{V}O_2$ kinetics do not. Journal of Sports Medicine and Physical Fitness 52 (3), 245–254.

Weltman, A., Katch, V., Sady, S., 1978. Effects of increasing oxygen availability on bicycle ergometer endurance performance. Ergonomics 21 (6), 427–437.

West, C.R., Leicht, C.A., Goosey-Tolfrey, V.L., Romer, L.M., 2015. Perspective: does laboratory-based maximal incremental exercise testing elicit maximum physiological responses in highly-trained athletes with cervical spinal cord injury? Frontiers in Physiology 6, 419.

Weston, M., Taylor, K.L., Batterham, A.M., Hopkins, W.G., 2014. Effects of low-volume high-intensity interval training (HIT) on fitness in adults: a meta-analysis of controlled and non-controlled trials. Journal of Sports Medicine 44 (7), 1005–1017.

Williams, C.J., Williams, M.G., Eynon, N., Ashton, K.J., Little, J.P., Wisloff, U., et al., 2017. Genes to predict $\dot{V}O_{2max}$ trainability: a systematic review. BMC Genomics 18 (S8), 831.

Winter, E.M., 2011. "Critical power": time to abandon. Medicine and Science in Sports and Exercise 43 (3), 552.

Wouters, M., Evenhuis, H.M., Hilgenkamp, T.I., 2017. Systematic review of field-based physical fitness tests for children and adolescents with intellectual disabilities. Research in Developmental Disabilities 61, 77–94.

Yoon, B.K., Kravitz, L., Robergs, R., 2007. $\dot{V}O_{2max}$, protocol duration, and the $\dot{V}O_{2max}$ plateau. Medicine and Science in Sports and Exercise 39 (7), 1186–1192.

Yoshida, T., Chida, M., Ichioka, M., Suda, Y., 1987. Blood lactate parameters related to aerobic capacity and endurance performance. European Journal of Applied Physiology and Occupational Physiology 56 (1), 7–11.

Zemková, E., 2014. Sport-specific balance. Journal of Sports Medicine 44 (5), 579–590.

Ziogas, G.G., Patras, K.N., Stergiou, N., Georgoulis, A.D., 2011. Velocity at lactate threshold and running economy must also be considered along with maximal oxygen uptake when testing elite soccer players during preseason. Journal of Strength and Conditioning Research 25 (2), 414–419.

Chapter | 13 |

Ultrasound imaging in groin injuries

Amanda Parry

In this chapter we discuss types of groin injuries that are prevalent in professional athletes, some of the pearls and pitfalls of using diagnostic ultrasonography (DUS), how it can be used to help aid diagnosis and when other imaging modalities are more appropriate. Ultrasonography is a modality requiring clinical expertise. Findings can be easily misinterpreted to an untrained eye, through poor machine manipulation and artifact, due to the nature of ultrasound physics. Individuals practising ultrasound should be qualified, or studying, to do so. Many courses are now available and encouragement to undertake a Consortium for the Accreditation of Sonographic Education (CASE)-accredited course is highly recommended before incorporating diagnostic ultrasound into practice.

Groin injuries are highly prevalent in sporting professionals, particularly in sports involving high-speed running, quick changes in direction and kicking. Elite athletes can be sidelined for a number of weeks or longer if they are not clearly and promptly diagnosed, treated and managed. Difficulty can lie in detecting the exact origin and extent of groin injury, as it is a complex area of soft tissue and bony anatomy. Thorough clinical examination is essential and always the first line of interrogation in any injury, allowing the clinician to narrow down the suspected area and mechanism for injury. This, however, is not a simple task, as groin pain can radiate from a number of different regions such as lumbar, abdominal, inguinal or hip. For further investigation, patients with groin pain are frequently referred for magnetic resonance imaging (MRI), which has its advantages and continues to be accepted as the gold standard, but is not without some limitations. With advancements in DUS technology and increasing knowledge and expertise of operators, the use of DUS by front-line sports practitioners is becoming more efficacious for accurate diagnosis. It is gradually becoming the *initial* imaging modality of choice for athletic groin pain.

The rule-out tool

Currently there is limited research available on DUS for the assessment of athletic groin pain. However, DUS is an area of imaging that has many advantages for groin assessment and its use is encouraged as a 'rule-out' tool before requesting further investigation. This imaging modality is mobile, meaning scans can be performed on site, which allows conference between various clinicians and other personnel involved at the time of the scan.

Optimal time to scan

Optimal time for scanning sports injuries is usually 48–72 hours postinjury. Although there are increasing pressures to diagnose players immediately postinjury, both from players themselves and other stakeholders involved with the athlete, it is still best practice to wait for this time period to achieve more accurate imaging. In the acute phase postinjury, swelling and oedema are present. This provides an added complication to imaging in that the superficial tissues have increased density and therefore the ultrasound beam is attenuated (i.e., weakened) through these tissues, resulting in poorer visualization of the underlying structures. Allowing the injury 48–72 hours to settle enables more accurate and dynamic assessment.

If surgery is to be considered, early diagnosis is advantageous. Better prognosis of recovery is recorded if surgery is performed in the early stages. The reasoning and rationale behind this is discussed further in Chapter 15.

Dynamic review

DUS is relatively inexpensive and generally quick to perform when compared to MRI. Sonopalpation, the use of transducer compression, can help to determine areas of pain in relation to what is demonstrated on an image and is a useful tool in assessing if what is visualized is actually symptomatic. It also enables the clinician to visualize what happens to the anatomical structure whilst manipulation is in progress. Dynamic review can aid diagnosis by opening out soft tissue tears, simply by the movement itself or by distension of fluid when moving the affected region, i.e., internal or external rotation of the hip may introduce fluid into an adductor tendon tear, thus making the injury more obvious. Dynamic assessment also aids the differential between full- and partial-thickness tears.

Full- vs. partial-thickness tears

If there is uncertainty whether a demonstrated tear is of partial or full thickness, flex/extend and rotate the affected limb. If a tendon is seen to move with manipulation of the insertional area, then a full-thickness tear may be ruled out; if it doesn't, a complete rupture is indicated. Full-thickness tears of the adductor longus tendon are usually obvious due to free fluid, a void in the ultrasound appearance of the fibrillar pattern and retraction of fibres. If further clarification is needed, scan the leg in a neutral position and an abducted frog-leg or figure-of-four position. The tear should be more obvious when abducted, as the tendon insertion has been stretched and therefore will pull the torn fibres apart.

Scanning planes

DUS has the ability to scan in any plane. Structures should always be visualized, assessed and imaged in two planes at 90 degrees to each other, in order to appreciate the full extent of the injury. To be able to view a tear along its complete length is advantageous but not essential to diagnosis. An extended field of view function is available on most machines.

Follow up

Follow-up scans are quick, simple and cheap with no risk to the patient. They are useful, as accurate measurements can be attainable from consistent landmarks, making it ideal to assess progression/regression of the injured structures.

Imaging

Plain radiographs: are they still helpful?

Yes. Sometimes, simple is not to be forgotten. If hip-related groin pain is suspected, then X-ray should still be first-line investigation. Although discrete bony changes are well visualized with ultrasound, it is not able to visualize the whole femoral head within the joint, which is advantageous for accurate diagnosis. X-ray assessment is essential to confirm the diagnosis and exclude bone or coxofemoral joint injuries or disorders (Pesquer et al., 2015).

Computerized tomography

Computerized tomography (CT) is not generally used for assessment of the hip and groin, due to MRI being able to give a more complete picture and also to the radiation dose involved, specifically to the gonad region of young adolescents and adults involved in professional sport.

Magnetic resonance imaging

MRI remains the reference standard for the imaging of many areas and the groin is no exception, especially when assessing for subtle abnormalities, intraarticular lesions and bony changes, such as bone marrow oedema (BMO). It is also useful in cases where no cause for symptoms has been identified using other imaging modalities but symptoms are persisting. MRI is superior in identifying subtle abnormalities, especially for pubic-related groin pain where there may be involvement of other structures such as nerves. MRI is more accurate for demonstrating neuropathies and if this is suspected, it is recommended the patient should be sent directly to MRI (Box 13.1).

Operator experience

The clinician undertaking DUS is the clinician reporting it, therefore the results and interpretation are very much operator dependant. This can be an advantage or disadvantage depending on clinician skillset. It is essential that practitioners are qualified to both perform the scan and interpret the results. Although there are likely to be small discrepancies between users, this should not be significant. Continuing professional development and peer review/audit can assist in making sure this is the case.

Box 13.1 **Comparison of MRI vs. ultrasound**

- *Imaging planes*: MRI can visualize anatomy in standard planes while ultrasound can visualize the area in almost any plane.
- *Imaging positions*: MRI is mostly performed in non-weight-bearing/nonprovocative positions, usually supine, in comparison to ultrasound in which the patient can be imaged in the position that replicates their symptoms or puts stress onto the affected area.
- *Dynamic assessment*: MRI is limited to a static view while ultrasound allows for dynamic assessment of the hip and groin complex.
- *Cost and availability*: MRI is expensive in comparison to ultrasound examination. Both are readily available for elite athletes but ultrasound has the benefit of being able to be on-site.
- *Interpretation*: MRI relies on an off-site radiologist, whilst ultrasound relies on a hands-on clinician who is involved as part of the multidisciplinary team.

Box 13.2 **Key points for optimal results when performing diagnostic ultrasound**

- Keep the ultrasound beam perpendicular to tendon/muscle fibres and fascia planes, where possible. This allows for better visualization and avoids anisotropy (an artificial void that is created when the ultrasound beam fails to be perpendicular to the desired imaging plane, i.e., tendon fibres, which can mimic tearing) (Sanders, 1998). Manipulate transducer position, pressure and heel–toe (gently putting more pressure onto one end) the transducer to achieve this.
- Use gentle pressure for musculoskeletal ultrasound, so as not to compress fluid/tears or neovascularity. However, there often needs to be a heavier pressure for the groin/hip region due to the increased depth of structures to be assessed and possibly body habitus.
- Use dynamic assessment to aid diagnosis, i.e., use Valsalva or straining to assess for herniation. Use hip flexion, extension, internal/external rotation to aid diagnosis by stretching and relaxing the tendon fibres and possibly introducing fluid into a torn interface.
- Consider dropping the frequency or changing transducers. The groin/hip region on any patient is challenging, particularly in larger patients, and penetration may be limited on a high-frequency linear transducer.
- Focal zones aid visualization of the region of interest. A focal zone corresponds to the narrowest width of the ultrasound beam. As the sound waves are closer together at this point, greater resolution is achieved; therefore your focal zone should be equal to the point of interest. This is now automatic on newer ultrasound machines.
- Be aware of artefact. There are many types of ultrasound artefact that could compromise your image and therefore your diagnosis. Artefact is an undesirable effect on an image and is due to one of three reasons:
  - Instrumentation – due to equipment not functioning as it should or the type of instrument being used.
  - Technique – due to lack of operator expertise and knowledge.
  - Tissue interaction – the way in which sound is affected by tissue type; these artefacts are unavoidable (Sanders, 1998).
- Always scan all anatomy in two planes to avoid many imaging pitfalls, particularly for dynamic imaging when the anatomical region will change in appearance.

Anatomical knowledge is key to getting accurate results from a musculoskeletal (MSK) ultrasound scan. Box 13.2 provides guidance for achieving optimal results when performing DUS.

The type and age of an ultrasound machine will also have an impact on the results obtained. It is, of course, preferable to use an up-to-date, high-end quality machine and to work together with the applications team to create settings that are suitable for your department's needs. Generally, for MSK ultrasound the higher frequency, linear transducer is the probe of choice, due to the superficial nature of most structures scanned. However, the groin and hip region can be the exception depending on patient habitus. A lower frequency linear transducer may be sufficient and in some cases, a curved transducer will be necessary – however, this is unlikely in sports professionals.

Ultrasound

A thorough examination of the groin and hip can be undertaken in a relatively short amount of time (compared to other techniques) and if the *suspected* injury is not demonstrated, ultrasound has the advantage of moving onto the adjacent area to rule out related injury. Ultrasound also has the ability to, quickly and without risk, compare any suspected abnormality to the nonsymptomatic side. This has a major advantage in working out what is clinically significant.

Suspected adductor-related groin pain

The most prevalent injuries in soccer players, and sports of a similar nature, are adductor related due to the quick change in direction, kicking and repetitive side-to-side movement. In order to rule out adductor-related groin pain (ARGP), a full examination of the adductor region should be performed, including assessment of the common aponeurosis where possible.

Things to consider:

- Is there a tear present? If so, is it partial- or full-thickness? Is free fluid present? A tear appears as a focal hypoechoic defect where tendon fibres have been disrupted.
- Is there evidence of tendinopathy? This will show as thickening of the tendon with loss of normal fibrillar pattern and often hypoechoic in nature. Vascularity (neovascularity) is not often identified in the hip region due to the depth of structures.
- Is there any myositis ossificans, enthesopathy or calcification present? Are there echogenic foci within the tendon fibres or bony irregularity?
- How does the symptomatic side compare to the non-symptomatic side?

Adductor protocol

The patient should be assessed initially in the supine position with ideally the leg abducted and externally rotated in a figure-of-four position. Here, the insertion of the adductor tendons can be more easily identified.

The anterior portion of the adductor longus tendon is reasonably small and is continuous with the rectus abdominis with a common sheath, the common aponeurosis. The rectus abdominis–adductor longus (RA–AL) aponeurosis blends with the underlying fibrocartilaginous disc and the capsule of the symphysis pubis. These anatomical findings reveal why pain can radiate from the affected structure and spread down into the thigh or up into the abdomen (Pesquer et al., 2015).

In a longitudinal plane of the tendon and muscles, scan from the adductor insertions into the muscle belly. Tearing and injury can occur at any point of the progression from tendon through the musculotendinous junction and into the muscle belly. The adductor longus tendon is noted superficially at the pubic tubercle and forms a hypoechoic triangle at the insertion. Care should be taken to not introduce anisotropy, which could be confused with tearing. The same region should then be assessed in the transverse scan plane of the tendon/muscle. Comparison with the other side will help to determine the significance of any irregularity, either of soft tissue structures or bone. Identifying the

exact location of injury along the tendon/muscle is important for the ongoing management and could make a difference to the return-to-play time. If there is an acute adductor injury, avulsion from the pubic bone may also be present, which will be clearly visible on ultrasound investigation as a small, echogenic area, possibly with some acoustic shadow, that appears to be within the tendon, adjacent to the insertion. Some surrounding reaction may also be identified, usually hypoechogenicity of tissues, some free fluid and possibly increased vascularity with colour or power Doppler imaging. Bony cortical irregularity is also often identified but is not always symptomatic, hence the need for comparison.

The common aponeurosis of the groin can be difficult to demonstrate but again ultrasound can be used as a rule-out tool for major injury in the region. Assessment can be made of the soft tissue area around the pubic symphysis, where the adductor tendon insertions become continuous with the rectus abdominis sheath. If abnormality is suspected, i.e., anything other than normal, such as any of the abnormalities listed, comparison to the contralateral side should be made. Adductor strains, in the first instance, may be scanned using ultrasound and if no cause for symptoms is identified or findings are inconclusive, MRI is recommended to assess for discrete lesions and intraarticular abnormalities.

Suspected inguinal-related groin pain

For sporting injuries, inguinal-related groin pain (IRGP) is not as common as adductor-related but still needs to be ruled out as a source of the problem if no other cause is found or if symptoms are persisting despite treatment. This is relatively quick and simple to do with ultrasound and has the added advantage of being able to be performed dynamically and allow for easy comparison to the contralateral side.

The ultrasound examination normally begins with the interrogation of the femoral and inguinal canal and the lower abdominal wall, in order to rule out hernia or any other abnormalities of the inguinal canal.

Things to consider:

- Is there a hernia identified? If so, is it femoral, arising in the femoral canal, or inguinal, arising either medially or laterally to the deep inguinal ring?
- If there is an inguinal hernia – is it a direct hernia, arising medially to the inferior epigastric vessels or an indirect hernia, arising laterally to the inferior epigastric vessels? A direct hernia is usually referred to as being mushroom shaped, whereas an indirect hernia follows the longitudinal line of the canal.

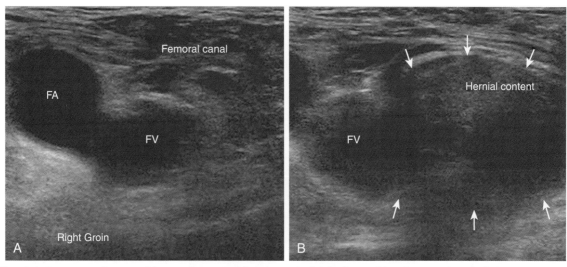

Fig. 13.1 Transverse ultrasound image demonstrating the typical right femoral hernia emerging medial to a compressed femoral vein with increased intraabdominal pressure. (A) was taken at rest and (B) during Valsalva. *FA*, Femoral artery; *FV*, femoral vein. (From Yoong, P., Duffy, S., Marshall, T.J., 2013. The inguinal and femoral canals: a practical step by step approach to accurate sonographic assessment. Indian Journal of Radiology and Imaging 23 (4), 391–395.)

- What does the hernia contain – bowel and/or omentum (abdominal fat)?
- Is it reducible? When compression is applied to the area, if the contents of the hernia can compress completely back through the defect then it is considered *reducible*. These hernias are less concerning for clinicians as there is less risk of incarcerated, or in extreme cases strangulated, bowel. If all or part of the herniation will not pass back through the defect, it is considered *nonreducible*.

Femoral region

The examination begins with the patient supine. A transverse plane is the best place to start and to work out orientation. Locate the femoral vessels. The femoral canal lies medial and superior to the superficial femoral junction. Assess the canal with Valsalva and at rest. With Valsalva, the femoral vein should dilate. If there is a femoral hernia present, the femoral vein will compress and bulging will be seen. The transducer can then be rotated through 90 degrees into a longitudinal plane and the hernia will be seen pushing along the canal. Femoral hernias are less common than inguinal hernias but can be a medical emergency if they become incarcerated, therefore accurate diagnosis is essential (Fig. 13.1).

Inguinal region

From the femoral canal, the transducer is moved superiorly to where the inferior epigastric vessels bifurcate from the external iliac vessels and track medially. The inferior epigastric vessels are a critical landmark for sonographic assessment of the groin. They originate from the external iliac artery and vein immediately above the inguinal ligament (Yoong et al., 2013). The inguinal canal is situated at the medial half of the ligament. The deep ring of the canal, therefore, sits just lateral to the inferior epigastric artery (IEA).

The transducer should be in a slightly oblique plane to view the length of the inguinal canal. Locate the deep ring, lateral to the IEA and just superior to the inguinal ligament. Again, assess the canal at rest and with Valsalva or straining. If there is an indirect hernia present, a mass of omentum/bowel or both will be seen moving medially through the deep ring and along the canal (Figs 13.2 and 13.3).

A direct hernia is seen medial to the IEA as it is a defect in the posterior wall. Slide the transducer, in the same plane, slightly medial and again ask the patient to Valsalva or strain. If there is a direct hernia present, a mushroom-type appearance is noted from deep to superficial through the posterior canal wall. The transverse plane is often usual in hernial assessment.

Hernias are often more clearly visualized with the patient standing. If no hernia is identified with the patient supine, an erect examination should be performed.

Suspected hip-related groin pain

Hip-related groin pain (HRGP) in athletes is less commonly seen but if there is no other cause for symptoms

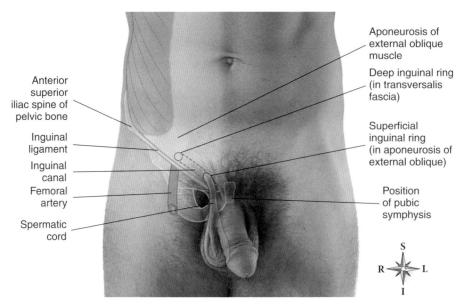

Anterior superior iliac spine of pelvic bone

Inguinal ligament

Inguinal canal

Femoral artery

Spermatic cord

Aponeurosis of external oblique muscle

Deep inguinal ring (in transversalis fascia)

Superficial inguinal ring (in aponeurosis of external oblique)

Position of pubic symphysis

Fig. 13.2 Inguinal region anatomy.

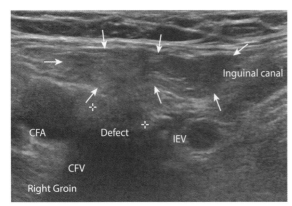

Fig. 13.3 Long axis ultrasound image through the right inguinal canal. The indirect inguinal hernia (*arrows*) emerges lateral to the inferior epigastric vessels (*IEV*) through the deep ring (*crosses*), passing over the vessels and down the canal toward the superficial ring. *CFA*, Common femoral artery; *CFV*, common femoral vein. (From Yoong, P., Duffy, S., Marshall, T.J., 2013. The inguinal and femoral canals: a practical step by step approach to accurate sonographic assessment. Indian Journal of Radiology and Imaging 23 (4), 391–395.)

identified, ultrasound can help to rule out hip structures as a cause of pain.

Things to consider:
- Is there evidence of tearing, or of inflammation of tendons (tendinopathy)?

- Is there any free fluid? Is there hip effusion in the anterior recess?
- Is there evidence of calcification?
- Remember to also dynamically assess the hip structures.

Hip region

A routine hip ultrasound examination begins with the patient in a supine position, legs extended and in a neutral position.

With the transducer in a longitudinal plane of the femoral neck, the anterior joint is assessed. Firstly, assess the contour of the acetabulum and femoral head and neck for any bony irregularities that would instigate further investigation of surrounding soft tissues. Bony irregularities, enthesopathy, increases the likelihood of tendon issues.

The anterior labral region can be assessed for labral cysts and fluid, which are easily visualized on ultrasound if there is adequate penetration and depth. Cysts appear as thin walled, anechoic (black) structures, either rounded or oval in appearance. Free fluid follows and fills the line of the joint. Following the femoral neck in the longitudinal plane, the joint capsule can be identified and evaluated for hip joint effusion at the femoral neck recess. Scan through the same area in a transverse plane also. Iliopsoas bursitis can be mistaken for hip joint effusion and vice versa on ultrasound. If there is communication with the hip joint – a defined track of fluid down into the joint – effusion is

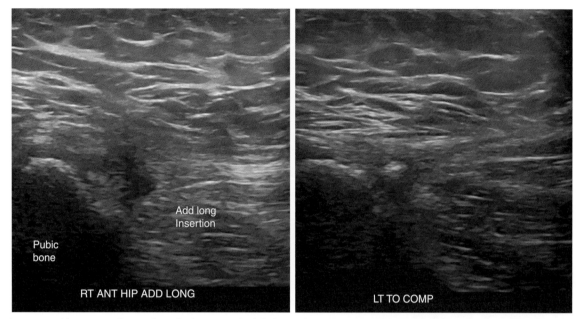

Fig. 13.4 Adductor tendinopathy. The image on the left shows the symptomatic right-sided adductor longus tendon insertion, which is thickened and hypoechoic with loss of normal fibrillar pattern as compared to the nonsymptomatic left side (right image).

present. No connection indicates bursitis rather than effusion.

Slide the transducer to the anterior inferior iliac spine (AIIS); the direct head of the rectus femoris can be visualized in the transverse and longitudinal planes. This can often be difficult to evaluate in the longitudinal plane due to anisotropy, and care needs to be taken to try to ensure the ultrasound beam is perpendicular to the fibres. Again, comparison to the nonsymptomatic side is useful to determine the significance of any findings. Colour or power Doppler may be introduced to check for any neovascularity, but this can also be difficult to visualize depending on patient habitus and machine set-up. The settings may not have been installed appropriately and may need to be manipulated. Keep the colour box as small as reasonably achievable in order to keep frame rate diagnostic.

In a transverse plane, follow the rectus femoris tendon distally and continue to interrogate the muscle. Come back to the proximal portion in order to assess the indirect rectus femoris tendon portion, looking for any thickening or adjacent tearing. A longitudinal view of the indirect head of the rectus femoris tendon can be obtained but is difficult to achieve without a superior quality machine. Adduct the affected leg, usually by crossing the ankles. With the transducer in the transverse plane, start at the AIIS and track inferiorly, slide the transducer laterally and angle back towards the hip joint to achieve the required view. The indirect tendon portion is noted as

a hypoechoic band. Firm pressure will reveal its fibrillar pattern. Suspected injuries to the indirect portion require MRI referral, but if ultrasound is available, it is, again, a good initial rule-out tool.

In the anterior hip view, the psoas muscle and tendon can be visualized along with the iliacus muscle. Other structures to consider around the hip joint are the lateral hip structures: the gluteal tendons and muscles, tensor fasciae latae and bursae in the region. The most common findings of the lateral hip are tendinopathy and bursitis. The European Society of Musculoskeletal Radiology (ESSR) provide guidelines for the hip ultrasound region (Beggs et al., 2010).

Appearances of common findings on ultrasound

Tendinopathy. This can be frequently seen at the adductor longus and rectus femoris tendon insertions. On ultrasound, the tendon appearance may look frayed, heterogenous (nonuniform) and hypoechoic. Some cystic degeneration may also be noted. The tendon may appear thickened and neovascularity may be identified, but not always (Fig. 13.4). It should be noted that there is no consensus on the pathophysiology of tendinopathy and that the above image findings can also be present in nonsymptomatic patients. In summary, it is important to treat the patient and not base your findings solely on imaging.

Tearing. This appears as a cleft or void within the muscle or tendon structure. In the acute phase, it is usually filled with fluid and therefore is hypoechoic on ultrasound. In the chronic phase, a tendon becomes thin. In a muscle, scar tissue may be noted. This appears as a hyperechoic area, with some irregularity to the muscle fibrillar pattern (Fig. 13.5).

Strain. There are varying degrees of muscle strain noted on ultrasound. It is usually depicted as an area of

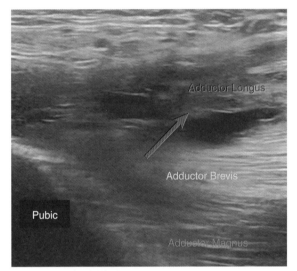

Fig. 13.5 Adductor tear. Longitudinal plane ultrasound image of the pubic bone and adductor group muscles demonstrates a tear and hematoma of the adductor longus with retracted tendon (*arrow*). (From McNally, E.G., 2014. Practical Musculoskeletal Ultrasound, second ed. Churchill Livingstone, Edinburgh.)

hyperechogenicity in the region of interest. There can be minimal fibrillar structure change.

Effusion. This is joint fluid and has a hypoechoic appearance on ultrasound. Debris within the fluid can sometimes also be identified. With an anterior hip effusion, a fluid collection would be observed over the anterior femoral neck region. Greater than 7 mm is considered a significant effusion (Fig. 13.6).

Calcification. Build up of calcification in tendons can be the result of repeated microtrauma. Echogenic areas are noted within the tendon. Shadowing is noted if it is hard calcification. Soft calcification is also recognized. It is still echogenic but not as bright and minimal, if any, shadowing is noted. These may be tiny flecks or substantial amounts. This is usually found in conjunction with tendinopathy. It is less common in the adductor longus and more frequently seen in the hamstring insertions (Fig. 13.7).

Avulsion. This describes where a small area of bone has been pulled away from the main bone as a result of tendon or ligamentous tear. A small echogenic area is seen as a separate entity and surrounding reaction is likely. This will vary depending on the age of the injury but may include hypoechoic fluid and retraction of fibres, i.e., a hypoechoic, flaccid tendon (Fig. 13.8).

Myositis ossificans. This is defined as the 'formation of bone tissue inside muscle tissue after a traumatic injury to the area' (www.marshfieldclinic.org). It appears as irregular echogenic, shadowing structures within the muscle tissue. They are common in the adductor longus region.

Conclusion

Groin injury is complex due to the anatomical make-up of the area. In order to aid a clinician to best

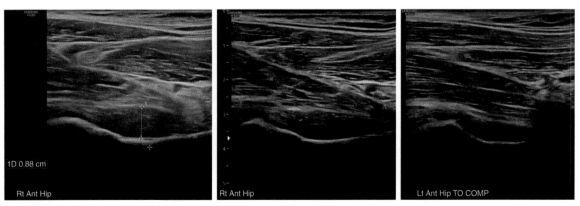

Fig. 13.6 Effusion. Image of a mild, anterior hip joint effusion seen in the anterior hip recess.

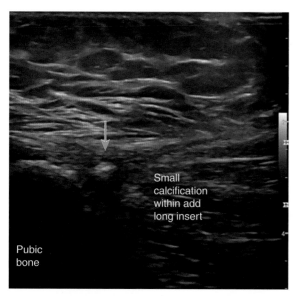

Small calcification within add long insert

Pubic bone

Fig. 13.7 Calcification. This image shows a small, echogenic focus in the adductor longus tendon at the insertion (*arrow*), consistent with a calcific deposit.

manage these types of injuries, various imaging techniques can be used. A combination of modalities may be needed for best results but ultrasound is becoming more commonly used as the initial imaging modality of choice due to its ease of availability, hands-on clinician input and ability to aid on-the-spot therapeutic techniques. However, it is essential that clinicians are trained appropriately or that they work closely with a multidisciplinary team including imaging practitioners to obtain optimal results. MRI remains the reference standard but with more sports medical facilities providing ultrasound imaging, there is no detriment to the patient by first performing an ultrasound examination as a method of rule-out.

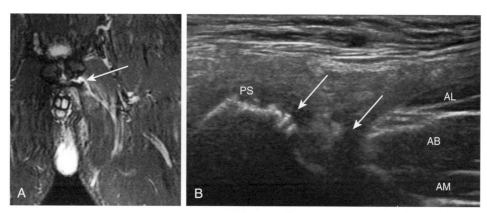

Fig. 13.8 Avulsion. Longitudinal ultrasound images of the adductor longus muscle and tendon (B) show a focal hypoechoic defect of the tendon at the insertion on the pubic bone consistent with a tendon tear (*arrows*). The axial fat-saturated T2 magnetic resonance image (A) more clearly demonstrates the partial avulsion of right adductor longus tendon (*arrowheads*). *AB*, Adductor brevis; *AL*, adductor longus; *AM*, adductor magnus; *PS*, pubic symphysis.

References

Beggs, I., Bianchi, S., Bueno, A., Cohen, M., Court-Payen, M., Grainger, A., et al., 2010. Musculoskeletal ultrasound technical guideline IV. Hip. European Society of Musculoskeletal Radiology. Available at: https://www.essr.org/subcommittees/ultrasound/.

Pesquer, L., Reboul, A., Silvestre, A., Poussange, N., Meyer, P., Dallaudiere, B., 2015. Imaging of adductor-related groin pain. Diagnostic and Interventional Imaging 96 (9), 861–869.

Sanders, R.C., 1998. Clinical Sonography: A Practical Guide, third ed. Lippincott Williams and Wilkins, Philadelphia, PA.

Yoong, P., Duffy, S., Marshall, T.J., 2013. The inguinal and femoral canals: a practical step by step approach to accurate sonographic assessment. Indian Journal of Radiology and Imaging 23 (4), 391–395.

Further reading

Books

McNally, E.G., 2014. Practical Musculoskeletal Ultrasound, second ed. Churchill Livingstone, Edinburgh.

Miller, M.D., Hart, J.A., MacKnight, J.M. (Eds.), 2019. Essential Orthopaedics, second ed. Elsevier, Amsterdam.

Online resources

www.ultrasoundtraining.co.uk.
www.theultrasoundsite.co.uk
www.jacobsonmskus.com.
www.essr.org.
www.aium.org.
www.bmus.org.
www.asum.com.au.
www.sonographers.org.

Chapter | **14** |

Conservative management of groin injuries: acute and chronic

James Moore and Michael Giakoumis

This chapter will focus on the conservative management of both acute and chronic groin pain. We will cover the differential diagnosis of groin pain; the incidence and epidemiology; the key diagnostic factors; provide an understanding of the areas that influence the function of the region; and equip you with the knowledge and framework that will allow you, the clinician, to be empowered with the necessary knowledge to appropriately rehabilitate the individual who presents with acute or chronic groin pain.

Introduction

Groin pain can be a debilitating injury in the sporting population. Often in chronic cases players can continue to train and play but with reduced performance output. For many years, groin injury has had more negative connotations than other types of sports injury, and is associated with the commonly used term 'osteitis pubis', which does not encompass the full spectrum of pathologies that can account for groin pain (Verrall et al., 2008).

The conservative management of the groin requires an appropriate understanding of the surrounding area, especially the role of the hip, which will not be discussed in this chapter. The reader should acknowledge its contribution in groin pain presentations and is directed to Chapter 16 for more information.

Incidence and epidemiology

Groin pain is common in athletes from a variety of football codes, skiing, hurdling, and hockey. These are all sports that involve high-speed torsion of the trunk, side-to-side cutting, kicking, sudden directional changes, running and sprinting, and that require specific use (or overuse) of the proximal musculature of the thigh and lower abdominal muscles. In a systematic review, it was noted that in football, groin pain accounted for 4–19% of all injuries with men being two times more likely to be affected than women (Walden et al., 2015). At the higher end of the results, a groin injury may occur 2.1 times per 1000 hours of training. It is worth noting that groin injury is likely to be underreported; as mentioned before, many athletes suffering with chronic groin pain can continue to play and train.

In football, 4 in 10 groin presentations will be of an acute nature (Hölmich et al., 2014). To highlight the prevalence of acute groin injuries in ice hockey, Mölsä and colleagues (1997) demonstrated that 43% of all muscle injures were in the adductor region. More recent studies have found that groin pain diagnosed as pubic bone stress injury (PBSI) or adductor-related groin pain, rarely occurs in isolation; rather, it is associated with concomitant pathology such as hip, psoas, abdominal, etc. (Bradshaw et al., 2008; Hölmich, 2007).

Unlike quadriceps injuries, which are often found during the start of preseason (Orchard, 2001), there is no associated seasonal trend to groin injuries. However the recurrence rate is high (Tyler et al., 2001; 2010) and in non-acute presentations it may be hard to treat, hence chronicity ensues.

Aetiology

The most common mechanism of injury, especially in an acute setting, is kicking (40%), followed by change of direction and stretching (17% each), and finally running/sprinting (15%). Of the adductor-related injuries, 93% involved the adductor longus (AL) whilst adductor brevis (AB) and pectineus were involved in 19% and 17% of cases, respectively (Serner et al., 2015). When presented with injuries involving brevis or pectineus, the clinician should note that this can be considered to be an unusual mechanism and, therefore, he/she should evaluate the associated joints for dysfunction and review the kinetic chain.

The aetiology of chronic presentations or acute-on-chronic presentations are often associated with an inability of the system to cope with the load presented – best summarized as 'exceeding capacity'. It is often related to many factors, not just the response of a pain-sensitized or pathological tissue.

Diagnosis

It is incredibly important that an appropriate diagnosis is established. The *Doha agreement meeting on terminology and definitions in groin pain in athletes* (Weir et al., 2015) has been a great advancement in establishing an accurate and consistent vocabulary; however, further work is needed to gain specificity in the diagnostic process. An acute, chronic or acute-on-chronic presentation cannot be treated the same way, even if it involves the same clinical entity. One would not rehabilitate patella–femoral pain and patellar tendinopathy the same way despite both being labelled as 'anterior knee pain'. Although the outcome of returning to sport at a high-performance level is the goal for both, the specific objectives and reasoning for them are heavily dependent on the correct diagnosis.

Table 14.1 provides a list of the musculoskeletal presentations that can present as groin pain with Table 14.2 presenting multiple differential diagnoses that can masquerade as groin pain. It is in this arena that extensive experience is valuable and often in these cases imaging and appropriate medical referral can aid in the correct diagnosis.

The subjective nature of the injury is pertinent to the examination process and formulates the majority of clinical reasoning. Listen closely to patient and to the choice of words, as this can often give an indication of the structures involved (joint, muscle, nerve). In general, a pain that is

---

Table 14.1 Musculoskeletal pathologies causing groin pain

Hip joint related	Pubic joint and adductor related	Abdominal related
Intraarticular – labral tear or rim lesion	Pubic stress response	Rectus abdominus tendinopathy
Delaminated acetabulum	Pubic stress fracture	Rectus and oblique myofascial
Osteochondral lesion or defect	Pubic disc degeneration	strains and tears
Osteochondral loose body	Pubic symphysitis	Abdominal nerve entrapment/
Cysts	Pubic instability	neuropathy
Ligamentum teres strain or rupture	Adductor enthesopathy or tendinopathy	'Inguinal ligament neuralgia'
Capsulitis or synovitis	Myofascial and myotendinous junction strains	True hernia
Periarticular ligament sprain or tear	Ligament sprain or tear	Gilmore's groin/posterior
Osteoarthritis	Secondary cleft injury	abdominal wall defect
Coxa saltans	PLAC injury	Iliopsoas-related pain
Iliopsoas and greater trochanter bursitis	Obturator neuropathy	
	Pubic apophysitis	

PLAC, Pyramidalis–anterior pubic ligament–adductor longus complex.

vague, deep and nonspecific (i.e., it covers an area) is likely to involve the joint (hip or pubic joint). A sharp pinpoint pain brought on by a specific movement may be indicative of a muscular (or tissue-specific) problem. Simply ask 'Can you put one finger on the problem?' If they can, this is more indicative of a specific-tissue problem or, for example, sportsman's groin, adductor or rectus tendinopathy. However, if they use the flat of their hand or cannot localize it, then this may indicate a deeper-seated problem from the joint, or overlapping clinical entities.

The age of the patient can be a significant indicator to the type of pathology. Different conditions occur in different age groups, e.g., pubic apophysitis <23 years of age. Always ask as to whether there was an incident or specific mechanism of injury. Often the injury has occurred during a sporting movement and thus the exact mechanism cannot always be recalled, or there has been a gradual onset or worsening of symptoms that has not precluded sporting involvement but has resulted in reduced performance. As a result, the patient may present some months (or even years) down the line. In these scenarios it is important to try and differentiate as much as possible.

Bradshaw et al. (2008) were able to show that different types of activity correlated to different pathologies. For example, in those involved in a kicking sport there is a greater incidence of pubic pathology. However, for athletes involved in a twisting sport (without kicking) or running in a straight line, the incidence of hip pathology is greater.

When trying to ascertain the irritability, do not just ask about aggravating and easing factors; be specific with your functional questions (see examples below). Try to find out about movements the patient avoids, those they feel a weakness or a loss of power when performing, or even just a lack of confidence. The patient may well have avoided certain movements for some time in order to function and they have

forgotten by the time they present for the consultation. Note that overuse injuries account for up to 80% of athletes presenting with hip and groin pain (Lloyd-Smith et al., 1985).

Ask specific questions about the following scenarios:
- Putting on socks and shoes/trousers – this is generally done at the same time every day, so gives a level of functional outcome, and will elucidate impingement of the hip and groin.
- Climbing up and down stairs – gives a functional outcome of single-leg stance and load on the hip and hemipelvis.
- Getting in and out of the car/bed – shows a possible inflammatory component if first thing in the morning, or just the mechanism of impinging the hip and tensile loading of the groin.
- Driving for long periods – indicates sustained compressive load on the hip, or overactivity of the hip flexors with relation to subtle pelvic dysfunction.
- Sleeping/rolling over in bed – problems here are classically related to the hip joint, but can be pubic joint in nature.
- Abdominal work, e.g., sit up/coughing – classically related to a sportsman's groin, but also can be associated with a pubic joint injury.
- Accelerated/unguarded movements – these are associated with groin disruption.
- Catching/giving way/'grasp sign' – classically associated with hip joint pathology.

The objective examination must be used to support or negate your hypotheses formulated during your subjective examination (Table 14.3). Hypothesis confirmation is built by clustering a number of tests to improve the probability that the null hypothesis is true. One cannot be 100% positive but can rather improve the probability of being positive. Following a good process and assessment has been shown to improve both intra- and interrater reliability to accurately diagnose different clinical entities (Hölmich et al., 2004). Be systematic and remember that more often than not there may be two or more pathologies present on examination (Bradshaw et al., 2008; Hölmich, 2007).

Despite the discussion around palpation and the lack of diagnostic factors in certain lower limb tendinopathies and pathologies, in the groin region good palpatory skill is necessary when looking to differentiate (Drew et al., 2016; Falvey et al., 2009). Falvey et al. (2009) use the term 'localize and recreate' and have been able to show a correlation with the location of pain in reference to the groin triangle and its association to the underlying pathology. In Michael Drew's PhD, those presenting with adductor-related pathology demonstrated mechanical hyperalgesia (Drew et al., 2016). To complicate things, when the AL was mechanically sensitized via a saline injection, subjects described a spread of symptoms along the superiolateral groin triangle that travelled along the inferior edge of the inguinal

Table 14.2 Non musculoskeletal pathologies causing groin pain

Benign neoplasms of bone or soft tissue	Primary hyperparathyroidism
Chondrocalcinosis	Psoas muscle abscess
Endometriosis	Psoriatic arthritis
Malignant neoplasms of bone or soft tissue	Reiter syndrome
Metastatic disease of bone	Rheumatoid arthritis
Osteomyelitis	Septic arthritis
Ovarian cyst	Spinal referred pain
Paget disease	Synovial chondromatosis
Peripheral vascular disease	Transient osteoporosis of the hip
Pigmented villonodular synovitis	

Table 14.3 Objective examination of groin pain

Pubic joint and adductors	Abdominals
Palpation: of bony landmarks, like superior and inferior pubic rami (tubercle), pubic joint line, superior and inferior pubic ligaments	**Palpation**: of all abdominal intersections – rectus insertion into the pubic bone, along the inguinal ligament, the oblique aponeurosis
Palpation: of muscle bellies, myotendinous junctions and tendon origins, especially adductor longus tendon origin, and adductor magnus consistency and cross-sectional area	**Resisted provocation tests**: sagittal plane dominant Resist bent knee and straight leg sit ups Resist double straight leg raise
Squeeze test: done in three positions 0 degrees: average male 200–220 mmHg 45–60 degrees: average male 220–240 mmHg 90 degrees: average male 200–220 mmHg (For female expect on avg. 20 mmHg less for each)	**Resisted provocation test**: transverse plane dominant In a sit-up position with 20 degrees rotation Resist right and left rotation on the right hand side and then repeat on the left hand side
Squeeze test: performed in a double straight leg raise at 30 degrees High-load provocation of PJI An anterior oblique sling test – also a criterion for return to running	**Scissor beats test**: lift both legs off the floor (approx. 15 cm) and then abduct and then adduct repeatedly for 1 min alternating the superior leg
Bent-knee fall out: for guarding Look for symmetry and smoothness of movement as well as range	**Thomas test hip flexion**: similar to an aspect of the PSST, the patient performs a small sit up and then produces hip flexion that can load the rectus abdominus as well as PLAC
Force capacity: measure force output in: Short lever outer range (FABER) Long lever outer range (EOR abduction)	
PSST: provocation in a modified Thomas test perform: Full passive hip extension Full passive hip extension and abduction resisted hip flexion in full passive extension Resisted adduction in full extension and abduction	

EOR, End of range; *FABER*, flexion- abduction-external rotation; *PJI*, pubic joint instability; *PLAC*, pyramidalis -anterior pubic ligament -adductor longus complex; *PSST*, pubic symphysis stress test.

line and in rare cases the lower abdomen (Drew et al., 2017). Therefore the clinician should be specific with their palpation to distinguish between pain-sensitive structures and subjective areas of symptoms as these may not be synonymous.

Evolution of the PLAC

Recently there have been increasing discussions and awareness of what was previously called the adductor aponeurotic plate, but termed here as the *pyramidalis–anterior pubic ligament–adductor longus complex* (PLAC). It was previously thought the tendons of rectus abdominis (RA) blended with the contralateral AL (Norton-Old et al., 2013). Injury to this structure has been previously annotated as secondary cleft or adductor traction injuries (Branci et al., 2013).

However Schilders and colleagues (2017) performed anatomical evaluations on cadavers and showed that this previously thought complex did not involve the RA tendon.

The pyramidalis is the only muscle anterior to the pubic bone and has attachments to the linea alba. From its anatomy alone, its role can be seen in providing tension and structure to the action of the RA and abdominal system, providing stiffness for the aponeurotic attachments of RA and obliques to work from. Therefore, it is the pyramidalis and AL whose tendons communicate to form the anterior pubic ligament. On the deep surface between the AL and pubic crest, a fibrocartilaginous structure is found. When disrupted it is this structure and the resultant fluid-filled cavity that is seen as a hyperechoic region on scanning.

The anterior pubic ligament provides an anchoring point for the obliques and is an integral structure to the mechanical stability of the pubic ring. It has been shown that most motion occurs in the transverse plane of the pubic joint, thus the PLAC acts as a stabilizer (Birmingham et al., 2012). Combining its role in stability with its role in transmitting and resisting high-tensional forces one can see it is an integral complex in the pelvic region.

Imaging

Imaging in this area can be tricky, as the anatomical findings do not always correspond to the clinical findings. Therefore, imaging is of great value in ruling out alternative or nonmusculoskeletal pathology. When able to provide a clear diagnosis then imaging is invaluable. However, it should always be used in conjunction with the clinical hypothesis from the physical examination and history. It is important to understand that many false positives are generated when imaging the pelvic region, as in the hip (Branci et al., 2015).

Research has so far provided varied results on the prevalence of pubic bone marrow oedema in asymptomatic individuals, but its presence was confirmed in 72% of young asymptomatic elite footballers in one cohort study (Lovell et al., 2006).There are a variety of options available to the clinician, this should always be discussed with the medical leads and radiologists to ascertain the most appropriate series of investigations needed.

Muscle function and myokinematics

As this chapter is focused on the conservative management of groin pain we will only address the muscles that cross the pubic joint complex.

Adductor muscle function

The primary focus of the adductor muscle group is across the adductor longus, magnus and gracilis; however, it should be acknowledged that meaningful adduction can be produced by the short adductors, psoas and medial hamstrings (Neumann, 2010).

All the adductors produce an adduction moment arm. However, when the thigh moves into hip flexion (>60 degrees) they all have an extension moment arm, with adductor magnus becoming the strongest extensor in hip flexion beyond 45 degrees (Vigotsky, 2016). When the thigh moves into extension, all of the adductors (except magnus) produce a flexion moment arm, with adductor longus being a key flexor behind iliopsoas. The adductor group also has the ability to produce a medial rotation moment arm about the hip.

Of all the adductors, adductor magnus has the largest cross-sectional area (CSA) and is the third largest muscle in

the lower limb. It has long fibre lengths and hence has the ability to produce high levels of force across a large range of motion. Adductor magnus can be divided into two or four distinct elements. Two elements are defined by different innervation: proximally by the obturator nerve and distally by the sciatic nerve. Four elements are defined by the different pennated angles, the compartments of muscle and subsequent actions (Takizawa et al., 2014). Therefore adductor magnus has both a lever arm for adduction, hip extension, knee flexion, and has a local stability role at the hip and pubic joint with its most proximal compartment.

Gracilis has the largest adductor moment arm as well as the second longest muscle fibre lengths in the lower limb, providing its ability to work at high velocity (Neumann, 2010; Ward et al., 2009).

The adductor longus has the largest flexion moment arm in the adductor muscle group which increases when placed into further hip extension, thus its role in hip flexion in running. It functions synergistically alongside the iliopsoas to produce hip flexion following the initiation of hip flexion. Adductor longus also works isometrically in midstance phase of gait in both walking and running to stabilize the pelvis in synergy with the gluteals. Finally AL has been shown to dampen the action of the abductors after propulsion; thus it has a large eccentric function about the hip to decelerate hip extension (Mann and Hagy, 1980).

As has been discussed, the adductors do not only contribute to adduction, which is the third strongest movement around the hip, but contribute extensively to the high flexion (second strongest) and extension (the strongest) torques that can be produced (Neumann, 2010).

Abdominal muscle function

In a similar way to the adductors, the abdominals, in particular the RA, play a key role in resisting extension-based torques. The RA, due to its linear (fusiform) nature and short muscle fibres, is better equipped to control the extension of the trunk and, alongside the hamstrings, resist anterior pelvic tilt during locomotion. The multipennated angle of the obliques (internal and external), together with their large cross-sectional area and lever arm, allows them to not only control, produce and resist rotation but also have a significant influence on trunk flexion, control posterior rotation of each ipsilateral innominate and provide stability to the pelvis through force closure.

Groin function in sport

The first thing to note is that the pelvis is a closed ring, providing a stable base for the spine and lower limbs and is an integral piece to the groin complex. It has been established that the axis of all motion at the pelvis occurs at the superior aspect of the pubic joint (Alderink, 1991). Through this it can be seen that its primary functional role is to transfer force. It provides support for the downward and forward thrust from the trunk, while at the same time absorbing the propulsive forces transmitted from the lower limbs in a reciprocal direction (Gracovetsky and Iacono, 1987). Therefore any instability, dysfunction or pain in the lumbopelvic region can overload the area leading to PLAC, bone or soft tissue injuries.

Kinetics and kinematics of sporting task

Running

Outside of in-step kicking, the adductors do not need to generate high levels of force in the coronal plane. Mann and Hagy (1980) showed that during jogging and running, the adductors were the only muscles to be working during and just prior to the toe-off period. In sprinting they were accompanied during this period by the RA. Hence their primary function during running is to control terminal hip extension and counteract the extension and external rotation torque produced during terminal stance by the gluteal musculature (Schache et al., 2011). They also have a role in helping to reaccelerate the thigh in the sagittal plane and act as synergists to the primary hip flexors, as is evident by the high levels of power produced during the initial swing phase (Schache et al., 2011). They also work synergistically with the abductors to maintain pelvic stability during the stance phase (Torry et al., 2006).

Change of direction

The way in which an individual cuts and turns will heavily influence the demands on the groin region. It has been shown in recent research that different individuals have a preferred change of direction (COD) movement pattern that results in varied kinematic outcomes (Franklyn-Miller et al., 2017).

During the turning motion it is shown that the iliopsoas and AL have important functions in either reorientating the swing leg or the orientation of the weight-bearing pelvis via opposing insertion-to-origin actions (Ventura et al., 2015).

One must consider the whole kinetic chain, especially the foot and ankle complex, in those presenting with groin pain in sports involving COD. It has been shown that the calf complex and in particular its ability to produce power (power = force × velocity) is the main physical determinant in COD performance (Marshall et al., 2014).

Kicking

The pelvic region becomes the primary generator of force as this becomes the pivot point for energy to be transferred from the proximal region to distal and is responsible for a large generation of torque. During kicking, the thigh moves at up to 500 degrees/s and of all the kinetic energy generated only 15% is absorbed by the ball; the rest of the forces are absorbed by the body (Barfield, 1998).

During the cocking phase, large amounts of traction and eccentric load occur on the groin coinciding with the fact that maximum activation occurs at peak hip extension (Charnock et al., 2009). The workload on the adductors during kicking in Australian rules football is further shown by Baczkowski et al. (2006). On average the AL underwent the second highest level of metabolic work in the adductor group behind gracilis and the highest metabolic change recorded was in the AL in one of their participants.

The technique employed during kicking in European football (in-step or side-step) dictates the spatial and temporal requirements on the AL. It has been determined that during the side-step kick, a greater level of activity is observed in the AL prior to impact; in contrast, the in-step kick demonstrates greater AL activity postimpact (Ikeda et al., 2011).

Other contributing muscles to the function of kicking include the iliopsoas, as peak hip torque generated during kicking coincides with peak iliopsoas activity; also contributing is the rectus femoris in its role in decelerating hip extension (Dörge et al., 1999). Given that the hip flexor muscles produce over 90% of the power generated during kicking, having the ability to not only generate but also tolerate these high levels of force is essential (Robertson and Mosher, 1985).

Medical intervention/pharmacotherapy

Injection therapy may be used as an adjunct to help pain management and elicit a change in the biochemical environment to evoke a better tissue response in the acute or chronic presentation of groin injury. Several options are listed below; however, it is beyond the scope of this chapter to discuss their value and relative merits. This issue must be discussed with your medical team or an appropriate medical referral made. Examples of possible injections include:

- cortisone
  - adductor 'sheath' injection
  - pubic cleft injection
- Traumeel
- autologous blood
- platelet-rich plasma
- bisphosphonates.

Rehabilitation

The rehabilitation and management of acute and persistent groin injury can be broken up into five key stages. These stages overlap, similar to the changing colours of a rainbow that cohesively blend with one another. As stages progress, exercise selection is often progressed from isolated actions to more global-based exercises and movements covering multiple planes of movement. The protocol for adductor muscle injury rehabilitation is shown in Fig. 14.1.

The first three stages are always present in an acute injury. However, they are not always present in persistent groin pain, unless the issue is an acute-on-chronic scenario or the clinician has deliberately initiated an inflammatory process by 'stressing' the tissue, for instance if they believe that there has been a failed tissue healing process from previous injury that is inhibiting the full return to play. The clinician should move fluidly through the stages depending on need and response.

Stages of management in acute setting

In the acute setting the use of pharmacotherapy can be extremely useful not only in the modulation of pain but also in regulating the biochemical response to injury and stimulating the right cytokines for repair.

It is important to understand the three primary phases associated with any tissue injury.

Stage 1: bleeding phase (0–48 hours)

This stage is one of the stages to which the saying 'less is more' applies. Appropriate management in this stage involves:
- avoiding the use of nonsteroidal anti-inflammatory drugs (NSAIDS)
- ice and compression
- early movement, but avoid stretching
- avoiding direct soft tissue work
- avoiding excessive travel.

At a biochemical level, this stage is characterized by an increase in neutrophil production to regulate the tissue damage. There is a whole chemical cascade behind this, but our focus should be directed towards two vital chemical mediators or cytokines: vascular endothelial growth factor (VEGF) and nitric oxide (NO). The former can help to regulate neurotransmitters of pain such as substance P and calcitonin gene–related peptide (CRGP), while the latter can help with noncontractile tissue pain and improve tissue repair.

Allowing the chemistry to regulate itself and find a homeostatic balance is critical, hence the strategies here are to 'offload' and allow the tissue trauma to 'settle'.

Stage 2: inflammatory phase (days 0–5/6/7)

The acute inflammatory response to injury is now settling and can be regulated with the use of NSAIDs or other pharmacotherapy. It is at this stage that there is likely to be residual swelling from stage 1 that will cause reflex inhibition and pain from both the pressure from the swelling (secondary hyperalgesia) and the chemical changes (primary hyperalgesia). This can result in reduced movement and range as well as muscle atrophy (a key risk factor in reinjury) and motor unit inhibition.

The key in this phase is to keep the area moving and under light load and restoring the range and compliance of the tissue and joint. Most importantly, there is a need to regain the recruitment thresholds at the motor unit. This can be facilitated with isometric loading that can allow for higher forces (which will recruit the motor unit) but with no movement and thus less strain to the tissue. Other adjuncts that are useful here are electrical stimulation devices such as Compex.

Stage 3: tissue conditioning/remodelling phase

In this phase, emphasis is placed on restoring the appropriate capacity to the tissue so that it can tolerate normal activities of daily living, followed by return to running and then sports-specific movements. When considering this continuum, it is important to vary the load on the tissue for their task as well as the demand that will be placed on them in their sport. The key principles here are to restore movement and force through range in the sagittal plane, followed by coronal, followed by transverse. Muscle function is best restored through isometric (through range) and concentric motions first, correcting for any motor unit loss and atrophy, before trying to restore eccentric function. We know that concentric-style movements may have more of an influence on the cross-sectional area of the muscle belly itself, while eccentric may have more of an influence on the muscle tendon unit and sarcomeres in series element.

Before we address the final two stages of rehabilitation, it is worth considering the appropriate principles of loading in both the acute and persistent groin pain patient. With persistent groin pain in particular, there may have been a failed tissue healing response. Therefore the tissue needs to be loaded beyond its normal physiological level to cause some micro- and possible macrotrauma to reinitiate appropriate healing that can be regulated and thus get better adaptation of the tissue to the load.

177

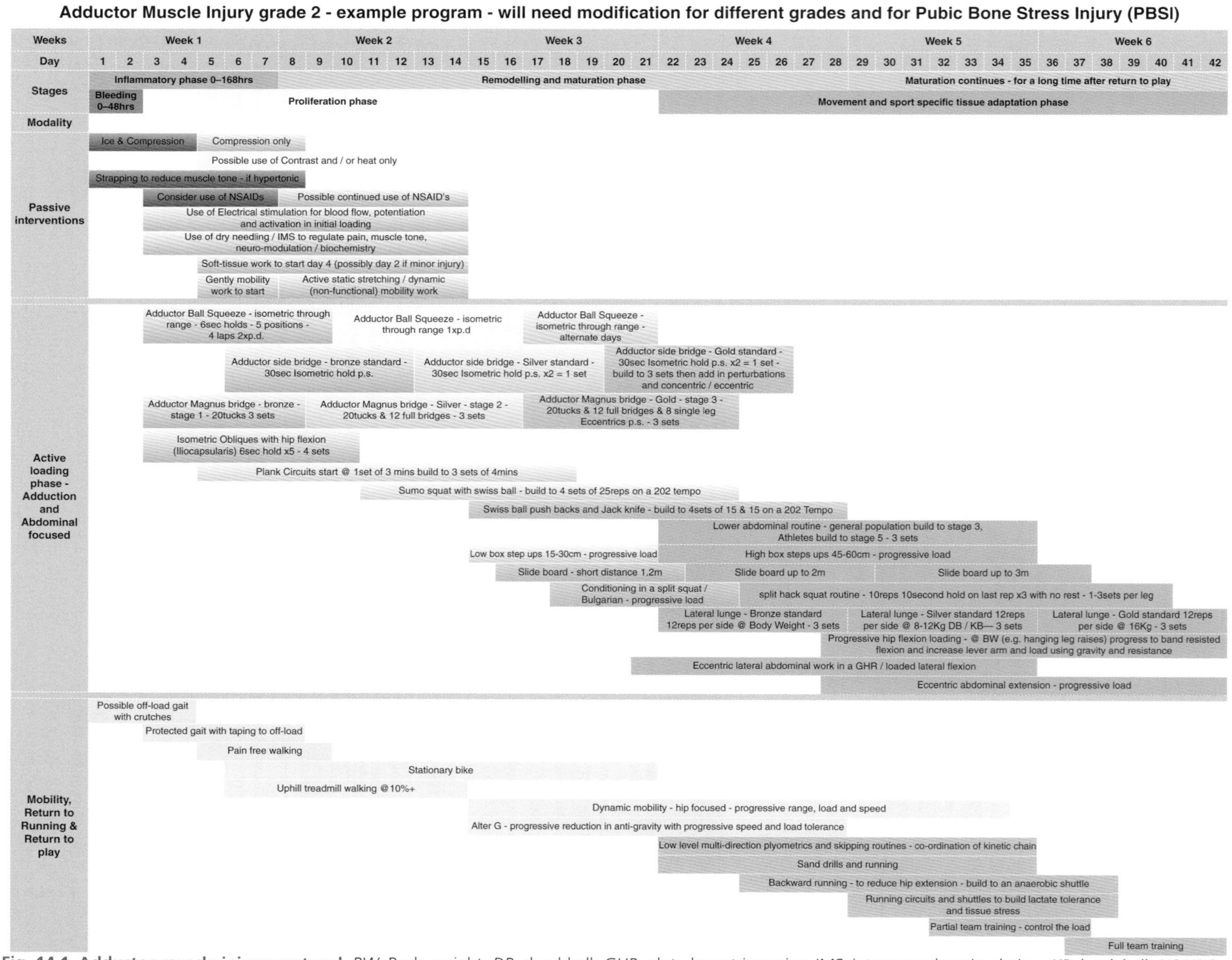

Fig. 14.1 Adductor muscle injury protocol. *BW*, Body-weight; *DB*, dumbbell; *GHR*, glute-hamstring raise; *IMS*, intramuscular stimulation; *KB*, kettlebell; *NSAIDS*, nonsteroidal anti-inflammatory drugs; *p.d.*, per day; *p.s.*, per set.

Differences in chronic/acute on chronic presentation

In chronic presentations adequate tissue adaptation often takes longer, hence a prolonged or continuing period of tissue conditioning may be required. This again does not stop progression as once milestones are reached progression can continue. Rather, understanding likely timeframes for adaptations to occur is key to long-term management success. One pitfall that can occur in this phase is that when a deconditioned athlete is progressed too quickly back to competition level, reinjury and chronicity are more likely.

Principles of loading

As described earlier, respecting the process and timeframe of tissue healing and ascertaining the right time to start loading and the appropriate level of loading is critical. It has been clear since Hölmich and colleagues' (1999) seminal paper that passive treatment does not evoke the required response or adaptation in those suffering with persistent groin pain; active progressive loading is required.

With this in mind, it is essential to understand the principles of loading and distinguish between loading for pain or loading for tissue restoration and capacity.

Despite the variations in loading principles for different tissues, the underlying process is that of mechanotransduction through mechanotherapy and its notion of progressive overload (Khan and Scott, 2009). Mechanotransduction describes the response of the extracellular matrix (ECM) to mechanical stimuli and the transformation of these cues into alterations in cell membrane permeability and consequent increases in cytokine proliferation in these cells. There are a number of different cytokines, but two key examples are vascular endothelial growth factor (VEGF) and nitric oxide (NO), as mentioned. These cytokines are most effectively expressed under certain conditions, namely a hypoxic environment for VEGF, or by using blood flow restriction training (BFR) for NO.

The principles of tissue loading need to be understood. The first aspect to consider is the length–tension curve (LTC). This curve describes the relationship between muscle length and tension/force. It illustrates that movement-orientated muscles generate optimal force in mid-range; however, they display reduced force capacity in outer range by being mechanically inefficient and in inner range by being physiologically inefficient. The efficiency relates to the approximation of the actin and myosin within an action–contraction coupling. Therefore the clinician is best advised to restore range, then build optimal force in mid-range and progress to force through range to balance the curve and allow for sporting movements, which frequently occur in the extremes of range.

Moving from the LTC, we now consider the stress–strain curve where stress represents load or force in Newton metres (NM) and strain is the percentage of tissue elongation under load. The gradient of the curve represents the Young's modulus, which is the measure of elasticity. As movement speed increases, so does the elastic component of the movement and as such the efficiency of movement, as elastic energy is more efficient than mechanical energy (see also Chapter 16). The clinician should progress the load within the available physiological range first, then start to increase the load and then progress the loading to outer range, as described above. This will increase the capacity of the curve and therefore the Young's modulus.

Hooke's law and Wolff's/Davis' law provide further guidance in terms of loading principles: the strain in a solid is proportional to the applied stress within the elastic limit of that solid (Hooke's law); the biological system's quality and orientation of the connective tissue adapts to mechanical stress to best resist external forces 'dynamic flexure' (Wolff's/ Davis' law). These laws tell us that as long as the clinician progressively loads the tissue within its physiological limits, it will continue to adapt and get stronger.

Finally, the clinician is wise to understand the force–velocity relationship, which can be seen as an extrapolation of a variety of LTCs. In short: the faster a movement, the less force can be generated. As most sport is conducted at high velocities (kicking at up to 500 degrees/s or sprinting at over 7 m/s) clinicians working with elite athletes need to retrain speed tolerance before progressing to sport-specific movements. Examples include backwards running for thigh speed as it reduces the extension moment arm, or leg swings without kicking for tissue tolerance.

Specific loading strategies can be seen below.

Adductor loading

The functionality of the adductors is quite varied and hence the loading required for certain muscles will vary too. It has been shown that the AL does not change recruitment whether there is weight-bearing or not, as increasing the load in a sagittal plane closed kinetic chain task from 10% to 50% bodyweight only increased the AL electromyography (EMG) output from 15% to 30%. However, when evaluating the adductor magnus (AM), the same increase in load resulted in an 80% jump in EMG recording from 60% to 140% of maximum voluntary contraction EMG (Hides et al., 2016). This means that in order to load AM one should perform weight-bearing exercises into flexion ideally past 45 degrees (like squat, split squat and lateral lunge), whereas adductor loading can be performed in a non-weight-bearing nature through adductor side bridges and ball squeezes.

It has been shown that the adductor ball squeeze elicits the highest EMG recordings of the AL bilaterally in comparison to a number of other exercises, especially the Copenhagen adduction exercise. This latter exercise has greater levels of activation throughout the lateral sling, with greater increases of load placed on the obliques and gluteals (Serner et al., 2014).

Both bench adduction (side bridge) and slide board (lateral skating) have been used in the progressive rehabilitation of young elite European football players during their return from pubic bone stress injuries. In unpublished data from the Australian Institute of Sport (AIS) it has been shown that the bench adduction has similar spatial characteristics to kicking, whereas the slide board has similar temporal characteristics. These exercises have relevance to the similar action of acceleration and skating and help to deliver eccentric adductor loading, which has been shown to be a differentiating factor in those with and without groin pain (Thorborg et al., 2014).

The reader is advised to remember that additional muscles have strong roles to play in working with the adductors. Therefore hip flexor loading in hip flexion ranges of >60 degrees (Yoshio et al., 2002) as well as hamstrings loading is recommended.

When considering further milestones, assessing the adduction-to-abduction ratio has been shown to be an important risk factor and should form a part of the tissue-conditioning phase and act as a milestone for the coronal plane. Tyler et al. (2001) demonstrated that, in ice-hockey players, those that went on to have subsequent adductor-related injuries had a ratio of <0.8 adductors-to-abductors, with those that did not having a ratio of close to 1. As the demand increases on the hip and groin, i.e., kicking or sprinting, there is evidence to suggest that the ratio needs to be weighted towards adduction, for example more adduction force may be needed to kick and run fast.

With persistent groin pain of adductor (or pubic joint) origin, the clinician is advised to think about alternative strategies to promote effective tissue adaptation. Suggested interventions might include: adductor offloading taping, compression shorts and sacroiliac belts (Mens et al., 2006) to reduce inappropriate muscle tone and improve synergistic muscle function; and soft tissue therapy, including the use of soft tissue mobilization and dry needling. In recalcitrant adductor pathology, one can induce an inflammatory process through the use of needles, especially in enthesopathy, to promote an increase in blood flow. It has been shown that the blood supply at the enthesis and mid-tendon is poor and may be one driver to chronicity (Davis et al., 2012).

Abdominal loading

To optimally load the abdominals, the reader should refer back to their function, physiology and architecture. Due to the varied fibre orientation of the obliques throughout their proximal-to-distal course, they need to be trained in multiple planes of movement. Being made up primarily of type 1

muscle fibres (Haggmark and Thorstensson, 1979) they have a high oxidative capacity and great ability to recover from bouts of exercise. In individuals presenting with inguinal-related pathology, the saying 'thicken or fail' applies; hence hypertrophy and therefore strain rate is key. The strength and conditioning literature has demonstrated that volume load is key for hypertrophy and even with low-magnitude loads hypertrophy can be achieved (Mitchell et al., 2012). Because of the physiological capacity this area can be trained daily and still recover and adapt to the loading stimulus.

The rectus abdominis however requires an extension moment to generate resistance in order to gain appropriate adaptation. This is where exercises may evolve from slow lowering during sit-ups to high-end activity such as roll outs or leg lowers to which the lever arm may be changed to progress difficulty.

Bone loading and noncontractile tissue

It is beyond the scope of this chapter to cover the principles of bone and noncontractile tissue loading in detail, but as groin pathology can involve pubic bone marrow oedema and noncontractile tissues (e.g., tendon; ligament and fascia), a brief summary of what is deemed optimal is provided in Table 14.4.

Stage 4 – sports-specific with return to running phase

Throughout this stage the clinician should start to address multiplanar movement. The key is regaining the extremes of sagittal plane movement, both in terms of force, control and speed. The next priority is the regaining of coronal

Table 14.4 Tissue loading parameters

Bone[a]	Tendon/connective tissue[b]
4–6 cycles per day	Maximum and submaximum isometric force
3–4 hour rest period	
Short cycles with longer rest periods	Isometric force through range
	Time under tension and strain
High magnitude and rate for most optimal osteoclast activation	Volume load key factor
	Can be loaded twice per day
	Following high-dose loading requires 72-hour response to reach homeostasis again
Nonlinear and nonrepetitive loads	

[a]Robling, A.G., Turner, C.H., 2009. Mechanical signaling for bone modeling and remodeling. Critical Reviews in Eukaryotic Gene Expression 19 (4), 319– 338.
[b]Magnusson, S.P., Langberg, H., Kjaer, M., 2010. The pathogenesis of tendinopathy: balancing the response to loading. Nature Reviews Rheumatology 6 (5), 262–268.

plane. Once these two planes are secured it will make restoring rotational control much easier. This will then allow the complexity of sports-specific movements to be achieved and mastered. At that point the clinician should incorporate speed, frequency, magnitude and direction of loading.

Stage 5 – integration back into full training

During this phase the clinician should consider the progressive and calculated return to full training and the required skills and movements to be performed. It is at this point that the tissue conditioning performed in previous stages provides the athlete with the capacity and level of resilience required to progress through the return-to-play criteria. Such criteria will include volume and intensity of distance, speed, change of direction and kicking/specific skills related to the sport. Avoid increasing multiple aspects at the same time as increasing speed and increasing kicking intensity or volume in the same session is doubling up on the demand of the groin region. In order to visualize and understand the progression of loading, the clinician may find it helpful to use the exponentially weighted acute-on-chronic moving average, the use of which is well established in sports science and medicine departments (Murray et al., 2017).

Further monitoring processes for the local tissues may incorporate the objective tests mentioned earlier with no exacerbation in symptoms and a <10% drop in groin squeeze scores posttraining. Groin squeeze scores are a product of the ability and willingness of the musculoskeletal system around the groin to transfer force and are *not* adductor force capacity tests. Although a nonpainful outcome may be produced, it may act as a sensitive measure as to whether the groin region is coping with the load.

Throughout the rehabilitative process the clinician must ensure a consistent and high level of fitness is maintained. Its imperative that the total system has enough aerobic capacity to not only withstand the rigours of returning to training so that onset of fatigue is sufficiently delayed and hence movement patterns are not altered, but also to ensure there is a greater ability to recover between bouts of exercise. Not only should conditioning cover cardiovascular fitness but it should also address the capacity of the anaerobic system and ATP-CP (adenosine triphosphate–phosphocreatine) system according to the demands of the sport. Additionally cross-training can be manipulated to provide an optimal hormonal environment to support other goals of tissue adaptation such as hormonal levels of growth hormone, insulin-like growth factor 1 (IGF-1), etc., that can positively influence the adaptations in connective tissue remodelling (Wang, 2006).

Understanding that muscles can act as force generators as well as force dissipaters is important for the nonreductionist view of the athlete. Other possible contributing factors identified during rehabilitation should be addressed throughout the stages as long as this does not excessively load the compromised tissue. For example, it may become apparent in an individual suffering from pubic bone stress that improving the capacity of the calf and quad complex may be advantageous. It is known that the ankle and then the knee are the first- and second-phase shock absorbers that help to absorb the forces (in all weight-bearing and dynamic movements) that are transferred up to the articular and bone structures of the pelvis (Zhang et al., 2000).

Summary

The acute or chronic management of groin pain can be difficult but is made easier with a systematic process of evaluation. The most important part is obtaining a correct diagnosis and being vigilant, being aware that there may be multiple pathologies present. It is key to ascertain which one is primary and which may be secondary or tertiary in the priority process; not deciding to address the issues in the correct order may limit progression. With a better understanding of the function of the groin region, exercise selection is made easier. Finally, knowing the athlete profile and the event or sport profile is key to understanding what criteria need to be met.

We encourage the reader to consider the use of strategies to optimize management. As with other interventions and treatment, ensuring the athlete understands the purpose of rehabilitation methods and has a level of autonomy, is a key factor to successful engagement.

References

Alderink, G.J., 1991. The sacroiliac joint: review of anatomy, mechanics, and function. The Journal of Orthopaedic and Sports Physical Therapy 13 (2), 71–84.

Baczkowski, K., Marks, P., Silberstein, M., Schneider-Kolsky, M.E., 2006. A new look into kicking a football: an investigation of muscle activity using MRI. Australasian Radiology 50 (4), 324–329.

Barfield, W.R., 1998. The biomechanics of kicking in soccer. Clinics in Sports Medicine 17 (4), 711–728, vi.

Birmingham, P.M., Kelly, B.T., Jacobs, R., McGrady, L., Wang, M., 2012. The effect of dynamic femoroacetabular impingement on pubic symphysis motion: a cadaveric study. The American Journal of Sports Medicine 40 (5), 1113–1118.

Bradshaw, C.J., Bundy, M., Falvey, E., 2008. The diagnosis of long-standing groin pain: a prospective clinical cohort study. British Journal of Sports Medicine 42 (10), 851–854.

Branci, S., Thorborg, K., Bech, B.H., Boesen, M., Nielsen, M.B., Hölmich, P., 2015. MRI findings in soccer players with long-standing adductor-related groin pain and asymptomatic controls. British Journal of Sports Medicine 49 (10), 681–691.

Branci, S., Thorborg, K., Nielsen, M.B., Hölmich, P., 2013. Radiological findings in symphyseal and adductor-related groin pain in athletes: a critical review of the literature. British Journal of Sports Medicine 47 (10), 611–619.

Charnock, B.L., Lewis, C.L., Garrett Jr., W.E., Queen, R.M., 2009. Adductor longus mechanics during the maximal effort soccer kick. Sports Biomechanics 8 (3), 223–234.

Davis, J.A., Stringer, M.D., Woodley, S.J., 2012. New insights into the proximal tendons of adductor longus, adductor brevis and gracilis. British Journal of Sports Medicine 46 (12), 871–876.

Dörge, H.C., Andersen, T.B., Sørensen, H., Simonsen, E.B., Aagaard, H., Dyhre-Poulsen, P., et al., 1999. EMG activity of the iliopsoas muscle and leg kinetics during the soccer place kick. Scandinavian Journal of Medicine & Science in Sports 9 (4), 195–200.

Drew, M.K., Lovell, G., Palsson, T.S., Chiarelli, P.E., Osmotherly, P.G., 2016. Do Australian football players have sensitive groins? Players with current groin pain exhibit mechanical hyperalgesia of the adductor tendon. Journal of Science and Medicine in Sport 19 (10), 784–788.

Drew, M.K., Palsson, T.S., Hirata, R.P., Izumi, M., Lovell, G., Welvaert, M., et al., 2017. Experimental pain in the groin may refer into the lower abdomen: Implications to clinical assessments. Journal of Science and Medicine in Sport 20 (10), 904–909.

Falvey, E.C., Franklyn-Miller, A., McCrory, P.R., 2009. The groin triangle: a patho-anatomical approach to the diagnosis of chronic groin pain in athletes. British Journal of Sports Medicine 43 (3), 213–220.

Franklyn-Miller, A., Richter, C., King, E., Gore, S., Moran, K., Strike, S., et al., 2017. Athletic groin pain (part 2): a prospective cohort study on the biomechanical evaluation of change of direction identifies three clusters of movement patterns. British Journal of Sports Medicine 51 (5), 460–468.

Gracovetsky, S.A., Iacono, S., 1987. Energy transfers in the spinal engine. Journal of Biomedical Engineering 9 (2), 99–114.

Haggmark, T., Thorstensson, A., 1979. Fibre types in human abdominal muscles. Acta Physiologica Scandinavica 107 (4), 319–325.

Hides, J.A., Beall, P., Franettovich Smith, M.M., Stanton, W., Miokovic, T., Richardson, C., 2016. Activation of the hip adductor muscles varies during a simulated weight-bearing task. Physical Therapy in Sport 17, 19–23.

Hölmich, P., Thorborg, K., Dehlendorff, C., Krogsgaard, K., Gluud, C., 2014. Incidence and clinical presentation of groin injuries in sub-elite male soccer. British Journal of Sports Medicine 48 (16), 1245–1250.

Hölmich, P., Uhrskou, P., Ulnits, L., Kanstrup, I.L., Nielsen, M.B., Bjerg, A.M., et al., 1999. Effectiveness of active physical training as treatment for long-standing adductor-related groin pain in athletes: randomised trial. Lancet 353 (9151), 439–443.

Hölmich, P., Hölmich, L.R., Bjerg, A.M., 2004. Clinical examination of athletes with groin pain: an intraobserver and interobserver reliability study. British Journal of Sports Medicine 38 (4), 446–451.

Hölmich, P., 2007. Long-standing groin pain in sportspeople falls into three primary patterns, a "clinical entity" approach: a prospective study of 207 patients. British Journal of Sports Medicine 41 (4), 247–252; discussion 252.

Ikeda, Y.Y., M, Sugawara, K., Katayose, M., 2011. The difference of hip adductor longus activity between side-foot kicks and instep kicks. British Journal of Sports Medicine 45 (4), 353.

Khan, K.M., Scott, A., 2009. Mechanotherapy: how physical therapists' prescription of exercise promotes tissue repair. British Journal of Sports Medicine 43 (4), 247–252.

Lloyd-Smith, R., Clement, D.B., McKenzie, D.C., Taunton, J.E., 1985. A survey of overuse and traumatic hip and pelvic injuries in athletes. The Physician and Sportsmedicine 13 (10), 131–141.

Lovell, G., Galloway, H., Hopkins, W., Harvey, A., 2006. Osteitis pubis and assessment of bone marrow edema at the pubic symphysis with MRI in an elite junior male soccer squad. Clinical Journal of Sport Medicine 16 (2), 117–122.

Mann, R.A., Hagy, J., 1980. Biomechanics of walking, running, and sprinting. The American Journal of Sports Medicine 8 (5), 345–350.

Marshall, B.M., Franklyn-Miller, A.D., King, E.A., Moran, K.A., Strike, S.C., Falvey, É.C., et al., 2014. Biomechanical factors associated with time to complete a change of direction cutting maneuver. Journal of Strength and Conditioning Research 28 (10), 2845–2851.

Mens, J.M., Damen, L., Snijders, C.J., Stam, H.J., 2006. The mechanical effect of a pelvic belt in patients with pregnancy-related pelvic pain. Clinical Biomechanics (Bristol, Avon) 21 (2), 122–127.

Mitchell, C.J., Churchward-Venne, T.A., West, D.W., Burd, N.A., Breen, L., Baker, S.K., et al., 2012. Resistance exercise load does not determine training-mediated hypertrophic gains in young men. Journal of Applied Physiology (1985) 113 (1), 71–77.

Mölsä, J., Airaksinen, O., Näsman, O., Torstila, I., 1997. Ice hockey injuries in Finland. A prospective epidemiologic study. The American Journal of Sports Medicine 25 (4), 495–499.

Murray, N.B., Gabbett, T.J., Townshend, A.D., Blanch, P., 2017. Calculating acute:chronic workload ratios using exponentially weighted moving averages provides a more sensitive indicator of injury likelihood than rolling averages. British Journal of Sports Medicine 51 (9), 749–754.

Neumann, D.A., 2010. Kinesiology of the hip: a focus on muscular actions. The Journal of Orthopaedic and Sports Physical Therapy 40 (2), 82–94.

Norton-Old, K.J., Schache, A.G., Barker, P.J., Clark, R.A., Harrison, S.M., Briggs, C.A., et al., 2013. Anatomical and mechanical relationship between the proximal attachment of adductor longus and the distal rectus sheath. Clinical Anatomy 26 (4), 522–530.

Orchard, J.W., 2001. Intrinsic and extrinsic risk factors for muscle strains in Australian football. The American Journal of Sports Medicine 29 (3), 300–303.

Robertson, D.G.E., Mosher, R.E., 1985. Work and power of the leg muscles in soccer kicking. In: Winter, D.A., Norman, R.W., Wells, R.P., Hayes, K.C., Patla, A.E. (Eds.), Biomechanics IX-B. Human Kinetics Publishers Inc., Champaign, IL, pp. 533–538.

Schache, A.G., Blanch, P.D., Dorn, T.W., Brown, N.A., Rosemond, D., Pandy, M.G., et al., 2011. Effect of running speed on lower limb joint kinetics. Medicine and Science in Sports and Exercise 43 (7), 1260–1271.

Schilders, E., Bharam, S., Golan, E., Dimitrakopoulou, A., Mitchell, A., Spaepen, M., et al., 2017. The pyramidalis–anterior pubic ligament–adductor longus complex (PLAC) and its role with adductor injuries: a new anatomical concept. Knee Surgery, Sports Traumatology, Arthroscopy 25 (12), 3969–3977.

Serner, A., Jakobsen, M.D., Andersen, L.L., Hölmich, P., Sundstrup, E., Thorborg, K., et al., 2014. EMG evaluation of hip adduction exercises for soccer players: implications for exercise selection in prevention and treatment of groin injuries. British Journal of Sports Medicine 48 (14), 1108–1114.

Serner, A., Tol, J.L., Jomaah, N., Weir, A., Whiteley, R., Thorborg, K., et al., 2015. Diagnosis of acute groin injuries: a prospective study of 110 athletes. The American Journal of Sports Medicine 43 (8), 1857–1864.

Takizawa, M., Suzuki, D., Ito, H., Fujimiya, M., Uchiyama, E., 2014. Why adductor magnus muscle is large: the function based on muscle morphology in cadavers. Scandinavian Journal of Medicine & Science in Sports 24 (1), 197–203.

Thorborg, K., Branci, S., Nielsen, M.P., Tang, L., Nielsen, M.B., Hölmich, P., et al., 2014. Eccentric and isometric hip adduction strength in male soccer players with and without adductor-related groin pain: an assessor-blinded comparison. Orthopaedic Journal of Sports Medicine 2 (2), 2325967114521778.

Torry, M.R., Schenker, M.L., Martin, H.D., Hogoboom, D., Philippon, M.J., 2006. Neuromuscular hip biomechanics and pathology in the athlete. Clinics in Sports Medicine 25 (2), 179–197, vii.

Tyler, T.F., Nicholas, S.J., Campbell, R.J., McHugh, M.P., 2001. The association of hip strength and flexibility with the incidence of adductor muscle strains in professional ice hockey players. The American Journal of Sports Medicine 29 (2), 124–128.

Tyler, T.F., Silvers, H.J., Gerhardt, M.B., Nicholas, S.J., 2010. Groin injuries in sports medicine. Sports Health 2 (3), 231–236.

Ventura, J.D., Klute, G.K., Neptune, R.R., 2015. Individual muscle contributions to circular turning mechanics. Journal of Biomechanics 48 (6), 1067–1074.

Verrall, G.M., Henry, L., Fazzalari, N.L., Slavotinek, J.P., Oakeshott, R.D., 2008. Bone biopsy of the parasymphyseal pubic bone region in athletes with chronic groin injury demonstrates new woven bone formation consistent with a diagnosis of pubic bone stress injury. The American Journal of Sports Medicine 36 (12), 2425–2431.

Vigotsky, A.D., Bryanton, M.A., 2016. Relative muscle contributions to net joint moments in the barbell back squat. 40 Annual Meeting of the American Society of Biomechanics, Raleigh, NC, USA, August 2–5, 2016.

Walden, M., Hagglund, M., Ekstrand, J., 2015. The epidemiology of groin injury in senior football: a systematic review of prospective studies. British Journal of Sports Medicine 49 (12), 792–797.

Wang, J.H., 2006. Mechanobiology of tendon. Journal of Biomechanics 39 (9), 1563–1582.

Ward, S.R., Eng, C.M., Smallwood, L.H., Lieber, R.L., 2009. Are current measurements of lower extremity muscle architecture accurate? Clinical Orthopaedics and Related Research 467 (4), 1074–1082.

Weir, A., Brukner, P., Delahunt, E., Ekstrand, J., Griffin, D., Khan, K.M., et al., 2015. Doha agreement meeting on terminology and definitions in groin pain in athletes. British Journal of Sports Medicine 49 (12), 768–774.

Yoshio, M., Murakami, G., Sato, T., Sato, S., Noriyasu, S., 2002. The function of the psoas major muscle: passive kinetics and morphological studies using donated cadavers. Journal of Orthopaedic Science 7 (2), 199–207.

Zhang, S.N., Bates, B.T., Dufek, J.S., 2000. Contributions of lower extremity joints to energy dissipation during landings. Medicine and Science in Sports and Exercise 32 (4), 812–819.

Chapter 15

The surgical management of sporting groin injuries

Simon Marsh

Introduction

The syndrome of groin disruption (Gilmore's Groin, sportsman's hernia, hockey groin) was first recognized by the London surgeon Jerry Gilmore in 1980 after the successful treatment of three professional footballers, all of whom had been unable to play for months because of undiagnosed groin pain (Dimitrakopoulou and Schilders, 2015; Paksoy and Sekmen, 2016).

The initial case was a Tottenham Hotspur player who had been unable to play for 17 weeks because of groin pain. In this case, there was a specific episode of an eversion injury causing the pain. The player described a characteristic pattern of pain when attempting to sprint, twist or turn and with coughing and sneezing. He had received three orthopaedic opinions, undergone X-rays, computed tomography (CT) scans and ultrasound scans with no obvious cause being found. Previous treatments included rest, manipulation and steroid injections, to no avail. When he was reviewed by Gilmore (his fourth opinion) there was no abnormality to see in the groin and nothing to find on palpation. In particular, there was no hernia. The crucial finding was a dilated superficial inguinal ring with a cough impulse and tenderness in the inguinal canal when compared with the other side. A similar pattern was observed with the second case: this individual also suffered an overstretching eversion injury and had been unable to play for 16 weeks. This patient was unable to do anything other than walk and experienced pain with jogging, kicking, sudden movements and also coughing and sneezing. The clinical findings were similar, with a dilated superficial inguinal ring and inguinal canal tenderness with a cough impulse when compared with the other side. The third patient had suffered groin pain for 72 weeks and been completely unable to play for 12 weeks. In this case, there was no specific injury but the symptoms and signs were similar to the other two cases.

All three underwent surgery to explore the groin and the characteristic findings of groin disruption (Gilmore's Groin) were found and repaired. In all three cases the findings at operation consisted of tears in the external oblique muscle, resulting in a dilated superficial inguinal ring, a torn conjoined tendon with the conjoined tendon and the internal oblique being pulled away from the inguinal ligament (dehiscence). The disruption was repaired with sutures. In each case, full training was resumed after the third week and top-level football was possible after 6 weeks, with one patient resuming international football at 7 weeks after surgery. There were no recurrences in the original cohort.

Incidence

Groin pain is a common presenting symptom for people with sports injuries (Gilmore, 1996; 1998; Renstrome, 1992). Whilst many of these cases will settle with conservative measures there are a significant number that will require surgery. Gilmore's Groin is most common in footballers, but can occur in many other sports including rugby (union and league), racquet games, athletics, cricket and hockey. Those simply undertaking general fitness training can also succumb (Table 15.1). Amateur sportsmen are now more aware of the potential treatments for injuries that formerly would have meant giving up their pastimes. Females make up 3% of those referred and 1% of those requiring surgery, reflecting the

Table 15.1 The different sports from which professionals have been treated at the Gilmore Groin and Hernia Clinic since 1980

Sport	% Patients
Association Football	56
Rugby Union and League	9
Athletics	5
Racquet games	4
Cricket	2
Field hockey	2
Other:	12
American football	
Australian rules football	
Gaelic football	
Handball	
Skiing	
Martial arts, including cage fighting	
Basketball	
Fencing	
Lacrosse	
Ice hockey	
Gymnastics	
Water polo	
'Strongman'	
Boxing	
Weightlifting	
No sport	10

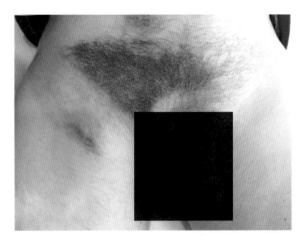

Fig. 15.1 The pattern of bruising that occurs in a severe groin tear. In this patient, a professional footballer, the bruising outlines the anatomical boundaries of the inguinal region, above the groin crease, as well as demonstrating a concomitant adductor tear with bruising at the upper part of the thigh. In cases such as this it is not appropriate to operate in the presence of significant bruising as the tissue planes will have been obliterated. In fact, this patient recovered completely over an 8-week period and did not require surgery.

different embryology and anatomy of the inguinal region (Schache et al., 2017).

Aetiology

The aetiology seems to involve a muscle imbalance between the abdominal muscles and those of the thigh. The strong hip flexors (the quadriceps) pull the pelvis down and the tilted pelvis stretches the abdominal muscles. The stretched abdominal muscle (the obliques) become weak and can no longer stabilize the pelvis, resulting in overuse injuries and recurrent tears leading to decompensated groin disruption. It is of note that with the advent of more rigorous core stability training in professional footballers the incidence of groin disruption is falling in this group (Walden et al., 2015). However, it is increasing in amateur sportsmen and in older people as they stay fitter and attempt to remain active and play sports for longer. The incidence in women is also increasing as women's football increases in popularity.

Presentation and diagnosis

Making an accurate diagnosis is fundamental to successful treatment (Bisciotti et al., 2016; Sheen et al., 2014). As in all medical conditions the diagnosis consists of evaluating the physical symptoms, examining for the clinical signs and performing specialized investigations. Fundamentally it is a sports injury and the typical patient is a young, active male who participates regularly in sporting activities. The primary symptom is of pain. Only in rare cases of coexisting hernia will there be a lump (Ekberg, 1981; Lovell et al., 1990; Smedberg et al., 1985). Very occasionally there may be bruising in the lower abdomen (Fig. 15.1). Previously the condition was rare over the age of 45 but is becoming more common in older people who continue active participation in sports for longer. The oldest patient to date to undergo successful operation was a 78-year-old, ex-international tennis player who resumed playing 3 weeks after surgery. In a third of patients there is a definite event that causes the pain, such as overstretching, excessive or miskicking, or abduction or eversion injuries. In two-thirds, there is no definite event and it seems to be an 'overuse' injury, where successive relatively minor injuries eventually result in the 'final straw that breaks the camel's back', so that the groin musculature can no longer perform its normal functions and pain results.

Box 15.1 **The symptoms of groin disruption that occur with exercise**

Pain in the groin increases with:
- Running
- Striding
- Sprinting
- Sudden movement
- Twisting and turning
- Side-stepping
- Jumping
- Dead ball kicking
- Long ball kicking

Box 15.2 **The symptoms of groin disruption that occur after exercise**

Pain in the groin increases with:
- Turning in bed
- Getting out of bed
- Getting out of a car
- Sit-ups
- Coughing
- Sneezing
- Sudden movements

Symptoms

The symptoms broadly fit into two groups: those during exercise and those afterwards (Boxes 15.1 and 15.2). During exercise, pain in the groin increases with running, striding, sprinting, twisting and turning, side-stepping and with sudden movements. Jumping, dead ball kicking and long ball kicking also cause pain. Commonly the patient is stiff and sore for a variable time after exercise. In addition, pain can occur with coughing, sneezing, rising from a low position (typically getting out of bed or out of a car) as well as turning in bed or with sudden movements.

Whilst the symptoms are relatively constant, different types of sport elicit characteristic patterns. The classical presentation for a footballer is someone who initially plays on a Saturday and is then stiff and sore for a couple of days, but can train midweek before playing again at the weekend. Then the stiffness and soreness after the game persists all week, so that no midweek training is possible, but the pain resolves by the weekend. Subsequently the pain comes on before the end of the game necessitating substitution. No midweek training is possible and at the next game substitution occurs earlier and eventually playing and training become impossible as pain occurs with

any form of exercise. Rugby union players have a similar pattern of symptoms, with the backs typically getting pain with sprinting, twisting, turning, accelerating, striding out, side-stepping and dead ball kicking, whilst the forwards also get pain when jumping or getting up after a tackle. In cricket, bowlers experience loss of pace and develop pain in the groin on landing. This is usually worse in the dragging leg compared with the landing leg. Batsmen get pain when running between the wickets and when twisting and turning and fielders experience groin pain with any sudden movement, pushing off, striding out and diving. The advent of the T20 form of the game has led to an increase in the incidence of groin injuries amongst cricketers. Athletes notice a loss of pace and long-distance runners particularly notice pain during the final sprint. There is also a loss of endurance and slower recovery. In field hockey, AstroTurf pitches may have increased the incidence of groin injuries and it particularly occurs in corner specialists, whilst in ice hockey goalminders are more prone to groin disruption. Conversely the incidence of groin disruption has fallen in Premier League footballers (by up to two-thirds) possibly as a consequence of adopting regular core stability exercises and eliminating inappropriate training methods (Whittaker et al., 2015).

Signs

On examination, there is usually nothing to see on inspection, although with severe, acute, tears, bruising may be apparent and often demarcates the anatomical regions of the groin and the adductor in those who also have adductor tears (see Fig. 15.1). The site of the pain is important. In a groin disruption, the patient will point to the area of the superficial inguinal ring. Other common areas where pain is experienced include the adductor origin on the inside of the thigh, indicating a possible adductor tear, or groin crease (sometime with radiation to the buttock), suggesting a hip problem (often femoroacetabular impingement). Flexion and internal rotation of the hip may produce stiffness that, again, may come from the hip. Squeezing the legs together against resistance may cause pain over the adductor origin in cases of adductor tears. In cases of groin disruption, straight-leg raising against resistance (with the physician leaning on the thighs) typically, but not always, causes pain over the affected superficial inguinal ring. The characteristic finding is of a dilated superficial inguinal ring, identified by invaginating the little finger into the back of the scrotum, and following the spermatic cord up to the superficial inguinal ring. Not only is the ring dilated, indicative of a tear in the external oblique muscle, but there is often exquisite tenderness in the inguinal canal itself with a marked cough impulse, demonstrating a lack of continuity in the posterior wall of the inguinal canal (Gilmore, 1992). Often the examination will bring on the pain experienced after exercise, which will then reduce with rest. All these findings must be compared with the normal side where they will be absent (except in the case of bilateral tears).

Adductor injuries

Up to 40% of patients with a groin disruption will have a concomitant adductor tear, although it may also present as an isolated injury (Pesquera et al., 2015). Whilst they will still experience pain with sprinting, twisting, turning and striding out, the pain is felt at the adductor origin on the inside of the thigh, below the inguinal ligament. There is tenderness at the adductor insertion on the affected side, with weakness and pain on resisted adduction (squeeze test). Whilst many of these cases can now be treated conservatively using image-guided injection techniques, around a quarter will require surgery to release the adductor tendon, resulting in decreased tension at the adductor origin. This is required in severe tears, or chronic tears not responding to conservative treatment. This can be performed at the same time as a groin reconstruction operation.

Investigations

Historically many different forms of imaging have been carried out to try and make the diagnosis more objective.

Plain X-rays

Whilst pain X-rays will not directly show the groin muscles they can pick up hip pathology. Plain X-rays will show changes of osteoarthritis or the abnormal anatomy of femoroacetabular impingement. There may even be an undisplaced femoral neck fracture or pubic ramus fractures. Stork views, where pelvic X-rays are obtained standing on one leg and then the other, may unmask the rare case of pubic symphysis instability with excessive movement seen at the pubic symphysis. Stress fractures of the pubic rami or of the femoral neck may also be seen.

Radionuclide bone scan

Abnormal radionuclide bone scans can pick up pubic bone stress injury (pubic osteitis) or stress fractures, as well as arthritic changes. Rarely metastatic cancer may be diagnosed.

Ultrasound scan

Ultrasound scans in the hands of an experienced musculoskeletal radiologist can sometimes show attenuation of the inguinal ligaments. A posterior wall bulge on ultrasound scan is an almost universal finding and does not add anything to the diagnosis. Similarly, many ultrasound scans purport to show a hernia when it is simply showing normal fat in the inguinal canal (Morley et al., 2016).

Magnetic resonance imaging

The gold standard investigation is a 3T magnetic resonance imaging (MRI) scan looking at the hips, groins and adductors (Cross et al., 2013; Omar et al., 2008). In cases of groin disruption this will almost always show a tear in the adductor longus–rectus abdominis aponeurosis with secondary clefts around the pubic tubercle (Murphy et al., 2013). It is vital that the MRI scans (or any imaging) are reported by an expert musculoskeletal radiologist with experience of groin disruption, or positive findings may be missed. Similarly, an expert centre is required to ensure the correct imaging sequences are obtained. Whilst a CT scan can give similar information to an MRI, the dose of X-rays required is too high to justify its routine use.

Differential diagnosis

The groin is a complex musculoskeletal junction between the leg and abdominal musculature. Whilst groin disruption will present with the typical symptoms, signs and MRI findings, there are multiple other pathologies that can produce similar symptoms (Corrigan and Stenstone, 1985; Ekberg et al., 1988; Hackney, 1993; Zimmerman, 1988).

Femoroacetabular impingement (FAI) is increasingly recognized as a potential cause of groin pain (Munegato, 2015). Usually this will present with pain in the groin crease, sometimes with radiation to the buttock, and there will be pain on compression and internal rotation of the hip. Cam- and pincer-type anatomical changes related to FAI are often seen on MRI scans but in many cases are simply coincidental and no treatment is needed. Osteoarthritis of the hip can also present with groin pain and there is a correlation between FAI and osteoarthritis in later life. Labral tears at the acetabulum can also produce similar symptoms and a hip arthrogram can be useful in making the diagnosis in these cases. It is not uncommon to see people whose symptoms are reminiscent of both hip and groin symptoms. In these cases a diagnostic hip injection can be a useful investigation to try to determine where the majority of the pain is coming from. A local anaesthetic injection into the hip (performed under image guidance) that relieves the pain would be diagnostic for primary hip pathology. In cases where the diagnosis is still equivocal, treating the groin first is appropriate as this is the more straightforward procedure with the quicker recovery time. These patients need to be warned that, in their case, surgery may not lead to complete resolution of their pain and further investigation may be needed. In younger patients Perthe's disease and slipped femoral epiphysis also need to be considered as possible diagnoses. Pelvic fractures, particularly around the pubic rami (and especially stress fractures), but also of the acetabulum, and even undisplaced femoral neck fractures, can also present with similar symptoms. Avulsion fractures can also occur, usually related to the adductor longus or the rectus femoris muscles.

At the symphysis pubis, disc degeneration and posterior protrusion can cause similar symptoms to adductor tears and also causes pain in the perineum, and osteitis pubis has long been recognized as a potential cause of pain in athletes (Harris and Murray, 1974). Whilst osteitis pubis undoubtedly can occur as a primary condition, in some cases it may be secondary to the stress caused by a groin disruption. In addition, although it is termed an 'itis' (inflammation), studies do not persistently show raised inflammatory markers. The term 'pubic bone stress injury' is therefore preferred. Pubic instability is a rare cause of more central suprapubic pain and can be diagnosed using stork-view X-rays. Movement at the symphysis of over 2 mm suggests instability. Pubic symphysis pain may also occur after trauma, including surgery, and it has been suggested there may be an infectious cause in some cases.

Other possible causes include nerve entrapment syndromes of the ilioinguinal, genitofemoral, iliohypogastric and obturator nerves and bursitis, particularly of the iliopsoas but also trochanteric. In addition, acute muscular strains of the rectus abdominis, adductors, rectus femoris and the iliopsoas need to be considered. An inguinal or femoral hernia and inguinal lymphadenopathy (secondary to infection, sexually transmitted infections and rarely lymphoma) can all present as groin pain and it is also important to remember that pain can be referred to the groin from the spine or from urological, testicular and gynaecological pathology.

Surgery

Surgery to repair a groin disruption is termed a *groin reconstruction* and is an anatomical repair of the torn groin muscles. An anterior, open approach is required since groin disruption affects the muscles of the anterior abdominal wall. No mesh is used since the aim is to restore normal anatomy and function. There is a suggestion that

implanting a mesh can stiffen the abdominal musculature and restrict hip flexion. In addition, simply placing a mesh patch over torn and disrupted muscles does not repair the primary pathology and may result in persistent pain, requiring further surgery to remove the mesh and reconstruct the groin.

Indications for surgery

For sports professionals, surgery is indicated if training and playing are inhibited, resulting in loss of speed and fitness. Many will already have had appropriate investigations and the club (or often the agent) will be requesting surgery.

For amateurs, surgery is indicated if the symptoms affect everyday life or if quality of life is affected by the inability to play sport. Patients with a moderate disruption can often continue to play using a combination of analgesics and nonsteroidal antiinflammatory medications until they suffer an acute episode or suffer the additional problem of an adductor tear. In all cases, surgery is indicated if conservative treatment methods have failed.

Surgical technique

The aim of surgery is to explore the groin and repair each element of the disruption, restoring normal anatomy and function. The operation is best carried out under general anaesthetic. In this group of patients, who are usually young and fit, local anaesthetic has no advantages and with general anaesthetic a degree of muscle relaxation can be induced to facilitate the repair, something that is impossible with local anaesthetic. Once general anaesthesia has been given, an ilioinguinal nerve block can be carried out under ultrasound guidance. This is placed laterally so it does not obscure the surgical planes and aids postoperative pain relief. A good block can last for up to 12 hours. For professionals, it is important that they receive a letter from the anaesthetist listing all the drugs that have been used during surgery so that this can be produced, if required, in the case of a random drugs test. The repair technique now used is based on the original, successful Gilmore technique with modifications (the Marsh modification of the Gilmore technique).

Groin reconstruction (Marsh modification of the Gilmore technique)

A 5-cm incision is used, placed in the groin crease below the 'belt-line' just within the area where the pubic hair can hide it. This should be marked preoperatively, with two dots at the extremes of the proposed incision with the patient standing, so that the patient can see where the incision will be and to ensure a good cosmetic outcome. Once in the operating room, the entire area is shaved. The incision is then made, per the preoperatively placed marks, and the subcutaneous fat incised down to the external oblique aponeurosis. This is then incised along the length of its fibres, for a length of approximately 4 cm, down to the superficial inguinal ring, and the upper and lower leaves reflected to reveal the spermatic cord (or the round ligament of the uterus in women). The cord is then mobilized to reveal the posterior wall of the inguinal canal and dehiscence of the internal oblique muscle and the inguinal ligament that will be present, along with tears to the conjoint tendon. In women, the round ligament of the uterus can be ligated and excised.

The first step of the repair is to perform an inguinal ligament tenolysis at the pubic tubercle to relieve the tension of the inguinal ligament. This also allows the primary 'anchor stitch' to be placed more laterally, and not in the pubic tubercle itself. This decreases the incidence of pubic tubercle pain postoperatively. The next stage is to plicate the lose tranversalis fascia, exposed by the internal oblique muscle dehiscence from the inguinal ligament and then the conjoint tendon and the internal oblique can be reattached to the inguinal ligament itself. These two layers are carried out with Vicryl sutures that dissolve in around 14 days. The next part of the repair is carried out with a longer-lasting suture. A loose darn is placed on the posterior wall to reinforce it and to maintain the integrity of the repair as the Vicryl sutures dissolve, before full physiological healing has occurred. Without such a suture, there is the danger that the dip in wound strength that naturally occurs at around 2 weeks could lead to the repair failing. The external oblique aponeurosis is then repaired with Vicryl, reconstituting and tightening the superficial inguinal ring before the subcutaneous layer (Scarpa's facia) is closed and a subcuticular, dissolvable stitch used to suture the skin (Fig. 15.2). The wound is dressed with Steri-Strips, a nonallergic dressing and a pressure dressing is applied for 24 hours. For many patients, the operation can be carried out as a day case, with a hospital stay of less than 24 hours.

The four major areas of disruption: the dehiscence (D), the inguinal ligament (I), the conjoint tendon (C) and the external oblique aponeurosis (E) can all be scored as mildly (1), moderately (2) or severely (3) disrupted, giving a total disruption (DICE) score out of 12. This allows the degree of disruption to be recorded objectively, aiding subsequent audit.

Adductor tenotomy

If adductor tenotomy is performed, this can be done through a small (2-cm) incision in the groin crease sited over the adductor tendon itself. This is marked preoperatively with the patient lying down and the hip and knee flexed and the leg externally rotated. The incision is deepened and the tendon sheath (peritenon) is opened longitudinally to exposed the tendons of adductor longus, adductor brevis and gracilis. The tendon is divided transversely to release the tension on the pubic tubercle from below, before the peritenon is repaired and the skin closed with a dissolvable subcuticular suture.

The physiology of wound healing

There has been much discussion about how quickly a patient can return to sport after surgery. Fundamentally this is related to how quickly surgical wounds heal and how long it takes for tissues to repair themselves after an operation. After an operation where the wound is sutured, healing is said to occur by 'primary intention'. The initial phase is characterized by *inflammation* and lasts for up to 10 days. Once haemostasis has occurred the blood vessels dilate to allow white blood cells, antibodies and cytokines (proteins that encourage healing) into the area. During this stage the wound is characteristically hot, red and painful. During the second stage, *proliferation*, collagen rebuilds the wound and new blood vessels grow into the area to increase the oxygen supply and granulation tissue is formed. This phase lasts up to a month. The final stage is *maturation*, where the normal structure and function of the tissues are established. The type of collagen changes from type III to type I and the number of blood vessels reduces. This phase begins after 3 days and whilst it may continue for 3 months, it is largely complete by 4 weeks (Ledingham and MacKay, 1988). The only part of a wound that is fully healed by 2 weeks is the skin. This understanding of wound healing elucidates why a period of 4 to 6 weeks is recommended for full recovery and return to sport.

Outcome and recurrence

In properly selected patients, 94% of professionals can resume their normal sporting activities (Choi et al., 2016; Gilmore, 1992; Hackney, 1993; Horsky et al., 1984; Polglase et al., 1991). Over a 5-year period 3% will get recurrent symptoms on the operated side and over a 10-year period 10% will present with pain on the opposite side. In these cases, the patients recognize the symptoms as being identical to the problem of the previous side and present requesting an operation knowing it will cure their symptoms. No operation has a 100% success rate.

Rehabilitation

The treatment of groin disruption does not end with the surgery. A strict rehabilitation programme is a fundamental

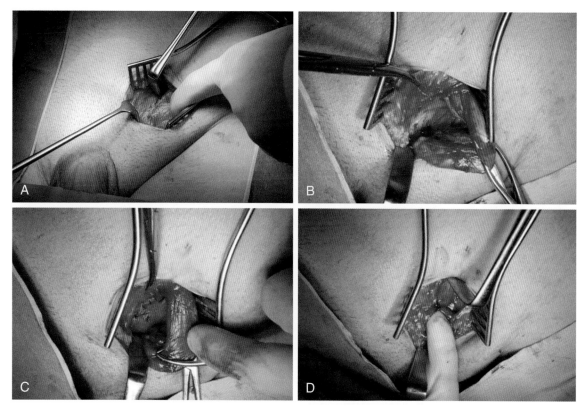

Fig. 15.2 Operative photographs during left groin reconstruction surgery. In all pictures the orientation is the same: the head is towards the top of the picture with the left leg towards the bottom right. (A) The attenuated external aponeurosis; (B) the spermatic cord being retracted laterally and inferiorly, and showing the posterior wall muscular disruption, seen as the white area to the left of the cord; (C) the same area after the posterior wall has been repaired – the internal oblique muscle has been reattached to the inguinal ligament so that the defect has been closed; and (D) the completed repair with the reconstituted superficial inguinal ring.

requirement for achieving a full recovery, in which the physiotherapist plays an integral role. Traditionally patients followed a 4-week programme devised to suit professionals with access to a full-time physiotherapist, many of whom are familiar with the condition and its treatment. Observing the operation is also encouraged since this can help with understanding the rehabilitation required. Professional sportsmen tend to be fitter than most at the time of surgery and this reduces recovery time. Classically, the first week is spent walking, with running and adductor exercises being added in week 2. Week 3 includes cycling and sprinting, with week 4 (for footballers) adding in twisting, turning and kicking, before return to playing after the fourth week. The efficacy of such a programme is well demonstrated by the fact that one England football captain was able to return to playing 20 days after bilateral groin reconstruction surgery.

To cater for those without access to full-time physiotherapy, and for amateurs, the standard 4-week programme has

been modified to reflect the fact that individuals recover at different rates and each patient is given a comprehensive written rehabilitation guide. Instead of using a specific time (a week), rehabilitation can be considered in stages, with each patient moving on to the next stage in their own time, as recovery allows. Broadly, the four stages are: mobility, flexibility and strength, followed by sport-specific training before returning to play. In the first stage, straight-line activities are encouraged and abdominal straining is avoided. Depending on the patient, appropriate activities include walking, front crawl swimming, static cycling and cross-training. In stage 2, bodyweight movements such as lunges, side lunges and partial squats can be added along with hip flexion and extension exercises. In stage 3, the intensity of the core stability work can be increased and change of direction at speed can commence, including box drills, cutting drills and figure-of-eight routines. When each stage has been completed, sport-specific training makes up the final stage before returning to play. For professionals, returning to sport in 3 to 4 weeks may be possible; however, for most people 6 to 8 weeks is more realistic. Addition of an adductor release adds around 2 weeks to the recovery period.

The multidisciplinary team

The association of groups of health professionals specializing in different aspects of sports medicine has improved the diagnosis and treatment of those with groin problems (Cross et al., 2013; Elattar et al., 2016). As well as general surgeons experienced in groin surgery, the team should have access to sports and exercise physicians specializing in nonoperative techniques, orthopaedic surgeons specializing in hip problems, physiotherapists and anaesthetists familiar with muscle relaxation, as well as pain specialists. An experienced consultant in musculoskeletal radiology is fundamental as there is no longer any place for surgeons carrying out and reporting their own imaging. Patients need access to information and advice at all stages and specialist nurses are also an important part of the team. All of those investigating and treating patients with groin problems should now be part of such an extended team.

Controversies

A number of other techniques have been described in an attempt to simplify the surgery, particularly as more surgeons attempt to undertake groin reconstruction. Some rely on reinforcing the weak posterior wall, whilst others focus mainly on the external oblique aponeurosis. All of them lack the robustness of the full repair. In some cases, ilioinguinal nerve entrapment in the external oblique aponeurosis may contribute to the pain (Ziprin et al., 1999). A neurolysis procedure (or even division of the nerve) may be appropriate in these cases. The role of the nerves in the aetiology of the pain is contentious. There are three nerves involved around the area of groin reconstruction. The ilioinguinal nerve runs with the spermatic cord and is easily controlled with the cord itself. The iliohypogastric nerve tends to run on the internal oblique muscle under the upper part of the external oblique aponeurosis and can be controlled by lifting it above the upper flap. The genital branch of the genitofemoral nerve tends to run on the surface of the spermatic cord, whilst the femoral branch runs under the inguinal ligament more deeply and laterally. Some surgeons feel that the cause of pain is always due to stretching of the nerve and so the nerves must always be divided. Whilst this might allow rapid return to pain-free sport, it risks the sportsman breaking down if an underlying musculotendinous disruption has not been repaired. In addition, the numbness caused by dividing the nerves can be distressing and nerve division can result in the formation of neuromas, which can actually increase postoperative pain (Minnich et al., 2011). Laparoscopic repair will reinforce the weak posterior wall but will not repair the anterior muscular disruption and this technique has largely been abandoned in Australia. Inguinal ligament tenolysis can be carried out laparoscopically and this does reduce pubic bone stress. It has been postulated that the inguinal ligament tenolysis may increase the incidence of femoral hernia, but this does not seem to be the case.

Summary

Groin pain in sportsmen remains a difficult clinical problem because of the number and variety of conditions that may be responsible (Bisciotti et al., 2016; Morales-Conde et al., 2010; Sheen et al., 2014; Weir et al., 2015). Today the more scientific approach to fitness and training focusing on balance and core stability has resulted in a reduced incidence of groin disruption. Whilst many groin injuries can be successfully treated conservatively, a significant proportion will not respond and will need surgical intervention (Garvey et al., 2010). The key to successful treatment is a thorough clinical examination, appropriate imaging and patient selection. If it is accepted that groin disruption is a complex musculotendinous injury, then an anatomical, functional and physiological repair is the logical approach to treatment, followed by a structured rehabilitation programme aiming for a rapid, but realistic, return to sport. The presence of a multidisciplinary team is fundamental (Cross et al., 2013; Elattar et al., 2016).

References

Bisciotti, G.N., Volpi, P., Zini, R., Auci, A., Aprato, A., Belli, A., et al., 2016. Groin Pain Syndrome Italian Consensus Conference on terminology, clinical evaluation and imaging assessment in groin pain in athlete. BMJ Open Sport & Exercise Medicine 2 (1), e000142.

Choi, H.R., Elatta, O., Dills, V.D., Busconi, B., 2016. Return to play after sports hernia surgery. Clinics in Sports Medicine 35 (4), 621.

Corrigan, B., Stenstone, B., 1985. Hip and groin problems in runners. Patients' Management 9, 33–42.

Cross, S.G., Rastogi, A., Ahmad, M., Carapeti, E., Marsh, S., Jalan, R., 2013. Sportsman's Groin: Importance of a Multidisciplinary Approach. ESSR 2013 Poster / P-0139. European Society for Musculoskeletal Radiology. Available at: https://doi.org/10.1594/essr2013/P-0139.

Dimitrakopoulou, A., Schilders, E., 2015. Sportsman's hernia? An ambiguous term. Journal of Hip Preservation Surgery 3 (1), 16–22. https://doi.org/10.1093/jhps/hnv083.

Ekberg, O., 1981. Inguinal herniography in adults: technique, normal anatomy and diagnostic criteria for hernias. Radiology 138 (1), 31–36.

Ekberg, O., Persson, N.H., Abrahamsson, P., Westlin, N.E., Lilja, B., 1988. Long standing groin pain in athletes. A multidisciplinary approach. Sports Med. 6, 56–61.

Elattar, O., Choi, H.R., Dills, V.D., Busconi, B., 2016. Groin injuries (athletic pubalgia) and return to play. Sports Health 8 (4), 313–323.

Garvey, J.F.W., Read, J.W., Turner, A., 2010. Sportsman hernia: What can we do? Hernia 14, 17–25.

Gilmore, J., 1996. A pain in the groin? Sports Med. 2, 1–3.

Gilmore, J., 1998. Groin pain in the soccer athlete: Fact, fiction, and treatment. Clinics in Sports Medicine 17, 787–793.

Gilmore, O.J.A., 1992. Gilmores' groin. Sports Medicine and Soft Tissue Trauma 3, 12–14.

Hackney, R.G., 1993. The sports hernia: a cause of chronic groin pain. British Journal of Sports Medicine 27, 58–62.

Harris, N.M., Murray, R.O., 1974. Lesions of the symphysis in athletes. British Medical Journal iv, 211–214.

Horsky, I., Huraj, E., 1984. Surgical treatment of the painful groin. Acta Chirugiae Orthopaedicae et Taumatologiae Cechoslovaca 52, 350–353.

Ledingham, IMcA., MacKay, C., 1988. Jamieson and Kay's Textbook of Surgical Physiology, fourth ed. Churchill Livingstone, Edinburgh.

Lovell, G., Malycha, P., Pieterse, S., 1990. Biopsy of the conjoint tendon in athletes with chronic groin pain. Australian Journal of Science and Medicine in Sport 22, 102–103.

Minnich, J.M., Hanks, J.B., Muschaweck, U., Brunt, L.M., Diduch, D., 2011. Sports hernia: Diagnosis and treatment highlighting a minimal repair surgical technique. American Journal of Sports Medicine 39, 1341–1349.

Morales-Conde, S., Socas, M., Barranco, A., 2010. Sportsmen hernia: what do we know? Hernia 14 (1), 5.

Morley, N., Grant, T., Blount, K., Omar, I., 2016. Sonographic evaluation of athletic pubalgia. Skeletal Radiology 45 (5), 689.

Munegato, D., 2015. Sports hernia and femoroacetabular impingement in athletes: a systematic review. World Journal of Clinical Cases 3 (9), 823.

Murphy, G., Foran, P., Murphy, D., Tobin, O., Moynagh, M., Eustace, S., 2013. "Superior cleft sign" as a marker of rectus abdominus/adductor longus tear in patients with suspected sportsman's hernia. Skeletal Radiology 42 (6), 819.

Omar, I.M., Zoga, A.C., Kavanagh, E.C., Koulouris, G., Bergin, D., Gopez, A.G., et al., 2008. Athletic pubalgia and "sports hernia": Optimal MR imaging technique and findings. Radiographics 28 (5), 1415.

Paksoy, M., Sekmen, U., 2016. Sportsman hernia; the review of current diagnosis and treatment modalities. Ulus Cerrahi Derg 32, 122–129.

Pesquera, L., Reboulb, G., Silvestre, A., Poussange, N., Meyer, P., Dallaudière, B., 2015. Imaging of adductor-related groin pain. Diagnostic and Interventional Imaging 96, 861–869.

Polglase, A.L., Frydman, G.M., Farmer, K.C., 1991. Inguinal surgery for debilitating chronic groin pain in athletes. Medical Journal of Australia 155, 674–677.

Renstrome, P.A., 1992. Tendon and muscle injuries in the groin area. Clinics in Sports Medicine 11, 815–831.

Schache, A.G., Woodley, S.J., Schilders, E., Orchard, J.W., Crossley, K.M., 2017. Anatomical and morphological characteristics may explain why groin pain is more common in male than female athletes. British Journal of Sports Medicine 51, 554–556.

Sheen, A.J., Stephenson, B.M., Lloyd, D.M., Robinson, P., Fevre, D., Paajanen, H., et al., 2014. 'Treatment of the sportsman's groin': British hernia society's 2014 position statement based on the manchester consensus conference. British Journal of Sports Medicine 48, 1079–1087. https://doi.org/10.1136/bjsports-2013-092872.

Smedberg, S.G., Broome, A.E.A., Elmer, O., Gullmo, A., Roos, H., 1985. Herniography in athletes with groin pain. The American Journal of Surgery 149, 378–382.

Walden, M., Hagglund, M., Ekstrand, J., 2015. The epidemiology of groin injury in senior football: a systematic review of prospective studies. British Journal of Sports Medicine 49, 792–797.

Weir, A., Brukner, P., Delahunt, A., Ekstrand, J., Griffin, D., Khan, K.M., et al., 2015. Doha agreement meeting on terminology and definitions in groin pain in athletes. British Journal of Sports Medicine 49 768–744.

Whittaker, J.L., Small, C., Maffrey, L., Emery, C.A., 2015. Risk factors for groin injury in sport: an updated systematic review. British Journal of Sports Medicine 49, 803–809.

Zimmerman, G., 1988. Groin pain in athletes. Australian Family Physician 17, 1046–1052.

Ziprin, P., Williams, P., Foster, M.E., 1999. External aponeurosis nerve entrapment as a cause of groin pain in the athelete. British Journal of Surgery 86 (4), 566–568.

Chapter | 16 |

The sporting hip

James Moore

Introduction

This chapter will focus on the role of the hip joint in sport, how it is the key to all sporting movement and how dysfunction and pathology can lead to pain and overload of a number of other structures.

In order to do this, we will concentrate on the structure, function and movement mechanics of the hip joint, and will provide indicators of where a practitioner can help to intervene and improve overall function as we explore each aspect. Finally, we will touch on pathology and incidence (which is well covered in a number of different texts), and what tests can be performed to ascertain the root cause of the problem. We will only discuss management through correct exercise prescription, as this is covered in more detail in Chapter 14.

Before starting, it is important to define that the sporting hip is primarily focused on a young athletic population with an age range of ~18 to 40/45 years. Prior to this, the hip is considered to be in an adolescent/developing range, and after this in a degenerative range.

> **Learning point**
>
> In order to understand the hip the clinician needs to consider the balance of relative contribution of three main pillars: structure; function; and movement

Structure

Joint shape

The hip joint is the best example of a ball and socket joint in the body. It is capable of taking very large forces, with the impact of eight times bodyweight being described in normal running (Mann and Hagy, 1980). The joint is generally regarded as one of the most stable joints in the body, which it gains through its bony configuration, the depth of the acetabulum and labrum and the strong capsular–ligamentous complex surrounding it.

The primary stability in the hip joint comes from the joint shape and how it covers the head of the femur. A normally orientated acetabulum faces laterally, inferiorly and anteriorly, and is concave with significant coverage superiorly and posteriorly, allowing good support for the femoral head in weight-bearing, particularly during heel strike to midstance in gait. However, the acetabulum has reduced coverage anteriorly and inferiorly due to the acetabular notch; this is perfect for allowing good range of motion into flexion and the ability to squat, lunge and crawl. This means that in extension, i.e., running and kicking, there is reduced coverage and bony support for the head of the femur (which is orientated medially, superiorly but also anteriorly) and thus there is a greater potential for anterior translation of the head within the socket engaging the anterior structures of labrum, capsule and myofascial tissue.

As described above, the joint surfaces do not quite fit in upright standing, with up to 30% of the head of the femur being exposed. This has led some anatomists to state that the hip joint is the joint that has not evolved and is best positioned to take load in a quadrupedal gait (flexion, abduction and external rotation of the femur on acetabulum), i.e., the loose-pack position of the hip.

The head of the femur is well supported by the acetabulum in flexion, abduction, adduction and internal rotation. Arthrokinematically, one can certainly observe that the primary constraint to adduction and internal rotation in flexion (femoroacetabular impingement) is engagement of the femoral neck on the anterior and superior aspect of the acetabulum. In extension and external rotation, the head of the femur becomes exposed and engages the labrum, periarticular structures and myofascial structures as contrasts to control motion.

The mechanics described above can significantly change with changes in the orientation of the head of femur and acetabulum, please see Radiology later in the chapter.

Learning point

Joint shape can significantly influence movement and muscle function and should be considered when devising all exercise and rehabilitation programmes.

Labrum

The acetabular labrum is a fibrocartilaginous structure, which deepens the socket, helping to cover an extra third of the femoral head. The labrum is richly innervated with unencapsulated free nerve endings; this means they can become sensitive to painful stimuli and are likely to refer in a sclerodomal pattern. The labrum creates a seal for the synovial fluid, which combined with the atmospheric pressure in the joint acts like a suction effect on the femoral head, enhancing stability.

Periarticular mechanics and microinstability

The capsular–ligamentous system can be considered as a continuous blended structure around the hip joint. The four primary ligaments to be considered here are: iliofemoral ligament (ligament of Bigelow); ischiofemoral ligament; pubofemoral ligament; and ligamentum teres. It is argued that the iliofemoral ligament is the strongest ligament in the body and, being a 'Y'-shaped ligament across the anterior aspect of the hip joint, it is best positioned to support the head of the femur in the acetabulum in upright standing, thus supporting the mechanics described above. The ligament resists extension and external rotation of the femur on the acetabulum. The superior band will also resist adduction and internal rotation in neutral at the hip joint. The anterior inferior aspects of the ligament will provide resistance to external rotation in a flexed and abducted position.

The ischiofemoral ligament provides resistance to internal rotation in both adduction with flexion, and abduction in extension. It provides little to no resistance to external rotation. The pubofemoral ligament provides a small amount of resistance to external rotation in extension with abduction; there is marginally more resistance to internal rotation in flexion with abduction. Ligamentum teres is stressed in abduction and external rotation, but it is intracapsular and has a synovial membrane. It has been likened anatomically and biomechanically to the anterior cruciate ligament in the knee.

The hip joint capsule is unique as well: It is not a uniform structure, with a significant increase in thickness (Philippon et al., 2014; Walters et al., 2014) (of millimetres) at 1–3 o'clock anteriorly (if you consider the acetabulum as a clock face), but still demonstrating thicker aspects inferiorly from 4–7 o'clock as well as at 12 o'clock. This can be seen to correspond to the lack of coverage of the acetabular surface. It has been argued that the thickness of the capsule provides increased stability to the hip joint and has some radiographic (magnetic resonance) evidence (Magerkurth et al., 2013) against laxity and hip joint stress. A thicker capsule not only provides support but also helps to control motion of the head of femur on the acetabulum.

An intact capsule can provide up to 200–400 N of force to prevent distraction of the head of femur on the acetabulum (Khair et al., 2017). However, following capsulotomy (of up to 8 cm) the force to displace the head of femur can drop to as low as 119 N; if repaired then the force goes back to 280–355 N. This implies that the one needs between 20 and 40 kg of force to displace the head of femur on the acetabulum in an intact capsule, but only 12 kg of force in a disrupted capsule.

Reduction in capsular integrity can lead to a number of issues (Wuerz et al., 2016): increase in range of motion (ROM) of up to 20%; increase in hysteresis area of up to 29%; and increase in neutral zone of up to 147%. Furthermore, any hip joint effusion has been shown to reduce rotational ROM in at 0 degrees and 90 degree flexion by tensioning the capsule, with the most significant loss occurring in external rotation (ER) at 0 degrees. Each individual detail highlighted above is interesting in its own right and provides the clinician with key aspects to function and movement. However, these structures should always be regarded as an integrated unit, and as such the reader's attention is directed to the notion of tensegrity. First described by architect Buckminster Fuller, in biological terms this refers to forces of tension (contractile and non-contractile) pulling on structures (articular) that helps keep the body both stable and efficient in mass and movement.

This concept is demonstrated by the fact that when the capsule and labrum are intact you need up to ~225 N of force to cause a 3-mm displacement of the head of the femur. However, if the capsule is removed and labrum intact it drops to ~125 N, and with both structures removed there is less than 5 N before displacement. Furthermore, it can be seen that the initial displacement of up to 3 mm is resisted by the labrum; however at 3.5 mm and further, the capsule begins to take the slack and provides the main resistance to displacement. This would imply that hip microinstability (Harris, 2016) during simple movements is primarily supported by the labrum, but as the ROM increases the capsuloligamentous system increases its contribution to the constraints of displacement (Nepple and Smith, 2015).

Finally, there is significant evidence that the capsular ligaments engage to prevent impingement, and that capsular rotational restraints guide the available ROM to these impingement-free positions (van Arkel et al., 2015).

The myofascial system is key in the structure of the hip joint; however, discussion of this aspect is incorporated into the coverage of function and movement, below, to make it more clinically applicable.

Learning points

- The capsuloligamentous system controls range of motion
- The capsule and labrum combine to provide tensegrity
- Loss of either constraint results in increase in joint play and microinstability
- Regaining and improving the integrity of the capsuloligamentous system helps to reduce impingement

---

Function

The hip joint is the key articulation from the lower limb to the spine via the pelvis. The pelvis is a closed ring providing a stable base for the spine and lower limbs, and acts to transfer force. It provides support for the downward and forward thrust from the trunk, while at the same time it absorbs the propulsive forces transmitted from the lower limbs in a reciprocal direction (Gracovetsky and Iacono, 1987). Therefore any instability or pain at one point can have a direct effect on another.

As such, the hip joint provides the key interface between the lower limb and the trunk, meaning that practitioners should always take a global view of the area, evaluating function from the top down and from the bottom up. The region should be regarded as a lumbopelvic–hip complex; any dysfunction within this complex may have a cumulative effect of hip mechanics and movement.

As mentioned above, in bipedal gait the hip joint is not best positioned to take load. This is highlighted by some gait laboratory work, where researchers showed that in the last 20% of stance (heel lift to toe-off), the head of the femur engages the anterior–superior acetabular rim and thus the labrum, placing a traction-type force on the labrum (Bergmann et al. 2001). The hip can be in extension longer during ambulation than when running; consequently, pain on terminal hip extension due to labral tensile strain may be more significant in normal ambulation and less in running.

Bringing the capsuloligamentous system into play, we can see how the iliofemoral ligament resists extension and external rotation in terminal stance phase (last 20%);

when combined with the ligamentum teres (which resists abduction and external rotation), you can see how both ligaments help to 'centre' the head of the femur on the acetabulum and thus support the labrum and anterior hip structures described above.

During ambulation (Lewis et al., 2007) the anterior and lateral forces at the hip joint reach up to 1 × bodyweight (BW) at approximately midstance. The superior forces can reach up to 4 × BW. This is made up of the vertical ground reaction force (VGRF) of 0.8–1.2 × BW and the muscular forces reaching up to 3 × BW. If the individual was to limit hip extension by shortening stride length, the anterior hip forces reduce. However, if hip extension is maximized then the anterior forces increase significantly. Based on the mechanics described above, it increases the relative strain on the labrum, anterior capsuloligamentous system (iliofemoral and ligamentum teres), as well as placing more demand on the myofascial system.

The lateral hip forces in midstance reach up to 1 × BW. The centre of mass (CoM) passes medially to the hip joint, with a lateral sinusoidal path causing a hip list; there is a large adductor moment arm about the hip joint. This is supported and controlled by the lateral hip structures as they eccentrically control this motion of the pelvis on the hip. The angle of the neck of femur on the shaft (coxa vara and valga) can influence the mechanical efficiency of the lateral hip structures. An abnormal angle is usually seen in children as a congenital deformity; it is worth noting in adults as it may influence efficiency of the lateral hip structures.

The primary forces at heel strike to midstance are absorbed at hip and knee. However as a person moves from heel lift to toe-off, we see a proportional demand on the ankle and hip providing an equal and opposite force in extension before the initiation of the swing phase. The hip undergoes a variety of different forces in the various activities of daily living (Table 16.1). It has been shown that with an increase in push-off compared to a natural push-off , there is earlier and increased activity in both medial

Table 16.1 Hip joint loads in activities of daily living

Movement	Percentage bodyweight load
Bicycling	25–50
Walking	80–120
Fast walking	220–270
Up stairs	300
Down stairs	350
Jogging	500
Stumbling	900

gastrocnemius and soleus, with a relative reduction in demand on iliopsoas (Lewis and Garibay, 2015). From this data, it is reasonable to extrapolate that the kinetic chain can influence the anterior hip load and function, and thus influence symptoms by reducing the strain on the anterior hip structures. Postsurgery for the hip joint the kinematics can change with a reduction in frontal and sagittal plane range of motion; smaller peak hip abduction and internal rotation moments; and decreased peak hip power (Brisson et al., 2013). Therefore, it is vital that the clinician understands normal ambulation forces and restores these either once the symptomatology has abated or postintervention.

The focus on functional mechanics has been on the hip articulation with the pelvis. It would be remiss not to mention the influence the pelvis and trunk has on the hip from a kinetic perspective. This is best described in the three planes of motion.

In the sagittal plane the whole pelvis can go into an anterior tilt, one innominate can become anteriorly rotated, or the lumbar spine can hyperlordose. Regardless of cause and initiation of movement, the resultant impact at the hip joint will be similar. The anterior acetabular rim will increase its coverage of the head of femur and thus provide more articular support/stability; this could be an active strategy to reduce anterior loads and reduce tensile strain on the anterior structures. The disadvantage of this is that there can be an increased tendency for impingement of the soft tissue structures around the anterior aspects of the hemipelvis (anterior superior iliac spine/anterior inferior iliac spine – ASIS/AIIS), and also increased load on the lumbar spine in extension.

In the coronal plane, the primary movement that will likely occur is an increase in list to the contralateral side in gait, thus increasing the excursion of the sinusoidal path. This movement will result in the ipsolateral hip staying in internal rotation longer and be seen as slight backward rotation of the lumbopelvic–hip complex in terminal stance. Again, this may reduce the tensile strain and instability on the anterior structures. The consequence of such a movement may increase the sheer force and adductor strain on the contralateral hip pubic joint and adductor muscle complex, as well as increase stress at the lumbosacral junction. Finally, the early weight shift may increase the relative eccentric load on the lateral structures of the contralateral hip, possibly predisposing to trochanteric stress and pain syndromes.

Transverse plane motion always occurs in conjunction with coronal plane movement, and so it is unlikely to see isolated rotation. If this does occur at the hip joint, it is likely to be driven from the ground up, with an increase in pronatory moment arm, or valgus and internal rotation of the femur. This will again reduce the load on the anterior hip joint structures but increase a corresponding load on the anterior and medial structures of the knee, and the plantar and medial structures of the foot.

Learning points

- The hip takes large forces in gait (superior 4 × bodyweight, anterior 1 × bodyweight)
- This can be influenced by joint shape and pelvic position
- Changing stride length can influence the anterior load on the hip
- Muscle function and timing can reduce the anterior load on the hip (improved push-off, through good calf function)

Movement in sport

In order to understand the hip in sporting movements we need to understand four key activities: jogging (i.e., slow-speed running <5.5 m/s, ~18 km/h); sprinting (i.e., high-speed running >7.0 m/s, ~24 km/h); change of direction; and kicking.

As we transition from walking gait to running, we move from a double-support to single-support phase. Walking is described as an inverted pendulum model, where the centre of mass reaches its high point in midstance phase and is described by periods of braking forces storing potential kinetic energy, and propulsion releasing kinetic energy. Conversely running is seen as a spring-loaded mass model, where centre of mass is at a low point in midstance. This time, braking is described by compression, which stores elastic energy, and propulsion by releasing the recoil of stored energy. It has been stated that running is 20% more efficient than walking as more elastic energy is used than mechanical energy.

Kinetically this looks like a shorter foot contact time, with much higher vertical forces, which is more likely to result in movement of the pelvis on the hip in stance phase. Thus, VGRF will produce a larger moment arm about the weight-bearing limb, increasing the load on the lateral structures. If there is positive running energy (the centre of mass is in front of the base of support) then there is an increased moment arm for the pelvis to be in anterior rotation and the lumbar spine to be lordosed, placing a greater demand on the abdominals, hamstrings and hip extensors (gluteals and adductors) to control the lumbo-pelvic–hip complex. Finally, the increase in arm drive will cause the pelvis to rotate towards the weight-bearing hip, placing much greater demand on torsional muscles like the obliques, gluteals and adductors.

Now let us consider the hip on pelvic movement during different speeds of running. The demands on the range of movement at the hip joint increase as one transitions through different speeds. Coupled with this is an increased demand on the passive constraints around the hip, from the labrum and to a greater extent from the capsuloligamentous complex. Also note that the shape of the hip joint will influence the range and muscle function utilized during all speeds of running.

For the purpose of this chapter we will focus on muscles that cross the hip joint. The reader is also referred to Chapter 14 for information on the influences of other muscles around the lumbopelvic–hip complex.

During slow walking we see the primary demand is at soleus, with gastrocnemius and gluteus medius closely following. As the individual moves through different speeds of walking from slow to fast, there is a proportional increase in demand on gluteus maximus, medius and gastrocnemius. As the individual moves from these walking speeds to slow running and preferred running, there is a marked increase in demand in the vasti in particular and soleus dominating the peak muscle force with up to 7 × and 5 × bodyweight respectively (Pandy and Andriacchi, 2010).

Interestingly, the demands at the hip during running (3.4–5.3 m/s, 12–19 km/h), certainly in the sagittal plane, are very low with only up to 2 × bodyweight being utilized by both psoas and the hamstring complex (Dorn et al., 2012). However, as soon as the individual gets over 7.0 m/s (25 km/h) the hip starts to take over, with hamstrings, psoas and the vasti contributing between 5–6 × bodyweight, while soleus is still dominant at nearly 9 x bodyweight. Once the individual is at very high velocities (9 m/s, 32.4 km/h) the hip is dominant, with soleus and vasti dropping to 7 × and 5 × bodyweight, respectively, while psoas and hamstrings are in the region of 9 × bodyweight (Pandy and Andriacchi, 2010).

With change of direction, the primary force comes from the ankle–foot complex (see Chapter 14). However, the hip has a key role to play, especially in relation to gluteus maximus and medius, as they control the creation of an abduction moment at the knee and allow the CoM to move away from the base of support.

In kicking, the hip has the highest net force with a ballistic impact, with reported forces around 450 N and acceleration prior to contact of 25.5 m/s (91 km/h); the thigh reaches an angular velocity of up to 500 degrees/s. However, despite these very high figures it is reported that only 15% of the kinetic energy is transferred to the ball (Barfield, 1998). The remaining force is lost at foot contact through ball deformation, lost as heat or dissipated through the body, increasing the traction and eccentric load on the lumbopelvic–hip complex. What is observed is that the maximum demand on the hip joint occurs in peak hip extension with maximum activation and peak eccentric load occurring on the myofascial complex here, especially adductor longus. Based on the mechanics described above, it follows that if there is any dysfunction or laxity in the hip joint, especially concerning the anterior structures, then the demand on the other myofascial structures, in particular adductor longus, will increase.

Learning points

- Different speeds of movement require different muscle firing patterns
- They can influence and be influenced by the kinetic chain
- The hip has a close connection to ankle–foot function
- Change in direction requires different function at the hip compared to straight-line running
- Kicking requires increased control into extension, with a greater demand on the anterior musculature
- Training and rehabilitation programmes require an understanding of the loads required for walking and running, and building capacity to tolerate these loads
- Consider a simple rugby kicking session involving 40–50 kicks out of hand; it is clear to see how the demand on the lumbopelvic–hip complex will rise significantly

Return to activity/sport

There are a number of different sport-specific aspects that need to be considered. However, the fundamentals for return to activity and sport do not change. In order to be able to function day to day, an individual first needs to tolerate the loads placed on the hip in normal gait and how this cumulatively builds during the day.

Let us use an 80-kg male as an example. Normal activities of daily living would have someone taking between 5000 and 10,000 steps per day. If we estimate that each lower limb represents 20% of bodyweight (16 kg), then in the swing phase there is a demand of between 40,000 and 80,000 kg of load. If we estimate the ground reaction force is 0.8–1.2 × BW per foot contact then the vertical force will be 1.6–4.8 mkg of load. Note that these figures are grossly exaggerated and only consider the mechanical energy in swing and stance phase, respectively, removing all other variables. This load will be greatly reduced when considering efficiency of movement, elastic energy transfer, stride length, footwear, surfaces, etc.

Let us now consider running at slow speed, again using the same 80-kg male with a moderate stride length of 1.5 m. It would mean that in 400 m there would be 266.66 strides (133.33 per side). We can estimate that VGRF will be 2–3 × BW per foot contact. Thus the following can be estimated per limb:

$$400 \text{ m} = 26,600 \text{ kg}$$

$$1 \text{ mile} = 106,400 \text{ kg}$$

$$5\text{K training session} = 666,666 \text{ kg}$$

(a simple rugby training session)

Box 16.1 **Hip joint–related hip pain**

- Intraarticular – labral tear or rim lesion
- Delaminated acetabulum
- Osteochondral lesion or defect
- Osteochondral loose body
- Cysts
- Ligamentum teres strain or rupture
- Capsulitis or synovitis
- Periarticular ligament sprain or tear
- Osteoarthritis
- Coxa saltans
- Iliopsoas and greater trochanter bursitis

These figures do not take into consideration fast jogging or high-speed running, and are purely mechanical load and follow the same principles of variable elimination described above.

If these are the fundamental demands on the human body to walk around for a day or to complete a single training session, then there are some basic force and force-endurance demands that need to be met in order to return to activity. Then we need to consider high-demand activities in daily living such as up and down stairs, sit to stand, or vice versa, the sporting demands of change of direction, high-speed running, or kicking. It is not surprising that if an individual has not met the basic requirements, as they return to daily life/sport they may break down as the activity demands increase.

Pathology

Differentiating the source of pain when a patient presents can become a diagnostic challenge (Box 16.1).

When assessing the sporting hip it is important to address the area using a structured, systematic approach. The practitioner should try and create a marriage between the history taken, the investigations ordered or received, and the physical examination. A detailed and thorough history is vital to help differentially diagnose the source of pain. The physical examination should be used to confirm or negate the underlying hypothesis for the pain and dysfunction that has already been formulated through the history and investigations.

A number of studies have shown that the hip can have ongoing (silent) pathology that may account for some of the pain in the majority of patients seen (up to 44%) (Bradshaw et al., 2008). The key is to ascertain if the hip is a primary or secondary problem, or sometimes even a red herring.

Generally hip pathology presents as a vague nonspecific deep achy pain, synonymous with somatic/sclerodomal pain, unlike adductor/inguinal pathology, which can be more superficial and specific/localized.

It has shown that all patients with primary hip articular pathology demonstrate deep inside groin pain that the patient cannot put a finger on. It is often demonstrated by the patient grabbing around the lateral and anterior aspects of the hip joint, known as a 'C-sign' due to the shape of the patient's hand as they grasp the region. It is also important to note that the hip joint can refer pain far and wide from the joint/groin itself, with up to 6.4 pain sites on average (Mitchell et al., 2003).

As part of the history taking, the specific sport the individual plays can be useful information to the clinician. While hip pathology is common in kicking sports, there is a much higher incidence of pubic/adductor-related pathology here, so the clinician would do well to differentiate this out. If the athlete is playing a twisting sport (squash, tennis, badminton, ice hockey) or running in a straight line (athletics/triathlon) then there is a greater incidence of hip joint pathology.

Work has been carried out looking at the incidence of hip joint versus other pathology in the sporting population. In males it was found that 45% had hip pathology, versus 77% in females. Furthermore, hip joint pathology occurred more frequently as an entity by itself, when compared with adductor- or pubic joint–related pain, which more likely occur with other pathology. The researchers were also able to show that the highest incidence of pathology in this region occurs in the 19–40-year age group, and that kicking sports (soccer and Gaelic) has the highest incidence of groin pathology (Rankin et al., 2015). These data illustrate that age and sport played are key determinants in the history taking.

When undertaking the physical examination to aid the rehabilitation process, the clinician is advised to break the goal of the physical examination into three parts:

1. Identifying the anatomical structural pathology that has the potential to be a source of pain
2. Identifying the likely pathophysiological process (inflammation vs. degeneration) that is causing the pain
3. Identifying the functional overload and contributing movement dysfunctions that may evoke continuous tissue stress and strain, thus perpetuating the above two.

Labral pathology is the most likely pathology that a clinician will come across in young athlete with hip pain. The labrum accounts for up to 63% of pathology seen on arthroscopy (Shetty and Villar, 2007).

When dealing with labral pathology, the clinician may find there is rarely a history of trauma; it is normally precipitated by repetitive stress, either through flexion and rotation (impingement) or through extension (traction on the labrum). The patient may complain of a clicking or catching sensation – this needs to be differentiated with coxa saltans (snapping hip syndrome) – or even a 'grasp' sign which is characterized by the sensation of 'missing a step'. Most commonly the pain is characterized by a vague, deep achy pain, usually in the groin crease that the patient cannot get to. It will be over a nonspecific area; rather than being able to point to the location with one finger, the patient will cup the hip joint between their index finger and thumb (the 'C-sign') and comment 'It is deep in there'. This is supported by a number of studies that have demonstrated that location of pain is key, depicting a 'groin triangle' (Falvey et al., 2009; Lovell, 1995).

For an overview of testing principles please see Table 16.2 (normal values are given); the testing process described is not exhaustive, but provides a suggestion of key tests.

When diagnosing hip pathology, the history (symptoms) and physical examination (clinical signs) are critical. There is good evidence to suggest that when these two sources of data are combined with radiological findings, there is a strong indication of source of pain (Peters et al., 2017). In the first instance plain radiographs are the most useful to elucidate cam or pincer morphology (Griffin et al., 2016).

Morphological changes such as cam or pincer (see below) that engage/approximate the acetabular surface with the neck of the femur dynamically on movement has been described as femoroacetabular impingement (FAI). However, this can happen in asymptomatic individuals and therefore the phenomenon of mechanical impingement should not be seen as pathology in isolation.

Studies have shown that over 55% of athletes will have a cam deformity (compared to general population at ~25%) and that ~50% of athletes have a pincer deformity (in the general population is closer to 80%). Most importantly, over 60% of both populations have a labral tear. In all cases in the populations sampled, these individuals were asymptomatic (Frank et al., 2015). Therefore the clinician must be aware that even though there may be signs of pathology in the hip, more information will be required before it can be confidently ascribed as the true cause of the presenting symptoms.

The reader is guided to the Warwick agreement (Griffin et al., 2016), which describes the triad of symptoms, signs and radiological features to provide a diagnosis of FAI syndrome (FAIS). Further weight to the diagnostic process can be added by enhancing the investigations to include cross-sectional imaging (magnetic resonance imaging; MRI, computed tomography; CT). There has been some further work done to look at functional movement and its association/correlation to FAIS. Provisional results indicate that there is some merit with doing tests such as a maximal squat in symptomatic patients; however more work needs to be done.

Learning points

- Differential diagnosis of hip pathology is complex; a systematic approach is required
- Balance the components of structure, pathophysiology and function
- Femoroacetabular impingement syndrome (FAIS) is diagnosed by symptoms, signs and radiology
- Function is to be clarified in the diagnostic process

Radiology

When examining a patient, it is important to refer to the all aspects of imaging that has been performed. It is beyond the scope of this chapter to go into detail about imaging; the reader is referred to other texts.

In order to better understand the structure (shape) of the hip joint and how this may influence pathology and symptoms, it is important to do a combination of weight-bearing and non-weight-bearing X-rays with or without a 3D CT scan. The clinician is then in a position to relate this to the function of the hip from the physical examination performed, so that the impact of the shape of the joint can be evaluated against the stability and mobility assessed.

Key angles to look for are: coxa profunda (depth of acetabulum); cross-over sign (retro/anteverted acetabulum); Tönnis angle (roof of acetabulum); lateral centre-edge angle (coverage of the head of femur); alpha angle (asphericity of the head of the femur; cam development). The shape of the joint is vitally important, as it has been found to be the cause of up to 73% of all labral injuries (Konrath et al., 1999).

An MRI and magnetic resonance arthrography can tell you a lot about the joint and structures that may be damaged. Any findings need to correlate with the physical examination and symptomatology. As mentioned previously, it is common to see pathology on imaging that do not relate to symptoms.

To aid with differential diagnosis, especially in a mixed pattern where there is concomitant pathology, examination under local anaesthetic (EULA) can be incredibly useful. If during the intervention the pain abates then the clinician can be relatively sure that the hip joint is a considerable contributor to the presentation (Frank et al., 2015).

Table 16.2 Testing procedure

Observation

Lower limb structure: Can affect overall hip and groin load	**Overall spinal posture**: Can indicate how muscles are functioning	**Direct visualization and inspection of the area**: Small areas of swelling and colour change can direct the examination

Movement screen

Squat: Look for symmetry at the hips and functional capacity to control the movement	**Lateral lunge or single-leg squat**: Look for symmetry at the hips and functional capacity to control the movement	**Open chain leg swing/running**: The former can tell a lot about muscle function and synergy

Supine tests – hip joint

Palpation of all bony prominences, and soft tissues that insert in and around the hip joint

ROM – full flexion – 130 degrees
Maintain sagittal plane motion with no deviation

ROM – full rotation
Normal ratio is 2:1 ER:IR
Rotational axis – 90 degrees = normal
<70 degrees = restricted; >100 degrees = mobile

ROM – abduction – 45–60 degrees
But also assess for guarding in the adductors

Dial test – quality and ROM of rotation in neutral/slight hip flexion – looking for signs of instability/laxity

Log roll – similar to the above but done with the leg resting on the plinth and assess 'spring back' of the lower limb
Anterior draw – in loose-pack position, apply a posterior–anterior glide to neck of femur (NOF)
Lateral draw - in loose-pack position apply a lateral glide to NOF

Femoroacetabular impingement tests
FADIR – flexion, adduction and IR and then flex – gentle test looking for provocation
FABIR – flexion, abduction and IR – looking for provocation – has a bias towards the superior acetabulum

Prone tests – hip joint

ROM – IR – both knees bent look for full passive IR
Normal = 30-35 degrees

ROM – ER
In slight abduction ER the hip
Normal = 60 degrees
At EOR apply a posterior–anterior glide to hip to provoke anterior structures

ROM – extension
Assess range – 15-60 degrees
Assess end feel of capsule

Provocation – EABERs - Extension, Abduction, External Rotation (ER)
at EOR apply a posterior–anterior glide to hip (greater trochanter) to provoke anterior structures

Passive constraint – EABERs and end feel
Same as above, but assess the end feel of the joint/iliofemoral ligament

ER, External rotation; EOR, end of range; IR, internal rotation; ROM, range of motion.

Rehabilitation

The shape of the joint is critical and affects both muscle recruitment patterns and movement at the joint. The clinician should always use radiology were available, even in asymptomatic patients, to help to guide the exercise selection.

Of particular note is the shape of the acetabulum (shallow, deep, anteverted or retroverted) and the shape of the femur, in particular, the neck of the femur (cam deformity or an anteverted neck). These variations can influence (enhance or inhibit) normal muscle function, as well as muscle function in a pathological state. Rehabilitation should not only focus on restoring functional movement and synergistic muscle activity, but also retrain muscles to compensate for the joint shape, the latter requiring more clinician experience.

If the acetabulum is shallow then effective recruitment of the deep hip rotators and adductors can help to stabilize it. If the hip is anteverted then the posterior hip musculature and in particular the gluteals need to have better capacity in outer range and eccentric control of the hip to decelerate the natural internal rotation axis, which is a movement bias consequence of having an anteverted hip.

Restoring normal rotational range of motion (to an equivalent level as the contralateral hip) should be a prerequisite of any hip and groin pathology. In particular, it is important to maximize the available internal and external rotational range of motion at the hip both in flexion and extension, not just from a passive capacity but making sure that there is effective rotational range of motion in a loaded position. The clinician should also note if the hip is generally restricted (70-degree total rotational axis or less), normal (~90-degree rotational axis), or mobile (>100-degree rotational axis), as this will effect the exercise prescription.

Finally, the clinician should focus on restoring normal myofascial compliance of both the contractile and non-contractile structures around the hip. This does not relate specifically to flexibility and stretch capacity, but more to extensibility, i.e., the ability of the tissue to actively lengthen without altering movement at a joint or region above or below the tissue in question. Once this has been restored in an unloaded active state, then the clinician should focus on restoration of this muscle capacity in an active loaded state, which is referred to as *tensile* capacity below.

When designing a hip rehabilitation programme it is common to think in terms of a typical rehabilitation paradigm with a linear progression; however, this is not always the best or optimal way to restore function. There is value in identifying the key areas that need to be addressed and applying different strategies simultaneously to evoke the response and adaptation around the joint. In short, the clinician should ask themselves which adaptions or changes in the hip will have the biggest impact on pain and function? Once ascertained, these areas should be prioritized in the decision-making process and appropriate exercises or treatment strategies assigned.

For example it is common practice for a clinician to restore the range of motion first, in particular with a focus on restoring rotation (taking into account the joint shape). While restoring the rotational axis of motion, it is also advisable to restore the appropriate amount of extension. Extension is a vital component of sport for producing an extension torque while sprinting, and to create a lever arm for a flexion force for kicking. It is important to note that the anterior hip force is greatest when the hip is in extension (Lewis and Garibay, 2015).

As mentioned, restoring the range early is usual practice; however, the clinician should note that sometimes what appears as a range restriction may be due to a loss of tissue extensibility under load, and appropriate recruitment and synergistic function about a joint. Therefore the strategy to restore range passively may vary from one of capacity of articular movement, to extensibility of tissues (neurological compliance) versus appropriate recruitment and coordinated function about a joint allowing the axis of movement to be maintained.

With that paradigm in mind, the clinician should think about the control of translation about a joint, as increased sheer forces within the joint can account for increase in tissue loading and therefore pain. A key strategy around this is placing the joint in an optimal position, i.e., loose pack; flexing, abducting and externally rotating the joint can do this. This position reduces the articular contact and increases the coverage of the head of the femur within the acetabulum. When the joint is in this position it allows the muscles around the joint to optimize the position sense and the cocontraction and coactivation needed to provide optimal stability. While in sport this is not a regularly held position, adopting it for exercises allows us to optimize tissue adaptation, i.e., the continuous muscular activity will stimulate the mechanoreceptors in the capsule and ligaments and thus modulate pain. Over time the periarticular tissue will adapt and increase in integrity thus providing greater passive stability to the joint.

Most rehabilitation programmes focus on weight-bearing exercises for hip function. However, as mentioned, the head of the femur can be exposed by up to one-third when in upright standing. The clinician is advised to construct exercises that adopt a variety of positions, especially in the early stages, such as frog-legged four-point kneeling and sumo squat–style positions, or positions that focus on closed chain activity in single-leg stance and slight trunk flexion. These positions reduce the attenuation of load on the anterior joint line and structures and thus help to restore the motor patterning and synergy around the hip.

While working on the range of motion and optimizing the motor patterning, the clinician can also be working on the strength balance around the hip simultaneously. This strength balance, especially in the coronal plane, is vital for sport as has been demonstrated in a number of papers. Ice hockey literature has looked extensively at this area and clearly shows that if the adduction force was ≤78% of the abduction force then the player was 17 times more likely to sustain a adductor muscle strain (Tyler et al., 2001). These results have been supported by similar research conducted on elite soccer players, which shows that the adduction isometric hip force is greater than that of abduction for both the dominant and nondominant sides and that there is no ratio difference between sides, but the ratio is significantly lower in players with groin pain (Thorborg et al., 2014).

While adduction-to-abduction ratio and balance on both the dominant and nondominant leg is a cornerstone of the rehabilitation process, this does not just mean the adductor muscles versus the abductor muscles. This is about total adduction force versus abduction force. So within this conceptual model of force vectors across the hip in the coronal plane, it is important to note that other muscles play an important role in helping to produce these force vectors, such as the hip flexors. O'Connor (2004), while studying groin pain, made reference to the fact that total hip strength involved the hip flexors, while Lewis et al., (2009) stated that a decrease in iliopsoas force contribution during flexion resulted in an increase in the anterior hip joint forces.

Once the clinician has restored the balance across the hip, it is time to consider ROM, especially rotation, force through range – especially coronal plane and extension, as well as synergistic muscle function across the axis of the joint. In order to return to full sporting activity, the clinician needs to transfer these methods to sports-specific activity and demands, whether that is at speed, in extremes of hip extension, or the specific endurance demands of the hip; it needs to be appropriate for the athlete and the sport.

Loading parameters around the hip and the groin are addressed in Chapter 14. However the reader should consider four key aspects in this regard, the role of the rotator cuff of the hip, the iliopsoas, the gluteals, and adductor magnus.

The deep hip rotators can be classified in many ways but are likely to make up a combination of gluteus minimus; the conjoined tendon of obturator internus with both superior and inferior gemelli; piriformis; quadratus femoris; obturator externus; rectus femoris (short head); and iliocapsularis. It is beyond the scope of the chapter to cover their function in detail. However, the author would like to draw the reader's attention to a few key aspects. Gluteus minimus communicates with the capsule superiorly, while obturator externus and the conjoint tendon on obturator internus and the gemeili (which flank obturator internus) communicates with the capsule posteriorly. Gluteus minimus, short head of rectus femoris and iliocapsularis all communicate with the capsule anteriorly. Therefore, regaining recruitment efficiency, control and appropriate tension can tension and control the capsule, which can guide the head of femur to impingement-free positions. Prolonged tension applied across the capsule can stimulate collagenous production and increase tensile strength and thus strain rate, improving the stability and movement patterns at the joint.

Rehabilitation strategies to help to stimulate the rotator cuff and capsule can be utilized by doing sustained submaximal isometric work in key tensile positions, and then holding these positions for periods of time to develop the tensile strain. Examples include four-point kneeing and a frog-legged or 'silverback gorilla' posture, and sumo squatting working in deeper ranges, by mobilizing from side to side. Particular reference is made to obturator externus (which interestingly also has an adduction moment); it has been shown to stabilize the head of femur in the socket and have selective external rotation moment at 0 degrees and 90 degrees. Again isometrics are key here as the muscle does not posses the muscle fibre length to produce excursion.

Iliopsoas has multiple roles, including axial (vertical) compression of the lumbar spine segments; eccentric control of lateral trunk flexion; control of the innominate, especially into posterior rotation; adduction moment arm at the hip (mainly psoas major); and then a large flexor moment at the hip in extension, especially as it uses the iliopectineal eminence as a fulcrum to increase the lever arm and mechanical efficiency in extension. However, as mentioned above, there is a partner muscle with iliopsoas in iliocapsularis, which sits directly over the anterior medial aspect of the capsule. This muscle has been shown to have selective activation in 90-degree hip flexion, where it tensions the capsule to avoid impingement.

Iliopsoas and its partners can be best loaded and activated with isometric hip flexion drills; recruitment threshold work from the spinal stability and 'drawing the hip into the socket' for local hip stability; static adduction loading at the hip (adductor side bridge); lateral trunk loading (side planks); and hip flexion loading.

The gluteals have a large variety of functions at the hip. Gluteus maximus is the largest force producer of extension, abduction and external rotation, with a large lever arm allowing it to influence excursion. While gluteus medius has a moment arm to abduct, its axis is close to that of the hip joint and as such does not posses the lever arm to efficiently produce abduction. Furthermore its muscle fibre length is very short, which implies that it cannot produce the excursion necessary. Rather gluteus medius is best designed to produce force into abduction or by decelerating/eccentrically controlling adduction. Gluteus maximus is therefore best trained with a variety of movements that involve both weight-bearing and non-weight-bearing, into all three planes of movement. However, gluteus medius may be best trained through heavy isometrics and resisting moments into adduction, like a single-leg dip, or lunging where the centre of mass produces an adduction moment arm at the hip.

Adductor magnus has been well described in Chapter 14. However, the key message at the hip is that its most proximal compartment (AM1) has a moment arm to approximate the head of the femur in the acetabulum and thus provide stability, drawing the head down and thus reducing the superior and anterior joint forces described above. Furthermore, due to its multipennated and multicompartment function, it has a large moment arm into hip extension and becomes a key component in acceleration drills, squats, split squats, lunges and step-ups.

Return to sport and full training/competition is beyond the scope of this chapter. However when designing such a programme it is useful to summarize and incorporate key components of the sport. Consider the following:

- Structure and design an appropriate programme that allows for the mechanics to be compensated for.
- Understand the functional loads at the hip and the different muscular support that can be provided from the deep and superficial structures, especially the capsule.
- Understand the extreme loads of running and kicking and allow enough time for adaptation in the tissues to tolerate these forces.
- Build appropriate balance across the hip primarily in the sagittal and coronal plane, so that there is at least a 1:1 ratio; the primary focus should always be in the sagittal and coronal plane, as rotational movement is tertiary and a combined movement with the coronal plane. Thus restoring coronal plane force vector balance will restore rotation. If special attention is needed for the deep rotators, this can be addressed but not at the expense of the former.

References

Barfield, W.R., 1998. The biomechanics of kicking in soccer. Clinics in Sports Medicine. 17 (4) 711-28.

Bergmann, G., Deuretzbacher, G., Heller, M., Graichen, F., Rohlmann, A.; Strauss, J., Duda, G.N.; 2001. Hip contact forces and gait patterns from routine activities. Journal of Biomechanics 34 (7), 859–871.

Bradshaw, C.J., Bundy, M., Falvey, E., 2008. The diagnosis of long-standing groin pain: a prospective clinical cohort study. British Journal of Sports Medicine 42 (10), 851–854.

Brisson, N., Lamontagne, M., Kennedy, M.J., Beaulé, P.E., 2013. The effects of cam femoroacetabular impingement corrective surgery on lower-extremity gait biomechanics. Gait Posture 37 (2), 258–263.

Dorn, T.W., Schache, A.G., Pandy, M.G., 2012. Muscular strategy shift in human running: dependence of running speed on hip and ankle muscle performance. The Journal of Experimental Biology 215 (Pt 11), 1944–1956.

Falvey, E.C., Franklyn-Miller, A., McCrory, P.R., 2009. The groin triangle: a patho-anatomical approach to the diagnosis of chronic groin pain in athletes. British Journal of Sports Medicine 43 (3), 213–220.

Frank, R.M., Lee, S., Bush-Joseph, C.A., Kelly, B.T., Salata, M.J., Nho, S.J., 2015. Improved outcomes after hip arthroscopic surgery in patients undergoing T-capsulotomy with complete repair versus partial repair for FAI; a comparative matched-pair analysis. The American Journal of Sports Medicine 42 (11), p2634–2642.

Gracovetsky, S.A., Iacono, S., 1987. Energy transfers in the spinal engine. Journal of Biomedical Enginering 9 (2), 99–114.

Griffin, D.R., Dickenson, E.J., O'Donnell, J., Agricola, R., Awan, T., Beck, M., et al., 2016. The Warwick agreement on femoroacetabular impingement syndrome (FAI syndrome): an international consensus statement. British Journal of Sports Medicine 50 (19), p1169–1176.

Harris, J.D., Gerrie, B.J., Lintner, D.M., Varner, K.E., McCulloch, P.C., 2016. Microinstability of the hip and the splits Radiograph. Orthopedics 39 (1), e169–e175.

Khair, M.M., Grzybowski, J.S., Kuhns, B.D., Wuerz, T.H., Shewman, E., Nho, S.J., 2017. The effect of capsulotomy and capsular repair on hip distraction a cadaveric investigation. Arthroscopy: The Journal of Arthroscopic and Related Surgery 33 (3), 559–565.

Konrath, G.A., Hamel, A.J., Olson, S.A., Bay, B., Sharkey, N.A., 1999. The role of the acetabular labrum and the transverse acetabular ligament in load transmission in the hip. The Journal of Bone and Joint Surgery 80 (12), 1781–1788.

Lewis, C.L., Garibay, E.J., 2015. Effect of increased pushoff during gait on hip joint forces. Journal of Biomechanics 48 (1), 181–185.

Lewis, C.L., Sahrmann, S.A., Moran, D.W., 2007. Anterior hip joint force increases with hip extension, decreased gluteal force, or decreased iliopsoas force. Journal of Biomechanics 40 (16), 3725–3731.

Lewis, C.L., Sahrmann, S.A., Moran, D.W., 2009. Effect of position and alteration in synergist muscle function contribution on hip forces when performing hip strengthening exercises. Clinical Biomechanics 24, 35–42.

Lovell, G., 1995. The diagnosis of chronic groin pain in athletes: a review of 189 cases. Australian Journal of Science and Medicine in Sport 27 (3), 76–79.

Magerkurth, O., Jacobson, J.A., Morag, Y., Caoili, E., Fessell, D., Sekiya, J.K., 2013. Capsular laxity of the Hip: findings at magnetic resonance arthrography. Arthroscopy: The Journal of Arthroscopic and Related Surgery 29 (10), 1615–1622.

Mann, R.A., Hagy, J., 1980. Biomechanics of walking, running, and sprinting. The American Journal of Sports Medicine 8 (5), 345–350.

Mitchell, B., McCrory, P., Brukner, P., O'Donnell, J., Colson, E., Howells, R., 2003. Hip joint pathology: clinical presentation and correlation between magnetic resonance arthrography, ultrasound, and arthroscopic findings in 25 consecutive cases. Clinical Journal of Sports Medicine 13,152–156.

Nepple, J.J., Smith, M.V., 2015. Biomechanics of the hip capsule and capsule management strategies in hip arthroscopy. Sports Medicine and Arthroscopy Review 23 (4), 164–168.

O'Connor, D., 2004. Groin injuries in professional rugby league players: a prospective study. Journal of Sports Science 22 (7), 629–636.

Pandy, M.G., Andriacchi, T.P., 2010. Muscle and joint function in human locomotion. Annual Review of Biomedical Engineering 12, 401–433.

Peters, S., Laing, A., Emerson, C., et al., 2017. Surgical criteria for femoroacetabular impingement syndrome: a scoping review. British Journal of Sports Medicine 51 (22), 1605–1610.

Philippon, M.J., Michalski, M.P., Campbell, K.J., Goldsmith, M.T., Devitt, B.M., Wijdicks, C.A., et al., 2014. Surgically relevant bony and soft tissue anatomy of the proximal femur. The Orthopedic Journal of Sports Medicine 2 (6), 1–9 DOI2325967114535188.

Rankin, A.T., Bleakley, C.M., Cullen, M., 2015. Hip Joint Pathology as a leading cause of groin pain in the sporting population; a 6 year review of 894 cases. The American Journal of Sports Medicine 43 (7), 1698–1703.

Shetty, V.D., Villar, R.N., 2007. Hip arthroscopy: current concepts and review of the literature. British Journal of Sports Medicine 41 (2), 64–68.

Thorborg, K., Branci, S., Nielsen, M.P., Tang, L., Nielsen, M.B., Hölmich, P., 2014. Eccentric and isometric hip adduction strength in male soccer players with and without adductor-related groin pain: an assessor-blinded comparison. Orthopaedic Journal of Sports Medicine 2 (2) 2325967114521778.

Tyler, T.F., Nicholas, S.J., Campbell, R.J., McHugh, M.P., 2001. The association of hip strength and flexibility with the incidence of adductor muscle strains in professional ice hockey players. American Journal of Sports Medicine 29 (2), 124–128.

van Arkel, R.J., Amis, A.A., Jeffers, J.R., 2015. The envelope of passive motion allowed by the capsular ligaments of the hip. Journal of Biomechanics. 48 (14), 3803–3809.

Walters, B.L., Cooper, J.H., Rodriguez, J.A., 2014. New findings in hip capsular anatomy: dimensions of capsular thickness and pericapsular contributions. Arthroscopy: The Journal of Arthroscopic and Related Surgery 30 (10), 1235–1245.

Wuerz, T.H., Song, S.H., Grzybowski, J.S., et al., 2016. Capsulotomy size affects hip joint kinematic stability. Arthroscopy: The Journal of Arthroscopic and Related Surgery 32 (8), 1571–1580.

Chapter | 17 |

Lumbopelvic dysfunction in the sporting population: the 'what', the 'why' and the 'how'

Neil Sullivan

Introduction

Throughout your career your treatment practices, methods and philosophies will inevitably evolve. This will be dependent upon influences such as courses, research, colleagues, expert opinion, experiences of positive outcomes and most definitely the experience of negative results. My own clinical practice was moulded very early in my career from spending time with a physiotherapist who taught me to question everything I did and everything I thought, which is, in essence, the crux of clinical reasoning. Watching the assessments and treatments and talking through the clinical reasoning in this practice provided great insight and deepened my desire to learn more about lumbopelvic dysfunction.

One chapter alone is not sufficient to provide comprehensive coverage of the function and pathology of the lumbopelvic region, including detailed anatomy and how this provides motion and stability. Instead, in this chapter I aim to provide guidance as to how to identify lumbopelvic dysfunction in the athlete. Objective tests and assessment techniques will be discussed enabling you to determine the manifestation of symptoms, their origin and, finally, find out why the problem might have occurred in the first place – essentially, the 'what', the 'why' and the 'how'.

The pelvis is the midway point in the human machine. It is a foundation for all that goes above and a significant platform for all that goes below. The structures that connect to the pelvis are vast and varied. They are essential to human locomotion, posture and function. The pelvis is often overlooked as a contributor to pain, dysfunction and injury. It is often easier to diagnose and treat other structures, rather than fix the root cause of the injury.

The lumbopelvic region is complex. It transfers load from the upper body and provides stability and dynamic control. It consists of the lumbar spine, two innominate bones (fused ilium, ischium and pubis) and the sacrum (Fig. 17.1). The sacrum and two innominate bones form the pelvic ring, with two sacroiliac joints posteriorly and the pubic symphysis anteriorly. The integrity of the pelvic ring is provided by force closure (active system using muscle and fascia) and form closure (passive system consisting of joints and ligaments). The anatomical landmarks that help clinicians in assessing and treating this are the anterior superior iliac spine (ASIS), posterior superior iliac spine (PSIS), iliac crests, inguinal ligament, ischial tuberosity and superior pubic ramus.

The key to successfully treating the patient with lumbopelvic issues is to widen the viewpoint from '*What* is the injured area in question?' to '*Why* has this problem occurred?' We need to look at the structures that can contribute to this problem and restore them to pain-free function. The final component of the process is the '*How* did this happen in the first instance?' Being able to find a contributor to the problem (the 'how') enables us as clinicians to fully appreciate the drivers behind the problem and educate the athletes accordingly. These drivers can be active training or competition related, or can be due to passive, habitual behaviours and/or postural positioning modifications. Understanding the *how* can ensure that we are more effective in our treatment of the athlete. It will enable us to advise athletes and then effectively treat with the confidence of achieving a positive outcome.

In professional football and rugby, and in private practice, lumbopelvic dysfunction can be a major contributor to many musculoskeletal presentations. Not every assessment of this area will be because of local symptoms. Experienced clinicians working in sport include examination of

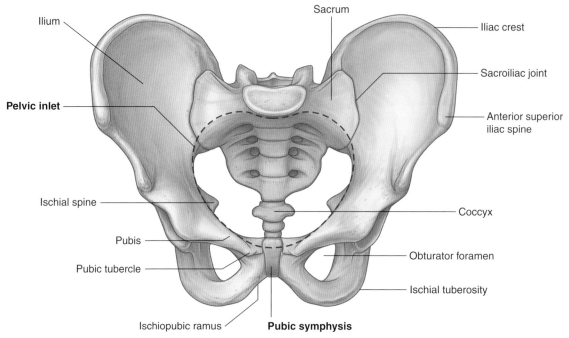

Fig. 17.1 The bony pelvis.

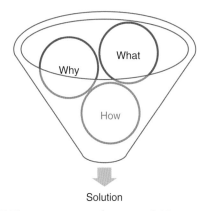

Fig. 17.2 The components of a successful intervention.

this area as part of the overall assessment process with several different presentations, especially if they are insidious or even chronic in nature. Specific pathologies, and conditions such as lower back pain, hamstring strains and groin pain also necessitate examining the lumbopelvic region as a contributor to a bigger picture. It may be the main driver or just a contributor to the athlete's dysfunction or pain, but either way, by including this as part of your overall assessment, as a clinician you are arming yourself with more information to address the issue.

For example, adductor-related groin pain is a commonly seen presentation in football. The adductor origin is found on the inferior pubic ramus, so it follows that any altered pelvic alignment could result with the pubis being in an altered position and therefore contributing to increased adductor tension and loading. A posterior rotation of one ilium could also be a contributor to anterior groin or pubic pain on the ipsilateral side, due to a potential increase in the strain on the inguinal ligament.

Transversely, an anterior rotation of the ilium will alter the position of the ischial tuberosity and therefore could contribute to increased tension of the hamstrings. Subtle positional changes of the pelvis or increases in tension of the structures that attach to and run off the pelvis can all have an effect on function (Fig. 17.2). Fascial trains proximal and distal to the pelvis can either contribute to altered function or positioning or be affected by the altered position of the lumbopelvic region.

Assessment – identifying the 'what'

Assessment should be methodical and strategic. If done in this way it should unearth clues that will enable an accurate diagnosis, and ultimately an effective treatment plan. The process should start with a detailed history, before moving on to a visual examination. The next stage is to put the patient through

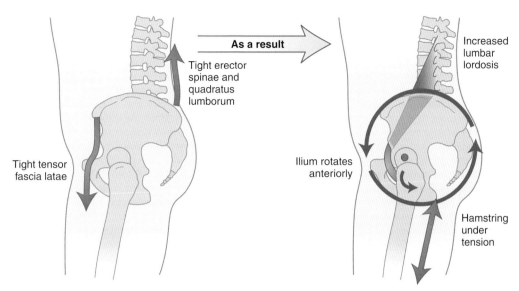

Fig. 17.3 The effects of tight musculature on the alignment of the pelvis.

some kinetic or movement tests, which are designed to high-light any movement deficiencies or dysfunction. Finally there is a physical assessment, where palpation and visual skills are used to confirm a diagnostic hypothesis that you have developed. The examination and assessment that follows has been developed over the years to suit my own clinical practice, and is a hybrid of courses and personal experiences.

Patient history

As with all good assessments, taking a detailed history from the athlete or patient is essential. In the sporting environment one often becomes familiar with the individual athletes' presentations. Maybe they are one-side dominant, have a known underlying condition or an injury history that predisposes them to a certain movement pattern or restriction. This is all relevant information. The most important thing to remember is that you are looking to decode the puzzle. The patient may report to the clinician with a hamstring injury; the clinician will then need to work out how it was likely to have occurred and whether the lumbopelvic region is a contributor. Here you can ask a series of structured questions to establish a picture:

- What was the mechanism?
- What was the activity at time of injury?
- How long has the patient been aware of the problem?
- What was the patient doing in the days leading up to that point that may have contributed (exercise and rest)?

Visual assessment and observation

Initial observation may reveal one of the classical abnormalities shown in Fig. 17.3.

With the patient standing there are often several clues which can be utilized to guide the rest of the assessment. Box 17.1 illustrates some visual assessment markers and gives detail that clinicians should look at.

Not every observation is relevant to lumbopelvic dysfunction, but each may provide a piece of the jigsaw that reveals the bigger picture. If you can link the pieces of the puzzle together, not only will you start to understand the presentation of the patient, but you may also be able to unearth the reasons why their lumbopelvic dysfunction manifested in the first instance.

The next step is to move onto kinetic tests. Unlike commonly used pain provocation tests, which are used to confirm sacroiliac joint (SIJ) pain, these tests are used to assess the movement quality of the lumbopelvic region and are key elements of the assessment. By assessing the movement quality, we can determine whether there is a dysfunction that is contributing to our patient's problem or one that may lead to a future problem. However, it is worth remembering at this point that there is limited evidence to support the reliability or validity of these tests in isolation when trying to identify an SIJ dysfunction. Laslett (2008) suggests that a reference standard for SIJ dysfunction tests has not been established, so validity of the tests for this disorder is unknown. However, by performing these tests in groups or clusters, some studies have found that reliability is increased (Laslett, 2008).

By performing the following tests regularly and collectively, we are able to start associating our test findings with our visual assessment. From here we can start to create a picture of which structures are involved and/or are contributing to the presentation. For example, a positive test (a test which shows altered movement) will direct the treatment process that follows. The positive side is not always the side that elicits pain and is often not even in the area where the patient perceives their symptoms are coming from, so bear that in mind. For example, in the past I have assessed many patients with hamstring symptoms. Sometimes it is easy to concentrate on the symptomatic area in question that the patient points to. By additionally examining the lumbopelvic region, it is easy to see how a dysfunction in this area can contribute to or be a causative factor in this presentation. By observing, understanding and correcting these dysfunctions, we can facilitate a successful outcome by speeding up recovery, aiding rehabilitation and even preventing future injury.

Before asking the patient to perform any of these movement tests, ensure that your patient or athlete is physically capable of performing these tests. Use your clinical reasoning skills to determine whether these tests will exacerbate any symptoms. There may be a case for performing only one or two of the tests rather than all of them. This may still be sufficient to provide you as the clinician with enough diagnostic information.

Tests in standing or kinetic tests

Trunk flexion assessment

Whilst performing this test, we are looking for any asymmetries in the amplitude and quality of the movement. We are assessing how well the sacroiliac joints move during this test. Other things to observe are the quality of lumbar spine flexion and thoracic tension or asymmetries. Further information about this test, its sensitivity and specificity is given by Tong et al. (2006).

Method. Ask the patient to stand facing away from you with feet hip-width apart. At this point you will need to palpate the PSIS. Hook the thumbs underneath these structures as this helps to eliminate many errors when monitoring the movement, and gives a much greater degree of feedback. Ask the patient to flex forwards as far as they comfortably can. Look for smooth and uniform movement of both PSIS as the patient flexes forwards. The amplitude and quality of the movements are key and should be symmetrical. If the PSIS on one side moves further than the other, this can suggest that the SIJ is hypomobile on that side. This assessment can provide a great deal of information to the clinician, but can also present some red herrings, so do not jump to conclusions too early.

Trunk extension assessment

For more detailed information about this test, its sensitivity and specificity, please see Gibbons (2017).

Method. Ask the patient to stand facing away from you and extend backwards whilst maintaining a hand position on their PSIS. You are looking for a slight inferior movement of the PSIS. The extension movement can sometimes

---

Box 17.1 Posture – visual assessment markers

Foot posture

Does the patient stand with equal foot posture? Pronation of the foot can suggest a compensation strategy for a longer limb length or an anterior rotation of the ilium (Fig. 17.4A). Supination can suggest a compensation strategy for a shorter limb length or a posterior ilium rotation (Fig. 17.4B).

Knee position

A patient standing with a flexed knee on one side could suggest a leg length discrepancy or an anterior rotation of the ilium (Fig. 17.4C).

Iliac crest alignment

If there is a visible difference in height, this can be caused by increased tone in lumbar paraspinals or quadratus lumborum. It can also suggest a leg length discrepancy – functional or structural (Fig. 17.4D).

Shoulder alignment

Here you are looking for any differences in shoulder heights. Does one side sit higher? If so is this due to localized tension or increased muscle bulk? It can also suggest a leg length discrepancy or lumbopelvic dysfunction (Fig. 17.4E).

Muscle bulk

Are there any obvious asymmetries in bulk? Some athletes will by the nature of their sport have asymmetries in bulk, so be careful not to assume that altered bulk is an abnormality.

Spinal alignment

Does the athlete stand with an increased lordosis or kyphosis? These postural changes may be longstanding if they are symmetrical and may be something to consider restoring over a period if they impact function and performance. More importantly though, is there any sign of a scoliosis? Any slight alteration or lateral deviation of the spine can suggest a structural or functional leg length discrepancy that will need to be addressed to get the best possible result (Fig. 17.4F).

Head and neck position

Look for any increased tone in the neck musculature, especially unilateral. This can indicate postural changes and increased tone in the superficial back line can alter the dynamics further down the chain.

Box 17.1 **Posture – visual assessment markers—cont'd**

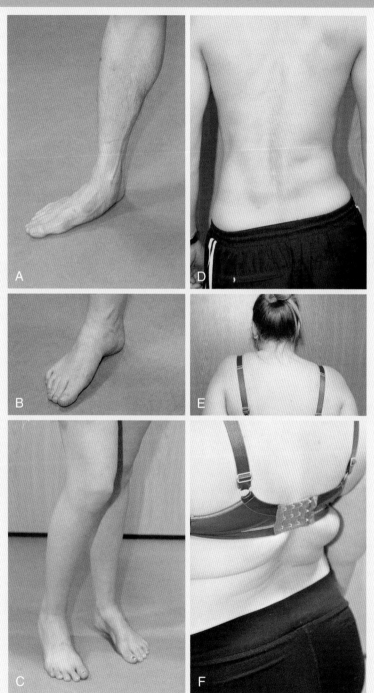

Fig. 17.4 (A) Pronated foot. (B) Supinated foot. (C) Knee flexion to accommodate leg length. (D) Raised iliac crest right side. (E) Elevated shoulder girdle left side. (F) Increased lumbar lordosis.

elicit pain and reproduce symptoms in some aetiologies, especially lumbar spine conditions such as discogenic pain or facet joint pain. This is also the time to perform Michelis' test (trunk extension with side flexion, whilst in single leg stance on the ipsilateral side) to assess the integrity of the pars interarticularis. A pars stress response is one of the most common causes of lower back pain in adolescent athletes. It is a chronic overuse condition which generally starts as a mild unilateral backache and progresses with activity. Progression of this condition can lead to a pars stress fracture; early identification of this presentation is key to management, as a delay can cause a permanent defect or spondylolysis.

Trunk side flexion

Further information about this test, its sensitivity and specificity is given in Gibbons (2017).

Method. The test will show how the sacrum moves in relation to the ilium. Place your thumbs on the PSIS, then move one thumb to the centre of the sacrum at the same level as the PSIS. Now ask the patient to side flex to the side that your thumb is palpating the PSIS. A subtle but smooth superior glide of the sacrum as the patient side flexes should be seen. A lack of superior movement when comparing one side to the other can, again, be suggestive of a hypomobile SIJ.

Gillet test or stork test

This commonly used test provides a great deal of information to the examiner when assessing the SIJ. Not only does it provide feedback on how the SIJ moves, but also how the stance leg performs to maintain pelvic alignment. Arab et al. (2009) provide further detail about this test, its sensitivity and specificity.

Method. To perform the test, stand behind the patient and palpate the PSIS by placing one thumb on the sacrum at the same level as the PSIS. Instruct the patient to stand on one leg whist raising the other leg into 90-degree knee and hip flexion. In this instance, if the patient is flexing the left hip, the examiner will have the left thumb on the left PSIS whilst the right thumb palpates the sacrum. Repeat the test on the other side and compare the movement amplitude and quality. A normal movement would show the PSIS glide inferiorly upon the sacrum. Any restriction in this movement in comparison to the other side suggests that the SIJ is hypomobile on that side.

Hip extension test

Gibbons (2017) provides further detail about this test, its sensitivity and specificity.

Method. Place one thumb on the PSIS and the other in the centre of the sacrum at the same level as the PSIS, in the same fashion as for the Gillet or stork test. Ask the patient to stand up straight and then stand on one leg whilst extending their hip taking their heel backwards towards you. A normal movement will show the PSIS glide in a superior direction. Compare left and right.

As with all of these tests, a positive test is determined if a movement is of smaller amplitude, of poorer quality or elicits pain. It does not matter if at this stage the patient does not have any positive kinetic tests (K+ve). Continue with the assessment process and build a complete picture of the patient's presentation and any pelvic dysfunction before considering treating the lumbar spine.

Palpation

Palpation skills are very important in the assessment process. Understanding the alignment of the bony points, tension in the musculature and restrictions of the tissues is essential to correctly diagnosing and treating the patient.

Supine

In this position you are looking to identify if there are any asymmetries in alignment: iliac crests, ASIS, superior pubic ramus, greater trochanter and medial malleolus. By including the medial malleolus, you are now able to consider if there is any leg length discrepancy present. This discrepancy may be either structural or functional and will need further investigation later to confirm.

Prone

With the patient or athlete lying on their front, you are now able to assess alignment of the iliac crests, PSIS, sacral sulcus, sacrotuberous ligament, ischial tuberosity and calcaneum. I would also, at this stage, perform an internal rotation comparison of the hips.

Sacral nutation, sacral counternutation or sacral tilt

As we know, the pelvis is comprised of three bones, two innominates and the sacrum. So far we have discussed tests used to identify alterations in the position of the innominates, but alterations in sacral position are also common presentations.

There are several ways to describe this next presentation. On occasion, a patient may present with a dysfunction during the standing kinetic tests but when they are on the plinth, there is very little to suggest any alignment variation. This is when the sacral position will need to be assessed by palpating the sacral sulcus. The simplest way to describe this, without going into detail about the anatomy of the pelvis and SIJ articulations, would be a tilt of the sacrum to one side or the other. We are now looking to assess how the sacral position maybe affecting the K+ve SIJ. The sacrum can appear higher or shallow (counternutated) on the K+ve side, in comparison to the functional side. Alternatively, the sacrum can appear to be lower or deep (nutated) on the K+ve side in comparison to the functional side.

Patient positioning

The technique used to assess for this presentation is with the patient lying in prone, to place the thumbs on top of both PSIS. One at a time roll the thumb over the PSIS medially and onto the sacrum. You are looking to compare the depth of the drop from the PSIS to the sacrum and see if there is a difference from left to right. This will require excellent palpatory skills. The difference will often be subtle, but you should try to feel the difference with your hands rather than visualize it with your eyes. This can also be assessed in lumbar extension by asking the patient to extend at the hips by resting on their elbows. Also, in lumbar flexion by asking the patient to sit back on their heels. These three testing positions will provide a clearer picture of this presentation.

Tests in supine lying

Active straight leg raise (SLR)

Ask the patient to lift one foot off the bed by 10 cm, then lower it back down again before lifting the opposite leg. Now ask the patient if one leg feels heavier than the other or if it elicits any pain. If the patient reports either of these symptoms then it may highlight a deficiency in force closure of the SIJ. There are two systems that provide structural integrity to the pelvic ring, force closure and form closure.

Form closure is a passive system utilizing joints and ligaments. In this instance, we are interested in the force closure, which is the active system comprised of muscle and fascia, and how that works to stabilize the SIJ. Further information about this test, it's sensitivity and specificity is provided by Mens, Vleeming, Snijders et al. (1999).

The test is then repeated with the clinician providing an equal bilateral pressure either side of the anterior, lateral or posterior aspect of the pelvis systematically. By adding this equal pressure whilst the patient performs the active SLR, this will give the clinician some important feedback as to whether the anterior, lateral or posterior structures are failing to aid the force closure of the pelvis.

Passive SLR

By raising the leg for the patient we are in theory biasing the neural structures rather than the contractile structures, but rather than assessing range of motion by asking the patient where they feel the tension, feel for tension through feedback from your hands to get a picture for whether there is a proximal or distal restriction.

Assessment findings – establishing the 'why'

The hardest part is to create a clear picture of what exactly you have discovered during the assessment. There are several presentations that you may discover, and we will now try to piece them together to help with treatment selections. We now need to associate any findings from the kinetic tests in standing with palpatory findings on the plinth. This is the time to rule out any structural leg length discrepancies. To accommodate for a leg length discrepancy, the human form will compensate in one way or another, and this can cloud the picture. Some of these presentations you may see during the examination such as foot pronation, knee flexion in standing, iliac crest in a superior position and anterior rotation of the ilium on the contralateral side. Table 17.1 shows the presentation on side of dysfunction.

Prevention – determining the 'how'

So, what causes a lumbopelvic dysfunction? Well, there are several different contributing factors to a lumbopelvic dysfunction and therefore several reasons why a lumbopelvic dysfunction can contribute to other injury presentations. Activities and sports that are unilateral in nature will cause a physical bias to a dominant side. But athletes are usually

Table 17.1 The presentation on side of dysfunction

Dysfunction	Iliac crest	ASIS	PSIS	Superior pubic ramus	Ischial tuberosity	Medial malleolus
Anterior rotation	Level	Inferior	Superior	Level	Superior	Inferior
Post rotation	Level	Superior	Inferior	Level	Inferior	Superior
Upslip	Superior	Superior	Superior	Superior	Superior	Superior
Downslip	Inferior	Inferior	Inferior	Inferior	Inferior	Inferior
Anterior rotation with upslip	Superior	Level	Superior	Superior	Superior	Level
Post rotation with upslip	Superior	Superior	Level	Superior	Level	Superior

ASIS, Anterior superior iliac spine; PSIS, posterior superior iliac spine.
Source: Gibbons, J., 2017. Functional Anatomy of the Pelvis and the Sacroiliac Joint. Lotus Publishing, Chichester, UK.

developed to function for the sport or activity that they perform. Structural imbalances such as leg length discrepancies are common enough and should be identified in the examination process before being addressed. Often, it is habitual postural positioning (which can lead to shortening of musculature) caused by the way athletes use their bodies away from the sporting environment which are often the significant precursors to dysfunction. These contributing factors away from the sporting arena can explain 'how' the problems manifest in the first instance. Athletes often have a lot of downtime to relax between training and competing, and how an individual spends their time away from their sport can be relevant to the presentation. These may seem to be obvious, but for the athlete who could be described as a repeat offender, we may need to look outside of the gym or the playing field and focus on other influences. If we as clinicians are thinking in this manner, then we can highlight to the athlete any potential red flags relating to postural change. Driving position, sofa or armchair posture, TV placement in relation to the sitting position, mobile phone usage, bedroom layout, gaming and excessive travel all have a role to play as contributing factors.

The role of imaging

From experience, I would suggest that imaging has a role in ruling out anything sinister in the lumbar spine, or if the patient fails to progress from treatment. Those patients with obvious lumbar spine presentations may need the extent of their injury to be confirmed. Athletic populations, especially in elite sports, often need a quick diagnosis to enable a speedy resolution by selecting the correct treatment or referral pathway. X-ray, magnetic resonance imaging and computed tomography imaging can provide a great deal of information to the referring clinician. But this information needs to be relevant to the presentation in question and the ability to marry up the clinical presentation with the findings on an image is extremely important.

Conclusion

Lumbopelvic dysfunction can contribute to many soft tissue presentations. There are a number of tests that have been shown to provide high levels of reliability in diagnosing SIJ pain. However, we are trying to diagnose movement dysfunction that will contribute to pain and/or injury. With regular management of pelvic and lumbar alignment, irrespective of symptomatic presentations, there is the opportunity to decrease the number of injuries that can be attributed to this region and limit chronic time-loss cases propagating into surgical cases. The problem is that quite often the athlete is not aware of any early alterations in alignment, so they do not seek treatment intervention. Those athletes who understand the link between habitual postural alignment and their signs and symptoms are the ones who seek regular maintenance and interventions. The key to successfully treating the patient is to widen the view point. We as clinicians need not only to focus on 'what' the symptoms of the injury are, but instead, ask ourselves 'why' has this problem occurred in the first instance? We need to start looking at the structures that can contribute to this problem and restore them to function before we can effectively overcome the injury. This, however, is not the end of the process. Understanding 'how' the dysfunction occurred in the first instance will enable us to make decisions that will change the outcome moving forward. Only once we can answer these three questions can we successfully treat the patient with the confidence of a long-term solution.

References

Arab, A.M., Abdollahi, I., Joghataei, M.T., Golafshani, Z., Kazemnejad, A., 2009. Inter- and intra-examiner reliability of single and composites of selected motion palpation and pain provocation tests for sacroiliac joint. Manual Therapy 14, 213–221.

Gibbons, J., 2017. Functional Anatomy of the Pelvis and the Sacroliliac Joint. Lotus Publishing, Chichester, UK.

Laslett, M., 2008. Evidence-based diagnosis and treatment of the painful sacroiliac joint. The Journal of Manual and Manipulative Therapy 16 (3).

Mens, J., Vleeming, A., Snijders, C., Stam, J.H., Ginai, A.Z., 1999. The active straight leg raising test and mobility of the pelvic joints. European Spine Journal 8, 469–473.

Tong, H.C., Heyman, O.G., Lado, D.A., Isser, M.M., 2006. Interexaminer reliability of three methods of combining test results to determine side of sacral restriction, sacral base position, and innominate bone position. Journal of the American Osteopathic Association 106 (8), 464–468.

Chapter | **18** |

Performance rehabilitation for hamstring injuries - a multimodal systems approach

Johnny Wilson, Paulina Czubacka and Neil Greig

Introduction

Hamstring injuries (HSIs) in elite football continue to be a challenging and complex conundrum. The progressively increasing incidence of HSIs over time, their tendency to recur upon return-to-play (RTP) and the evident lack of consensus in both assessment, rehabilitation and RTP criteria may lead to suboptimal management.

HSIs remain the most prevalent injury within professional football, contributing approximately 12% of all recorded injuries (Ekstrand et al., 2013). This increasing trend (4% per year) places a large burden on professional football clubs, with around 18 training days and three games missed per player per season (Woods et al., 2004). Alarmingly, up to 33% of these injuries recur, with over 50% of these reinjuries occurring within 30 days of the player's initial RTP (Ekstrand et al., 2013). When observing that recurrence rates have not improved over the past three decades, it is suggested that poor outcomes may be related, in part, to inadequate rehabilitation, premature RTP and a lack of consensus on best practice (Orchard et al., 2013).

These factors, allied to the purported increasing physical demands of the sport at the elite level demonstrate the need for an evidence-informed and appropriately structured multidisciplinary team (MDT) approach when rehabilitating HSIs. In reality, however, despite the aforementioned complexities, the management of football players suffering HSIs, and their subsequent RTP, is influenced by a far wider group of stakeholders than simply those with a medical background – many of whom may have competing interests in a specific player returning to the field ahead of prognosis. Although the sports clinician and player themselves may be best placed to measure and monitor the achievement of RTP criteria, the influence of coaches, the stage of the season, agents and contractual terms, etc., all suggest that a wider consensus should be sought for final RTP decisions (Van Der Horst et al., 2017). Ultimately, an athlete-centred model, incorporating the views of those who directly influence medical risk management may serve to improve outcomes.

From a clinical perspective, gaining consensus on the most valuable objective criteria with which progress can most effectively be gauged, has proven a challenge that is yet to be fully overcome. Commonly used generic terms such as, 'absence of pain', 'nullity of clinical signs', 'similar strength and flexibility' and 'good neuromuscular function' lack any degree of specificity upon which the assessing clinician can rely. Achieving 'similar strength' in isolation, for example, may cloud decision-making, particularly when considering that around 70% of successfully rehabilitated HSIs still demonstrate isokinetic strength deficits of greater than 10% following RTP (Tol et al., 2014). Similarly imaging in isolation, whilst a valuable diagnostic tool, does not demonstrate great value when predicting RTP (De Vos et al., 2014; Reurink et al., 2015). These vagaries have led to an absence of consensus and wide variations in assessment and management between cases and may contribute to the high recurrence rates. In practical terms, no single clinical or physical criterion alone is likely to be specific or sensitive enough to predict a safe RTP. More reliable, perhaps, is the understanding that a battery of clearly defined clinical, gym- and field-based objective markers specific to the individual case, along with subjective player feedback, can offer meaningful insight in a well-constructed RTP rehabilitation plan. These objective markers will be discussed in-depth in this chapter.

Sporting anatomical demands

As a complex biarticular muscle group, the hamstrings' primary function is to flex the knee and/or extend the hip (Petersen and Hölmich, 2005). In performance sport, this group of three (or four when considering the assistance of adductor magnus) muscles are placed under the greatest physical demand whilst sprinting, in comparison to walking and jogging (Schache et al., 2009). Peak eccentric force and stretch occur in the hamstrings during the late swing phase of the gait cycle, as they work eccentrically to control knee extension and oppose the activity of the quadriceps (Schache et al., 2012). At ground contact and during the stance phase, the hamstrings change function, contracting concentrically to extend the hip and propel the body forward, before generating large eccentric forces during deceleration in order to resist forward motion of the trunk (Chumanov et al., 2012; Schache et al., 2012).

Classification of hamstring injuries

Given the demands discussed, it is reasonable to expect that there will be large variations between injury types, location and severity, not to mention the subsequent rehabilitation. At least two distinctly different types of HSIs are discussed within the literature (Brukner, 2012). The more common type I occurs predominantly during high-speed running, whilst the less frequently seen type II tends to occur during loaded lengthening of the muscles, as seen with high kicking and slide tackling and may occur at slower speeds (Askling and Thorstensson, 2008; Woods et al., 2004). Type I injuries usually involve the laterally located long head of biceps femoris at the proximal muscle–tendon junction (MTJ) and commonly recover well. In contrast, type II injuries typically involve the proximal free tendon of the semimembranosis muscle and result in a prolonged recovery (Brukner, 2012). With this in mind, the judicious sports clinician tasked with managing athletes suffering with HSIs should consider how their management plan supports athletes' recovery, given the wide variations in injury type, location, involved tissues and the differing demands of their specific sport and/or playing position.

The importance of adequate rehabilitation

Inadequate rehabilitation is an often-cited reason for the high recurrence rates associated with HSI (De Visser et al., 2012; Wangensteen et al., 2016). The aim of this chapter, therefore, is to offer an evidence-informed, but applied, overview of the key aspects of performance rehabilitation for HSIs. The multivariate nature of HSIs should lead the clinician away from rehabilitation programmes that fail to account for the nuances of the injury, towards an equally multivariate approach. The physical demands of professional football, risk factors associated with HSIs, strength and conditioning approaches to exercise selection and the field-based demands of performance rehabilitation will all be discussed. Considering this overview, the authors aim to stimulate the reader into critiquing and evolving their current practice, in order to return their athletes to field with the capability to perform at elite level.

Creating a performance-enhancement environment

There is no perfect rehab. A wise clinician can expect to compromise when agreeing RTP timeframes, adapt to unrealistic demands from players, managers and stakeholders, cope with the pressures of working in an elite sporting environment and be prepared for scenarios such as setbacks throughout the rehabilitation period and early recurrence of the injury upon RTP. We, as a group of authors, take the view that clinicians should relish these adverse situations and use them as an opportunity to improve their clinical practice. This chapter critiques current research and expert opinions and discusses the aspects that we feel are imperative to prepare athletes to physically and psychologically tolerate the attritional demands of professional football. Fundamental to performance rehabilitation is the notion that rehabilitation sessions are intentionally designed to cater for the most demanding match-day scenarios. By adopting this methodology, athletes are enabled to adapt to unexpected stressors during competition, are robust enough to cope with 60 games over a 10-month period and have developed a resiliency through ultra-preparedness during the rehabilitation journey.

Performance-enhancing rehabilitation philosophy

Below are listed the main tenets that underpin this rehabilitation philosophy.

Improving athletic ability

Time spent while recovering from injury is time that can be effectively used to address deficits that cannot be addressed or are difficult to target inseason. Every athlete has areas to improve – human performance has not yet reached its genetic ceiling.

Reducing risk of future injury

Injury recurrence is rife in professional sport; therefore an important aspect of performance rehabilitation is to mitigate the risk of reinjury upon RTP. Given the high loads associated with football performance, efficacious rehab incorporates a global approach, targeting most commonly injured areas associated with significant time loss per season, namely hamstring, groin, knee and ankle injuries.

Optimizing athlete engagement

Athlete engagement is crucial when delivering efficacious rehabilitation. This can be facilitated through improving the player's understanding of how rehabilitation translates to a game situation – in effect empowering athletes through education. Rehabilitation strategies should be motivationally sensitive and compliance to the rehabilitation journey can be improved by making the process novel, fun and competitive. The clinician must possess a high level of emotional intelligence to cultivate an effective working relationship where the athlete and the therapist are both creators, managers, programmers and reflective learners (Mulvany and Wilson, 2018). Finally, incorporating outcome measures that are relevant and meaningful to the athlete can improve athlete engagement.

Performance rehabilitation: strength

Developing a variety of hamstring strength qualities

As highlighted in the introduction, HSIs often occur due to excessive peak eccentric forces placed upon them during high-intensity ballistic sporting activities such as sprinting, decelerating, kicking and stretching. Therefore, if a muscle has the strength characteristics to withstand these forces, the likelihood of getting injured is reduced. As a consequence, a well-planned individually prescribed strength training program designed around specificity and progressive overload is fundamental to our rehabilitation philosophy, as it produces the required physiological adaptations within the muscle to reduce the risk of injury. Strength underpins power and power underpins speed, and speed is 'king' in professional soccer.

Principles underpinning hamstring strength rehabilitation philosophy
Specificity

The first fundamental concept we adhere to when designing a strength programme for our athletes is to incorporate specificity to their individual needs and the sport they play. Specificity was first coined as far back as 1945 by DeLorme (1945). In essence, it refers to a method whereby we rehab

the athlete in a specific manner to produce desired specific adaptation, further discussed by Todd et al. (2012), for example implementing Nordics as a stimulus to improve eccentric strength or prescribing high-speed running to improve the athlete's contraction velocity during peak eccentric forces. Playing the game itself is indeed a form of strength training and provides the greatest opportunity to improve sport-specific strength and should play a major role when designing the strength programme.

Progressive overload

In the time-impoverished environment of rehabilitating hamstrings for professional sport, increasing the intensity and/or speed of an exercise, rather than the volume or frequency (number of sessions per week) is generally the most efficient way of applying the principle of 'progressive overload' to achieve improvements in strength qualities (Bruton, 2002). This simply means that we need to continually expose the athlete to a greater stimulus than they are used to (e.g., increasing weight, running at a higher speed, increasing difficulty of the task) throughout the rehab phase and upon their RTP. By applying this principle correctly one can avoid overtraining and maximize the effect of the strength stimulus during their RTP (Bompa and Haff, 2009).

To achieve long-term strength improvements needed to tolerate the demands of competing in nearly 60 games over a season, integrating two basic scientific principles: Hooke's law and Wolff's law is very beneficial indeed. These laws state that if you apply an external load (strength exercise) to a solid object (bone, tendon, ligament or muscle) it will adapt specifically to the imposed demands (specific adaptation to imposed demands – the SAID principle). Therefore, if one is to continually progress the external stimulus (exercise), the object (hamstring) will continue to adapt. However if you fail to progress the stimulus, then not only will strength gains plateau, they will also eventually start to decline (Bruton, 2002). Therefore, given that the time period from onset of injury to RTP is so brief, it is imperative that athletes continue to progress the intensity of their strength programme for at least 4–6 weeks following their RTP. Subsequent to that time period they then begin a new phase: a sustainability strength programme to mitigate future injury risk.

Note: it has been argued that we all have a genetic ceiling for strength capacity. However, few athletes are ever really near their genetic ceiling, especially in team-based sports such as soccer, hence the need to continually progressively load players.

Exercise selection

Exercises are individually prescribed to reflect a player's idiosyncratic needs and are dependent on many factors, a few examples being training status, period of season, injury history, risk analysis of exercise, strength testing results, eccentric profile. Variety of exercises and movement qualities are essential in developing strength to reduce risk of reinjury (Mendiguchia et al., 2017). Exercises such as isometric deadlift pull (Fig. 18.1), single leg Romanian deadlift variations (Figs 18.2 and 18.3), hamstring sliders using slide board (Fig. 18.4), hip thrusts (Fig. 18.5) and Nordics (Fig. 18.6) are some examples we can use.

It is essential to provide variation to challenge the hamstring complex in many ways: perturbation, single leg, double leg, knee dominant, hip dominant and proprioceptively. Variety of stimuli flood this highly dense area rich with information-receiving structures. Nevertheless, research is highly focused on the importance of eccentric strength. Recent studies show that increasing fascicle length may be imperative to successful hamstring rehabilitation although, there is some conflicting evidence in relation to this topic (Bourne et al., 2017; Fukutani and Kurihara, 2015).

Eccentrically lengthening the hamstrings increases fascicle length, cross-sectional area and peak muscle output and is thought to be essential for efficacious rehabilitation of HSIs (Timmins et al., 2016). This intervention has been shown to reduce inseason hamstring injury incidence in many running-based sports (Evans and Williams, 2017; Van Der Horst et al., 2015) as well as increasing performance markers (Clark et al., 2005).

The Nordic is a simple eccentric exercise that can be executed without expensive equipment and requires minimal proficiency. The athlete can work through large ranges of movement at the knee under a steady pace so the muscular time under tension increases. Although used as part of our rehab strategy, Nordics are never used in isolation as the recovering hamstring needs exposure to diverse stimuli to develop immunity for fast-paced soccer game demands.

Our strength programme is shown in Table 18.1.

Explosive strength: plyometrics

As already mentioned, hamstring injuries commonly occur during explosive movements when the muscle in exposed to high-velocity loads. Therefore exposing this muscle group to the explosive actions of plyometric training will help habituate the hamstrings to tolerate hazardous activities by improving their ability to effectively decelerate the limb during high-speed actions. As well as reducing future injury risk there is a strong body of evidence that suggests that plyometric training is also very effective at enhancing speed characteristics such as

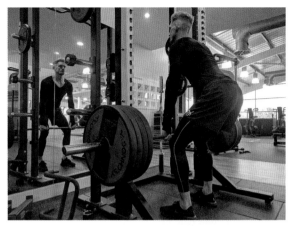

Fig. 18.1 Isometric deadlift pull.

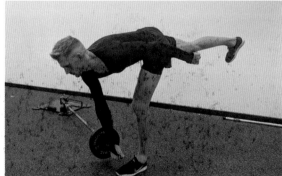

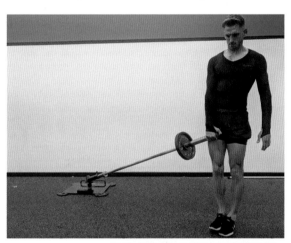

Fig. 18.2 Single leg Romanian deadlift with barbell.

acceleration, maximal velocity and agility (Manouras et al., 2016; Sáez de Villarreal et al., 2015). To run at speed, jump explosively and change direction, players needs to combine horizontal, vertical and lateral forces to generate

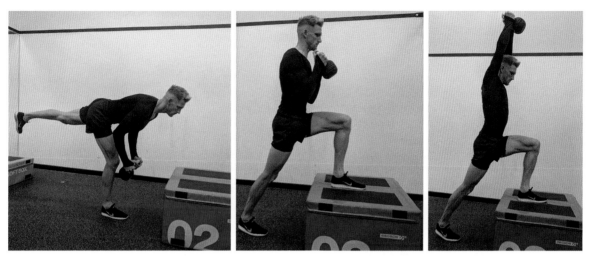

Fig. 18.3 Single leg Romanian deadlift with a knee drive and with overhead press.

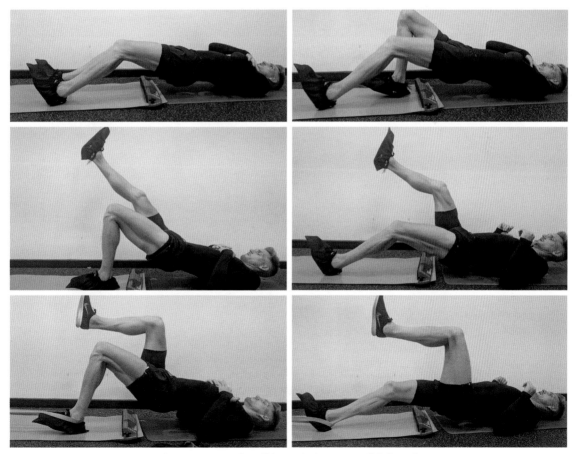

Fig. 18.4 Hamstring slider variations on a slide board.

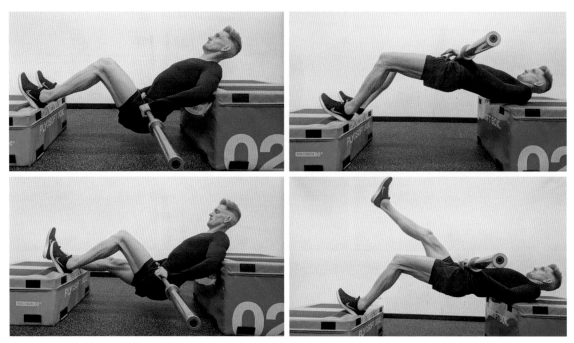

Fig. 18.5 Double leg and single leg hip thrust.

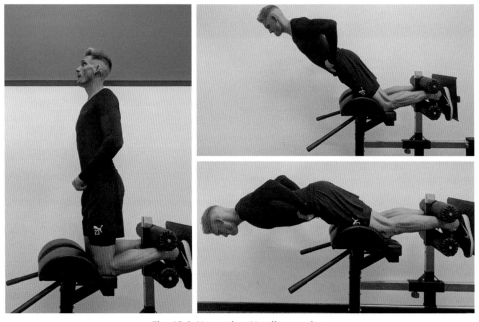

Fig. 18.6 Hamstring Nordic exercise.

Table 18.1 Examples for strength exercise selection

Exercise	Variations	Set range	Rep range	Load range
Focus: Isometrics - Increase peak isometric fibre stress by increasing number of actin–myosin cross-bridges per fibre and strength per cross-bridge. As a consequence this will lead to an increase in maximal voluntary contraction and rate of torque development				
Bridge holds	BW, bilateral, unilateral, inner range, outer range, elevated, resisted, perturbation			
Isometric deadlift pull (Fig. 18.1)	Bilateral, unilateral, mid range, resisted	1–3	6 × 6-s hold	Max contraction
Nordic/glute-ham machine holds	Assisted, BW, resisted, inner range, outer range			
Focus: General strength - Increase muscle cross-sectional area (sarcomeres in parallel) and strength. Improved synchronization of motor unit pattern recruitment and firing. All exercises to be completed through range.				
Bridge variations	BW, bilateral, unilateral, inner range, outer range, elevated, with ankling, resisted			
Reverse lunge	BW, resisted, jammer press, to a step up	1–3	6–8	60–85% 6RM
Split squat variations	BW, resisted, Bulgarian split squat, perturbation			
Focus: Eccentric loading - Increase the number of sarcomeres in series, fascicle length and pennation angle. Eccentric action to be slow and controlled				
RDL	BW, resisted, bilateral, unilateral (Fig. 18.2)	1–3	4–6	60–85% 6RM
Nordic variations	Assisted, unassisted (Fig. 18.3), resisted	1–3	6–10	BW
Slide board eccentrics (Fig. 18.4)	Bilateral, alternate, unilateral, resistance	1–3	8–12	BW to 30% 6RM
Focus: Power - Increase the rate of force development by influencing motor unit activation/recruitment to increase muscle force output				
Hip thrust (Fig. 18.5)	BW, resisted, bilateral, unilateral			
Single leg RDL (Fig. 18.6)	BW, resisted, bilateral, unilateral, with overhead press or rotation knee drive, step up	1–3	4–6	≤30% 6RM
Kettlebell swings	Loaded	1–3	12–20	≤30% 6RM

BW, Bodyweight; *RDL*, Romanian deadlift; *RM*, repetition maximum.

Table 18.2 Examples for plyometric exercise selection

Exercise	Variations	Set range	Rep range	Load range
Focus: Landing mechanics/low-threshold plyometrics. Improving muscle activation strategies and stretch reflex excitability through neuromuscular adaptations to sensory and motor control systems				
Jumps	Hydro, BW, with a turn of various degrees, perturbation	1–3	4–6	BW to 30% 6RM
Leaps	Hydro, BW, perturbation			
SL hop to stick	Hydro, BW, with a turn of various degrees, perturbation			
Triple hop to stick	Hydro, BW			
Drop jump	BW, bilateral, unilateral			
Focus: High-threshold plyometrics. Utilizing stretch–shortening cycle and improving intermuscular coordination to increase rate of force development				
Vertical jump	BW, resisted, eccentrically loaded, combined	1–3	4–6	BW to 30% 6RM
Horizontal jump				
Hurdle jump	Unilateral, multidirectional			
Hurdle hop	BW, bilateral, unilateral, combined, lateral, multidirectional			
Split squat jumps	Switches, Bulgarian split squat, eccentrically loaded, off-the-box split squat jump			
Single leg RDL to single leg box jump	BW, eccentrically loaded, resisted			

BW, bodyweight; *RDL*, Romanian deadlift; *RM*, repetition maximum.

these powerful movements. Therefore, horizontal, vertical and lateral plyometrics form important components of our rehab philosophy.

Low-threshold plyometrics

We start our athletes off by introducing them to low-threshold plyometrics in the pool, which allows us to introduce jumping activities as early as three days postinjury while still respecting the constraints of the healing tissue. Water buoyancy allows for a reduction of gravity acting on the body and reduces weight-bearing and shearing forces through the affected muscle. We progress these activities to land very quickly (usually the next day), where submaximal exercises such as the squat jump, broad jump (jumping forwards), leaps (jumping sideways from one foot to the

other) and single leg hops (jumping and landing on the same leg), are introduced if tolerated by the athlete.

High-threshold plyometrics

The next stage of the rehab is to introduce the player to high-threshold plyometrics with the aim of developing strength, maximal power output and rate of force development to enhance explosive athletic abilities. Research has shown that horizontal plyometric exercises have a greater transference to improving acceleration qualities, whilst vertical plyometrics have more of an effect on maximal velocity performance over 30–40 m (Loturco et al., 2015). Therefore we expose our athletes to a combined stimulus of horizontal and vertical plyometrics throughout their rehabilitation. Ideas for plyometric progressions for hamstring rehab can be seen in Table 18.2.

Performance rehabilitation: importance of lumbopelvic–hip strength

Lumbopelvic–hip complex

Core strength and neuromuscular control are associated with decreased risk of developing a lower limb injury (Willson et al., 2005). The coordinated action of stabilizing and mobilizing muscle groups about the lumbar, pelvic and hip regions enable effective energy transfer throughout the body to allow for optimal movement during activities like running, jumping, changing direction and kicking (De Blaiser et al., 2018). It has also been suggested that weakness about this anatomical region can have a negative effect on lower limb alignment through inability to control hip internal rotation, resulting in knee valgus collapse, which can predispose the player to increased injury risk (Wilkerson and Colston, 2015). Conversely improved neuromuscular control of this region allows for greater control of body position during cutting actions, running and jumping (Zazulak et al., 2007).

Scientific investigation shows that the gluteal muscles, in particular gluteus maximus (GM) (responsible for hip extension) and the superficial trunk muscles – specifically erector spinae (ES), can reduce the risk of hamstring injury (Schuermans et al., 2017) The GM and ES also act as important stabilizers of the hip, especially in single leg stance (Lieberman et al., 2006), providing a stable base for the hamstring to generate meaningful force during hip extension. This is essential for explosive movements vital for success in soccer. Like the hamstrings, GM and ES are designed to absorb and generate a significant amount of force for hip extension so that the total burden of this vital action during running is not solely borne by the hamstrings themselves (Lieberman et al., 2006). In effect, they help stress-shield the hamstring against the high forces associated with high-speed running, sprinting, changing direction powerfully, maximally jumping and forcefully kicking, activities that may otherwise damage the hamstrings. Lumboplevic–hip stability, strength and neuromuscular control play a vital role in hamstring rehabilitation (Chumanov et al., 2007; Huxel Bliven and Anderson, 2013).

Neuromuscular control (NMC) and neurodynamics

For successful RTP elite level athletes need to be able to accomplish complex motor tasks that replicate the demands of the sport. NMC training results in more efficient muscle firing patterns, improved dynamic joint stability and is fundamental to learning or relearning of movement patterns and skills essential for football.

We propose two NMC exercises: windmill (Fig. 18.7) and diver (Fig. 18.8) as key components of hamstring rehabilitation. We incorporate these exercises due to their multijoint and multiplanar nature; they require a whole host of muscle groups to work in unison to link various body parts. Both exercises are highly specific to football and focus on dynamic balance in single leg stance with the aim of improving control when transitioning from triple flexion to triple extension at the hip, knee and ankle. These NMC exercises challenge the athlete in the transverse plane, which is the plane in which most HSIs occur. The athlete is required to control external rotation in a transverse plane when executing said NMC exercises.

Following a hamstring injury, branches of sciatic nerve can become sensitized and as a result can lead to increased neural tension in the posterior chain muscles (Turl and George, 1998). Neurodynamic exercises such as the stability ball neural sliders (Fig. 18.9) facilitate alternate distal and proximal gliding of the neural tissue chain, with the aim of either maintaining or improving neural mobility when moving through myofascial structures.

Performance rehabilitation: running exposure

Typically, professional soccer players in the English Football League will, on average, cover 300–1000 m running at a speed above 6.3 ms^{-1} at intermittent bursts during a game. This has the potential to injure the hamstring muscles (Bradley et al., 2013). Given the hazardous nature of running fast, it is important to expose players to this type of stimulus as early as possible as a 'vaccination' against hamstring injuries, as discussed by Malone et al. (2017). Players are introduced to running as early as day 3 postinjury in the pool, progressing onto land by day 4 (steady-state jog). The intensity and volume of the running is progressed to high-speed running, resisted runs and sprinting as soon as the player is able to tolerate the forces involved with explosive activities. Ideally prior to their return to training, players are exposed to running loads that exceed match demands to ensure they are capable of tolerating the demands of training and playing. However, in the pressurized environment of professional football, this does not always occur and players are returned to training prematurely. Sharp spikes in intensity and volume for high-speed running should be avoided and instead a gradual build-up of running load is needed to effectively transition the player through their rehabilitation. In order to provide the best 'immunity' against reinjury, the aim is to apply an optimal dose of running-based activities. Some of these these activities include:
- pool-based running
- resisted running

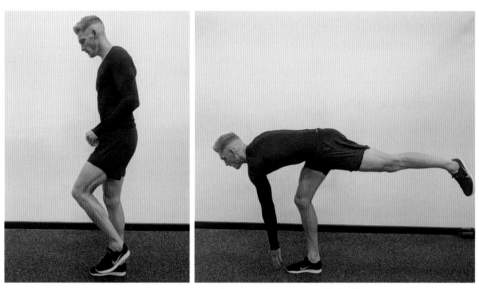

Fig. 18.7 Neuromuscular control exercise: windmill.

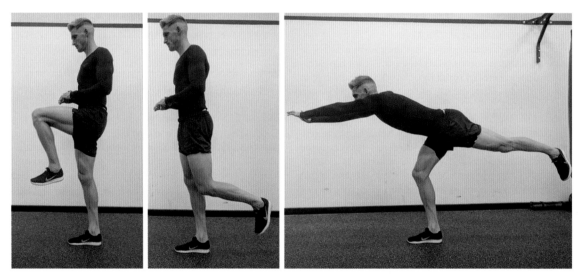

Fig. 18.8 Neuromuscular control exercise: diver.

- assisted running
- explosive change-of-direction running
- high-speed running and sprinting.
  See Fig. 18.10 for an example of our running prescription.

Pool running: the battle with time begins …

The majority of players with hamstring injuries in professional football will generally RTP 18–24 days from initial injury (Dinnery and Wilson, 2018). Immediately upon their RTP they will be expected to run at high speed, repeatedly sprint, change direction at pace, accelerate, decelerate, jump maximally and strike the ball forcefully hundreds upon hundreds of times, not only in games but also in consecutive training sessions. Therefore, their 'RTP stopwatch' starts the moment they clutch the back of their thigh in agony. Clinicians are tasked with the unenviable mission of making the most out of every second to help mastermind a successful transition back into the volatile, high-paced, action-packed arena of professional football within a short period of time.

Hydrotherapy has been conjectured to reduce RTP timescales via a whole host of processes. It allows for the early restoration of function as the natural buoyancy of

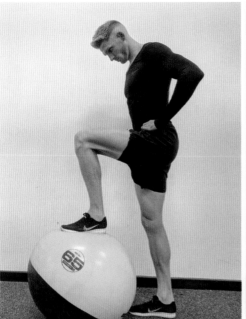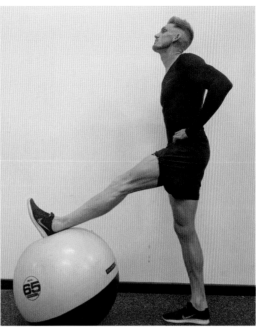

Fig. 18.9 Neurodynamics: stability ball neural sliders.

water reduces the amount of weight-bearing forces through the hamstring, enabling early mobilization and tissue loading to help align newly formed collagen with the existing muscle tissue (Kim and Choi, 2014; Nualon et al., 2013). Gait re-education can begin as early as 48 hours post incident in the pool and systemically, it can be utilized throughout the whole rehabilitation period to maintain $\dot{V}O_{2max}$ levels and improve lactate threshold via swimming (arms only in the early stages).

Pain is very commonly used as a guide for progression through rehabilitation and as such it can act as a significant barrier to progression in rehabilitation. Therefore, we use the pool as early as 24 hours postinjury to help reduce pain levels via the effect of temperature and pressure from the water on thermoreceptors and mechanoreceptors, respectively (Konlian, 1999). This load-optimized environment helps ease the transition to land-based running and jumping, both physically and psychologically.

Resisted runs and how much resistance is enough?

Perhaps the most important parameter in resisted running is the level of load applied to the athlete. High loads can potentially alter running technique and have been theorized to have a negative effect on sprint performance. Petrakos et al. (2016) advocated the use of heavy (20% body mass) sled loads to improve initial acceleration where velocity is slow and resistive forces are high, and a lighter

load (>10% body mass) to improve maximal velocity. Multiple methods of applying resistance exist and consideration for resisted running methods are further discussed in Table 18.3.

Assisted runs

Assisted running can provide a training stimulus to improve maximal speed by utilizing external force to drive the athlete forward where assistance may be provided by elastic cord, resistance band or environmental adaptation, such as running downhill. Assisted running has been proven to be effective in increasing maximal running speed and acceleration. Salient literature recommends a slope of 3.4–5.8 degrees as optimal to develop this quality (Ebben et al., 2008). The assistance when using any of the methods allows the athlete to achieve faster acceleration to peak speed through gravitational or externally applied force. The increase in acceleration and running speed may be a consequence of increased stride length and frequency while performing assisted running and through athlete exposure to supramaximal running.

Change of direction and agility

During a soccer game players are exposed to cognitively challenging scenarios that require fast movement and change of direction (COD) in response to various stimuli in and out of ball possession. The ability to accelerate,

Example plan for running progressions

Type of stimulus	Frequency	Progression criteria				
		Phase 1	Phase 2	Phase 3	Phase 4	Running based RTT
Hydrotherapy	2–3 sessions	Gradual build up to 8mins continuous run.		Later stages – used as recovery modality		
Jogging 7.2–14.3 km/h	3–4x week	Jog/walk 30secs on/off 2x8				
Running 14.4–19.7 km/h	3–4x week	Jog/walk 1min 1:1 W:R ratio x8 (4mins x 3–4; 1mins rest)	20secs 1:1 W:R ratio 8x2 (3mins rest)	30secs 1:1 W:R ratio 8x2 (4mins rest)		
HSR 19.8–25.1 km/h	3x week			<22secs pitch length 8x2	<20secs pitch length 10x2; 1:1 W:R ratio	<18secs pitch length 10x2; 1:1 W:R ratio
Sprinting > 25.1 km/h	2x week				Sprints 10m x4, 20m; Full recovery	Sprint 30m 2x4; GPS ≥95% max velocity; 1:1 W:R ratio
Resisted runs: sled	1–2x week			Sled run 10% BW 15m 2x4; Sled run 20% BW 5m 2x6; Recovery 60secs	Sled run 15% BW 15m x4; Sled run 25% BW 5m x4; Recovery 45secs	Sled run 15% BW 15m 2x4; Sled run 25% BW 15m 2x4; Recovery 45secs
Asisted runs: decline run	1–2x week		1x3x15m	1x3x20m	1x3x25m to a 10m deceleration	1x3x25m to a 5m deceleration
Change of direction	3x week	e.g., slalom run, turning on a curve, lateral shuffle 1x4x10m	e.g., cutting, 90° turn 1x4x10m; 180° turn (half pitch/full pitch); progression cones every 20–10m	e.g., acceleration/deceleration drills + turning in multiple planes, various angles; ('Y','L','T' and 'zig-zag', 'modified 505' test variations (2–3drills per session) 1–2x4 1:1 W:R ratio	Reactive agility drills – introduction of cognitive components and ball work e.g. 'shadows', 'cone field drills (2–3 drills per session) 1–2x4 1:1 W:R ratio; Agility drills – incorporation of sprinting (2–3 drills per session) 1–2x4 (recovery <60secs)	Sport/position-specific agility drills e.g 1v1, turn/receive under pressure (recovery <60secs)
Repeated sprints	2x week					5x6secs max sprint; GPS ≥95% max velocity

Warm up: Sport-specific warm up + running mechanics, marching, bounding, skipping variations

Subjectively: asymptomatic OR able to complete with minimal symptoms not affecting task

Guidelines for progressions	Phase 1	Phase 2	Phase 3	Phase 4	Running based RTT
	Normal running gait				
	Able to tolerate low pace Introduction to COD activities	Able to tolerate turning at various angles	Able to tolerate fast-paced multidirectional tasks	COD test score within 10% of baseline	During rehab session cover distance corresponding to distances covered during the game for: total distance, high-speed running and sprinting (GPS data)
	Able to complete bridge matrix : double and single leg, inner range	Able to complete bridge matrix : double and single leg outer range	SL elevated bridge >30 reps and within 20% LSI	SL elevated bridge >30 reps and within 10% LSI	Able to tolerate sport specific/position-specific drills replicating game demands
	AKE within 10% LSI		Isometric SL HS strength test-blood pressure cuff; score within 10% LSI	SL power scores within 10% LSI	Achieve >90% of max velocity from baseline data

Transition through the rehab stages is always athlete led and decisions about moving forward or remaining in the current phase comes down to athlete's mental readiness. Athlete should be given enough information about progression guidelines to allow them to make informed decisions about their rehabilitation process. Physical outcome measures alone are insignificant if athlete is not psychologically ready to advance in their rehabilitation journey.

AKE, Active knee extension; BW, body weight; COD, change of direction; GPS, global positioning system; HS, hamstring; HSR, high-speed running; LSI, limb symmetry index; RTP, return-to-play; RTT, return to training; SL, single leg; W:R ratio, work to rest ratio.

Fig. 18.10 Example plan for running progression.

Table 18.3 Resisted running method considerations

Method	Load (% BW)	Drawbacks	Aim
Rationale: Creating overload and increasing lower limb strength as well maximizing propulsion forces during initial stages of sprint; promoting forward lean and greater hip, knee and ankle flexion degree; developing strength endurance and power; improving anaerobic qualities			
Resistance band/ elastic cord	Resistance applied should allow athlete to propel forward with a forward lean and complete moderate speed run without negatively affecting running mechanics	Hard to objectively quantify the load applied Relying on band and on resistance applied by person holding the resistance band	To improve acceleration and maximal velocity
Weighted vest	8–20% BW	May negatively affect running mechanics; reduced hip extension Forward lean may be avoided by athlete (centre of mass translated anteriorly during forward lean with vest may put athlete off-balance)	
Parachute	Size depending on athlete's BW and environmental conditions, e.g., wind if completing runs outdoors	Hard to control load applied, parachute size vs. athlete's BW vs. environment. Larger distance runs only to allow parachute to open fully	
Sled runs	>20% BW	May negatively affect running mechanics if load used is too high	To improve initial acceleration
	10–20% BW		To improve max velocity

BW, Bodyweight.

decelerate and change direction at speed through a series of movements in multiple planes and in response to a stimulus is defined as agility (Sheppard and Young, 2006). These explosive moments can decide the outcome of the game, e.g., beating an opponent to the ball in a goal-scoring opportunity. More often than not, these explosive activities are also the aetiology for many HSIs. Therefore agility is a highly important component of performance in soccer and a significant risk factor for HSI. Improving an athlete's agility performance forms an integral part of our HSI rehabilitation philosophy.

Deceleration and turning

For effective COD, athletes need to possess the ability to decelerate and break rapidly. Athletes who can decelerate quickly will also be able to change direction quickly, as deceleration directly influences the time needed to redirect the force to a new plane of movement. This allows the

athlete to be a step ahead of and dominate their opponent. High-velocity COD movements are generated by GM while the short external rotators work to stabilize the hip joint. With one foot planted and the hip in a stable position, the action from the contralateral external rotators of the hip (predominantly GM) allows for efficient combination of extension and rotational movement creating a cutting and propulsion action; a COD during running (Neumann, 2010). Eccentric hamstring strength seems to be a key performance predictor to decelerate effectively (Naylor and Greig, 2015). For COD activities, the lateral hamstring muscles (biceps femoris) play a major role in propelling the athlete forward by their ability to produce high horizontal ground reaction forces (Morin et al., 2015).

During deceleration movements we adopt more of an erect posture and posterior lean, which moves the centre of mass posteriorly in relation to base of support allowing for generation of greater horizontal breaking forces (Dintiman and Ward, 2003). The hip and knee flexion and ankle dorsiflexion during deceleration help dissipate the eccentric impact force. The foot strikes the ground with the heel to prolong the ground contact time, resisting the forward momentum of the body. During this end-stage braking action, all the muscles of the lower limb are working eccentrically to absorb and disperse the load through the lower limb (Hewit et al., 2011). During soccer games, players are completing these activities repetitively for a duration of 90 minutes or more; they need to possess great 'braking' abilities to withstand high external forces and maintain joint stability through the series of explosive actions.

Acceleration

Soccer players require great acceleration capacity; research suggests that the hamstring muscles play a significant role in the acceleration phase of sprinting, as the horizontal ground reaction force during sprint accelerations is associated with greater biceps femoris activation prior to ground contact and eccentric knee flexor peak torque necessary to propel the athlete forward (Morin et al., 2015). This provides the rationale for its inclusion during rehabilitation. Body position during the acceleration phase of running is adjusted to allow for the production of greater horizontal forces and to maximize propulsion (Morin et al., 2015). These adaptations include a forward lean, a preference for forefoot ground contact (minimizing braking), powerful arm movements (balancing angular momentum of the legs) and minimal flight time (as more time in air will lead to a decrease in velocity) as discussed by Hewit et al. (2011), Dintiman and Ward (2003) and Kreighbaum and Barthels (1996). More specifically to hamstrings and their contribution to the acceleration phase of sprinting, research has shown that individuals who are capable of generating high-level horizontal ground reaction forces possess high torque production capacity for hip extension and highest hamstring electromyographic activity during the end-of-swing phase of acceleration sprint (Morin et al., 2015). The hamstring muscle group also contribute to a net transfer of power from proximal to distal joints during explosive leg extension (Jacobs et al., 1993) directly influencing the energy transfer through the kinetic chain.

Implementing acceleration drills in rehab will challenge hamstrings to produce this high-intensity action. A gradual increase in intensity and volume is required to prepare an athlete for the repeated acceleration sprints they will be exposed to upon RTP. Accelerations in soccer are not solely initiated from a stationary position, therefore the athlete needs to have an ability to complete a 'moving' start acceleration, where they change the plane of movement through a series of multiplanar actions at various speeds.

Agility

Agility training forms an integral role during performance rehabilitation. The focus of this intervention is to develop the connection between the physical and psychological systems necessary to carry out complex multidirectional tasks in response to a stimulus with the aim of improving the mind–body connection when processing signals and cues from the environment (Sheppard and Young, 2006). Challenging an athlete's mental processing speed during sport-specific tasks reinforces reaction learning and allows them to initiate movement faster and/or with the most appropriate timing to achieve the best outcome (Pojskic et al., 2018). To influence the perceptual and decision-making components of agility, reactive drills, small sided games or 1v1s can help to reduce the total response time, by influencing the time needed to react to a stimulus (processing of the sensory input) and duration of time needed to perform the movement (motor-control response) (Serpell et al., 2011; Young et al., 2015; Young and Rogers, 2014). For a more in-depth discussion on how to train agility, see Chapter 33.

High-speed running and sprinting

High-speed running (HSR) and sprinting accounts for 8–12% of total running distance covered in soccer, with 90% of all sprints not exceeding a 5-s in duration. Forward players having significantly greater exposure to HSR and sprinting throughout the game (Andrzejewski et al., 2013; Bradley et al., 2013). Every 3–5 s during a soccer match, players are exposed to ~1200 unpredictable changes in activity, which include multiple sprints, tackles and jumps (Mohr et al., 2003), turns (Bloomfield et al., 2007) and various other explosive actions such as kicking and dribbling. Healing hamstring muscles need a gradual build-up of running intensity exposure to progress to high-speed running and sprinting where the majority of hamstring injuries occur (Askling et al., 2007).

HSR exposure, especially under fatigue, is an important component of end-stage hamstring rehabilitation as research indicates that fatigue may reduce hip flexion and knee extension angles as well increase anterior pelvic tilt during late swing phase, which in turn may increase the strain on the hamstrings during running (Small et al., 2009).

Return to play

The rehabilitation process does not end when the athlete declares fit and returns to training and competition. Monitoring HSR exposure on a weekly basis, ensuring the player completes HSR drills (>95% max velocity) will help mitigate against future hamstring injury occurrence (Malone et al., 2017). Due to variability of match and training demands, players may not always achieve sufficient exposure to HSR during these activities; therefore it is important to introduce drills that allow athletes to reach their top-end speed

Table 18.4 Considerations for hamstring injury outcome measures upon return to play

Clinical testing			
No tenderness to palpation	Asymptomatic on slump	Straight leg raise R = L Asymptomatic	Active knee extension R = L
Strength-based testing			
Bridge matrix: Inner range DL and SL Outer range DL and SL	Isometric hamstring strength: (blood pressure cuff) within 10% LSI General strength: Reverse Lunge 3 × 6 (75% 1RM) SL elevated bridge 3 × 6 (75% 1RM) or SL elevated bridge max reps >30 within 10% LSI	Eccentric strength: Nordic 3 × 6 with 10-kg weight Weighted hamstring slider 3 × 8 (75% 1RM)	Explosive strength: SL hip thrust 3 × 6 (30% 1RM) Countermovement jump DL and SL or vertical jump test within 10% LSI Triple hop for distance within 10% LSI
Field-based testing			
Sprint time in comparison to baseline: 10 m 30 m Tolerate 2 weeks of full squad training before RTP	COD test time in comparison to baseline: Modified 5-0-5 test T-test	Repeated sprint ability: 6 × 6 max sprints with 24 s recovery between each sprint and achieve fatigue index of 85%+	Maximal aerobic speed: Distance covered in comparison to baseline match data 1600-m MAS test GPS achieve 130% of HSR in 3 rehab sessions prior to RTP
Lumbopelvic–hip stability and neuromuscular control			
Deadbug 20 reps with 20-kg weight	Maintain stability during: windmill, diver, SEBT using single-leg loading qualitative assessment tool (QASLS)		

Most tests will be compared against baseline data (if available) or uninvolved limb test result.
COD, Change of direction; *DL*, double leg; *GPS*, global positioning system; *HSR*, high-speed running; *LSI*, limb symmetry index; *MAS*, maximal aerobic speed; *QASLS*, qualitative analysis of single leg squat; *RM*, repetition maximum; *RTP*, return to play; *SEBT*, star excursion balance test; *SL*, single leg.
Useful tools for objective strength measurements: Norbord®, hand held dynamometer, isokinetic testing.

regularly to maintain the adaptations achieved through rehab. We also recommend this approach as an injury risk–mitigation strategy for all players, with or without a history of hamstring injury. Athletes need regular exposure to HSR which replicate the demands that they will encounter on the pitch; tolerating sprinting in a fatigued state provides effective translation from rehab to competition.

Outcome measures

Outcome measures can help determine a player's readiness to return to competition. RTP testing may vary from clinician to clinician based on available resources and time constraints (Zambaldi et al., 2017). Athletes should be given sufficient information about progression guidelines and objective criteria to allow them to make informed decisions. Physical outcome measures alone are not meaningful if the athlete is not psychologically ready to return to competition. Multiple outcome measures should be considered when returning to play post–hamstring injury to minimize the chances of reinjury. See Fig. 18.10 and Table 18.4 for how we use objective markers as part of our running progression and for RTP outcome measures.

Conclusion

Performance rehabilitation aims to prepare athletes both physically and psychologically by creating a flexible rehab environment catering for individual athletes' needs. To date, there is still no consensus for assessment, rehabilitation and RTP criteria for HSIs. The architectural complexity of hamstrings and the increasing demands athletes place on this muscle group create a challenge for clinicians attempting to safely return their athletes to play.

Effective hamstring rehabilitation needs to be multimodal in nature to replicate game demands, with the 'RTP stopwatch' being switched on the moment injury occurs. Well-planned individually prescribed multimodal programmes designed around specificity and progressive overload is fundamental to our rehabilitation philosophy. A wide spectrum of exercises needs to be considered to cater for individual athletes' needs and there is no one prescription that fits all. Eccentric strength profile as well as exposure to high-speed running are two significant components when treating HSIs. However, many more sub components need to be targeted for successful and safe RTP following HSI and as clinicians we need to be able to adapt and cope with setbacks, recurrences and unusual cases.

The goal of performance rehabilitation is to build the athletes' physical and mental resilience, improve athletic ability, mitigate future injury risk and optimize engagement. No single intervention or clinical or physical outcome measure is likely to be specific or sensitive enough to predict a safe RTP – given the hazardous nature of soccer – and a battery of clinical, gym- and field-based objective markers specific to the individual, along with subjective player feedback, can offer more meaningful information when making RTP decisions.

Acknowledgements

This author group would like to acknowledge contributions from Andy Mitchell of Blackburn Rovers FC, Mike Edwards of Notts County FC, Simon Mulvany, Dave Orton of Leicester Tigers RFC and Lee Taylor of Peterborough United FC in the writing this chapter.

References

Andrzejewski, M., Chmura, J., Pluta, B., Strzelczyk, R., Kasprzak, A., 2013. Analysis of sprinting activities of professional soccer players. Journal of Strength and Conditioning Research 27, 2134–2140.

Askling, C.M., Tengvar, M., Saartok, T., Thorstensson, A., 2007. Acute first-time hamstring strains during high-speed running: a longitudinal study including clinical and magnetic resonance imaging findings. American Journal of Sports Medicine 35 (2), 197–206.

Askling, C., Thorstensson, A., 2008. Hamstring muscle strain in sprinters. N. Stud. Athl. 23, 67–79.

Bloomfield, J., Polman, R., O'Donoghue, P., 2007. Physical demands of different positions in FA premier League soccer. Journal of Sports Science and Medicine 6 (1), 63–70.

Bompa, T.O., Haff, G.G., 2009. Periodization: Theory and Methodology of Training, fifth ed. Human Kinetics, Champaign, Il, pp. 259–286.

Bourne, M.N., Duhig, S.J., Timmins, R.G., Williams, M.D., Opar, D.A., Al Najjar, A., et al., 2017. Impact of the Nordic hamstring and hip extension exercises on hamstring architecture and morphology: implications for injury prevention. British Journal of Sports Medicine 51 (5), 469–477.

Bradley, P.S., Carling, C., Diaz, A.G., Hood, P., Barnes, C., Ade, J., et al., 2013. Match performance and physical capacity of players in the top three competitive standards of English professional soccer. Human Movement Science 32, 808–821.

Brukner, P., 2012. Brukner & Khan's Clinical Sports Medicine. McGraw-Hill, North Ryde, Australia.

Bruton, A., 2002. Muscle plasticity: response to training and detraining. Physiotherapy 88 (7), 398–408.

Chumanov, E.S., Schache, A.G., Heiderscheit, B.C., Thelen, D.G., 2012. Hamstrings are most susceptible to injury during the late swing phase of sprinting. British Journal of Sports Medicine 46 (2), 90.

Chumanov, E.S., Heiderscheit, B.C., Thelen, D.G., 2007. The effect of speed and influence of individual muscles on hamstring mechanics during the swing phase of sprinting. Journal of Biomechanics 40 (16), 3555–3562.

Clark, R., Bryant, A., Culgan, J.-P., Hartley, B., 2005. The effects of eccentric hamstring strength training on dynamic jumping performance and isokinetic strength parameters: a pilot study on the implications for the prevention of hamstring injuries. Physical Therapy in Sport 6, 67–73.

De Blaiser, C., Roosen, P., Willems, T., Danneels, L., Bossche, L.V., De Ridder, R., 2018. Is core stability a risk factor for lower extremity injuries in an athletic population? A systematic review. Physical Therapy in Sport 30, 48–56.

De Visser, H., Reijman, M., Heijboer, M., Bos, P., 2012. Risk factors of recurrent hamstring injuries: a systematic review. British Journal of Sports Medicine 46, 124–130.

De Vos, R.J., Reurink, G., Goudswaard, G.J., Moen, M.H., Weir, A., Tol, J.L., 2014. Clinical findings just after return to play predict hamstring re-injury, but baseline MRI findings do not. British Journal of Sports Medicine 48 (18), 1377–1384.

Delorme, T.L., 1945. Restoration of muscle power by heavy-resistance exercises. Journal of Bone and Joint Surgery 27, 645–667.

Dinnery, B., Wilson, J., 2018. Return to Play Timeframes Following Hamstring Injury in the Premier League. www.premierinjuries.com/betting.php?.

Dintiman, G., Ward, B., 2003. Starting and stopping. In: Sports Speed, third ed. Human Kinetics, Champaign, IL, pp. 212–217.

Ebben, W.P., Davies, J.A., Clewien, R.W., 2008. Effect of the degree of hill slope on acute downhill running velocity and acceleration. Journal of Strength and Conditioning Research 22, 898–902.

Ekstrand, J., Hägglund, M., Kristenson, K., Magnusson, H., Waldén, M., 2013. Fewer ligament injuries but no preventive effect on muscle injuries and severe injuries: an 11-year follow-up of the UEFA Champions League injury study. British Journal of Sports Medicine 47, 732–737.

Evans, K., Williams, M., 2017. The effect of Nordic hamstring exercise on hamstring injury in professional rugby union. British Journal of Sports Medicine 51, 316–317.

Fukutani, A., Kurihara, T., 2015. Comparison of the muscle fascicle length between resistance-trained and untrained individuals: cross-sectional observation. SpringerPlus 4, 341.

Hewit, J., Cronin, J., Button, C., Hume, P., 2011. Understanding deceleration in sport. Strength and Conditioning Journal 33 (1), 47–52.

Huxel Bliven, K.C., Anderson, B.E., 2013. Core stability training for injury prevention. Sports Health 5 (6), 514–522.

Jacobs, R., Bobbert, M.F., van Ingen Schenau, G.J., 1993. Function of mono- and biarticular muscles in running. Medicine & Science in Sports & Exercise 25 (10), 1163–1173.

Kim, E., Choi, H., 2014. Aquatic physical therapy in the rehabilitation of athletic injuries: a systematic review of the literatures. Journal of Yoga and Physical Therapy 5.

Konlian, C., 1999. Aquatic therapy: making a wave in the treatment of low back injuries. Journal of Orthopaedic Nursing 3, 181.

Kreighbaum, E., Barthels, K.M., 1996. Biomechanics: A Qualitative Approach for Studying Human Movement. Allyn and Bacon, Boston, MA.

Lieberman, D.E., Raichlen, D.A., Pontzer, H., Bramble, D.M., Cutright-Smith, E., 2006. The human gluteus maximus and its role in running. Journal of Experimental Biology 209 (Pt 11), 2143–2155.

Loturco, I., Pereira, L.A., Kobal, R., Zanetti, V., Kitamura, K., Abad, C.C.C., et al., 2015. Transference effect of vertical and horizontal plyometrics on sprint performance of high-level U-20 soccer players. Journal of Sports Sciences 33, 2182–2191.

Malone, S., Roe, M., Doran, D.A., Gabbett, T.J., Collins, K., 2017. High chronic training loads and exposure to bouts of maximal velocity running reduce injury risk in elite Gaelic football. Journal of Science and Medicine in Sport 20, 250–254.

Manouras, N., Papanikolaou, Z., Karatrantou, K., Kouvarakis, P., Gerodimos, V., 2016. The efficacy of vertical vs. horizontal plyometric training on speed, jumping performance and agility in soccer players. International Journal of Sports Science & Coaching 11, 702–709.

Mendiguchia, J., Martinez-Ruiz, E., Edouard, P., Morin, J.-B., Martinez-Martinez, F., Idoate, F., et al., 2017. A multifactorial, criteria-based progressive algorithm for hamstring injury treatment. Medicine & Science in Sports & Exercise 49, 1482–1492.

Mohr, M., Krustrup, P., Bangsbo, J., 2003. Match performance of high-standard soccer players with special reference to development of fatigue. Journal of Sports Sciences 21, 519–528.

Morin, J.-B., Gimenez, P., Edouard, P., Arnal, P., Jiménez-Reyes, P., Samozino, P., et al., 2015. Sprint acceleration mechanics: the major role of hamstrings in horizontal force production. Frontiers in Physiology 6, 404.

Mulvany, S.T., Wilson, J., 2018. Complex-Adaptive Modeling in Sports Science & Sports Medicine. https://wilsonmulvany.wordpress.com/2018/10/18/model-number-1-neuromuscular-systems-conditioning-nsc-advantaged-stacked-over-preparedness-for-sport-specific-demand/

Naylor, J., Greig, M., 2015. A hierarchical model of factors influencing a battery of agility tests. Journal of Sports Medicine and Physical Fitness 55, 1329–1335.

Neumann, D.A., 2010. Kinesiology of the hip: a focus on muscular actions. Journal of Orthopaedic & Sports Physical Therapy 40, 82–94.

Nualon, P., Piriyaprasarth, P., Yuktanandana, P., 2013. The role of 6-week hydrotherapy and land-based therapy plus ankle taping in a preseason rehabilitation program for athletes with chronic ankle instability. Asian Biomedicine 7, 553–559.

Orchard, J.W., Seward, H., Orchard, J.J., 2013. Results of 2 decades of injury surveillance and public release of data in the Australian Football League. American Journal of Sports Medicine 41, 734–741.

Petersen, J., Hölmich, P., 2005. Evidence based prevention of hamstring injuries in sport. British Journal of Sports Medicine 39, 319–323.

Petrakos, G., Morin, J.-B., Egan, B., 2016. Resisted sled sprint training to improve sprint performance: a systematic review. Sports Medicine 46, 381–400.

Pojskic, H., Åslin, E., Krolo, A., Jukic, I., Uljevic, O., Spasic, M., et al., 2018. Importance of reactive agility and change of direction speed in differentiating performance levels in junior soccer players: reliability and validity of newly developed soccer-specific tests. Frontiers in Physiology 9, 506.

Reurink, G., Whiteley, R., Tol, J.L., 2015. Hamstring injuries and predicting return to play: 'bye-bye MRI?' British Journal of Sports Medicine 49 (18), 1162–1163.

Sáez De Villarreal, E., Suarez-Arrones, L., Requena, B., Haff, G.G., Ferrete, C., 2015. Effects of plyometric and sprint training on physical and technical skill performance in adolescent soccer players. Journal of Strength and Conditioning Research 29, 1894–1903.

Schache, A.G., Dorn, T.W., Blanch, P.D., Brown, N.A., Pandy, M.G., 2012. Mechanics of the human hamstring muscles during sprinting. Medicine & Science in Sports & Exercise 44, 647–658.

Schache, A.G., Wrigley, T.V., Baker, R., Pandy, M.G., 2009. Biomechanical response to hamstring muscle strain injury. Gait Posture 29, 332–338.

Schuermans, J., Van Tiggelen, D., Witvrouw, E., 2017. Prone hip extension muscle recruitment is associated with hamstring injury risk in amateur soccer. International Journal of Sports Medicine 38, 696–706.

Serpell, B.G., Young, W.B., Ford, M., 2011. Are the perceptual and decision-making components of agility trainable? A preliminary investigation. Journal of Strength and Conditioning Research 25 (5), 1240–1248.

Sheppard, J.M., Young, W.B., 2006. Agility literature review: classifications, training and testing. Journal of Sports Sciences 24, 919–932.

Small, K., Mcnaughton, L., Greig, M., Lohkamp, M., Lovell, R., 2009. Soccer fatigue, sprinting and hamstring injury risk. International Journal of Sports Medicine 30, 573.

Timmins, R.G., Bourne, M.N., Shield, A.J., Williams, M.D., Lorenzen, C., Opar, D.A., 2016. Short biceps femoris fascicles and eccentric knee flexor weakness increase the risk of hamstring injury in elite football (soccer): a prospective cohort study. British Journal of Sports Medicine 50 (24), 1524–1535.

Todd, J.S., Shurley, J.P., Todd, T.C., 2012. Thomas L. DeLorme and the science of progressive resistance exercise. Journal of Strength and Conditioning Research 26, 2913–2923.

Tol, J.L., Hamilton, B., Eirale, C., Muxart, P., Jacobsen, P., Whiteley, R., 2014. At return to play following hamstring injury the majority of professional football players have residual isokinetic deficits. British Journal of Sports Medicine 48 (18), 1364–1369.

Turl, S.E., George, K.P., 1998. Adverse neural tension: a factor in repetitive hamstring strain? Journal of Orthopaedic & Sports Physical Therapy 27, 16–21.

Van Der Horst, N., Backx, F., Goedhart, E.A., Huisstede, B.M., 2017. Return to play after hamstring injuries in football (soccer): a worldwide Delphi procedure regarding definition, medical criteria and decision-making. British Journal of Sports Medicine 51 (22), 1583–1591.

Van Der Horst, N., Smits, D.-W., Petersen, J., Goedhart, E.A., Backx, F.J.G., 2015. The preventive effect of the Nordic hamstring exercise on hamstring injuries in amateur soccer players: a randomized controlled trial. American Journal of Sports Medicine 43, 1316–1323.

Wangensteen, A., Tol, J.L., Witvrouw, E., Van Linschoten, R., Almusa, E., Hamilton, B., et al., 2016. Hamstring reinjuries occur at the same location and early after return to sport: a descriptive study of MRI-confirmed reinjuries. American Journal of Sports Medicine 44, 2112–2121.

Wilkerson, G.B., Colston, M.A., 2015. A refined prediction model for core and lower extremity sprains and strains among collegiate football players. Journal of Athletic Training 50, 643–650.

Willson, J.D., Dougherty, C.P., Ireland, M.L., Davis, I.M., 2005. Core stability and its relationship to lower extremity function and injury. JAAOS - Journal of the American Academy of Orthopaedic Surgeons 13, 316–325.

Woods, C., Hawkins, R., Maltby, S., Hulse, M., Thomas, A., Hodson, A., 2004. The Football Association Medical Research Programme: an audit of injuries in professional football—analysis of hamstring injuries. British Journal of Sports Medicine 38, 36–41.

Young, W., Rogers, N., 2014. Effects of small-sided game and change-of-direction training on reactive agility and change-of-direction speed. Journal of Sports Sciences 32 (4), 307–314.

Young, W.B., Dawson, B., Henry, G.J., 2015. Agility and change-of-direction speed are independent skills: implications for training for agility in invasion sports. International Journal of Sports Science and Coaching 10 (1), 159–169.

Zambaldi, M., Beasley, I., Rushton, A., 2017. Return to play criteria after hamstring muscle injury in professional football: a Delphi consensus study. British Journal of Sports Medicine 51 (16), 1221–1226.

Zazulak, B.T., Hewett, T.E., Reeves, N.P., Goldberg, B., Cholewicki, J., 2007. Deficits in neuromuscular control of the trunk predict knee injury risk:prospective biomechanical-epidemiologic study. American Journal of Sports Medicine 35, 1123–1130.

Chapter | 19 |

The management of gastrocnemius and soleus muscle tears in professional footballers

Paul Godfrey, Mike Beere and James Rowland

Introduction

It is beyond the scope of this chapter to discuss all causes of calf pain in the professional football player. Instead we discuss common calf injuries seen within this population and that is the strain or tear to the soleus and gastrocnemius muscles. There is a paucity of research relating to these types of injuries within the elite sport setting and even less relating to professional football. Of the research that can be found on the subject (Dixon, 2009; Pedret et al., 2015), there are none that would be considered of a high-quality research design, i.e., double-blind randomized controlled trials, and therefore much that has been written should perhaps be viewed with considerable caution.

The authors, who work at the 'coal face' in professional football and other elite sports, have treated many calf muscle injuries over the years and have successfully reduced such injuries over the course of a professional football season(s). This chapter, therefore, represents many years of combined experience, during which the authors have trialled various approaches to the management of calf muscle tears. The authors present what works from these various approaches and have outlined here a comprehensive management strategy. The case studies given later in the text show examples of how elements of this strategy work when applied to an individual's circumstances.

This chapter also covers when to expect such injuries during a season, the possible causes of such injuries – including the commonly considered 'myths' and the poor rehabilitation that results from such myths. An approach to the assessment and rehabilitation of these muscle tears using tried and tested methods as utilized by the authors is presented. The chapter clarifies the meaning of such terms

as 'load', 'overload' and 'load management' and aim to give the reader a better understanding of what each of these terms means in the context of calf tears. The text analyses what these engineering terms really mean and why they should not be confused with the now-common concept within the sport science profession of acute versus chronic load.

The chapter looks at what the reported differences are in anatomy, muscle fibres and function of each muscle, and if such differences do exist, how rehabilitation should differ for each muscle and different training methods applied.

Finally, the authors also discuss how the professional football environment and the pressures placed on the players and staff working in the field often influences the use of radiological imaging, the rehabilitation process and ultimately the effectiveness of such rehab. In reality an 'ideal approach' to rehabilitating soleus and gastrocnemius tears such as discussed in this chapter is not always possible, much to the detriment of all concerned.

Stress/strain concept

Any clinician who has studied muscle physiology will be familiar with the engineering concept of stress/strain and the curve that depicts how human tissue responds to any given *force* or *load*, i.e., how tissue lengthens or compresses to tolerate a weight that is placed upon it (Fig. 19.1).

Every tissue in the body (e.g., ligament, tendon, muscle, bone) has properties that are common to all tissues – the properties of *elasticity* and *plasticity*. Elasticity relates to a tissue's ability to stretch (or compress) under loading and return to its original state when the load is removed (denoted by the black line A to B in Fig. 19.1). Plasticity

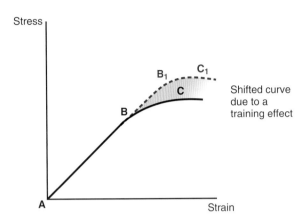

A–B: Elastic properties
B–C: Plastic properties
Beyond C: Tissue failure/rupture
- - - - : Denotes increased elasticity (A–B₁) in a tissue
▨ : Shaded area under red dashed line denotes the increased robustness in tissue caused by appropriate loading from correct training

Fig. 19.1 Simplified stress/strain curve relating to human tissue and a training effect.

in a tissue is a point at which the force/load being applied is so great that the tissue can no longer accommodate it and the tissue loses its ability to return to its original state – it remains in its deformed (lengthened or compressed) state. This indicates where microtrauma to the tissue has occurred and the tissues, recoil properties have been exceeded (denoted by the black line B to C in Fig. 19.1). Symptoms at this point would include mild inflammation and some degree of discomfort – a very low-grade strain maybe diagnosed.

Complete failure of a tissue occurs when the amount of force/load or *overload* exceeds both the tissue's elastic and plastic properties causing the tissue to significantly break, i.e., ranging from a sizeable tear to a complete rupture (denoted by the point beyond C in Fig. 19.1). Symptoms from this would be high levels of pain, considerable inflammation and a significant loss of function in the affected tissue.

It falls to the medical and sports science departments within a football club to assist the management in the concept of *load management*, i.e., to provide information on the amount of work being assigned to each player during training and what the accumulative work or load is as the training week develops. The idea is to try and determine the optimal amount of work/load or stimulus to produce a training effect to improve cardiovascular fitness, strength, power, ability to recover and repeat. Furthermore, these departments should also advise how much *off-load*

is needed to allow players' tissues to recover and respond to the stimulus, without reaching the critical failure point of any one tissue or overtraining as a whole. The ultimate goal in terms of the stress/strain curve is to move the curve upwards and to the right (denoted by the red dashed line in Fig. 19.1 and the new points B_1 and C_1). This suggests that a good training response via appropriate repeated stimulus/loading causes human tissue to respond by increases in its robustness (denoted by the shaded area in Fig. 19.1) to withstand bigger forces/load before the tissue becomes injured, achieved by optimal load management.

Incidence of tears and the football calendar

There are periods in a football season when there is the potential for a higher incidence of soft tissue injuries, especially muscle tears – specifically to muscles of the posterior chain (the hamstring and calf muscle groups; Woods et al., 2002). Why these specific muscle groups are more at risk is not well understood; however, it is the opinion of the authors that this could be due to the role these muscles play in shock attenuation and propulsion during the gait cycle. Furthermore, these muscles have to deal with vast forces or load whilst in lengthened positions as they cross the hip and knee or knee and ankle.

The two distinct periods in question are preseason (July and early August) and towards the end of the season (March, April, May). The former is defined by the introduction of an increased demand or workload in the lead up to the start of the season. Preseason always follows a summer period (May and June) of a much reduced workload, where players have been on holiday and had a period of relative rest, allowing the muscles to become deconditioned because of the reduced exercise undertaken. July sees a sudden spike in demand being placed on the leg muscles as they attempt to regain this lost fitness and conditioning in a short period of time, i.e., usually 6 weeks. This increased workload, if too great and applied too soon, massively overloads the muscles causing them to fail (tear) as they cannot cope with the demand expected of them. However, the modern day professional footballer is aware of the consequences of not exercising enough during their summer break and are (in the main) happy to follow the close season programme set for them by their club's medical and sports science departments in an attempt to maintain a level of conditioning that negates the likelihood of injury during the preseason.

Despite this period being known as a potential injury 'hot spot', there are still some players who would rather run the risk of preseason injury by taking a longer than advised rest from exercise in the summer and they often pay the price during preseason.

- Did the pain/stiffness felt in the posterior lower leg start suddenly or gradually?
- Is there pain/discomfort on walking?
- Is there pain with active non-weight-bearing (NWB) ankle dorsiflexion? With knee straight and/or knee flexed?
- Is there pain with passive NWB ankle dorsiflexion? With knee straight and/or knee flexed?
- Can the player perform a heel raise? With knee straight and/or knee flexed?
- Can the player hop?
- What symptoms are elicited with palpation and where?

The other period for heightened injury risk, particularly for muscle tears, is the end of the season months. These are characterized by players having a higher level of accumulative fatigue and this fatigue results from inadequate training or overtraining volumes set by the coaching staff and/or poor recovery strategies not allowing players to rest enough and to allow muscles to prepare for the next bout of exercise. This means players go into the final few months of the season (when pressure to perform and the overall stakes are highest) in a less-than-ideal state to play, meaning that muscles are at a higher risk of not being able to withstand the workload being asked of them, so they fail and tear.

However, it must also be noted that if players are not trained appropriately when they enter the preseason period (i.e., worked hard enough), and if this lack of stimulus is continued into the season, players are then trying to play competitive matches in a deconditioned state. This means soft tissue injuries can and will invariably occur at anytime throughout the season and not just during the two periods highlighted.

Assessment and use of radiological imaging

There are many tests stated in various texts (Brukner and Kahn, 2012) on how muscle injuries should be assessed to diagnose a muscle tear and perhaps even establish the extent of the tear. However, in reality, soleus and gastrocnemius tears need only a few questions to be asked when performing a few simple tests to assist in the diagnostic process (Box 19.1).

For a muscle tear to be diagnosed, most of the tests mentioned above need to be positive for producing pain. Symptoms produced with a predominately flexed knee but not when the knee is straight, suggest more of a soleus

involvement; the converse is true for the gastrocnemius muscle. The ability to perform a heel raise and/or hop suggests less muscle compromise than a player who is unable to heel raise or hop at all due to pain and this then suggests a sizeable tear in one of the two main calf muscles.

In the authors' experience, the more tests that are positive and the more sudden the onset, the more severe the tear is likely to be. However, in professional football, due to the pressures to get players back playing in as little time as possible, medical departments are expected to confirm this type of injury using radiological imaging, either an ultrasound or a magnetic resonance imaging (MRI) scan. At this point, the scan tends to be routine to appease the player and management, who have come to expect imaging as part and parcel of the diagnostic process. Very few experienced clinicians need a scan to confirm what their clinical assessment has told them; the scan merely corroborates the diagnosis from the clinical assessment.

Scanning an injury does not, in the main, influence how an injury is treated; it should always be the symptoms that dictate the treatment. However, an injured player and/or the management at a club tends to be more reassured if a scan has been carried out and it would seem that clinicians working in professional football simply must accept this.

Commonly considered causes

Flexibility

A lack of flexibility (perhaps more outside of elite sport) is often considered to be a possible underlying cause as to why a muscle tear occurred. The notion exists that if the soleus and/or gastrocnemius muscles lack sufficient range of movement, they will lack the necessary ability to lengthen far enough or fast enough to stop the muscle from tearing when force/load is placed upon them and, as a result, the muscle tears.

Anatomical ankle range is deemed to be ~0–50 degrees of plantar flexion and 0–20 degrees of dorsiflexion (Standring, 2015). It is this ~20 degrees of dorsiflexion that gives rise to a knee-to-wall (KTW) test with a range of 8 cm or more being the aim (Fig. 19.2). Unless a professional footballer has sustained a previous ankle injury that may limit his dorsiflexion, most players easily achieve an ≥8-cm KTW test score and even those that do not, rarely go on and sustain a soleus or gastrocnemius muscle tear.

Flexibility and its possible relationship to muscle injury has been studied in more detail than many other factors thought to contribute to muscle injury (Cornwall et al., 2002; Ettema et al., 1996; Kubo et al., 2002; van Mechelen et al., 1993; Wilson et al., 1992; Witvrouw et al., 2003; 2004). However, the research does not appear to support the widely held notion that lack of flexibility predisposes

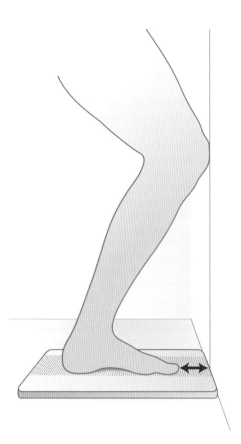

Fig. 19.2 Knee-to-wall (KTW) test position. The arrow denotes the distance being measured from big toe to wall, with the knee touching the wall and heel remaining in contact with the floor.

an individual to muscle tearing. This is echoed by the authors' own experiences to date. The clear majority of professional footballers that sustain soleus or gastrocnemius tears do so with no adverse loss to that muscle's flexibility and this suggests that there are other aetiological factors.

Strength inadequacies

Coupled with a lack of perceived flexibility, a lack of strength or a weakness in the gastrocnemius/soleus complex is another commonly believed reason for these muscles to tear. Unlike flexibility as a cause, it is the experience of the authors' that if a player is unable to generate enough strength and power to perform all the actions required in professional football, e.g., run, sprint, jump, land, the

forces placed upon these muscles when such activities are undertaken can cause one or both of these muscles to fail and tear. (See Gym rehabilitation to return to play below for a discussion on how to rectify this deficiency.)

Foot mechanics and orthotic use

If the foot is not functioning as it should and not transferring force from the ground upon impact during gait up through the ankle and into the lower leg, then other structures in the region can be overloaded to failure.

The foot's structures should hold their form, but have enough give to deal with the ground reaction forces placed upon them during the gait cycle – the foot acting as a shock attenuator during the stance phase of gait and ensuring those forces are pushed up the lower leg. Equally, the foot's structures should also be solid enough to transfer propulsion forces down from the soleus and gastrocnemius muscles and into the ground, aiding effective movement through to the push-off phase of gait so that maximal power transfer is achieved.

However, many professional footballers do not have 'ideal' foot mechanics for various reasons ranging from genetic predisposition to previous foot injury and/or surgery. The authors believe that this lack of appropriate foot function causes an increased loading of the soleus and gastrocnemius, and that if allowed to occur repeatedly without correction can lead to these muscles being overloaded to the point of failure; tearing of these muscles being one possible outcome.

One solution to poor foot mechanics is the prescription of custom-made orthotic devices. These are bespoke to the individual player and are considerably more than just an 'arch support'. The orthotic offers proprioceptive and structural support to the failing foot structures in an attempt to optimize the functioning of the foot. It might include a heel raise, rear foot wedging or first metatarsal phalangeal (MTP) cut out, all aimed at improving the role the foot plays during gait and effectively offloads excessive force being placed through the calf muscles that might lead to muscle failure.

Once prescribed, the orthotics are placed into the players trainers and boots to ensure uniformity in foot function at all times – not just during training or matches. The challenge is to find a podiatrist that can make different types of orthotics to fit trainers and especially a player's boots. Quite often players wear their boots very tight (possibly even a half-size too small), leaving no room for a corrective device to be inserted; therefore these players will simply not wear these devices in their boots and so will not benefit from their correction during key times. Some players have the opportunity to work with their boot manufacturer and have an orthotic device incorporated into the boot design, negating the above issues (Box 19.2).

A 34-year-old professional footballer had a history of recurrent calf tears, both soleus and gastrocnemius, over a 12-month period and an inability to run any distance without a cramping-type pain in his calves. This player had good calf and ankle mobility and had been treated with various soft tissue techniques, a Compex machine to stimulate muscle contraction and blood flow, and a strength programme in the gym to increase isometric, concentric and eccentric muscle strength. Despite all of this, he was still experiencing calf muscle tears. This player was sent to see a podiatrist who assessed his foot function and felt that an orthotic device was required, including a heel raise to reduce the stretch through the calf complex during the gait cycle. Within a week of wearing the orthotics, this player's calf symptoms abated completely, allowing him to run without restriction. To date he has suffered no further calf muscle tears.

Many clinicians take the view that if a player is born with a foot type that might be considered 'faulty' and so have always walked and run on that foot type, then the suggestion that this is a cause of any soleus or gastrocnemius tear is ridiculous as that player has had a lifetime to condition his lower limbs to the way his feet perform. Although one might take the view, 'If it's not broken, don't fix it', once a tear occurs to the soleus or gastrocnemius caused by internal forces, i.e., not a direct blow from another player but from repeated overload, then foot mechanics are a worthwhile area to assess as part of the rehabilitation process.

Less commonly considered causes

Hydration and its effects on muscle elasticity

There is much research (Baker et al., 2014; Nuccio et al., 2017) on the effects of dehydration on sporting performance – specifically, the effects of inadequate hydration prior to, during and after exercise. It is clear that sporting performance is dramatically impaired both cognitively and physiologically by an athlete being dehydrated when they compete. One study by Cleary et al. (2005) looked at the issue of delayed onset muscle soreness (DOMS) and hydration. The researchers found that athletes that were dehydrated during exercise suffered an increase in DOMS postexercise when compared to the hydrated control group.

Whilst DOMS is not considered a tear to a muscle(s), it is a form of muscle damage. If, as has been shown, hydration plays a very important role in preventing DOMS during exercise, it is postulated that the lack of elasticity in a tissue caused by dehydration may increase the likelihood that tissue could fail completely, i.e., tear or rupture. However, there is currently a paucity of research looking at the relationship of dehydration and its role in muscle tears, such as those in the soleus and gastrocnemius muscles.

It is the authors' considered opinion from their own clinical experiences that dehydration and muscle tears are closely related in some professional footballers. Whilst all professional football clubs understand the need for a hydration protocol for their players when training and playing, it is invariably implemented for its effect on overall performance and not specifically for injury prevention. Such hydration protocols will often be of a 'one protocol fits all' type, and all players are expected to follow this with equal results. This contrasts with a greater individualization of other areas of players' training regimes. Players are not expected to follow the same strength training programme in the gym, as it is well recognized that every player needs a programme that reflects their own needs. The authors question why this same approach is not being taken with the issue of hydration.

One of the authors' current clubs has recently instigated a sweat profiling policy, where every player has been sweat tested to gauge not only the total amount of fluid lost during exercise but also the electrolyte balance of their perspiration. What is apparent from testing a squad of 25 professional first team footballers is that at least 5 of this squad are considered to be 'high sweaters', meaning that for every millilitre of sweat lost, these players are also losing a higher than normal amount of electrolytes as part of this sweat loss.

If this electrolyte deficit is not replenished correctly, these players run the risk of the detrimental effects of electrolyte imbalance, perhaps in spite of replenishing the total fluid volume lost. It is the authors' view that electrolyte imbalance more than any total loss of fluid makes muscles more prone to damage, increasing the risk of muscle tears due to reduced muscle elasticity and increased fatigue. Electrolytes like sodium and calcium are essential for muscle contraction. Therefore, any deficit or imbalance means muscle function is suboptimal and the tissue may not withstand the rigours of exercise (Box 19.3).

Poor training load management

Load management (see Stress/Strain concept, above), i.e., monitoring the amount of work assigned to a player and team on a daily and weekly basis in order to optimize training and ensure players are in the best possible physical shape come match day has become the 'holy grail' of sports science in recent years.

Box 19.3 **Case study 2**

A 27-year-old professional footballer who plays at international level had a history of intermittent soleus muscle tears and regular episodes of bilateral cramping in his calves in the last 30 min of matches. He had been seen by a podiatrist for foot function assessment and wore orthotics. He had undertaken a strength programme in the gym and built his calf strength up to being able to lift multiples of bodyweight during heel raising and had good ankle joint and calf muscle mobility. He was also very conscientious about following the club's rehydration protocols posttraining and for games. Yet still he suffered from soleus tears.

This player was sweat tested at the beginning of the season (see Hydration and its effects on muscle elasticity) and found to be one of five players deemed to be a 'high sweater', both in terms of volume of sweat lost and electrolyte content. He was started on a specific rehydration drink that provided the correct electrolyte replenishment; within a week he reported noticing his calf cramps had disappeared during training and at the end of games. He reported feeling much fresher the following day postgame, with minimal delayed onset muscle soreness. To date he has not suffered another soleus tear.

This has much to do with the work of Dr. Tim Gabbett and his research relating to the acute/chronic load relationship (Gabbett, 2016). Gabbett postulated that if athletes are exposed to sharp spikes in excess loading during training or a match, then they are at higher risk of injury (e.g., muscle tears) than those that maintain a high volume of consistent loading, as the latter group are much more prepared for the demands of a bout of intense exercise, e.g., during a match.

However, Gabbett's concept of load relates to all exertion placed upon an athlete's body during training and matches and the perceived effort each athlete feels they were exposed to. For the purpose of this chapter, however, the authors utilize the concept of load management specifically as the amount of force (load) applied to the soleus and gastrocnemius muscles during resistance training and its ability to bring about the desired isometric, concentric, eccentric strength and power increases needed to perform at the highest level of professional football on a repeated basis and without failure, i.e., injury.

Rehabilitation

Treatment room to gym

Baseline screening becomes important when assessing how a player is improving following any type of injury. Some examples of outcome measures commonly used in clinical practice while monitoring calf injuries are given below.

Knee-to-wall test/weight-bearing lunge test

The knee-to-wall (KTW) test is used to assess for ankle dorsiflexion range of motion deficits (Fig. 19.2). Achieving 8 cm appears optimal amongst footballers with any significant restriction being associated with altered knee and ankle kinematics. This can lead to high-risk movement patterns commonly linked to noncontact injuries.

Powden et al. (2015) described the KTW test as the weight-bearing lunge test (WBLT). They demonstrated consistent intra- and intertester reliability in measuring ankle dorsiflexion, albeit generally utilizing a healthy population. However, these results are easily translatable into the sporting population. iPhone applications for measuring ankle dorsiflexion are appearing and one has been studied by Balsalobre-Fernandez et al. (2018). Whilst these researchers conclude that the app easily, accurately, and reliably evaluates weight-bearing ankle dorsiflexion, small sample sizes make their findings unreliable.

Although there is no literature linking poor KTW/WBLT and calf injuries, immediate measurements postinjury and throughout the rehabilitation process can indicate progress. To begin outdoor running, we would expect the athlete to have returned to their baseline measurement and have <2 cm asymmetry, in addition to considering other markers discussed later in the chapter.

Muscle work capacity/calf endurance test

A muscle work capacity (MWC)/calf endurance test can be used to assess the functional capacity of the triceps surae musculature. Using a 2-s concentric and eccentric phase appears to obtain the most accurate results, based on the authors' personal experience. In the applied setting, this test requires careful examination to ensure no compensations take place to achieve false scores. An inability to fully complete the concentric/eccentric phase and/or excessive inversion/eversion would indicate stopping the test.

To participate in outdoor running sessions the athlete should be able to complete >25 reps with over 90% score on the limb symmetry index. This type of test is advantageous as it is performed in a weight-bearing position, making it, arguably, a more relevant outcome measure than isokinetic dynamometry. It is often used for baseline screening, often completed in preseason, to ensure an athlete is working to their optimal physical capabilities and can return to play/competition safely. It can highlight athletes who are at more risk by displaying asymmetries or low scores that may increase the risk of suffering a calf injury. Although calf endurance deficits have been noted post–Achilles tendon repair (Bostick et al., 2010), further research is required to better identify athletes in the sporting population at higher risk of developing a calf injury.

Handheld dynamometry (HHD)

Handheld dynamometry (HHD) can be useful in measuring maximum voluntary isometric contraction (MVIC). However, the current evidence base indicates that there are some reliability issues. Clarke et al. (2011) demonstrated moderate-to-excellent intratester reliability in contrast to relatively poor-to-moderate interrater reliability using the MicroFET3 device. In the personal experience of the authors, these measurements can be used periodically throughout the rehabilitation process to indicate progress and right-to-left asymmetries. By altering the knee angle, practitioners may argue that they can isolate the soleus compared to a straight knee positioning biasing the gastrocnemius. This clearly requires further longitudinal study in professional athletes to standardize testing procedures. In spite of that, the MicroFET3 has been useful in identifying strength deficits and asymmetries when rehabilitating long-term injuries.

Alongside capacity testing, HHD can start to create an athlete profile, identifying their strength and conditioning needs. By collecting this data, bodyweight:strength ratios can also be developed and interlimb asymmetries calculated. It is unreasonable to expect an athlete weighing 70 kg to produce the same MVIC as an athlete weighing 90 kg. This can be made proportionate by using weight categories. Whether HHD scores correlate with MWC scores is yet to be established.

AlterG protocol

The AlterG treadmill is a novel piece of equipment utilized in most high-performance sporting environments. It uses differential air pressure technology to enable athletes to load as little as 30% of their bodyweight, allowing an earlier return to normal function, which can reduce recovery times.

When an athlete can tolerate isometric holds with a straight and bent knee at 30% of their bodyweight in the gym we begin the AlterG return to outdoor running protocol. For a grade 1 calf lesion, 4 sessions may be suitable. By comparison, a grade 2 lesion may require 6–8 progressive sessions. When a player can tolerate 85–90% bodyweight for 4 × 4 minutes at 16 km/h, it is deemed appropriate to begin physiotherapy-led, on-field sessions. Recently it has been shown that running speed largely affects plantar forces created on the AlterG (Thomson et al., 2017). This allows an objective progression of plantar loading during rehabilitation. For example, running at 16 km/h at 80% bodyweight produces 2.11 multiples of bodyweight. This enables the strength and conditioning coaches to plan their strength programme accordingly and helps us understand how much load the athlete can tolerate safely.

The AlterG is all about increasing the chronic workload to prepare the athlete for on-field conditioning. In addition to running, plyometric training can be initiated using a variation of pogo jumps, countermovement jumps and drop landings.

An athlete will very often describe a 'flat tyre' effect when initially running outdoors. The AlterG allows us to condition the triceps surae complex and improve ankle stiffness. From experience, athletes very often complain of calf tightness during the early stages of outdoor rehabilitation. By increasing the muscle work capacities of the gastrocnemius and soleus to tolerate these loads we can eradicate these issues and create a more fluent rehabilitation process.

What and who are we rehabilitating?

Different muscle fibre types exist within the gastrocnemius and soleus, affecting their roles in locomotion. Human studies indicate that soleus consists of a higher percentage of slow-twitch oxidative fibres (type I) compared to fast-twitch (type II) fibres (70:30%). Findings also reveal that the number of type II fibres is much higher in gastrocnemius compared to soleus, with no difference between the medial or lateral head. How does this affect how we rehabilitate?

Soleus injuries require increased endurance training and are predominantly responsible for locomotion up to around 18 km/h or 5 m/s. Gastrocnemius is more explosive, requiring power/strength training to be able to sustain repeated sprint efforts at >18 km/h and powerful triple extension of the posterior chain.

The soleus muscle generates greater isometric and dynamic strength during running (Blazkiewicz et al., 2017) compared to the gastrocnemius. It works eccentrically during midstance to control the body's centre of gravity; it is argued that by improving the soleus' force-absorbing efficiency running economy can be improved. Soleus will typically absorb 6–8 × bodyweight during running and produces the highest peak force compared to other lower limb muscles. Heavy strength training must commence as soon as it can be tolerated.

Rehabilitation is a complex process in which many variables, intrinsic and extrinsic, need to be considered. Take for instance, a central defender compared to an attacking wide player. How do their games differ?

A 6'6″ central defender who predominantly wins headers operates in straight lines compared to a skilful winger who needs to be able to change direction at high speed and make explosive runs repeatedly. But how do we know what is 'normal'?

Global positioning systems (GPS) are regularly used and available in elite sport. They enable the sports medicine team to see the total distance covered, high-intensity metres >19 km/h and number of sprints >25 km/h. This information can be used in a variety of ways, for example when considering extra training, tapering down and high-lighting potential overtraining or overreaching athletes.

Transitioning an athlete from the gym to on-field rehabilitation should take into account a number of considerations:

- Has the athlete got full range of motion?
- Does the athlete have >90% peak power scores, with no asymmetries?
- Is he able to complete a unilateral heel raise and hop, continually and pain free, in straight/flexed knee positions?
- Can the athlete absorb load, produce force and complete plyometric challenges?

If the answer is 'yes' to all the above, then we can clinically reason that this athlete is ready to increase their physical demands.

Physiotherapy-led sessions need to cover all angles to ensure safe handover to sports science/rehabilitation fitness staff. At this point, the athlete should be able to complete high-speed running up to 80% maximum speed, change of direction at pace, position-specific plyometric efforts and technical/ball work drills based on their position. A low-grade/grade 1 lesion may require 2–3 sessions whereas a grade 2 lesion or above may need extra care and 4–6 sessions.

Intensive and extensive conditioning is the focus of the rehabilitation fitness coaches at this stage. The soleus is responsible for ~80% of the load at lower speed levels; therefore the focus is less on explosiveness but more about robustness of the soleus and its ability to tolerate chronic workloads. In contrast, repeated and reactive speed testing needs to be covered following a gastrocnemius injury. An example of this could be 6 × 50-m sprints working at 1:1 work:rest ratio. This can be progressed to a reactive, position-specific scenario including a 1v1 situation with the ball. This removes the predictability element and requires the athlete to respond to random movement patterns.

Are there other factors that we need to consider? Recurring injury? Mechanism of injury? The psychological aspect of rehabilitation always merits consideration. Have maladaptations taken place within the triceps surae resulting in neuromuscular inhibition? Can we recreate the mechanism to instil confidence, to prevent any fear–avoidance strategies in running style or movement patterning?

As a multidisciplinary team, it is important to discuss these factors and involve the athlete in the decision-making process. This can improve compliance and enables the athlete to buy-in to your thought process and planning. This should lead into a pre- and posttraining routine and help to reduce the risk of recurrence. As in most elite environments, the time spent outside of the training facility outweighs the time spent within, highlighting the importance of education on physical preparation, regeneration and recovery.

Gym rehabilitation to return to play

There is no single factor that determines return to play (RTP) after a muscle injury (Benito et al., 2014; Ekstrand et al., 2012). However, increased local and global muscle strength and power capabilities are key determining factors in a successful RTP. In particular reference to the calf (gastrocnemius and soleus) many return to training (RTT) or RTP programmes often neglect the key determining functions of the individual muscle and fail to provide sufficient stimulus for adaptation.

During running, the calf and ankle complex absorb and produce forces of 5–13 × bodyweight (Burdett, 2012). Without sufficient progressive loading, the returning athlete is at risk of reinjury not only to the calf but also potentially to the Achilles tendon.

A lot of rehabilitation programmes ignore the fact that the calf musculature responds to heavy loading, and they often prescribe bodyweight-only exercises or stretching. The danger of this bodyweight, low-load only approach is that it does not sufficiently and effectively prepare the athlete for the demands of the forthcoming gym-based plyometric exercises, and more importantly the return-to-running protocol on the pitch.

Despite the common misconception that the gastrocnemius is the main force producer during running, research has shown that it is, in fact, the soleus, which produces up to 50% of the total vertical force (Albracht et al., 2008). The soleus has the largest force-producing ability due to its large physiological cross-sectional area. The soleus can produce actual forces of around 8 × bodyweight in comparison to the gastrocnemius producing 3 × bodyweight (Albracht et al., 2008). The fact that the soleus is such a large force contributor lends its self to the notion that heavy resistance training is required to adequately train the calf musculature.

Coupled with heavy-resistance training, RTP programmes should also aim to incorporate plyometric exercises. These should follow a controlled, progressive plyometric programme paying attention to force-absorption exercises (e.g., drop landings), force-production exercises (e.g., jumps) and continuous reactive jumps (e.g., pogos, skipping or rebound jumps). Plyometric exercises, especially the continuous reactive jumps should only be performed once the returning athlete has completed the desired strength programme and reduced any strength inadequacies and imbalances.

In the authors' opinion, during rehabilitation and once an athlete begins to regain full range of motion, a logical progressive RTP should follow three steps, although there is overlap and continuity between these stages: (1) restore

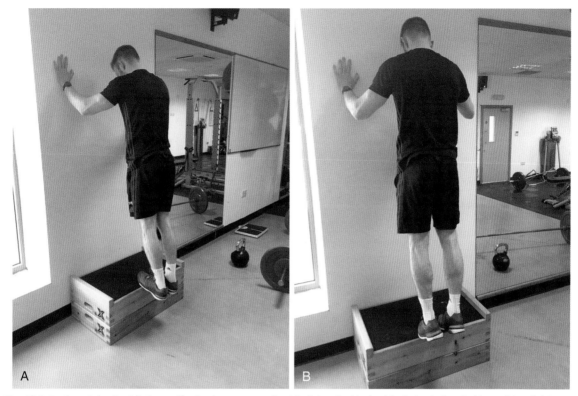

Fig. 19.3 Bodyweight double leg calf raise (gastrocnemius bias). Load with dumbbells, barbell or Smith machine. (A) Start of the movement, (B) end of the movement.

concentric muscle strength, (2) restore eccentric muscle strength, (3) restore high-speed and power capabilities. Each stage requires a progression from bodyweight-only to higher external loads, bilateral to unilateral loading, increases in total volume and increases in speed.

How an athlete progresses through these stages will depend on a number of factors such as severity of injury, preinjury strength, previous injury, previous training age/exposure and pain-free tolerance.

How to load

As previously mentioned, to adequately rehabilitate an injured muscle, progressive loading is required. Traditional guidelines for strength training suggest that loading to >85% 1-repetition maximum (1RM), 4–6 repetitions, 4–6 sets, with 3–5-min recovery periods (Fleck and Kraemer, 2003). In the authors' opinion and experience, this is just part of the way to help increase muscle strength and successful RTP. Due to the involvement of the calf in nearly all movements on the football pitch (jogging, running, jumping, etc.) the calf not only needs maximal strength but also

strength endurance and rate of force development (RFD) training to help prevent risk of injury. Therefore, higher repetition training, e.g., 10–15 reps, or increased volume, e.g., 8–12 sets, maybe also be required for adequate strength gains, as well as quicker, more powerful movements for RFD.

Considering the increase in research into the injury prevention and performance benefits of eccentric exercises and isometrics, especially in the hamstrings, it would be remiss of any strength and conditioning coach or physiotherapist to ignore these types of exercises when strengthening or rehabbing a calf-related injury.

Eccentric exercises aim to strengthen the muscle when it is at its weakest and longest length. At these end-range positions, muscles are often at the greatest risk of tearing. Eccentric strategies to emphasize eccentric force generation and eccentric movement control may be important in normalizing muscle function and strength, as well as injury-related movement behaviour. Strengthening the muscle in these eccentric movements also helps prepare the athlete for the forthcoming plyometric and especially drop landing exercises. Research shows that eccentric exercises are

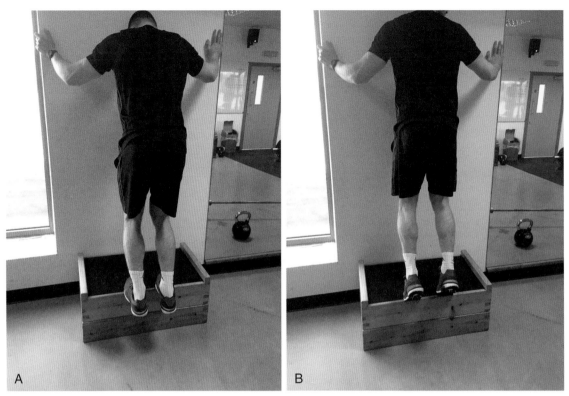

Fig. 19.4 Bodyweight double leg bent knee calf raise (soleus bias). Load with dumbbells, barbell or Smith machine. (A) Start of the movement, (B) end of the movement.

superior to other forms of rehabilitation when dealing with Achilles tendon injuries, and by association help with RTP after calf injuries (Allison, 2009).

Isometric training is a training method that has been around for a long time, yet is not practiced by many. Like eccentric training, research into isometric training often focuses on hamstring training (Van Hooren and Bosch, 2018). However, research has shown huge benefits to isometric loading in Achilles tendinopathy (Cook, 2009) and anecdotal evidence supports its use in training the calf musculature for improving sprint performance. Isometric training is essentially holding muscle tension in a specific position for a desired amount of time, ideally with maximal contraction of the muscle being trained.

The success of isometrics is based on the time-under-tension (TUT) notion and serves to improve neural efficiency, muscle activation, agonist and antagonist interaction as well as high-frequency muscle firing and thus rate of force development. The two main types of isometric training are often referred to as isometric holds and isometric pushes/pulls. Isometric holds refer to supporting or holding body mass and an external load in a static position for a set period of time (6–40 s).

Isometric pushes/pulls refer to application of very high pushing/pulling forces against an immovable object, e.g., often seen in a mid-thigh pull test. The intention is to apply force rapidly up to individual maximum for a short period of time (4–6 s) before resting.

Although an athlete should be eccentrically strong in order to get the most out of isometric training, isometric loading can be of great benefit to injured athletes due to the limited range of motion required and the lack of residual muscle soreness (or DOMS) generated, which would potentially aggravate already-injured tissue. In the authors' opinion, therefore, sensible early loading via isometrics can serve the injured athlete well.

Once strength, muscle endurance and firing rate have reached a desired level, the rehabilitation of the calf should focus on returning to high speed, power and RFD exercises, namely plyometric exercises. Initiation of plyometric exercises should follow a controlled, progressive programme, paying attention to force-absorption exercises (e.g., drop landings), force-production exercises (e.g., jumps) and continuous reactive jumps (e.g., pogos, skipping or rebound jumps).

244

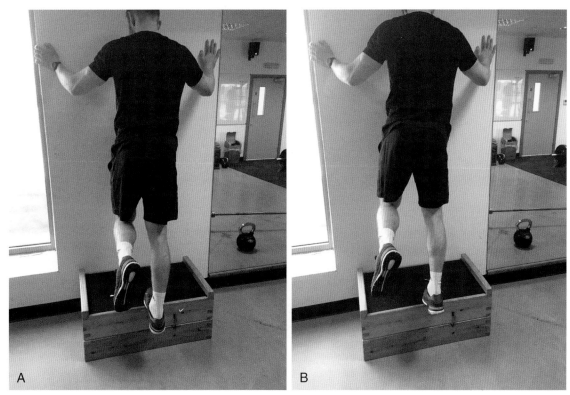

Fig. 19.5 Bodyweight single leg calf raise (gastrocnemius bias). Load with dumbbells, barbell or Smith machine. (A) Start of the movement, (B) end of the movement.

Force-absorption exercises are a logical functional progression from eccentric exercises, as they provide an overload of eccentric force due to gravity acting upon the body. Before an athlete can produce force at speed (power), it is essential for them to be able to safely absorb their maximal braking force. Linear and lateral drop landings from progressive box heights is a key starting point.

It is beyond the scope of this chapter to give a detailed review of the stretch–shortening cycle (SSC; see also Chapters 1 and 4) but its importance to strengthening, prevention and rehabilitation of a calf injury is of vital importance. The calf and ankle encounter huge forces, and the reapplication of these forces at speed when running. Ensuring an athlete can perform both double and single leg jump from the floor to a small to medium–height box (15–45 cm) in both a squat and countermovement jump movement is an essential test for an athlete returning from a calf muscle tear.

The final stage of a successful plyometric programme is reactive/continuous jumps, such as skipping or pogo jumps, and finally reactive drop jumps. These exercises combine the functions of all the previous ones by utilizing eccentric strength and concentric power production under great load and speed. In the authors' opinion it is these exercises that help the returning athlete lose that 'flat tyre' feeling often associated with calf and ankle injuries.

Calf raises, isometrics and eccentric exercises are commonly completed in two knee positions of varying angles of knee flexion in an attempt to isolate and target both of the calf muscles. This often stems from Alfredson's original training regime (Alfredson et al., 1998). Whilst several researchers have reported the inhibition of gastrocnemius with increasing knee flexion angles there are limited reports of alterations to soleus activity by biasing certain knee angles (Reid et al., 2012). Essentially, soleus works equally (measured as a percentage of its maximal voluntary contraction) in either knee flexion or extension. Reid et al. (2012) concluded that there appeared to be no benefit of using flexed knee eccentric rehabilitation as the soleus worked equally hard during extended knee rehabilitation. However, Price et al. (2003) reported that the medial gastrocnemius muscle appeared significantly more active during the fully extended knee position trial, while the soleus muscle activity was significantly less. However, the soleus muscle activity appeared significantly greater during the bent knee (90 degree) condition compared to the gastrocnemius.

Although it is unclear if soleus activity increases with great knee flexion, there is a suggestion that the dominance

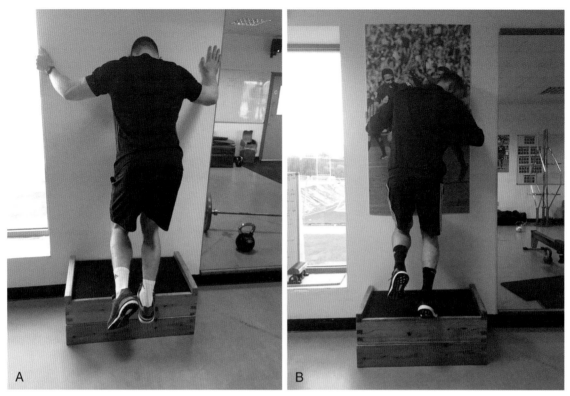

Fig. 19.6 Bodyweight single leg bent knee calf raise (soleus bias). Load with dumbbells, barbell or Smith machine. (A) Start of the movement, (B) end of the movement.

of the gastrocnemius diminishes with these greater knee flexion angles, suggesting a rationale for utilizing a variety of knee flexion angles to target specific calf injuries.

Ultimately it is a combination of these strength training factors, working the full spectrum of strength ranges, the force–velocity curve, knee flexion angle and a manipulation of the RTP scheduling that will provide the greatest chance of a successful RTP (Figs 19.3–19.8).

Red flags

When considering lower limb conditions, it is important to rule out serious pathologies that, although rare, can exist in the sporting population. Therefore, it is necessary to ensure that red flags are ruled out based on subjective history and objective examination.

Deep vein thrombosis

Deep vein thrombosis (DVT) is a blood clot that develops within a deep vein in the lower leg and can present as pain,

swelling and tenderness in the calf. This can lead to serious complications such as pulmonary embolism. Aching, heat and redness are other symptoms that may present with this scenario. DVTs may be seen postsurgically in an athlete, during periods of inactivity or following trauma to a blood vessel. In female athletes, some contraceptive medications can cause the blood to clot more easily. DVTs are usually diagnosed using an ultrasound scan by an experienced radiologist; treatment consists of anticoagulant medications such as warfarin. Although a DVT is often as a result of surgery or inactivity, it is important to rule out this pathology in patients who have vague calf pain symptoms and no mechanism of injury.

Tumour

Soft tissue masses such as a tumour (malignant or benign) can occur in elite athletes. Often these have an insidious onset and may be associated with a palpable lump and swelling. Importantly, tumours can mimic conditions such as a Baker's cyst or synovial sarcoma, highlighting the importance of magnetic resonance imaging (MRI) or other tests to confirm diagnosis. It is important to consider family history, as well as symptoms such as general malaise,

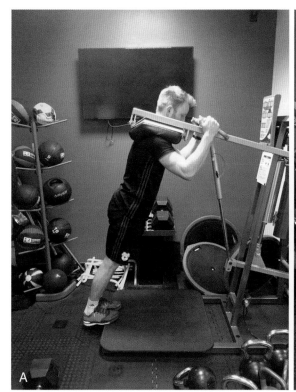 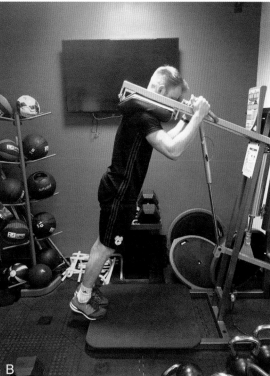

Fig. 19.7 Double leg isometric holds (using the Keiser machine, but barbell or Smith machine are also options). (A) Start of the movement, (B) end of the movement.

unexplained weight loss and unknown causes when considering malignant tumours.

Stress fractures

Stress fractures of the lower limb tend to occur within the tibia. Symptoms usually include pain on the lower third of the tibia with occasional localized swelling and tenderness over the fracture site. Athletes may be predisposed to stress fracture following a period of inactivity or running extraordinary long distances compared to their usual loads. Tenderness will usually be present directly on palpation of the tibia and is important when differentiating between medial tibial stress syndrome. Early X-rays may miss a stress fracture, with MRI being the gold standard. Bone marrow oedema evident on an MRI scan may indicate a stress fracture. Computed tomography (CT) scanning can also be utilized if required.

Popliteal artery entrapment syndrome (PAES)

Popliteal artery entrapment syndrome (PAES) is an uncommon pathology in athletes. It is a rare vascular disease that can particularly affect young athletes. It can be caused by a developmental defect in the calf or popliteus muscle, or occur over time as a result of triceps surae muscle hypertrophy compressing the popliteal artery. Often these cases are bilateral, with symptoms including calf muscle pain, cramping and numbness of the feet. Investigations include MRI scanning and postexercise compartment pressure testing. Importantly, an examination by an experienced vascular specialist is required if PAES is suspected.

Summary

Calf pathology and injury management have been rather overlooked in the literature to date. However, there is emerging empirical evidence indicating the importance of the soleus muscle and its role in locomotion.

Using a battery of tests, we can build athlete profiles that identify if there are subtle differences/deficits in gastrocnemius compared to soleus strength, as well as limb asymmetries. We can utilize this information to implement strength and conditioning programmes to increase the robustness

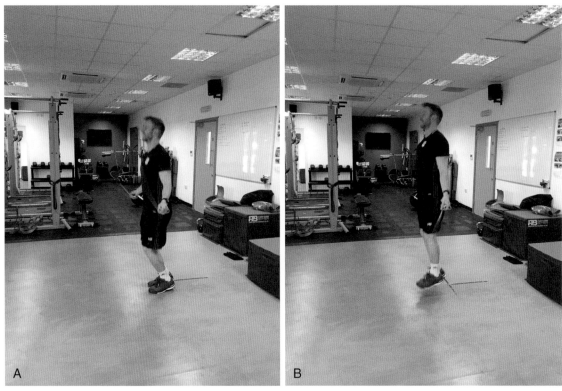

A   B

Fig. 19.8 Skipping (rate of force development, plyometric). (A) Start of the movement, (B) end of the movement.

of the triceps surae musculature. It is key to tailor each reha-bilitation programme to the individual, ensuring they meet or exceed their baseline markers and continue postinjury. Developing isometric resilience, concentric triple extension power production, eccentric control and optimal ankle stiffness can contribute to the overall demands required to compete in a fast-paced, multidirectional contact sport such as football.

To sum up, the authors' approach to gastrocnemius and soleus muscle tears is as follows:

- A simple, but thorough assessment is needed to diag-nose a calf muscle tear, although in professional foot-ball it often expected that some form of imaging is 'needed' to confirm the clinician's diagnosis.
- Flexibility is not a cause of muscle tears.
- A lack of strength and power does make muscles more susceptible to failure, but improving these elements

requires good programme design and considerably more overload than most would undertake in a gym setting.
- Dehydration reduces a muscle's elastic properties, mak-ing it more prone to failure. Individually sweat profile your players so individual replenishment plans can be implemented.
- Orthotics aid in the optimization of foot mechanics and therefore promote good force transfer up and down the lower leg.
- Optimal training load management is key to reducing the risk of muscle injury by making the tissue more ro-bust and increasing its elastic properties. Too little load-ing leaves a player undertrained and too much training leaves a player fatigued; both scenarios increase a play-er's susceptibility to muscle tearing.
- Always rule out potential 'red flags' as part of the differ-ential diagnosis for calf muscle tears.

References

Albracht, K., Arampatzis, A., Baltzopoulos, V., 2008. Assessment of muscle volume and physiological cross-sectional area of the human triceps surae muscle in vivo. Journal of Biomechanics 41 (10), 2211–2218.

Alfredson, H., Pietila, T., Jonsson, P., Lorentzon, R., 1998. Heavy-load eccentric calf muscle training for the treatment of chronic Achilles tendinosis. American Journal of Sports Medicine 26 (3), 360–366.

Allison, G.T., Purdam, C., 2009. Eccentric loading for Achilles tendinopathy strengthening or stretching? British Journal of Sports Medicine 43 (4), 276.

Baker, LB., Jeukendrup, AE., 2014. Optimal composition of fluid-replacement beverages. Comprehensive Physiology 4 (2), 575–620.

Balsalobre-Fernandez, C., Romero-Franco, N., Jimenez-Reyes, P., 2018. Concurrent validity and reliability of an iPhone app for the measurement of ankle dorsiflexion and inter-limb asymmetries. Journal of Sports Sciences 37 (3), 1–5.

Benito, L., Ayan, C., Revuelta, G., Maestro, A., Fernandez, T., Sanchez, M., 2014. Influence of the soccer players' professional status on the frequency and severity of injuries: a comparative pilot study [in Spanish]. Apunts Medicine Esport 49 (181), 20–24.

Blazkiewicz, M., Wiszomirska, I., Kaczmarczyk, K., Naemi, R., Wit, A., 2017. Inter-individual similarities and variations in muscle forces acting on the ankle joint during gait. Gait & Posture 58, 166–170.

Bostick, G.P., Jomha, N.M., Suchak, A.A., Beaupre, L.A., 2010. Factors associated with calf muscle endurance recovery 1 year after Achilles tendon rupture repair. Journal of Orthopaedic & Sports Physical Therapy 40, 345–351.

Brukner, P., Kahn, K., 2012. Brukner & Khan's Clinical Sports Medicine, fourth ed. McGraw Hill Australia, Sydney, pp. 761–775. Chapter 36.

Burdett, R., 1981. Forces predicted at the ankle during running. Medicine & Science in Sports & Exercise 14, 308–316.

Clarke, M., Nimhuircheartaigh, D., Walsh, G., Walsh, J., Meldrum, D., 2011. Intra-tester and inter-tester reliability of the MicroFET 3 hand-held dynamometer. Physiotherapy Practice and Research 32, 13–18.

Cleary, M.A., Sweeney, L.A., Kendrick, Z.V., Sitler, M.R., 2005. Dehydration and symptoms of delayed onset muscle soreness in hyperthermic males. Journal of Athletic Training 40 (4), 288–297.

Cook, J.L., Purdam, C.R., 2009. Is tendon pathology a continuum? A pathology model to explain the clinical presentation of load-induced tendinopathy. British Journal of Sports Medicine 43 (6), 409–416.

Cornwell, A., Nelson, A.G., Sidaway, B., 2002. Acute effects of stretching on the neuromechanical properties of the triceps surae muscle complex. European Journal of Applied Physiology 86, 428–434.

Dixon, J.B., 2009. Gastrocnemius vs. soleus strain: how to differentiate and deal with calf muscle injuries. Current Reviews in Musculoskeletal Medicine 2, 74–77.

Ekstrand, J., Healy, J.C., Walden, M., Lee, J.C., English, B., Hagglund, M., 2012. Hamstring muscle injuries in professional football: the correlation of MRI findings with return to play. British Journal of Sports Medicine 46, 112–117.

Ettema, G.J.C., 1996. Mechanical efficiency and efficiency of storage and release of series elastic energy in skeletal muscle during stretch-shortening cycles. The Journal of Experimental Biology 199, 1983–1997.

Fleck, S.J., Kraemer, W.J., 2003. Designing Resistance Training Programs, third ed. Human Kinetics, Champaign, Il.

Gabbett, T.J., 2016. The training–injury prevention paradox: should athletes be training smarter and harder? British Journal of Sports Medicine (50), 5.

Kubo, K., Kanehisa, H., Fukunaga, T., 2002. Effects of resistance and stretching training programmes on the viscoelastic properties of human tendon structures in vivo. The Journal of Physiology 538, 219–226.

Nuccio, R.P., Barnes, K.A., Carter, J.M., Baker, L.B., 2017. Fluid balance in team sport athletes and the effect of hydration on cognitive, technical and physical performance. Sports Medicine 47, 1951–1982.

Pedret, C., Rodas, G., Balius, R., 2015. Return to play after soleus muscle injuries. Orthopaedic Journal of Sports Medicine 3 (7), 2325967115595802.

Powden, C.J., Hoch, J.M., Hoch, M.C., 2015. Reliability and minimal detectable change of the weight-bearing lunge test: a systematic review. Manual Therapy 20, 524–532.

Price, T.B., Kamen, G., Damon, B.M., Knight, C.A., Applegate, B., Gore, J.C., et al., 2003. Comparison of MRI with EMG to study muscle activity associated with dynamic plantar flexion. Magnetic Resonance Imaging 21 (8), 853–861.

Reid, D., McNair, P.J., Johnson, S., Potts, G., Witvrouw, E., Mahieu, N., 2012. Electromyographic analysis of an eccentric calf muscle exercise in persons with and without Achilles tendinopathy. Physical Therapy in Sport 13 (3), 150–155.

Standring, S., 2015. In: Gray's Anatomy 41st Edition, The Anatomical Basis of Clinical Practice. Elsevier.

Thomson, A., Einarsson, E., Witvrouw, E., Whiteley, R., 2017. Running speed increases plantar load more than per cent body weight on an AlterG® treadmill. Journal of Sports Sciences 35, 277–282.

Van Hooren, B., Bosch, F., 2018. Preventing hamstring injuries - Part 2: There is possibly an isometric action of the hamstrings in high-speed running and it does matter. Sport Performance & Science Reports.

van Mechelen, W., Hlobil, H., Kemper, H.C., Voorn, W.J., De Jongh, H.R., 1993. Prevention of running injuries by warm-up, cool-down, and stretching exercises. American Journal of Sports Medicine 21 (5), 711–719.

Wilson, G.J., Elliott, B.C., Wood, G.A., 1992. Stretch-shortening cycle performance enhancement through flexibility training. Medicine and Science in Sports and Exercise 24, 116–123.

Witvrouw, E., Danneels, L., Asselman, P., D'Have, T., Cambier, D., 2003. Muscle flexibility as a risk factor of developing muscle injuries in professional male soccer players. American Journal of Sports Medicine 31 (1), 41–46.

Witvrouw, E., Mahieu, N., Danneels, L., McNair, P., 2004. Stretching and injury prevention – an obscure relationship. Sports Medicine 34 (7), 443–449.

Woods, C., Hawkins, R., Hulse, M., Hodson, A., 2002. The Football Association Medical Research Programme: an audit of injuries in professional football – analysis of preseason injuries. British Journal of Sports Medicine 36 (6), 436–441.

Chapter | 20 |

Knee injuries in professional football

Jon Fearn, Paco Biosca, Dimitris Kalogiannidis and Jason Palmer

Introduction

In this chapter, we will aim to give the reader an insight into our experience in professional football and into the types of knee injuries we are exposed to in an elite football environment, i.e., the reality of football medicine. We will introduce the Chelsea Football Club Medical Department philosophy of approach, discuss some specifics of our functional rehabilitation progression and finally discuss in a little more detail specific knee injury types. We acknowledge that there are many ways to successfully deliver injury rehabilitation programmes.

Knee injuries are a common occurrence in a multidirectional sport such as football (Majewski et al., 2006), where the unique movements and loads placed on the knee complex can challenge the knee joint's integrity. Knee injuries are sustained through direct contact such as when tackling or being tackled, or during noncontact incidents such as when a player jumps and lands awkwardly, during pivoting and change-of-direction movements.

Epidemiology

The key to an effective injury rehabilitation approach is to record results and outcomes. It is important to document clearly the types of injuries sustained and how they are managed. The information below represents knee injury data from the Chelsea FC first team squad's injury audit between the 2011/12 and 2016/17 seasons. It is worth noting that under our audit criteria, a 'knee injury' refers to knee pathology where a player is unavailable to play or train for more than 48 hours.

Audit data review during the six seasons noted above showed that knee injury was the most common (n = 66) area to be injured, representing 23% of all injuries

sustained over those six seasons. The second most common injury type was thigh muscle injuries (n = 65) including hamstrings and quadriceps.

It is generally believed that ankle injuries are one of the common musculoskeletal injuries in football, but they only make up 11% of injuries at Chelsea FC and 13% in Union of European Football Associations (UEFA) Champions league football clubs. Knee articular structure injuries form the majority of knee injuries sustained (84%), with ligament (36%) and meniscal injuries (1%) being the most prevalent (Table 20.1).

Injury burden is a combined measure of the frequency (injury rate) and severity (days' absence) of injuries giving the burden of injury for the player and the consequences for the team. Injury burden is usually expressed as the number of days of absence/1000 hours of exposure. Example: Team A with 10 injuries in 5000 hours, each resulting in an absence of 10 days on average, has an injury burden of 20 days/1000 h. Team B with 20 injuries in 5000 hours, each resulting in an absence of 5 days on average, also has an injury burden of 20 days/1000 h.

The burden of knee injuries varies considerably with injury type and degree, varying between just a few days of time loss with minor issues, to several months in the more severe cases. For example, of the 17 medial collateral ligament (MCL) injuries sustained, the days where training was missed as a consequence varied from 2 to 16 days. In contrast, with more severe knee injuries such as anterior cruciate ligament (ACL) injuries (n = 4), time loss was between 146 and 193 days.

The Chelsea FC Medical Department philosophy

In our experience, key to a quality service for managing all injuries is to have a logical, progressive and

Table 20.1 Knee injuries sustained in Chelsea FC's first team squad between June 2011 and May 2017

Season	MCL[a]	LCL	ACL[a]	PCL	PLC[a]	Meniscus[a]	Patellar tendon	Patellofemoral joint	Synovium/ effusion[a]	Other
2011–12	4[b]	-	1	-	-	2	-	1	1	2
2012–13	2	-	1	1	1	2	-	-	-	-
2013–14	8	1	1	-	-	-	-	2	1	2
2014–15	-	-	-	-	1	2	1	-	1	2
2015–16	2	-	1	-	1	2	-	-	1	1
2016–17	1	2	-	-	1	-	1	-	1	1
Total	17	3	4	1	4	8	2	3	5	NA

The main structure involved is noted as the diagnosis tissue, though other structures may have also been involved.
[a]Most common knee injuries sustained.
[b]Indicates one reinjury.
ACL, Anterior cruciate ligament; LCL, lateral collateral ligament; MCL, medial collateral ligament; PCL, posterior cruciate ligament; PLC, posterolateral corner.

multidisciplinary approach that all staff understand and adhere to. This, combined with experienced multidisciplinary and multiskilled staff and excellent facilities, permits us deliver our rehabilitation service.

An overriding theme to our medical philosophy is to keep things as simple as possible. The more complex a process, the more chances there are for things to go wrong, so we try to not complicate things. Other aspects that underpin our departmental philosophy are:

- To work as a multidisciplinary team.
- To have an experienced medical staff, with a varied skill mix.
- To achieve an accurate diagnosis; this is essential to ensure that the correct management plan is implemented.
- To perform the assessment and decide on a diagnosis with multiple staff, including at least one doctor and one physiotherapist.
- To deliver one agreed diagnosis: After the group assessment, the player is asked to leave the room while the staff members discuss the findings and agree a single diagnosis and treatment plan. The player is then invited back into the room and is given a single 'team' diagnosis and a plan which the player can then also ask questions about and contribute to as they wish.
- Further investigations (magnetic resonance imaging (MRI) etc.) are carried out as necessary but are not always essential.
- A physiotherapist then leads the implementation of the injury-management plan.
- Regular feedback and communication with the medical team regarding progress, challenges and management is discussed daily, with group reviews being undertaken as required.

Chelsea FC's philosophy
'Pain-free movement is therapeutic.'

Once a diagnosis has been agreed, the goal of any rehabilitation programme is to return the individual to their previous level of function as soon as is safely possible with minimal risk of reinjury. According to our philosophy, rehab is functionally specific and therefore football-specific movement patterns are introduced as soon as is safe to do so.

Starting with simple pain-free movement patterns, our functional rehabilitation–biased approach progresses through more complex patterns as pain and the pathology permit, culminating in full injury-specific, football-specific and position-specific challenges. Again importantly, all progressions are to be performed without pain, but once, for example, 'stage 7' can be performed pain-free, we start with 'stage 8'. This approach is used by the medical staff for all players, i.e., in all squads, at all ages (professional squad, academy system from U9 to U23, women's squads) and simply adapted to the individuals accordingly.

Treatment structure

In our treatment approach, specific knee treatment is complemented with global functional movement in different modalities and environments. Players are closely supervised and progressed in these environments in a logical manner, which allows gradual and controlled load progression and therefore challenge to the healing tissue.

Methods of adapting loading include:
- aquatic therapy, where varying depth of submersion and underwater treadmills can adapt loading
- antigravity treadmills, which permit control of relative weight-bearing status
- on-field rehabilitation, where attention to drill structure can permit controlled progression.

Most players begin their functional movement progression in the water, where its qualities create a safe and productive way for the players to progress. One such water quality is that of buoyancy, which acts to reduce the relative weight-bearing status of an individual according to depth submerged. This effect has a linear relationship, whereby the greater the depth of submersion, the greater the degree of relative weight-bearing offload. Therefore, often players start walking in water at shoulder depth, which equates to approximately 20–25% weight-bearing. As comfort and quality of functional pattern improve at one water level, then the water depth is reduced, thus increasing relative weight-bearing and therefore progressing the individual towards full weight-bearing functional movement. As soon as the player can walk effectively and is symptom-free in the water at 40–50% weight-bearing, they are then progressed onto running drills, which may begin with deeper water once again, to reduce relative weight-bearing for the start of that progression. During this process the clinical presentation of the knee is closely monitored by the medical team. Early mobilization in the water not only allows the knee to move functionally in a safe and stable environment but also allows early proprioceptive stimulation to occur, which can accelerate the player's ability to progress with confidence.

Methods of functional progression

There are different ways to progress functional movement. Some examples are listed below:
- Progress from partial weight-bearing in the aquatic environment to full weight-bearing.
- Movement pattern progression: a progression may start with linear (straight line) movements in order to protect the affected knee structures before progressing onto lateral, rotational or multidirectional movements that require more knee control.
- Progress session and drill time, movement speed and movement intensity: starting with a less challenging format and progressing as the player's tolerance to the movement permits.

Again, it is important to regularly monitor the injured area's response to the intervention. This monitoring may involve looking at any pain during or after the drills, changes in swelling/effusion, monitoring knee mobility and adapting session content in the future accordingly.

This 'functional rehabilitation' approach is combined daily with manual therapy, electrotherapy techniques, proprioceptive neuromuscular control exercises and on specific occasions we may use platelet-rich plasma (PRP) injection therapy. This will depend on the site of the injury, the tissue type involved and the degree of damage sustained (see Medial collateral ligament injuries for further information on PRP injection).

A typical day for an injured player can involve 4–5 hours of work, and normally includes one-to-one attention from a member of the medical team. Each day could include:
- a multidisciplinary team assessment review
- manual therapy
- functionally based rehabilitation (e.g., in the pool, on-field with the ball, in the gym)
- proprioceptive exercises
- electrotherapy.

> ### Chelsea FC's philosophy
> 'The best prevention from football injuries is to play football.'

Our philosophy is based on the principle that the sooner the player is performing football-specific functional movement the better. This concept sits well with the theories that the best prevention strategies are very specific to the intended activity. Nothing is more specific to playing football, than playing football.

By following a comprehensive 'football function'-biased rehabilitation process for knee injuries, where gradually increasing demand is placed on the player executing functional movements, the player is best prepared for competitive return to play. We believe this approach is effective at minimizing the risk of further injury and cases of instability, and reduces the need for surgical intervention. Over the six-season period discussed, we have only had one minor reinjury (ligament injury), which also reassures us that our approach is not excessively aggressive.

'Knee-specific' targeted interventions

Following a thorough examination and an agreed diagnosis, key areas to be taken into consideration in developing a treatment plan are:
- the level and extent of anatomical injury sustained, to plan the direction of treatment, e.g., conservative or surgical

- the player's morphotype (e.g., ectomorph, mesomorph, endomorph) and the consequent pathomechanics (e.g., pes cavus, genu varum) which may have predisposed the individual to knee injury
- mobilization of the knee joint complex together with other surrounding structures involved to gain optimal range of movement
- strengthening of the muscles that can affect knee function, including those around other joints that will be involved in the lower limb kinetic chain
- neuromuscular control and proprioception of the knee, pelvis and lower limb.

Improving neuromuscular control can start with drills in controlled environments such as the pool. By making functional movements more dynamic, such as progressing walking to running and changing movement patterns from linear to multidirectional, can increase the proprioceptive demand to the knee and lower limb.

Treatment interventions need to vary according to the stage and state of the healing tissue. For example, different interventions are necessary at different healing stages and will vary in their effectiveness, but small advances can collectively help overall progression. Some examples of these include:

- Manual therapy to improve joint and soft tissue mobility.
- Rest/passive therapy to allow the tissue to heal but enhance joint mobility, e.g., continual passive motion (CPM) machines.
- Electrotherapy to optimize the healing and manage the inflammatory response for example:
  - Shortwave diathermy and magnetic therapy in the acute stages (Peres et al., 2002).
  - Therapeutic ultrasound during the proliferative and remodelling phase, particularly on superficial collagenous structures such as the MCL and lateral collateral ligament.
  - Transcutaneous electrical nerve stimulation (TENS) for pain control (Atamaz et al., 2012).
- Exercise therapy to improve proprioception, neuromuscular control and strength of the knee and lower limb (Aman et al., 2018).
- Local muscle electrical stimulation for muscles at risk of atrophy such as quadriceps. This can be combined with dynamic exercises such as cycling, straight leg raises, squats or leg press (Feil et al., 2011; Taradaj et al., 2013).
- Intermittent pneumatic compression device to reduce excessive swelling and enhance lymphatic drainage (Goats, 1989).
- Thermal therapy to either dampen the inflammatory response in the initial stages (e.g., cold/ice) or further facilitate healing response accordingly, depending on stage of healing.
- Medication use for pain control including nonsteroidal antiinflammatory drugs (NSAIDs), particularly to facilitate effective function by reducing pain in the early stages (Ong et al., 2007).
- Injection therapy – specifically PRP therapy, to facilitate the healing response (Miranda-Grajales, 2017). For example, all MCL injuries sustained at Chelsea FC returned to training within 16 days and, of these individuals, several had PRP injections included in their rehab plan. We find the use of PRP injections as an adjunct to the rehabilitation process very effective.

Common knee injuries

Following analysis of the knee injuries sustained within the first team squad over the past six seasons, the four most common knee injuries are the medial ligament, anterior cruciate ligament, meniscus and posterolateral corner.

Other structures that may become injured about the knee complex include the lateral collateral ligament, posterior cruciate ligament, patellar tendon, patellofemoral joint and synovium, as well as contusion injuries. These are relatively rare occurrences with only one or two incidents per season in the squad. Also many only stop the player from participating for a few days. Therefore we will concentrate on the more commonly seen knee injuries.

It should be noted that, in most knee injuries, there can be multiple structures involved, but we will concentrate on the main problem and diagnosis agreed.

Medial collateral ligament injuries

These have consistently been the commonest type of knee injury sustained in the first team squad over the past six seasons. The majority of kicking manoeuvres and tackles a player executes is with the instep of their foot, which puts more stress on the medial compartments of the lower limb. Injury to the MCL usually occurs because of a tackle with an opponent or an unfamiliar kicking movement excessively stressing the medial aspect of the knee.

In the early stages of an MCL injury the usual rehabilitation fundamentals are followed (as described above), i.e., restoring full knee mobility, maximizing knee strength and proprioception and maximizing the player's level of function while the injured tissue is healing. In addition to this process, with nearly all MCL injuries we perform a series of weekly PRP injections (Box 20.1 and Table 20.2). We believe this is very effective in facilitating a prompt recovery following injury.

In the case of recovery from an MCL injury, even after a relatively brief period of time, the player is able to perform pain-free linear (forward and backward) movements with ease as the MCL is not excessively stressed by these movements. These may initially be performed in the pool but they can quickly be progressed onto the field, albeit with some restrictions of space, speed and movements in a lateral or rotational direction. Over time, this can be progressed further, once the injured tissue can sustain greater and more varied loads. A player will still be performing specific exercises in the pool or gym aimed at pain-free stressing of the MCL, together with functional movements on the field (as discussed later). It is essential to differentiate between instability, that is likely to require surgical intervention, and laxity.

As the MCL recovers, the two most provocative movements that require specific attention are kicking the ball and running on a bend where the medial aspect of the knee is excessively stressed and opened. Ironically, short-distance and sometimes fast-feet manoeuvres on the field can be pain-free to execute relatively early on in their recovery, but the longer S-bend or circle runs can be troublesome. Starting kicking drills with a light volleyball or smaller, size 3 ball can be a novel way of stimulating the medial complex during the action of kicking without pain, and over time this can be built up to the full size 5 ball. This is done initially with short 'punch' passing drills and progressing to longer passing, crossing and shooting drills when the player is able.

Anterior cruciate ligament injuries

Within many professional football squads at least one player will sustain an ACL injury in any given season. They usually occur as a noncontact injury where the player moves or lands awkwardly excessively rotating and stressing the ACL complex.

In the Chelsea first team squad we have sustained four ACL injuries in six seasons. They all required surgical reconstruction, but interestingly, one player who returned to full fitness and first team–level match play did so with an ACL-deficient knee, i.e., at some point from surgery to investigation, which covered an 18-month period, the ACL graft had failed. Despite the ACL being torn, he was able to play and compete at a high level of football with no knee symptoms. These types of patients are often referred to as 'copers', versus 'non-copers' where the ACL-deficient knee is not able to cope with functional load and results in episodes of instability.

Due to the multidirectional demands of football and the excessive stresses placed on the knee joint, most players have surgery with the aim of restoring the functional anatomy of the ACL ligament and stabilizing the knee complex. In many sports, particularly those that do not put as much rotational stress on the knee, athletes can cope without having the ACL reconstructed and do not have episodes of instability or giving way while performing their given sports.

In nearly all cases of ACL injury, not only is the ACL torn but other structures are often involved. Damage to the meniscus or articular cartilage, as well as other ligaments such as the posterior cruciate ligament (PCL), MCL and posterolateral ligament complex, may also have occurred. It is important to plan the management of all aspects of the injury and decide on what interventions are appropriate. This may have a reflection in the time to return to training.

Box 20.1 What is platelet-rich plasma?

Platelet-rich plasma (PRP) is isolated from blood via a centrifuge. The proposed mechanism of action of PRP is that it assists in the healing process of an injured tendon. Tendon connective tissue has poor blood supply and, hence, decreased healing properties. Platelets contain endogenous growth factors. These growth factors are: transforming growth factor-β1 (TGF-β1), insulin-like growth factors (IGF) 1 and 2, vascular endothelial growth factor (VEGF), basic fibroblast growth factor (BFGF) and hepatocyte growth factor (HGF).

Miranda-Grajales, H., 2017. Platelet-rich plasma. In: Pope, J., Deer, T. (Eds.), Treatment of Chronic Pain Conditions. Springer, New York, NY.

Table 20.2 Recovery time for MCL injuries receiving platelet-rich plasma injections at Chelsea FC

Season	No. of MCL injuries	Days out	Average days out
2011–12	4	3:7:16:13	10
2012–13	2	5:4	4
2013–14	8	15:5:15:4:13:15:7:2	9
2014–15	0	-	-
2015–16	2	13:16	14
2016–17	1	5	5

MCL, Medial collateral ligament.

In a relatively straightforward ACL injury with no or minor meniscal involvement we would expect a player to return to training at around 5 months; however, with more complex injuries it may take considerably longer due to more structural damage to the knee.

The rehabilitation of an ACL injury does take time as the knee is heavily compromised. Every player responds to surgery differently and therefore the rehabilitation of a player with an ACL injury is different in every case. We have compiled an ACL rehabilitation protocol (Appendix 1) to guide clinicians as to our approach when managing this type of injury. This guide is used for all squads within the club.

Meniscus injuries

It is worth noting that it is not uncommon to identify meniscal issues on clinical examination of the knee and commonly seen in investigations such as MRI scans (Fig. 20.1). Many of these findings are old chronic meniscal changes that have been present without any symptoms for some time and do not require any intervention. They definitely do not require surgery. It is accepted practice now when dealing with meniscal disruption (i.e., the presence of tears or degeneration) to avoid performing surgery unless clinically indicated, for example in a knee locked due to meniscal disruption. Unnecessary surgery may render the player vulnerable to premature articular cartilage damage, and in the case of a young player can be career threatening within a few years of surgery.

Once a meniscal injury is diagnosed by clinical examination, which may or may not be supported by MRI findings, the medical team decide on the management approach indicated. Over the past six seasons, we have sustained eight meniscal injuries, five of which resulted in arthroscopic surgery (either resection or repair) and these players missed between 21 to 78 days. Of the remaining three meniscal injuries treated conservatively, all had PRP injections, which we believe accelerates the healing response and players' return to play. Players managed conservatively returned to play in 3 to 8 days. The decision as to whether conservative or surgical intervention was required was based on the clinical examination and the extent of the damage to the meniscus.

The rehabilitation approach is fundamentally the same as with all other knee injuries, i.e., reducing swelling/effusion, restoring full knee mobility, normalizing strength and proprioception around the knee complex and progressing the functional capabilities of the knee specific to football and the players' positional demands. During the rehabilitation of meniscal injuries, particular attention is given to the presence or extent of an effusion within the knee or any loss of knee mobility. This may give a clear indication as to whether the knee is coping with the level and progress of the rehabilitation process.

Posterolateral corner injuries

The posterolateral corner (PLC) has a complex anatomical structure with muscles such as the popliteus, tendons including the biceps femoris and ligaments such as the arcuate ligament and popliteofibular ligament all contributing to its ability to control knee extension, lateral rotation and varus stress.

Injuries usually occur as a result of the PLC complex restraint being overstretched during forceful open or closed chain activities such as tackling or landing awkwardly (Fig. 20.2).

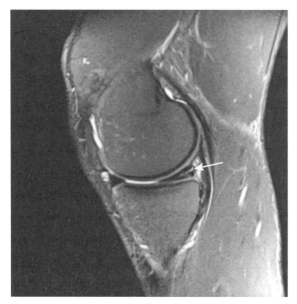

Fig. 20.1 MRI scan of the right knee showing a meniscal tear (arrow).

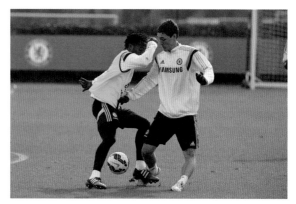

Fig. 20.2 Hyperextension of the knee is a common mechanism of posterolateral corner injuries.

Rehabilitation of PLC injuries essentially follows a logical, conservative management process as described previously with care not to overmobilize the damaged structures. This excessive mobilization may lead to laxity of the PLC complex and problems during functional activities. In our experience, many of these injuries recover within a few weeks. One case took 46 days to return to training but this was complicated with an associated partial tear to the biceps tendon.

On-field rehabilitation

If the player is unable to train or perform their normal sporting activities it is important they optimize the 'functional rehabilitation' recovery process in a more controlled environment. This may take the form of on-field rehabilitation.

As soon as the player is able to complete quality movement patterns in a reduced–weight bearing environment such as the water, then both you and the player will have confidence making the transition to full–weight bearing function. If you have not been able to do this, then you need to introduce the activity in its most basic form and build up the complexity as they tolerate each step.

Although the functional movement approach aims to focus on function rather than the pathology, the nature and type of movement you are going to include in your first sessions on the grass will be influenced, in part, by the pathology you are dealing with.

Again, as per the functional movement philosophy, as soon as you can do something you should. If, for example, you have been doing light multidirectional movements in the water and the player has tolerated these well, then you can introduce low-intensity versions of these movements early, even in the first session on land.

The sessions are then progressed accordingly by increasing the intensity or speed of the exercises, the amount of time spent on field and the increasing complexity and stress on the knee structures.

As previously mentioned, start with linear, straight-line drills at a low pace, which ensures the knee complex is protected and the neuromuscular control progressed. Fig. 20.3 is an example of an early linear drill that a player may execute on the field.

The player is then progressed onto lateral cutting or rotational movements with increasing speed. Also, introducing external cues and obstacles such as the ball provides subtle ways of increasing the complexity and demand of the exercise.

Fig. 20.4 is an example of a more advanced, controlled on-field drill for an attacking footballer. With problem-free execution of drills such as this, the player will be close to return to modified training.

The Injury-Prevention Unit at Chelsea FC

We are currently compiling a 'Prevention Unit' to ensure our injury-prevention philosophy is mirrored throughout the Football Club. This involves all squads at all ages to include professional, academy and ladies, as well as the foundation and developmental squads.

The Unit will be multidisciplinary, involving doctors, physios, coaches, fitness coaches and sport scientists representing all the squads involved.

As a club there is a common message for all players to be educated in the importance of health essentials such as nutrition, sleep, lifestyle and mental and physical wellbeing. It is the Prevention Unit's role to look at ways to improve a player's locomotor control and performance.

By having a Prevention Unit delivering the same message, we hope to ensure our philosophy is followed from the first team squad down to the youngest age group (8-year-olds) throughout the club and ensure our players are able to play and enjoy their football as much as possible.

It is worth noting that within the first team squad, due to players' playing commitments for both club and country with regular periods where there is only 2–3 days between competitive games, having the time to implement injury-prevention strategies can be challenging.

Conclusion

There are numerous articles, research papers and books dedicated to the epidemiology and management of knee injuries. These tend to come from academic institutions or hospitals, which are far removed from the reality of our experiences in professional football. Our experience shows that scientific methodology of injury management is generally not a true reflection of what happens within a professional football club.

We believe that a logical, progressive, functional approach is the most effective management for knee injuries in football. This essentially starts with an accurate diagnosis involving all members of the medical team following a thorough and comprehensive examination. The player's injury is then managed with local or knee-specific targeted interventions together with early functional loading strategies in safe, controlled environments. The ultimate goal is completing football-related tasks relevant to the individual player's position to a sufficient speed, intensity and duration to allow them to return to the training environment. On many occasions when returning to the squad training environment, there may be a period of modification where the player's involvement is adapted according to their requirements. This obviously requires close discussion with the management and coaching staff and may or may not always be necessary. Having said that, there is no alternative when preparing to return to playing professional football than to play professional football: The random, unexpected movements and decisions that occur in the training and match environment cannot be replicated in any other way.

Linear Function Drill

Simple linear functional drill

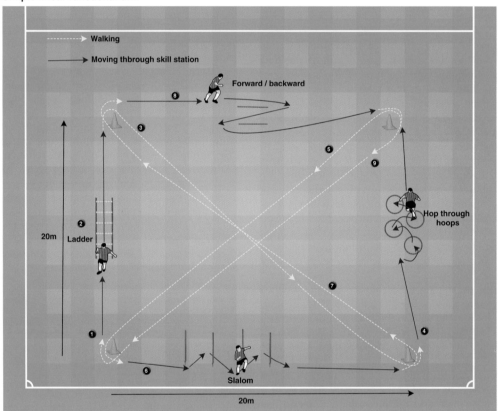

Linear Functional Movement Drill (no ball):
- The player starts at one cone (1) and then moves through the first drill station (2).
- Once the player reaches the cone at the other end, they slow down turn around the cone, walking across the grid to the next cone (3).
- At the next cone the player turns and moves through the next drill station (4), repeating the cycle of turning and walking across the grid (5) for recovery.
- This cycle continues until all 4 drill stations have been performed. This drill could be performed at varying intensities during the work phase, and could be repeated 2-3 times as a single cycle of 4 stations with 60-90 seconds rest between each cycle, or the player could perform the circuit 2-3 times in a row as their function and rehab progress.

Fig. 20.3 Diagram showing an early linear drill.

Attacking drill

Complex attacking drill

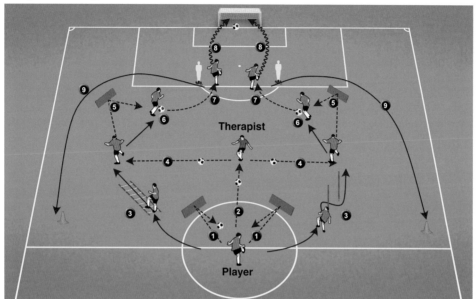

Attacking drill: Player stands in the centre circle and alternates passes off the 2 bounce boards near him/her (1). After 5-8 seconds the therapist calls "left" or "right" and the player reacts by passing the ball to the therapist (2) and moves in the direction nominated through the skill station without the ball (3). As the player comes out of the skill station, the therapist passes the player the ball (4). The player controls the ball and passes the ball off the second bounce board (5), controls the rebounding ball (6) then attacks the nearest mannequin (7), shooting as they pass it (8). Then immediately after shooting, the player runs at pace back to the cone near the halfway line (9).

This drill can be performed 4-6 times in varying directions, with a good recovery period (60-90 seconds) between each performance so that quality and intensity of performance are optimised.

Fig. 20.4 Diagram showing a more advanced controlled on-field drill for an attacking footballer.

Acknowledgements

The content of this chapter is a reflection of the team approach we have in the Chelsea FC Medical Department. We have a very experienced medical team representing differing backgrounds, opinions and skills but we aim to deliver an agreed approach by the collective. We, the authors, would like to acknowledge the contribution of the whole medical team to this chapter.

References

Åman, M., Larsén, K., Forssblad, M., Näsmark, A., Waldén, M., Hägglund, M., 2018. A nationwide follow-up survey on the effectiveness of an implemented neuromuscular training program to reduce acute knee injuries in soccer players. Orthopaedic Journal of Sports Medicine 6 (12), 2325967118813841.

Atamaz, F.C., Durmaz, B., Baydar, M., et al., 2012. Comparison of the efficacy of transcutaneous electrical nerve stimulation, interferential currents, and shortwave diathermy in knee osteoarthritis: a double-blind, randomized, controlled, multicenter study. Archives of Physical Medicine and Rehabilitation 93 (5), 748–756.

Feil, S., Newell, J., Minogue, C., Paessler, H.H., 2011. The effectiveness of supplementing a standard rehabilitation program with superimposed neuromuscular electrical stimulation after anterior cruciate ligament reconstruction: a prospective, randomized, single-blind study. The American Journal of Sports Medicine 39 (6), 1238–1247.

Goats, G.C., 1989. Pulsed electromagnetic (short-wave) energy therapy. British Journal of Sports Medicine 23 (4), 213–216.

Majewski, M., Habelt, S., Steinbrück, K., 2006. Epidemiology of athletic knee injuries: a 10-year study. The Knee Journal 13 (3), 184–188.

Miranda-Grajales, H., 2017. Platelet-rich plasma. In: Pope, J., Deer, T. (Eds.), Treatment of Chronic Pain Conditions. Springer, New York, NY.

Ong, C.K.S., Lirk, P., Seymour, R.A., 2007. An evidence-based update on nonsteroidal anti-inflammatory drugs. Clinical Medicine & Research 5 (1), 19–34.

Peres, S.D., Knight, K., 2002. Pulsed shortwave diathermy and prolonged long-duration stretching increase dorsiflexion range of motion more than identical stretching without diathermy. Journal of Athletic Training 37(1), 43–50.

Taradaj, J., Halski, T., Kucharzewski, M., Walewicz, K., Smykla, A., Ozon, M., et al., 2013. The effect of neuromuscular electrical stimulation on quadriceps strength and knee function in professional soccer players: return to sport after ACL reconstruction. BioMed Research International 2013, 802534.

UEFA Champions League Injury Audit Data 2011–2017. Chelsea FC unpublished data.

Chapter | 21 |

The sporting ankle: lateral ankle sprain, the most commonly incurred lower limb musculoskeletal injury

Eamonn Delahunt

Introduction

Ankle joint injuries are commonly sustained by athletes who participate in field and court sports. The most frequently sustained ankle joint injury by athletes participating in these sports is a lateral ankle sprain. Due to the high prevalence, injury incidence rate and injury burden of lateral ankle sprains, it is essential that clinicians working with field and court sport athletes are 'experts' in ankle joint injury assessment, diagnosis and rehabilitation. This chapter details a case study of a semiprofessional football (soccer) player who sustained an acute ankle joint injury. This case study details the clinical assessment and clinical reasoning processes associated with an injury diagnosis and the development of an impairment-based rehabilitation framework.

Case description

A 22-year-old male semiprofessional association football player (Player A) sustained a traumatic contact ankle joint injury. At the time of injury he was in possession of the football and was running at high speed towards the opposing team's 18-yard box. In an effort to prevent him from penetrating the 18-yard box, a defending player performed a sliding tackle but missed the football and instead made contact with Player A on the inside of his shin just above the medial malleolus. This physical contact resulted in a substantial inversion and internal rotation of Player A's ankle/foot

complex. As a result of this injury, Player A was substituted; however, he was able to ambulate off the pitch with minor assistance from the team Chartered Physiotherapist.

Injury epidemiology

Ankle joint injuries account for 13% of all injuries sustained by elite European football players (Walden et al., 2013). The injury incidence rate for ankle joint injuries is 1/1000 hours; this means that a professional football team with a 25-player squad will incur seven ankle joint injuries per season. Ankle sprain injuries account for 68% of all ankle joint injuries, with an injury incidence rate of 0.7/1000 hours, which means that a professional football team with a 25-player squad will incur five ankle sprain injuries per season. Up to 75% of all ankle sprain injuries involve injury to the lateral ligament complex, with only 5% of injuries being classified as 'high ankle sprains'. The average time loss due to ankle joint injury is 16 days; however 'high ankle sprains' have a substantially longer average time loss of 43 days. Foul play has been reported to contribute to 40% of match-related ankle joint sprains. Thus, it clear that ankle joint injuries are a substantial concern in football.

Mechanism of injury

Establishing the mechanism of injury is a fundamental component of all clinical assessments. It gives clinicians an indication as to the anatomical structures which are likely to have incurred injury and hence, what tissues should be prioritized during the physical component of the clinical assessment.

To develop a comprehensive understanding of the mechanisms of ankle joint injuries and, in particular, ankle sprains in football, Andersen and colleagues (2004) evaluated videotape recordings of 26 ankle sprains in Norwegian and Icelandic elite football from the 1999–2000 seasons. They reported that one of the most common injury mechanisms included player-to-player contact, with impact by an opponent on the medial aspect of the leg just before or at foot strike resulting in a laterally directed force causing an inversion and internal rotation of the ankle/foot complex. Therefore, based on one published article in the peer-reviewed literature, the mechanism of injury described in the case description above is common in football.

Clinicians should suspect injury to the lateral ligaments of the ankle joint if a patient reports that the injury mechanism included a contact-based or noncontact-based sudden rapid inversion and internal rotation loading of the ankle/foot complex. The mechanisms of injury associated with 'high ankle sprains' are less clear, but typically include external rotation of the foot and hyperdorsiflexion of the ankle joint.

Clinical assessment: the essentials

Fracture

As described in the case description, Player A was able to ambulate off the pitch with minor assistance from the team chartered physiotherapist. This indicates that it was unlikely an ankle joint fracture was sustained. A specific criterion of the Ottawa ankle rules relates to the weight-bearing status of the patient immediately after injury and upon clinical assessment (Stiell et al., 1993). If instead, Player A had been unable to weight-bear immediately after injury or at the time of clinical assessment then the probability of ankle joint fracture would have been heightened. Nonetheless, due to the traumatic contact nature of the mechanism of injury, it would be prudent to undertake the Ottawa ankle rules clinical assessment (Stiell et al., 1993). In this instance, the primary objective would be to assess for bone tenderness located along the distal posterior 6 cm of the medial or lateral malleolus, which specifically replicates or recreates Player A's 'known pain'. At the time of clinical assessment, no bone tenderness replicating Player A's 'known pain' was observed, hence negating the need for an X-ray of the ankle joint. This finding of no specific bone tenderness replicating his 'known pain' coupled with his ability to ambulate immediately after the injury (albeit with assistance) means that an X-ray was not warranted, as the probability of ankle joint fracture in this instance was less than 1%.

Ligaments

The mechanism of injury outlined in the case description indicates that injury to the lateral ankle joint ligaments is highly likely. As such, the anterior talofibular ligament and calcaneofibular ligament should be prioritized during the physical component of the clinical assessment. Ankle sprain injuries account for 68% of all ankle joint injuries in football, with 75% of these involving tissue damage to the lateral ankle joint ligaments (Waldén et al., 2013).

The anterior talofibular ligament should be palpated and stretched (passive plantar flexion of the ankle joint combined with passive inversion and internal rotation of the foot). Replication or recreation of Player A's 'known pain' on palpation or stretching of the anterior talofibular ligament is indicative of tissue damage to this ligament. In this instance, both palpation and stretching of the anterior talofibular ligament recreated Player A's 'known pain', indicating tissue damage to this ligament. In addition to palpation and stretching of the anterior talofibular ligament, the anterior drawer test can be performed. This is a clinical assessment test that can be utilized to determine whether the anterior talofibular ligament is completely ruptured. Note that the sensitivity and specificity of the anterior drawer test is optimized if this clinical assessment test is performed 4–6 days postinjury (van Dijk et al., 1996). In this instance, no sulcus sign was observed on clinical assessment during the performance of the anterior drawer test, indicating that Player A had not sustained a complete rupture of his anterior talofibular ligament.

The calcaneofibular ligament should be palpated and stretched (passive inversion of the rearfoot with the ankle joint in a dorsiflexed position). Replication or recreation of Player A's 'known pain' on palpation or stretching of the calcaneofibular ligament is indicative of tissue damage to this ligament. In this instance, palpation and stretching of the calcaneofibular ligament did not recreated Player A's 'known pain', thus indicating no tissue damage to this ligament.

Although the mechanism of injury outlined in the descriptive case is not in keeping with that of a 'high ankle sprain', due to the traumatic contact nature of the injury, it would nonetheless be prudent to undertake a clinical assessment of the ankle joint syndesmosis ligaments. The two most important clinical assessment tests include palpation of the anterior inferior tibiofibular ligament (most sensitive) and the squeeze test (most specific). The combined findings of these clinical assessments can guide a clinician in determining whether a patient is likely to have sustained tissue damage to the ankle joint syndesmosis ligaments. If tissue damage of the ankle joint syndesmosis ligaments is suspected, diagnostic imaging (typically magnetic resonance imaging) can be utilized to confirm or refute the suspicion. In the case of Player A, palpation of the anterior inferior tibiofibular ligament did not recreate his 'known pain', nor did the squeeze test. These combined negative clinical assessment findings indicate that tissue damage to the ankle joint syndesmosis ligaments was unlikely.

Physical component of the clinical assessment: the summary

Integrating the information about the mechanism of injury and the primary findings of the clinical assessment detailed above, it was concluded that Player A sustained an isolated injury of his anterior talofibular ligament. Diagnostic medical imaging was not utilized as there were no indications from the clinical assessment that this was necessary.

Rehabilitation of the footballer's ankle

The primary objective is to return Player A to his preinjury level of performance without putting him or others at undue risk of injury, whilst simultaneously mitigating his risk of future injury. To achieve such an objective, it is essential that clinicians consider the paradigm of injury-induced sensorimotor insufficiencies.

Sensorimotor insufficiencies: the theory

The sensorimotor system is the biological system that controls the contributions of the dynamic restraints (i.e., muscles) for the maintenance of functional joint stability. It comprises all the afferent, efferent and central integration and processing components involved in preserving functional joint stability. A constant flow of afferent impulses (i.e., somatosensory input) from articular, cutaneous and musculotendinous mechanoreceptors enter the spinal cord via the dorsal root and are projected to higher-order processing centres including the brainstem, cerebellum and somatosensory cortex. An appropriate coordinated motor response (i.e., efferent response) with the objective of maintaining functional joint stability is developed in response to the afferent impulses from these aforementioned mechanoreceptors. As an example, following joint perturbation (e.g., unexpected sudden supination of the foot due to placing the foot in a divot on a football pitch whilst running), articular, cutaneous and musculotendinous mechanoreceptors are stimulated. In response, there is neural transmission of afferent signals to the central

nervous system with processing of these signals occurring at higher-order centres. The resultant efferent signals initiate muscle activation and force production in order to maintain functional stability of the ankle joint and prevent injury. Ankle joint injury can injure articular, cutaneous and musculotendinous tissues. Hence, it is logical to conclude that somatosensory input to the sensorimotor system is disrupted following ankle joint injury.

The safe and efficient performance of motor tasks is dependent upon the synchronous interaction of preprogrammed sensorimotor efferent and afferent feedback mechanisms. Disturbance of this synchrony, as may occur upon disruption of somatosensory afferents, may have the capacity to distort the preprogrammed motor task–specific coordination and movement strategies 'stored' by the sensorimotor system. For example, the organismic constraints (e.g., pain, swelling, tissue injury) induced by an ankle sprain injury have been proposed to interrupt the flow of impulses from the mechanoreceptors in the injured tissues to the central nervous system. This, in turn, may trigger adaptive patterns of sensorimotor reorganization, 'resetting' previously established coordination and movement strategies in the adoption of new coordination and movement patterns. These alterations may then manifest either in a continuum of residual symptoms that compromise functional joint stability and that heighten the risk of future injury. Of particular note is that these alterations do not resolve quickly and continue to manifest in the weeks and months after injury, unless a specific, targeted and appropriate sensorimotor intervention is implemented.

Clinical assessment of sensorimotor insufficiencies

The following sections outline the rationale and some proposed evidence-supported mechanisms for undertaking a comprehensive clinical assessment, with the objective of establishing the presence of sensorimotor impairments.

Pain

Player A's self-reported ankle joint pain could be quantified using an appropriate patient-oriented outcome measure. A number of options exist for assessing ankle joint pain in clinical environments. A numeric rating scale for pain, which can be administered both verbally and in writing, could be easily utilized to quantify his pain during the performance of various motor tasks. The quantification of Player A's self-reported ankle joint pain could be used as a clinically oriented outcome measure to guide the progression of an exercise-based rehabilitation intervention. For example, in performing an anterior

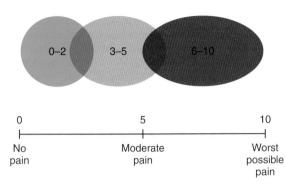

0   5   10

No   Moderate   Worst
pain   pain   possible
pain

Fig. 21.1 'Traffic light' numeric pain rating scale. Green, likely safe to continue the exercise; orange, caution warranted as the exercise may exceed the tolerance of the loaded tissues; red, likely unsafe to continue the exercise as the tolerance of the loaded tissues is likely exceeded.

hopping drill, the distance of the required hop should not be progressed until the patient can perform the required hop distance with minimal pain. If, for example, Player A noted an increase in his ankle joint pain in response to a specific exercise progression involving an increase in hopping distance, then it would be logical to conclude that this exercise progression is excessively loading the injured tissues and may not be appropriately aligned to the phase of tissue healing. In these instances, a 'traffic light system' could be integrated with the numeric rating scale for pain, allowing for unambiguous guidance of exercise progression (Fig. 21.1). The quantification of Player A's self-reported ankle joint pain serves another purpose. It could also be used to assess the efficacy of any treatment implemented, thus helping to guide the appropriate choice of therapeutic interventions.

Swelling

Ankle joint swelling can alter the flow of afferent impulses into the central nervous system, with the primary manifestation being the development of arthrogenic muscle inhibition. This, in turn, can compromise functional joint stability via an alteration in muscle activation and consequent force production.

The magnitude of swelling of Player A's injured ankle joint could be assessed clinically using the figure-of-eight mechanism and then used as a clinically oriented outcome measure to guide the progression of an exercise-based rehabilitation intervention. For example, during the rehabilitation of jump landing technique, an increase in ankle joint swelling (greater than the minimum detectable change that has been established for the figure-of-eight: 9.6 mm) (Rohner-Spengler et al., 2007) following the progression from double leg landings to single leg landing on the

injured ankle would indicate that this progression is premature. Therefore, in this instance, it may be more appropriate to add an 'environmental constraint' (e.g., having Player A control a football on his chest and pass it back to the clinician immediately following landing or having Player A perform a heading task with a double leg landing), rather than changing the 'task constraint' (i.e., performing a single leg landing on the injured ankle).

Quantifying the magnitude of swelling of Player A's injured ankle serves another purpose. Similar to that described in the paragraph above for pain, quantifying the magnitude of swelling could also be used to assess the efficacy of any treatment implemented, helping to guide the appropriate choice of therapeutic interventions.

Range of motion: osteokinematics and arthrokinematics

Ankle joint range of motion is dependent upon the interaction of osteokinematics and arthrokinematics. Osteokinematics refers to the movements that occur around a centre of rotation, namely the joint axis. In relation to the ankle joint, the primary osteokinematic movements include plantar flexion/dorsiflexion. Since the axis of rotation of the ankle joint is not situated in a cardinal plane, the motions occurring at the ankle joint are typically described as triplanar; plantar flexion is associated with inversion and internal rotation whilst dorsiflexion is associated with eversion and abduction. In contrast, arthrokinematics refers to the movement of joint surfaces, with normal joint surface motion being integral to long-term joint integrity. Joint surfaces move with respect to one another by simultaneously rolling, gliding and spinning. Relative to the ankle joint, posterior glide of the talus occurs during dorsiflexion with the opposite glide (i.e., anterior glide) occurring during plantar flexion.

A common finding following ankle joint injury and in particular lateral ankle sprain injury is a temporary or long-term restriction in dorsiflexion range of motion. This is particularly relevant and warrants considerable attention, as dorsiflexion range of motion has been reported to explain up to 28% of the variance in dynamic postural balance performance as assessed by the anterior reach direction of the star excursion balance test (Hoch et al., 2011). Player A's ankle joint dorsiflexion range of motion could be assessed using the valid and reliable weight-bearing lunge test (Langarika-Rocafort et al., 2017). To determine whether an associated dorsiflexion deficit is primarily osteokinematic or arthrokinematic, the clinician could perform a series of anterior-to-posterior mobilizations applied to the talus. In this instance, if the dorsiflexion deficit was primarily arthrokinematic, then such a series of mobilizations would result in an immediate improvement in dorsiflexion range of motion.

Table 21.1 Isometric ankle joint strength scores for Player A's noninjured and injured ankle joints as assessed via handheld dynamometry

	Noninjured ankle joint	Injured ankle joint	Mean difference
Isometric inversion (N)	95	80	15
Isometric eversion (N)	92	79	13
Isometric dorsiflexion (N)	159	140	19
Values are measured in Newtons (N)			

Player A's weight-bearing lunge test score for his injured ankle joint was 13 cm. Immediately following the application of two 2-min sets of Maitland grade III anterior-to-posterior talocrural joint mobilizations with 1 min of rest between sets, his weight-bearing lunge test score improved by 2 cm. This indicated that his restriction in dorsiflexion range of motion was primarily arthrokinematic in nature.

Muscle strength

The ankle joint muscles constitute the dynamic restraints for the maintenance of functional joint stability. During the contractile process, musculotendinous units generate stiffness, which contribute to the dynamic protection of the joint upon which they act. A deficit in ankle joint strength could compromise the integrity of the ankle joint to withstand sudden injurious movements. Therefore, the clinical assessment of ankle joint strength is important to consider following ankle joint injury. A handheld dynamometer can be used in clinical settings to reliably and objectively quantify ankle joint strength (Kelln et al., 2008).

Player A's isometric ankle joint strength values as assessed using a handheld dynamometer are detailed in Table 21.1.

Static and dynamic postural balance

Postural balance refers to the ability of an individual to control the position of their centre of mass relative to their base of support to prevent falls. Decreased postural balance is commonly reported as a primary risk factor for sustaining noncontact lower limb musculoskeletal injuries. Therefore, following musculoskeletal injury, if a primary objective is to mitigate the risk of recurrent injury, then it is logical to conclude that the assessment of both static and dynamic postural balance should be routinely incorporated into any clinical assessment.

Player A's static postural balance performance could be assessed by having him perform each of the six constituent tests of the Balance Error Scoring System (BESS) (Fig. 21.2). Assessing Player A's performance in each of these six tests could provide useful information for the development of the static postural balance exercise component of his rehabilitation programme.

Player A's static postural balance performance could be assessed by having him perform specified reach directions of the star excursion balance test (Fig. 21.3). The three most commonly utilized reach directions are the anterior, posterior-lateral and posterior-medial reach directions. In each instance, the reach distance is normalized relative to the patient's leg length (as measured from anterior superior iliac spine to distal tip of medial malleolus) and multiplied by 100, producing a score that represents a percentage of leg length (Eq. 21.1). Additionally, a composite score can also be calculated (Eq. 21.2).

$$\text{Normalized reach distance (\% leg length)} = \frac{\text{reach distance achieved (cm)}}{\text{leg length (cm)}} \times 100 \qquad \text{Eq. 21.1}$$

$$\text{Composite normalized reach distance (\% leg length)} =$$
$$\frac{[\text{anterior (cm)} + \text{posterior} - \text{lateral (cm)} + \text{posterior} - \text{medial (cm)}]}{\text{leg length (cm)} \times 3} \times 100$$
$$\text{Eq. 21.2}$$

Player A's performance on these reach directions could then be utilized as a clinically oriented outcome measure to assess the efficacy of any treatment implemented and also to monitor the recovery of his dynamic postural balance performance.

Table 21.2 summarizes the number of 'errors' made by Player A when performing each of the constituent tests of the BESS. Table 21.3 summarizes the normalized reach distance scores (i.e., percentage leg length) achieved by Player A when performing the anterior, posterior-medial and posterior-lateral reach directions of the star excursion balance test.

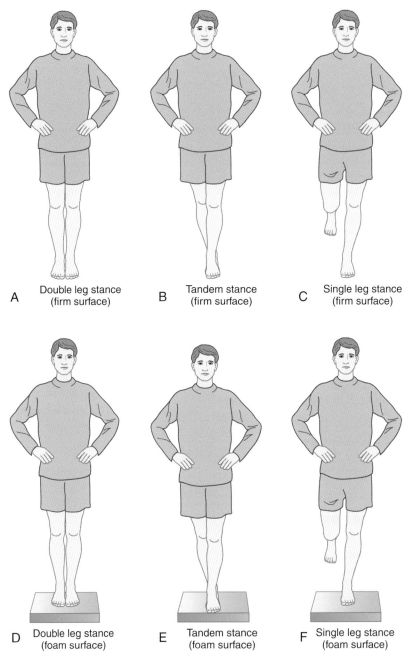

A Double leg stance
(firm surface)

B Tandem stance
(firm surface)

C Single leg stance
(firm surface)

D Double leg stance
(foam surface)

E Tandem stance
(foam surface)

F Single leg stance
(foam surface)

Fig. 21.2 The six constituent tests of the Balance Error Scoring System. (A) Double leg stance (firm surface). (B) Tandem stance (firm surface). (C) Single leg stance (firm surface). (D) Double leg stance (foam surface). (E) Tandem stance (foam surface). (F) Single leg stance (foam surface). All tests are initiated and last for 20 s when the patient closes his eyes.

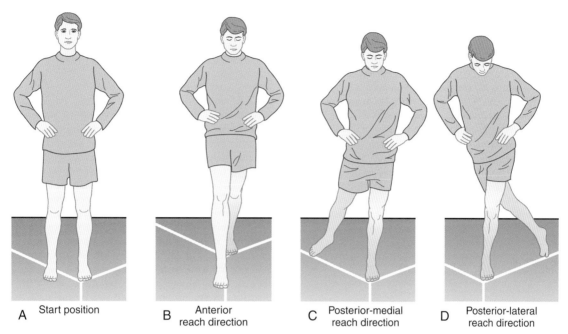

| A | Start position | B | Anterior reach direction | C | Posterior-medial reach direction | D | Posterior-lateral reach direction |

Fig. 21.3 The star excursion balance test. (A) Start position. (B) Anterior reach direction. (C) Posterior-medial reach direction. (D) Posterior-lateral reach direction.

Table 21.2 Balance errors made by Player A as assessed via performance on the Balance Error Scoring System

	Double leg stance (firm surface)	Tandem stance (firm surface)	Single leg stance (firm surface)	Double leg stance (foam surface)	Tandem stance (foam surface)	Single leg stance (foam surface)
Errors	0	2	5	2	5	10

Table 21.3 Normalized reach distance scores achieved by Player A on three of the reach directions of the star excursion balance test

	Anterior reach direction	Posterior-medial reach direction	Posterior-lateral reach direction
Normalized reach distance (% leg length)	58	94	83

Therapeutic interventions for and rehabilitation of identified sensorimotor insufficiencies

The goal of any postinjury therapeutic intervention and rehabilitation programme should be to return the injured athlete to practice or competition without putting him/her or others at undue risk for injury, whilst concomitantly mitigating the risk of reinjury. In the case description

presented, a number of sensorimotor insufficiencies were identified on clinical assessment using objective, valid and reliable methodologies. These sensorimotor insufficiencies should be utilized to guide any planned therapeutic interventions and exercise-based rehabilitation.

Range of motion: osteokinematics and arthrokinematics

Using a clinical reasoning approach, it was determined that Player A's restriction in dorsiflexion range of motion was primarily arthrokinematic. As such, utilization of joint mobilizations with the specific purpose of improving posterior glide of the talus should be implemented as a therapeutic intervention. There are a number of manual therapy techniques that are supported by peer-reviewed literature, including Maitland anterior-to-posterior talocrural joint mobilizations (Hoch et al., 2012; Hoch and McKeon, 2011), as well as dorsiflexion mobilizations with movement (Collins et al., 2004; Vicenzino et al., 2006). The weight-bearing lunge test should be used to clinically evaluate Player A's response to the application of any manual therapy techniques. In this instance the objective would be to minimize any between-limb asymmetry in dorsiflexion range of motion. Note that weight-bearing dorsiflexion should continue to be evaluated during the later stages of rehabilitation, as anecdotally, arthrokinematic deficits in dorsiflexion range of motion can reemerge when ankle joint loading increases during the performance of sport-specific motor tasks.

Muscle strength

As detailed in Table 21.1 it was determined using hand-held dynamometry that Player A had impairments in isometric strength of his injured ankle joint. Strength training has been reported to influence motor unit recruitment, selective activation of agonist muscles and their motor units and antagonist coactivation (Komi and Sale, 1992). Additionally, when considering the performance of dynamic and sport-specific exercises, a fundamental level of musculotendionous stiffness is necessary for optimal utilization of the stretch–shortening cycle process. As such, multiplanar ankle joint strengthening exercises should be incorporated as an integral part of an exercise-based rehabilitation programme. Numerous exercise-based rehabilitation programmes have been detailed in the published literature, which include ankle joint strengthening exercises (Docherty et al., 1998; Hall et al., 2015).

Static and dynamic postural balance

The results obtained from the clinical assessment of Player A's static (see Table 21.2) and dynamic (see Table 21.3) postural balance performance could be utilized to develop the initial foundation for the exercise-based postural balance component of his rehabilitation programme. Regarding the interpretation of the static postural balance performance scores outlined in Table 21.2, the following would be an appropriate clinical reasoning approach. No errors were made by Player A when completing the double leg stance (firm surface) task. Hence, this task will not challenge the sensorimotor system and

its incorporation into a rehabilitation programme would be redundant. Player A made two errors whilst completing the tandem stance (firm surface) task and the double leg stance (foam surface) task. This low number of errors would suggest that these tasks should only constitute a minority component (i.e., small percentage) of the total time devoted to postural balance exercises. Player A made five errors whilst completing the single leg stance (firm surface) task and the tandem stance (foam surface) task. This is a substantial number of errors for each of these tasks and suggests that they are appropriately challenging the sensorimotor system, i.e., they are not so easy such that he can complete them with minimal errors, but they are not so difficult such that he cannot complete them at all. Therefore, it would be prudent to include these tasks as key exercises of the postural balance component of his rehabilitation programme. Player A made 10 errors (i.e., the maximum number of errors) whilst completing the single leg stance (foam surface) task. This suggests that this task is too challenging (at this time point) for the sensorimotor system and should not be included as an initial exercise of the postural balance component of his rehabilitation programme.

Regarding the interpretation of the dynamic postural balance performance scores outlined in Table 21.3, the following would be an appropriate clinical reasoning approach. All of the normalized reach distance scores are lower than what would be expected of a noninjured semiprofessional soccer player (Butler et al., 2012; Stiffler et al., 2015), hence Player A presents with substantial impairments in dynamic postural balance performance. The star excursion balance test should not just be considered as a clinical assessment methodology, rather it should also be considered as a dynamic postural balance rehabilitation exercise. Performance of the different reach directions of the star excursion balance test challenge multiple components of the sensorimotor system (Gabriner et al., 2015).

Athlete profile

In assessing Player A's readiness to return to sport, it would be necessary to ensure that he is adequately prepared for the physiological, tactical and psychological demands of his sport. As stated before, the primary objective of any therapeutic intervention and rehabilitation programme would be to return Player A to his preinjury level of performance without putting him or others at undue risk of injury, whilst simultaneously mitigating his risk of future injury. As such, it is vital that clinicians have a comprehensive understanding of the physiological, tactical and

Table 21.4 Characteristic features of other ankle joint injuries experienced by field and court sport athletes

Injury	Characteristic patient-reported injury symptoms	Typical clinical assessment findings
Posterior ankle impingement	Pain experienced at end-range plantar flexion	Pain reproduced on forced plantar flexion
Midportion Achilles tendinopathy	Morning stiffness localized in the midportion of the Achilles tendon	Pain localized in the midportion of the Achilles tendon with activities that load the tendon, such as hopping
Insertional Achilles tendinopathy	Morning stiffness localized in the insertion region of Achilles tendon	Pain localized in the insertion region of the Achilles tendon with activities which load the tendon
Achilles tendon rupture	Sudden disabling sensation felt in the Achilles tendon. An audible sound or feeling like being kicked in the back of the leg is often described	Positive calf squeeze test
Chronic ankle instability	Self-reported multiple lateral ankle sprains. Reporting that the ankle joint feels unstable. Self-reported episodes of 'giving way' of the ankle joint	A combination of mechanical (pathological laxity, hyper/hypomobility) and functional (impairments in postural balance, strength, proprioception and neuromuscular control) insufficiencies
Sinus tarsi syndrome	Pain experienced on the lateral aspect of the ankle joint anterior and inferior to the lateral malleolus	Tenderness and swelling at the sinus tarsi. Pain with inversion of the rearfoot
Anterior ankle impingement	Pain experienced at end range dorsiflexion	Pain reproduced on forced dorsiflexion
Plantar heel pain	Pain experienced under the heel with the 'first step' in the morning	Tenderness at medial tuberosity of the calcaneus

psychological demands of the sport. Such an understanding will reduce the risk of Player A being inappropriately exposed to demands that he is ill prepared for.

Other ankle joint injuries: a brief commentary

Although lateral ankle sprains are the most frequently incurred ankle injury by field and court sport athletes, clinicians should be aware of the characteristic features of other ankle joint injuries. Recognition of the characteristic features of these injuries can assist clinicians in appropriately targeting their clinical assessment towards those tissues/structures that are most likely to be injured. A brief overview of some of these other ankle joint injuries along with their characteristic features are outlined in Table 21.4.

Conclusion and summary

Lateral ankle sprains are one of the most prevalent injuries sustained by athletes participating in field and court sports. As such, it is vital that clinicians working with athletes participating in these sports are 'experts' in the assessment, diagnosis and rehabilitation of ankle joint injuries and in particular lateral ankle sprain injuries. Of particular concern following lateral ankle sprain injury is the propensity to develop a range of sensorimotor impairments, which can result in the persistence of long term injury–related symptoms. A structured clinical assessment following acute lateral ankle sprain injury that assesses sensorimotor impairments is an imperative first step towards the development of an appropriate management pathway. Such an assessment will allow clinicians to focus the design and progression of treatment and rehabilitation programmes around objectively identified impairments.

References

Andersen, T.E., Floerenes, T.W., Arnason, A., Bahr, R., 2004. Video analysis of the mechanisms for ankle injuries in football. The American Journal of Sports Medicine 32 (1 Suppl. l), 69S–79S.

Butler, R.J., Southers, C., Gorman, P.P., Kiesel, K.B., Plisky, P.J., 2012. Differences in soccer players' dynamic balance across levels of competition. Journal of Athletic Training 47 (6), 616–620.

Collins, N., Teys, P., Vicenzino, B., 2004. The initial effects of a Mulligan's mobilization with movement technique on dorsiflexion and pain in subacute ankle sprains. Manual Therapy 9 (2), 77–82.

Docherty, C.L., Moore, J.H., Arnold, B.L., 1998. Effects of strength training on strength development and joint position sense in functionally unstable ankles. Journal of Athletic Training 33 (4), 310–314.

Gabriner, M.L., Houston, M.N., Kirby, J.L., Hoch, M.C., 2015. Contributing factors to star excursion balance test performance in individuals with chronic ankle instability. Gait & Posture 41 (4), 912–916.

Hall, E.A., Docherty, C.L., Simon, J., Kingma, J.J., Klossner, J.C., 2015. Strength-training protocols to improve deficits in participants with chronic ankle instability: a randomized controlled trial. Journal of Athletic Training 50 (1), 36–44.

Hoch, M.C., Andreatta, R.D., Mullineaux, D.R., English, R.A., Medina McKeon, J.M., Mattacola, C.G., et al., 2012. Two-week joint mobilization intervention improves self-reported function, range of motion, and dynamic balance in those with chronic ankle instability. Journal of Orthopaedic Research 30 (11), 1798–1804.

Hoch, M.C., McKeon, P.O., 2011. Joint mobilization improves spatiotemporal postural control and range of motion in those with chronic ankle instability. Journal of Orthopaedic Research 29 (3), 326–332.

Hoch, M.C., Staton, G.S., McKeon, P.O., 2011. Dorsiflexion range of motion significantly influences dynamic balance. Journal of Science and Medicine in Sport 14 (1), 90–92.

Kelln, B.M., McKeon, P.O., Gontkof, L.M., Hertel, J., 2008. Hand-held dynamometry: reliability of lower extremity muscle testing in healthy, physically active, young adults. Journal of Sport Rehabilitation 17 (2), 160–170.

Komi, P.V., Sale, D.G., 1992. Neural adaptation to strength training. In: Strength and Power in Sport. Blackwell Scientific Publications, Oxford, pp. 249–265.

Langarika-Rocafort, A., Emparanza, J.I., Aramendi, J.F., Castellano, J., Calleja-González, J., 2017. Intra-rater reliability and agreement of various methods of measurement to assess dorsiflexion in the Weight Bearing Dorsiflexion Lunge Test (WBLT) among female athletes. Physical Therapy in Sport 23, 37–44.

Rohner-Spengler, M., Mannion, A.F., Babst, R., 2007. Reliability and minimal detectable change for the figure-of-eight-20 method of measurement of ankle edema. Journal of Orthopaedic & Sports Physical Therapy 37 (4), 199–205.

Stiell, I.G., Greenberg, G.H., McKnight, R.D., Nair, R.C., McDowell, I., Reardon, M., et al., 1993. Decision rules for the use of radiography in acute ankle injuries. Refinement and prospective validation. Journal of the American Medical Association 269 (9), 1127–1132.

Stiffler, M.R., Sanfilippo, J.L., Brooks, M.A., Heiderscheit, B.C., 2015. Star excursion balance test performance varies by sport in healthy division I collegiate athletes. Journal of Orthopaedic & Sports Physical Therapy 45 (10), 772–780.

van Dijk, C.N., Lim, L.S., Bossuyt, P.M., Marti, R.K., 1996. Physical examination is sufficient for the diagnosis of sprained ankles. The Journal of Bone and Joint Surgery. British Volume 78 (6), 958–962.

Vicenzino, B., Branjerdporn, M., Teys, P., Jordan, K., 2006. Initial changes in posterior talar glide and dorsiflexion of the ankle after mobilization with movement in individuals with recurrent ankle sprain. Journal of Orthopaedic & Sports Physical Therapy 36 (7), 464–471.

Waldén, M., Hägglund, M., Ekstrand, J., 2013. Time-trends and circumstances surrounding ankle injuries in men's professional football: an 11-year follow-up of the UEFA Champions League injury study. British Journal of Sports Medicine 47 (12), 748–753.

Chapter | **22** |

The rehabilitation of the rugby shoulder: a proposed approach to management

Keith Thornhill and Marc Beggs

Introduction

The purpose of this chapter is to present a progressive and flexible rehabilitation model that can be adapted and used with a variety of athletes at differing stages of their return to play (RTP) following injury. A significant challenge in professional sport is returning injured athletes to play as quickly and as safely as possible while at the same time promoting shoulder health to assist in reducing injury risk of uninjured athletes. This has driven the evolution of our approach.

Not all clinical guidelines and postoperative protocols typically used focus on elite sporting environments and not all research involves elite sporting populations. As a result, our rehabilitation approach has been created, applied and developed in elite-level rugby union, and has evolved largely based on clinical experience, with support from best available research.

Task-based/criterion-based model

Although it is necessary to give accurate timeframes based on previous clinical experiences to work towards when returning from an injury, it is essential that both the player and the coaching staff are aware that the injury process is led by the player meeting exit criteria and milestones during the RTP process rather than by dictating timeframes.

The injured player is set progress goals along the rehabilitation pathway and should meet these in order to progress to the next stage. The prognostic timeframe given is fluid and can be amended depending on how the player progresses through the rehabilitation journey. It is important

to ensure that the player knows that this timeframe may also be accelerated if they are progressing well; for instance if every week of a 14-week injury they are 1 day ahead of the planned targets, then they essentially are 14 days ahead of schedule.

Rugby union and its demands on the shoulder

Incidence of shoulder injuries in rugby union is 13 per 1000 hours of content (Usman et al., 2014). To understand how to successfully rehabilitate a shoulder, it is necessary to understand the global demands a shoulder will have to tolerate during rugby union. On average, 116 contacts of all types (tackle, collision and falling) are observed in a rugby union match (Hendricks et al., 2014). For each positional group, forward or back, each individual is subjected to between 33 and 42 contacts as a forward, or 10 and 23 contacts as a back (Reardon et al., 2017).

In terms of the forces exerted in the tackle scenario, Seminati et al. (2016) observed that forces between 1.78 kN and 1.96 kN will be exerted on the tackler and ball carrier, respectively. On field, forces of up to 2 kN will be experienced by the tackler (Usman et al., 2014). Another aspect of game demands that is important to understand is the scrum. Quarrie and Wilson (2000) observed forces between 6210 and 9090 N collectively produced in the scrum.

There should also be a good understanding of the positional demands of each player, as this will dictate how rehabilitation is progressed. For example, a hooker will need the ability to reach overhead to perform a line-out throw, while a backline player needs to ensure they have adequate shoulder and cuff strength at outer ranges as a large proportion

Table 22.1 Correlation between shoulder movement and rotator cuff bias

Movement	Cuff bias
Flexion	Posterior cuff
Extension	Anterior cuff
Abduction	Cocontraction

of their tackling situations are likely to be performed while reaching to tackle an opponent who is attempting to side-step to evade the tackle at speed.

Healthy shoulders

To understand symptomatic shoulders, we must first understand how shoulders function when they are asymptomatic. We know from previous research (Escamilla et al., 2009) that the rotator cuff is largely responsible for maintaining joint stability and controlling humeral head translation.

The rotator cuff

Wattanaprakornkul et al. (2011a,b) have shown via electromyography (EMG) that the rotator cuff is recruited depending on the direction of arm movement. Specifically, during shoulder flexion–based movements the posterior cuff (supraspinatus, infraspinatus, teres minor) is more active than the anterior cuff (subscapularis); during shoulder extension–based movements the anterior cuff is more active; during shoulder abduction movements there is a relative cocontraction occurring between anterior and posterior cuffs (Table 22.1).

Assessment

There is no consistent evidence that any examination procedure used in shoulder assessments has acceptable levels of reliability (May et al., 2010). A systematic review in 2007 revealed that the diagnostic accuracy of Neer's test for impingement, the Hawkins–Kennedy test for impingement, and the Speed's test for labral pathology is limited (Hegedus et al., 2007).

Shoulder tests may show benefit when used in clusters or when ruling out certain pathologies, but there is a lack of specificity and sensitivity when performing these tests in isolation. Clinically, we place value in clustering instability tests when indicated by the mechanism of injury. A proposed assessment algorithm is shown in Fig. 22.1.

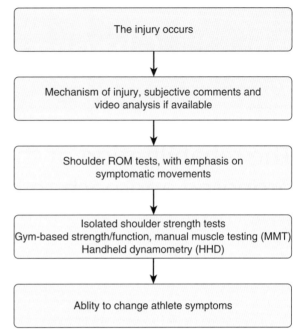

Fig. 22.1 Assessment algorithm for examination of the shoulder. ROM, Range of motion.

Knowing that during shoulder flexion–based movements the posterior cuff is more active, our aim here is to provide a stimulus which increases the activity of the posterior cuff with the goal of eliciting positive changes in symptoms. Two potential ways of increasing posterior cuff activity are via hand grip (Sporrong et al., 1995; 1996) or by the addition of a resisted isometric external rotation force to the flexion-based symptomatic or meaningful task.

Subsequently, during shoulder extension–based movements the anterior cuff is more active; our aim here is to provide a stimulus which increases the activity of the anterior cuff with the goal of eliciting positive changes in symptoms. We postulate that this may be achieved by the addition of a resisted isometric internal rotation force.

During shoulder abduction–based movements there is a cocontraction of the anterior and posterior cuff (Wattanaprakornkul et al., 2011a,b). This cocontraction provides a compression of the humeral head into the glenoid (Reed et al., 2018) and reduces humeral head translation (Wattanaprakornkul et al., 2011a,b).

This may be reproduced by the addition of an externally applied compressive force by compressing the humeral head into the glenoid during the symptomatic or meaningful task. This compressive force can also be achieved by performing weight-bearing activities through the upper limb (e.g., four-point kneeling position) and assessing whether

Table 22.2 Additional activities undertaken during clinical assessment

Symptomatic movement	Additional activity	Action
Flexion	Handgrip	Increase posterior cuff activity
	External rotation resistance	
Extension	Internal rotation resistance	Increase anterior cuff activity
Abduction	Compression	Replication of cocontraction via compression
	Weight-bearing	

Table 22.3 Accessory activities undertaken during clinical assessment

Movement	Accessory activity	Action
All	Reduce lever length	Decrease workload of the cuff
	Kinetic chain activity	Increase cuff activity via feedforward mechanism[1]
	Scapular assistance	Assists axial scapular muscle activity

[1]From McMullen, J., Uhl, T. L., 2000. A kinetic chain approach for shoulder rehabilitation. Journal of Athletic Training 35 (3), 329–337; Sciascia, A., Cromwell, R, 2012. Kinetic chain rehabilitation; a theoretical framework. Rehabilitation Research and Practise 1–9.

this positively affects the symptomatic movement or meaningful task (Table 22.2).

The use of an additional activity, as described above, during the assessment can be complemented by the addition of any number of accessory activities which are not directionally specific to shoulder movements.

Reducing the lever length (e.g., arm) by maintaining elbow flexion during a symptomatic movement or meaningful task, where possible, will reduce the demand placed upon the shoulder and rotator cuff. The addition of a kinetic chain activity, such as adding a lower body–dominant movement (e.g., lunge or a step-up) during the symptomatic movement or meaningful task will increase cuff activity via a feedforward mechanism. The manual application of a scapular assistance test throughout range will assist axial scapular muscle activity. The aim of adding these accessory activities to the addition activities is to further positively affect change in the symptomatic movement or meaningful task (Table 22.3).

Based on the outcomes of the assessment, the athlete will generally fall into one of four broad categories shown in Table 22.4.

The role of imaging in the sporting shoulder

The use of medical imaging, painkillers and nonsteroidal antiinflammatory drugs (NSAIDs), and steroid and local injections in the management of shoulder issues in professional rugby must be viewed as being distinct to the normal management of a nonsporting, amateur or semi-professional population. There are some instances where these avenues are used. These adjuncts can assist in the clinical decision-making process by helping to provide an early diagnosis. Additionally, they may also be used to help reduce rehabilitation timeframes to enable players to return to play as quickly but as safely as possible. If these avenues are utilized, the player is still required to meet the return-to-play criteria to be available to train and play.

Furthermore, these adjuncts may help with clinical decisions about whether a conservative or nonconservative rehabilitation is most appropriate.

In general, imaging is reserved for those who have a traumatic aetiology and clinical presentation suggesting a dislocation or subluxation. For those injuries with clinical features primarily around pain, magnetic resonance imaging (MRI)/magnetic resonance arthrography (MRA) may not be warranted, as these cases tend to be managed conservatively regardless of the underlying pathology, as they generally respond to NSAIDs and low-level rehabilitation.

The adolescent shoulder

Young athletes who fall into category 2 (see Table 22.4) present distinct challenges. Following dislocation, athletes

Table 22.4 Four broad categories to classify sporting shoulder injury

Category 1: 'Banged up Monday morning shoulder'	
Mechanism of injury	No clear MOI. Likely to have completed game; presents postgame/next day with pain/dysfunction
Shoulder range of movement	Active ROM (AROM) >70% with minor to moderate pain
Isolated shoulder strength	Ability to provide a moderate to good level of resistance on testing with presence of pain and/or weakness/inhibition
Functional shoulder strength	Likely to be able to complete a modified UB gym session with use of regressed UB lifts (e.g., press-up instead of bench press)
Ability to change athlete's symptoms	Use of an additional activity and/or an accessory activity provides a positive change to their symptomatic movement or meaningful task
Prognosis	Likely to complete modified training throughout the week and be available to play within 1–2 weeks. Unlikely to have structural abnormalities; does not require further investigation (e.g., MRI)
Category 2: Short to medium–term injury	
Mechanism of injury	Clear and suspicious MOI; immediately painful, likely to have been removed from play immediately or within a few minutes if symptoms did not improve
Shoulder range of movement	AROM <70% with moderate pain
Isolated shoulder strength	Ability to provide low to moderate level of resistance on testing with moderate levels of pain and/or weakness/inhibition
Functional shoulder strength	Unable to complete a modified UB gym sessions with use of regressed UB lifts
Ability to change athlete's symptoms	Poor to minimal changes in symptomatic movement or meaningful task
Prognosis	Unable to train. Likely to become a short to medium term injury, with unavailability for selection of 2–8 weeks. Possible structural abnormalities; does not require further investigation currently
Category 3: Failed category 2 rehabilitation	
Mechanism of injury	As category 2
Shoulder range of movement	
Isolated shoulder strength	
Functional shoulder strength	
Ability to change athlete's symptoms	
Prognosis	Player may be managed during the season to allow availability for selection, will require surgery postseason. This will require highly modified training weeks. Will require further investigation (e.g., MRI, MRA, orthopaedic consultation). If unable to be managed inseason will require surgery as soon as possible. Will become a category 4 shoulder
Category 4: Long-term postoperative rehabilitation	
Mechanism of injury	Clear and suspicious MOI – possible dislocation/subluxation. Immediately painful and dysfunctional; removed from play immediately
Shoulder range of movement	Very limited AROM, may be unwilling to attempt AROM due to pain or apprehension
Isolated shoulder strength	May be unwilling to attempt testing due to pain or apprehension. Likely to be very weak and painful if test performed

Table 22.4 Four broad categories of sporting shoulder injury—cont'd

Functional shoulder strength	Not suitable to perform due to pain, dysfunction and/or apprehension
Ability to change athlete's symptoms	None to poor changes in symptomatic movement or meaningful task. May not be appropriate to assess
Prognosis	High indication of a significant structural abnormality; high indication for further investigation (e.g., MRI, MRA, surgical consult) which will require surgical intervention

AROM, Active range of movement; *MOI*, mechanism of injury; *MRA*, magnetic resonance arthrography; *MRI*, magnetic resonance imaging; *UB*, upper body.

under the age of 18 have a high incidence of reoccurrence following conservative management (Boileau et al., 2006). Arthroscopic surgery for these athletes also presents a challenge, with up to a 70% failure rate at 31 months postinjury. A recent study compared recurrence rates following primary arthroscopic stabilization in rugby players grouped as: <16 years, 16–17 years and 25 years. It showed very high percentages of failure in the under-18s (Torrance et al., 2018). Management decisions for these athletes should consider:
1. participation level: recreational or elite pathway athlete
2. bony injury: presence of Hill–Sachs lesion and/or glenoid loss
3. number and frequency of previous dislocations: two or more previous shoulder dislocations may be an indication for surgery.

These cases should be assessed on an individual basis before any decision is made with the involvement primarily of the player, parent/guardian, physiotherapist, doctor and consultant.

Rehabilitation of the injured shoulder

Following assessment and categorization of the athlete postinjury, the individual rehabilitation pathway is layered to suit the needs of the athlete, their specific injury and any additional goals or targets. We have listed below the pillars of rehabilitation which we deem important during the postinjury return-to-play (RTP) process. These pillars allow for a structured, logical progression throughout the RTP process, allowing for gradual, graded exposure to increasingly demanding aspects of rugby. An important aspect of this process in elite rugby union is ensuring that the rehabilitation is all-encompassing.

The pillars not only focus on the rehabilitation of the specific shoulder injury but also address the athlete as a whole, to allow them to return to play and perform with the physiological and psychological abilities required in elite rugby union. This ensures that a holistic and progressive

task-/criterion-based approach is taken by multiple departments in the organization (e.g., physiotherapy, strength and conditioning, rugby coaches, nutrition).

Rehabilitation pillars

1. **Active assisted range of movement (AAROM).** Generally, these ranges are used primarily with regard to shoulder flexion as a marker to indicate when progression may be appropriate.
2. **Active range of movement (AROM).** Generally, these ranges are used primarily with regard to shoulder flexion as a marker to indicate when progression may be appropriate.
3. **Isometric rotator cuff activation.** Production of force via the rotator cuff without a change in muscle length or shoulder movement occurring (Mullaney et al., 2017).
4. **Off-feet conditioning.** Non-weight-bearing aerobic and anaerobic training (e.g., Wattbike).
5. **Rotator cuff endurance exercises.** Exercises that target the rotator cuff with the aim to increase endurance capacity.
6. **On-feet conditioning.** Weight-bearing aerobic and anaerobic training (e.g., running).
7. **Closed kinetic chain exercises.** Exercises that are performed whilst the upper or lower limbs are in contact with a fixed object (De Mey et al., 2014).
8. **Eccentric rotator cuff strength exercises.** Exercises that specifically target the eccentric component of rotator cuff strength.
9. **Open kinetic chain exercises.** Exercises that are performed whilst the upper or lower limbs are not in contact with a fixed object and are therefore free to move (De Mey et al., 2014).
10. **Upper body maximum strength exercises.** Gym-based strength programme to target global upper body strength.
11. **Rotator cuff reactive strength.** Exercises that are aimed at increasing the speed at which the shoulder

275

AAROM/PROM (in shoulder flexion)	AROM (shoulder flex)	Cuff isometric activation		Off feet	Cuff endurance	On-feet	Closed kinetic chain	Cuff strength
		ER	IR					
0	0							
0–30	0	Outer range ER	Belly press	Bike spin				
30–60	0–30	ER @ 0 / Neutral ER / Inner range ER	IR @ 0 / Neutral IR / Outer range IR	Time trial for Distance longer duration / No max efforts / No standing on bike	(Mid range, outer range, inner range, full range) ER @ 0 / Side lying external rotations / 1. 3 × 45–60 seconds / 2. 3 × 10–12 / 3. 3 × 8–10 — (Inner range, gradual increase to full outer range) IR @ 0 / Standing banded IR / 1. 3 × 45–60 seconds / 2. 3 × 10–12 / 3. 3 × 8–10 / Elbow supported progressing to elbow unsupported	Speed tech (no arm use - hands on hips/cross arms)	Standing weight shifts (leaning on table) / Standing GB banded roll out with mini squat	ER @ 0 / Sidelying eccentric ER — IR @ 0 / Sidelying/standing eccentric IR / Elbow supported progressing to elbow unsupported
60–90	30–60	ER @ 45 / Neutral ER / Outer range ER / Inner range ER	IR @ 45 / Neutral IR / Inner range IR / Outer range IR	Middle distance / No standing / No max high Intensity efforts	(Mid range, outer range, inner range, full range) ER @ 45 / 1. 3 × 45–60 seconds / 2. 3 × 10–12 / 3. 3 × 8–10 — (Inner range, gradual increase to full outer range) IR @ 45 / Elbow supported progressing to elbow unsupported	Speed tech plyos (no arm use - hands on hips/cross arms)	Progress range from above	ER @ 45 / Elbow supported progressing to elbow unsupported — IR @ 45
90–120	60–90	ER @ 90 / Neutral ER / Outer range ER / Inner range ER	IR @ 90 / Neutral IR / Inner range IR / Outer range IR		(Mid range, outer range, inner range, full range) ER @ 45 / 1. 3 × 45–60 seconds / 2. 3 × 10–12 / 3. 3 × 8–10 — (Inner range, gradual increase to full outer range) IR @ 45 / Elbow supported progressing to elbow unsupported	Intro to running walk/jog / Tempo / MAS running / Intro to speed and agility training	4pt kneeling weight shift / 4pt kneeling shoulder taps / Bear crawl position / Bear crawl position shoulder taps / Bear crawl – linear / Bear crawl – linear + lateral / Bear crawl rotations ± linear/lateral	
120–150	90–120			Any bike session	ER @ 90 prone ER / 1. Mid to outer range — IR @ 90 prone IR / 1. Mid to inner range	Conditioning running speed and agility	Wall walk / GymBall stir the pot / GymBall walk out / Inverted pike holds / Inverted pike walk outs	ER @ 45 / Elbow supported progressing to elbow unsupported — IR @ 45
From	120–150				Supine ER / 1. Mid to inner range / 2. Increase outer range as able — Supine IR / 1. Mid to inner range / 2. Increase outer range as able	Sport/position specific conditioning sessions	GB pike / GB pike with shoulder taps inchworm	ER @ 90 / Supine/prone eccentric ER sidelying bastard / Elbow supported progressing to elbow unsupported — IR @ 90 / Supine/ prone eccentric IR
	From				Standing ER / 1. Mid to inner range / 2. Increase outer range as able — Standing IR / 1. Outer range to full as able / Elbow supported progressing to elbow unsupported		Wall handstand / Wall handstand with alternate hand lifts (and variations) / Handstand / Handstand walk	

Fig. 22.2 Shoulder rehabilitation pathway. AAROM, Active assisted range of movement; AROM, active range of movement; BB, barbell; DA, double arm; DB, dumbbell; ER, external rotation; GB, gymball; IR, internal rotation; KB, kettlebell; MAS, maximal aerobic speed; OKC, open kinetic chain; PROM, passive range of motion; SA, single arm; TGU, Turkish get up; UB, upper body.

Open kinetic chain	UB strength — Horizontal Push	UB strength — Horizontal Pull	UB strength — Vertical Push	UB strength — Vertical Pull	Reactive cuff strength	Sports specific skills/rehab (forwards) — Forwards	Sports specific skills/rehab (forwards) — Backs	Contact	Rugby
Turkish get up body rolls	**Level 1 horizontal:** Isometric push-up holds (various degress of elbow flex); Cable horizontal press	**Level 1 horizontal:** DA cable row; SA cable pull	**Level 1 vertical:** Jammer press	**Level 1 vertical:** SA high-low cable pull	Neutral ball slap; Neutral ball slap to stop ball throw/catch	Passing with physios; Scrum tech; Tackle tech	Passing with physio; Kick/catch with physio; Passing with coaches; Tackle tech kick/catch with coaches; Rugby skills/noncontact units	Rolling patterns; fending close combat pummeling/wrestling (controlled); intro falling; Level 1 contact	Noncontact rugby; Bag contact rugby
1/4 TGU; Position-specific OKC exercise	**Level 2 horizontal:** BB floor press; DB floor press; DB bench; BB bench (limited range) press-up	SA KB/DB row	**Level 2 vertical:** SA DB / KB shoulder press	**Level 2 vertical:** SA cable lat pull down; DA cable lat down	45 ball slap; 45 ball slap to stop catch/reload	Intro to line-out lifting (physios); Level 1 scrums; Maul tech	Noncontact units; Noncontact rugby	Level 2 contact	Full rugby
1/2 TGU; Position-specific OKC exercise	**Level 3 horizontal:** Weighted press-up; DB/KB bench press; BB benchpress	**Level 3 horizontal:** BB prone bench pull; KB / DB prone bench pull	**Level 3 vertical:** BB military press	**Level 3 vertical:** Chins	90 ball slap; 90 ball slap to stop supine ball catch/reload 1/2 kneeling catch/reload	Line-out lifting/catching; Line-out contesting; Level 2 scrums; Live mauls; Level 3 scrums; Full rugby	Full rugby	Level 3 contact	
Full TGU; Position-specific OKC exercise									

Fig. 22.2, cont'd.

musculature can change from absorbing forces eccentrically to generating forces concentrically

12. Sport-/position-specific skills/rehabilitation. Gradual, progressive exposure to rugby-based skills.

13. Contact skills. Gradual, progressive exposure to contact-based skills used to replicate the demands of rugby union.

14. Rugby. Gradual, progressive exposure to rugby training sessions (Fig. 22.2).

Category 3 and 4 injuries

With category 3 and 4 shoulder injuries, the approach that we commonly take generally flows from left to right of the shoulder rehabilitation pathway (see Fig. 22.2). This enables commencement of rehabilitation early, whilst still in sling postoperation. Progression from this point is guided by active and active assisted range of movement (ROM), generally guided by shoulder flexion, and progression is determined by completion of and competency performing the specific pillar. This task-/criterion-based approach allows for a waterfall effect towards the pillars to be employed throughout the rehabilitation of the athlete. A snapshot of how the rehabilitation pillars interact with each other is shown in Fig. 22.3.

For instance, typically when the AAROM is between 60–90 degrees of shoulder flexion, the AROM will be between 30–60 degrees shoulder flexion. This means we can focus our isometric rotator cuff activation at 90 degrees, commencing with elbow supported. Our rotator cuff endurance rehabilitation is now focused at 45 degrees flexion, we have commenced closed kinetic chain (CKC) exercises in the current available AROM and our eccentric rotator cuff strength at 0 degrees shoulder flexion can be commenced. Essentially, this enables us to train rotator cuff endurance, strength and, at a later point, reactive strength at the same time, but individually at different ranges. This ensures that we are targeting the shoulder and rotator cuff at multiple ranges, as early and as safely as possible with appropriate exercise selections.

Although, for ease, ranges have been indicated to remain at 0 degrees, 45 degrees and 90 degrees when exercising the rotator cuff, in practice the shoulder is placed in various ranges to ensure that the shoulder is trained throughout full range.

Fig. 22.4 is a macro-representation of how we would layer this waterfall effect with regard to specific exercise-based rehabilitation pillars throughout the rehabilitation pathway.

Category 1 and 2 injuries

With regard to the rehabilitation of category 1 and 2 shoulder injuries, the assessment process will dictate where the athlete starts the rehabilitation process. Each athlete's programme is designed in conjunction with their individual needs.

The overall goal for the category 1 injury is to minimize time lost to the injury. As a result, rehabilitation should be viewed more as a regression-based approach. The first goal with a category 1 injury is to ensure selection for rugby within 1–2 weeks, therefore placing rugby session as the priority.

As the second goal, the restoration of shoulder health and function then becomes the driver to allow the athlete to safely return to full training and therefore be available for game selection. Practically, this results in all other components of the rehabilitation becoming modifiable in order to meet these two goals. Theoretically, this is accomplished by regressing from the endpoint of the rehabilitation pathway (i.e., from the right of the pathway) until the athlete can tolerate and perform the components of a specific rehabilitation pillar with competency. This then becomes the starting point in the rehabilitation process and is progressed back to rugby as appropriate.

As mentioned above, the starting point for category 1 injuries will be dictated by their assessment. For example, an athlete, having completed a fixture, presents 1-day postgame with no clear mechanism of injury with pain throughout full range of motion shoulder flexion. His isolated shoulder strength appears to be inhibited by pain. However, functionally his is able to complete a full-range press up but with pain. Use of an additional activity and/or an accessory activity provides a positive change to his presentation.

A simple three-stage approach is proposed:

1. Integrate. Integrate additional and/or accessory activities that proved effective during the assessment to their symptomatic movement.

2. Isolate. Isolate their direction-specific cuff exercises. For example, this athlete has presented with pain with shoulder flexion. Additional and/or accessory activities improved the symptomatic movement (e.g., reduced pain). Therefore, we can postulate that by further challenging the posterior cuff with isolated rehabilitation exercises we hope to improve the player's presentation (e.g., reduce pain).

3. Potentiate. Potentiate the shoulder complex. Modifications of the upper body (UB) gym programme can be used as appropriate to ensure a strength stimulus is maintained whilst still challenging the athlete.

For category 2 injuries, this is essentially a condensed version of the category 3/4 rehabilitation. The athlete may not need to regress fully to the start of the pathway, their starting point, similar to category 1 injuries is specific to their presentation. The main difference with these injuries is that initially, they are unable to complete rugby

AROM (shoulder flexion)	Isometric rotator cuff activation		Off feet conditioning	Rotator cuff endurance exercises		Joint position sense	Eccentric rotator cuff strength exercises	
	External rotation	Internal rotation		External rotation	Internal rotation		External rotation	Internal rotation
30–60°	Commenced at 90° scaption 1. External rotation holds	1. Internal rotation holds	No max efforts No standing on bike	Commenced at 45° scaption 1. Low to high rotation	1. High to low rotation	1. Floor slides with targetting 2. Laser ER / IR at 45° abduction 3. General OKC laser targetting drills	Commenced at 45° scaption 1. Sidelying/ standing eccentric ER	1. Sidelying/ standing ecccentric IR

Fig. 22.3 Rehabilitation pillars. AROM, active range of movement; ER, external rotation; IR, internal rotation; OKC, open kinetic chain.

Pillar	Rehabilitation focus								
Isometric rotator cuff activiation	0°	45°	90°	Pre-stim activation (if required)					
Rotator cuff endurance	nil	0°	45°	90°	Pre-stim activation				
Eccentric rotator cuff strength	nil	nil	0°	45°	90°	Address deficits		Maintain	Gain
Plyometric / reactive rotator cuff strength	nil	nil	nil	0°	45°	90°	90°/90°	Address deficits	
Upper body (horizontal push / pull	nil	nil	nil	Intro to	Hypertrophy	Strength	Max strength	Power	Gain
Upper body (vertical push / pull)	nil	nil	nil	nil	Intro to	Hypertrophy	Strength	Max strength	Power

Fig. 22.4 Waterfall concurrent training table.

sessions, therefore rehabilitation becomes their primary focus.

Isometric rotator cuff activation

Isometric activation of the rotator cuff can commence from very early in the rehabilitation pathway. This provides a low level of stimulus for the rotator cuff musculature (Fig. 22.5).

Postoperatively, while still in sling, isometric internal and external rotation exercises can be completed with the contralateral side providing low-level resistance. As the exercise is dictated by the athlete's perceived exertion and comfort this can be a safe way of beginning rehabilitation. This exercise can be progressed throughout multiple ranges as appropriate. This becomes a precursor to commencing low-level rotator cuff endurance.

Rotator cuff endurance exercises

As mentioned previously, the rotator cuff plays an important functional and stability role in the shoulder joint. Without an appropriately functioning rotator cuff that possesses the required endurance, strength and power characteristics, it is likely to be exposed to during sport and the risk of injury is increased. Before developing rotator cuff strength and power characteristics it is important to first ensure that the rotator cuff has developed a solid endurance capacity. Essentially, this endurance capacity is the keystone upon which the performance characteristics of rotator cuff and global strength and power will be built during the rehabilitation of the athlete (Fig. 22.6).

When setting up and performing the exercise it is important to ensure that the athlete is aware that the

279

Isometric rotator cuff activation exercises							
0° Shoulder flexion/abduction		0° Shoulder flexion		45° Shoulder scaption		90° Shoulder scaption	
External rotation	Internal rotation	External rotation	Internal rotation	External rotation	Internal rotation	External rotation	Internal rotation
Exericse selection							
1. Outer range ER iso hold	1. Belly press isometric (inner range IR)	1. External rotation holds	1. Internal rotation holds	1. External rotation holds	1. Internal rotation holds	1. External rotation holds	1. Internal rotation holds
Performed in sling		Performed when out of sling					
Exercise progresson							
Not applicable		1. Mid range ER 2. Inner range ER Start with elbow supported, progress to unsupported	1. Mid range IR 2. Outer range IR	1. Mid range ER 2. Inner range ER 3. Outer range ER Start with elbow supported, progress to unsupported, progress to 45° shoulder abduction/flexion		1. Mid range ER 2. Inner range ER 3. Outer range ER Start with elbow supported, progress to unsupported, progress to 90° shoulder abduction/flexion	
Exercise prescription							
1. 3×10 second hold 2. 3×20 second hold 3. 3×30 second hold Increase resistance as appropriate							
Any combination of relevanat accessory or additional activites, if appropriate can be added if needed, but should be ceased before progressing							

Fig. 22.5 Isometric rotator cuff activation exercises. ER, External rotation; IR, internal rotation.

Rotator cuff endurance exercises					
0° Shoulder flexion		45° Shoulder scaption		90° Shoulder scaption	
External rotation	Internal rotation	External rotation	Internal rotation	External rotation	Internal rotation
Exercise selection					
1. Sidelying external rotations	1. Standing/sidelying internal rotations	1. Low to high rotation	1. High to low rotation	1. Supine rotations 2. Prone rotations 3. Archer 4. Standing exernal rotations	1. Supine rotations 2. Prone rotations 3. Standing internal rotations
Exercise progression					
1. Mid range 2. Mid to inner range 3. Increase outer range as able Start with elbow supported, progress to unsupported		1. Mid range 2. Mid to inner range 3. Increase outer range as able Start with elbow supported, progress to unsupported commence in 45 degrees of scaption, progress to horizontal abduction		1. Mid range 2. Mid to inner range 3. Increase outer range as able Start with elbow supported, progress to unsupported commence in 45 degrees of scaption, progress to horizontal abduction	
Exercise prescription					
1. 3×20–30 seconds 2. 3×30–45 seconds 3. 3×15–20 repetitions Increase weight/resistance as appropriate					
Any combination of relevant accessory or additional activites, if appropriate, can be added if needed, but should be ceased before progressing					

Fig. 22.6 Rotator cuff endurance exercises.

Joint position sense		
AROM 0–30⁰	AROM 30–60⁰	AROM 60–90⁰+
Exercise selection and progression		
1. Table slides with targetting 2. Laser ER/IR targetting drills at 0⁰ 3. General OKC laser targetting drills	1. Floor slides with targetting 2. Laser ER/IR targetting drills at 45⁰ abduction 3. General OKC laser targetting drills	1. Standing wall slide with targetting 2. Laser ER/IR targetting drills at 90⁰ abduction/scaption 3. General OKC laser targetting drills

Fig. 22.7 **Joint position sense.** AROM, Active range of motion; ER, External rotation; IR, internal rotation; OKC, open kinetic chain.

relevant area is worked; for instance, when preforming an external rotation exercise the primary movers should be the posterior cuff (teres minor, supraspinatus, infraspinatus). Therefore, the individual should be able to identify a deep burn within the posterior cuff region, rather than feeling the posterior deltoid or upper trapezius primarily engaging. If the posterior cuff is not felt, then addressing the set-up, reducing the resistance or minimizing the range of motion can be helpful in engaging the cuff. It is important to get this feedback from the athlete as failure to do so may result in either overactivity in another muscle group, promotion of further dysfunction or a delay in the RTP process. Furthermore, any combination of accessory and/or additional activities that were found to have a positive effect on the individual's symptomatic movement or meaningful task can be added if need.

In line with the aim of building endurance, the exercise prescription requires the athlete to essentially be able to perform multiple repetitions of a low-load exercise. With increased competence and improved endurance, the timeframe will reduce and be replaced with specific repetition ranges – typically this occurs in line with an increase in load lifted. This assists with the transition and a shift in focus towards developing rotator cuff strength characteristics during the rehabilitation process.

Joint position sense (proprioception)

Proprioception is the sense of the relative position of one's body parts. Research and clinical experience suggest that shoulder joint position sense (JPS) or proprioception is altered in contact sports (Herrington et al., 2008; Morgan and Herrington, 2013). Contact results in reduction in the feedback from mechanoreceptors at outer ranges following tackling. These sensorimotor deficits potentially increase the risk of injury in rugby players due to the repeated contact demands of the sport. During the rehabilitation process

is it necessary to develop this characteristic by challenging the JPS systems in order to help create a more robust athlete (Fig. 22.7).

During the rehabilitation process, especially for those with long-term injuries or chronic ongoing issues, care must be taken to ensure that this area is not overlooked. Simple assessment of JPS and proprioception such as internal/external rotation targeting drills can be used both as an assessment tool and treatment intervention. These drills are typically introduced as a closed chain exercise where the individual has to target certain markers, firstly with their eyes open, and then after several repetitions their eyes are closed and they are asked to move their hand to a specific point. This can be objectively measured simply by measuring the distance from the target to a certain point on their hand (e.g., second finger). Similarly, during external rotation/internal rotation (ER/IR) movements a laser can be added with the individual being asked to perform the rotational movement while aiming the laser to a fixed point. This can be progressed by the addition of compound shoulder movements at various ranges to challenge the athlete further.

Closed kinetic chain exercises

Closed kinetic chain (CKC) or closed chain exercises are exercises performed where the hand (for arm movement) or foot (for leg movement) is fixed in space and cannot move. The extremity remains in constant contact with the immobile surface, usually the ground or the base of a machine. The opposite of CKC exercises are open kinetic chain exercises (OKC).

CKC exercises are a vital facet of rehabilitating the rugby shoulder. This is most beneficial when dealing with an unstable shoulder and can be progressed from CKC to OKC and into sport-specific training easily (Fig. 22.8). CKC exercises increase the compressive forces at the glenohumeral joint, which in turn increases joint proprioception. There is

Closed kinetic chain exercises			
0–60° Shoulder flexion	60–90° Shoulder abduction	90–120° Shoulder abduction	120°–FROM Shoulder flexion
Exericse selection			Exercise selection and progression
1. Standing weight shifts (leaning on table)	1. 4-point kneeling weight shifts	1. Wall walk and/or 2. Gymball roll out from knees	1. Mini inchworm 2. Gymball pike 3. Gymball pike with alternate shoulder taps 4. Full inchworm 5. Pike position holds 6. Pike with alternate shoulder taps 7. Pike position push-up 8. Wall supported handstand hold 9. Wall handstand with alternate hand lifts 10. Unsupported handstand 11. Handstand walk
Exercise progressions			
1. Add gymball roll out (Increase ROM - actively) 2. Add isometric band holds (Increase posterior cuff activity) 3. Add mini squat (Increase ROM - passively) Increase range/resistance as able	1. Alternate shoulder taps 2. Clockface taps 3. Linear crawl 4. Lateral crawl 5. Multidirectional crawls 6. Reactive crawls Starting position on knees, progress to on toes (bear crawl position)	1. Add isometric band holds 2. a. Complete on toes b. Add isometric band holds	
Exercise prescription			
	1. 3 × 10–20 seconds 2. 3 × 20–30 seconds 3. 3 × 30–45 seconds		Due to variety of exercise progressions used, this is difficult to define. Typically, exercises start with fixed durations for the holds (e.g., 10 seconds), specific repetition ranges (e.g., 6–8) for the taps/lifts and set distance for the walk (e.g., 5 meters). These are progressed as appropriate.

Fig. 22.8 **Closed kinetic chain exercises.** FROM, Full range of motion; ROM, range of movement.

also improved muscle activation, primarily in the posterior rotator cuff musculature. Care must be taken when utilizing these exercises with athletes who experience posterior instability; however, this is not a contraindication.

CKC exercises can begin from the initial stage of rehabilitation when the athlete has minimal AROM into shoulder flexion. Standing weight shifts on a bed (Fig. 22.9A) can be commenced and progressed as per the table below. Ground-based training is also a good option for progression when the athlete has 90 degrees of AROM in shoulder flexion. For us, this begins as four-point kneeling exercises and is progressed into bear-crawling positions (see Fig. 22.9B). Incorporating weight shifts and single arm variations of bear-crawling helps improve single arm (SA) control in weight-bearing. Adding shoulder taps (see Fig. 22.9C) and adding in an unstable surface for the athlete's legs/feet (such as a gym ball) are good options to increase the difficulty of the exercise. This will be progressed from static bear-crawling positions to linear and lateral moving bear-crawls and eventually to multidirectional bear-crawls, including rotations.

As the athlete's range increases to >120 degrees we progress the athlete to inverted positions such as a pike position and eventually onto wall handstand with the aim of achieving a full unsupported handstand. Some athletes will progress onto handstand walking. This is a good aim and challenge for the athlete – although they will never be in that position when competing, it provides the athlete with confidence, knowing they can support and control their bodyweight above their head in a handstand walking exercise.

Eccentric rotator cuff strength

Once the endurance capacity has been progressed, strength development is required to enable the shoulder to be able to produce and absorb the forces that it will be exposed to during a demanding high-contact game of rugby union. These rotator cuff strength characteristics will assist with increasing the stability of the shoulder while also providing the foundation from which general shoulder strength can be developed.

When focusing on strengthening the rotator cuff, we focus on the eccentric component of the movement as a quicker method to develop strength. When carrying out standard concentric/eccentric movements the maximum weight lifted is always limited by the concentric component, with forces generated by the eccentric component of a muscle contraction

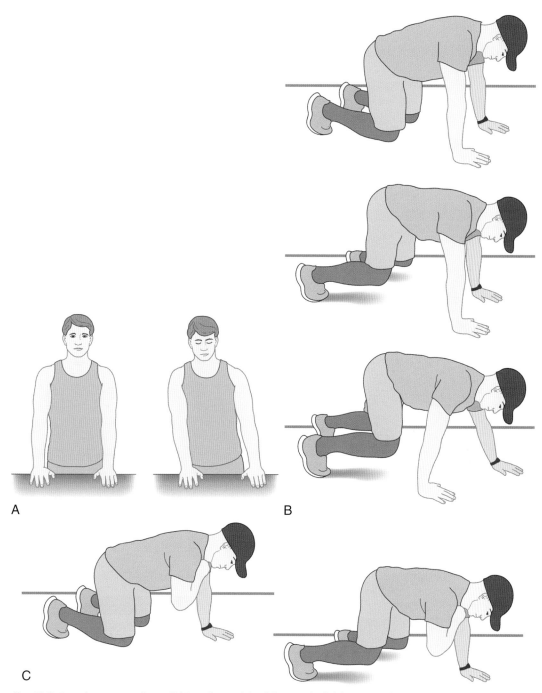

Fig. 22.9 Exercise progressions. (A) Standing weight shifts on a bed. (B) Bear-crawling positions. (C) Shoulder taps.

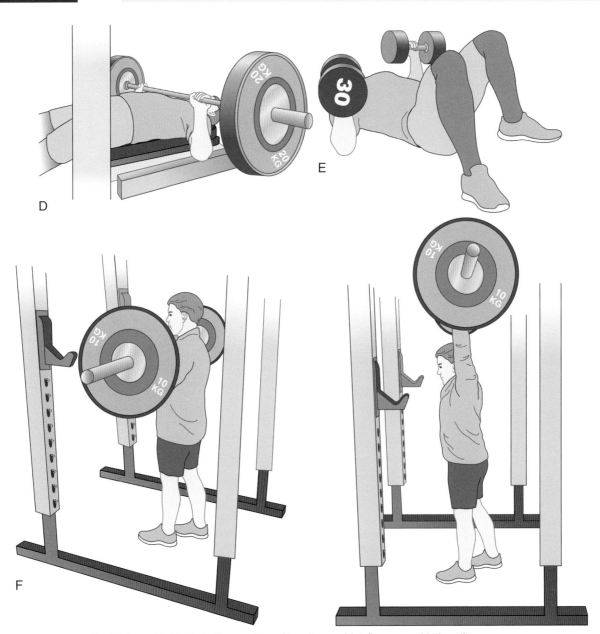

Fig. 22.9 cont'd (D) The bottom position of bench press (E) A floor press. (F) The military press.

being as much at 50% greater than that of the concentric component (Hortobágyi et al., 2001). Eccentric-only training provides a quicker pathway to regaining or developing concentric strength (Brandenburg and Docherty, 2000) (Fig. 22.10).

We have also noted that eccentric training reduces the potential for compensatory strategies to occur and the challenge presented to the athlete improves compliance. This is likely to be the first exercise since the onset of the injury

where the athlete feels they are being maximally challenged. As one would expect, a professional rugby player loves being challenged, especially physically, so the addition of eccentric strength provides an outlet for this.

An important consideration for eccentric strength training is the placement of the session. The introduction of eccentric cuff strengthening is typically introduced around the mid-stages of rehabilitation, once sufficient cuff endurance is

Eccentric rotator cuff strength exercises					
0⁰ Shoulder flexion/abduction		45⁰ Shoulder scaption		90⁰ Shoulder scaption	
External rotation	**Internal rotation**	**External rotation**	**Internal rotation**	**External rotation**	**Internal rotation**
Exericse selection					
1. Sidelying /standing eccentric ER	1. Sidelying /standing ecccentric IR	1. Low to high rotation	1. High to low rotation	1. Supine eccentric ER 2. Prone eccentric ER 3. Standing eccentric ER 4. Eccentric archer 5. Sidelying straight arm lower	1. Supine eccentric IR 2. Prone eccentric IR 3. Standing eccentric IR
Exercise progressons					
1. Mid range 2. Inner to mid range 3. Increase outer range as able Elbow supported progressing to elbow unsupported		1. Mid range 2. Inner to mid range 3. Increase outer range as able Elbow supported progressing to elbow unsupported Commence exercise in scaption, progress to horizontal abduction (at 45⁰ or 90⁰)			
Exercise prescription					
1. 3 × 6–8 Reps 2. 3 × 4–6 Reps 3. 4 × 4–6 Reps 5 Second lower Starting twice weekly, increasing to three times weekly		1. 3 × 6–8 Reps 2. 3 × 4–6 Reps 3. 4 × 4–6 Reps 5 Second lower Starting twice weekly, increasing to three times weekly		1. 3 × 6–8 Reps 2. 3 × 4–6 Reps 3. 4 × 4–6 Reps 5 Second lower Starting twice weekly, increasing to three times weekly	

Fig. 22.10 Eccentric rotator cuff strength exercises.

evident. The planning and placement is easier at this stage when rugby training is not involved. As an introduction to eccentric-based cuff strength training, 2 days per week is typically a good starting point in order for the athlete to recover between sessions. Once the athlete becomes accustomed to the challenge of eccentric exercises, alternate days can be introduced, thus allowing for 3 days of strength training per week. This is important for a number of reasons, but primarily to create a more robust and durable athlete, reducing the likelihood of further injury but also assisting in creating a more dominant athlete on the rugby field.

The approach we take and the exercises we typically use complement the endurance cuff work. We try not to complicate things and simply load the cuff endurance exercises and follow standard strength training parameters and periodization. This is beneficial as, following completion of the cuff endurance programme, we know that the athlete has completed multiple repetitions of the same or similar exercise. Because of this familiarity, we can be confident that they can maintain good technique, the exercise does not aggravate the underlying injury and furthermore it provides a gauge to quantify progression since commencing rehabilitation. With this approach, by isolating the cuff while adding heavy load, we are confident that we are able to specifically target the rotator cuff more than targeting global shoulder prime movers. However, it is important to ensure you continue to

ask the player questions like 'What do you feel is working?' or 'Where is the burn?' If they are feeling other structures (e.g., posterior deltoid) working harder than the posterior cuff during an external rotation exercise, for instance, then the exercise set-up should be altered or load modified.

The eccentric exercise selection, as discussed, aims to mirror the endurance exercise selection. Care must be taken to ensure the full range is achieved – that the athlete is working eccentrically from full external rotation to full internal rotation while controlling the lowering or eccentric action. This rest time can be used productively, with the athlete completing either another shoulder rehabilitation exercise or a lower body exercise. This helps ensure that the rehabilitation session does not become prohibitively long and helps with adherence.

Due to the demands of the exercise, the rehabilitator must work as a motivator to continually encourage the athlete to control the eccentric phase. It is not unusual to work close to failure with this type of training, so the rehabilitator must gauge the quality of the repetitions and respond appropriately by:
1. increasing encouragement to the athlete (intent)
2. reducing the requested repetitions during the set
3. selecting a lighter weight before commencement of the next set
4. increasing the load.

Open kinetic chain exercises			
60–90° Shoulder flexion	**90–120° Shoulder flexion**	**120–150° Shoulder flexion**	**FROM shoulder flexion**
Exercise selection and progressions			
1. Unweighted Turkish get up (TGU) body rolls	1. 1/4 TGU	1. 1/2 TGU	1. Full TGU
2. KB TGU body roll	2. Position specific OKC exercise entry in available range	2. Position specific OKC exercise progressions in available range	2. Position specific OKC exercise progressions through range
3. Bottoms up KB TGU body roll			

Fig. 22.11 Open kinetic chain exercises. *FROM*, Full range of motion; *KB*, kettlebell; *OKC*, open kinetic chain.

Table 22.5 Rugby positions, related game demands and strengthening rehabilitation activities

Position	Game demand	Rehabilitation activity
Prop	Line-out lifting	Banded squat into overhead press
Second row/flanker	Line-out catching	Overhead bottoms up kettlebell carry
Scrum half	Passing from the ground	Lateral lunge to medicine ball throw
Winger	Hand off during line break	Forward lunge to cable press

Open kinetic chain exercises

Although a large proportion of shoulder rehabilitation exercises focus on developing endurance and strength in isolation, it is important to incorporate the open kinetic chain exercises during the rehabilitation process. This type of intervention challenges the player's ability to control an unfixed weight throughout their lift. These exercises challenge integration of rotator cuff and global shoulder function, which assists in the preparation of the athlete's shoulder for the uncontrolled nature of the sport (Fig. 22.11).

Practically, this would involve having the player perform an activity in a rehabilitation setting which mirrors a rugby-specific task. The approach used typically commences with a simple OKC exercise and is progressed as appropriate to continually challenge the athlete. The goal is to gradually and increasingly expose the player to a sport-specific task in a highly controlled environment as a precursor to carrying out the activity in a controlled scenario (e.g., rugby skills, return to contact) before exposing the player to the uncontrolled chaotic scenarios that occur during rugby training and games.

Creation of the exercise involves understanding the role and demands of the position in question, an example of which is demonstrated in Table 22.5. Integration of rehabilitation exercises that reproduce a game task allows sports-specific intent to be added to the exercise.

Upper body strength

One of the key aims of any rehabilitation is to return the athlete to full function as quickly and safely as possible. Upper body strength is vital in the management of shoulder injuries to allow them to withstand the demands of the game. Prompt reintegration, when able, into a modified UB gym programme is important, which then is progressed to return the athlete to a full gym programme. This is where good multidisciplinary collaboration plays a fundamental role.

From the outset, once the athlete returns to UB strength, the aim should be to return them to their preinjury strength levels as well as their preinjury UB lifts of choice (e.g., horizontal push – bench press, horizontal press – barbell (BB) bench pull). This can be achieved by following the regression/progression model (Table 22.6), typically starting with the most regressed exercise and progressing exercise selection as appropriate.

Horizontal push

Bench press remains the main horizontal press exercise in most gym programmes. In terms of regressing this, we would look at the dumbbell (DB) bench press as a viable

Table 22.6 Regression/progression model

Level of difficulty	Horizontal push	Horizontal pull	Vertical push	Vertical pull
Difficult	BB bench press	KB bench pull	Military press	Chin-ups
↑	DB bench press	BB bench pull	DA DB/KB shoulder press	DA cable pull down
	Weighted press-up	SA DB/KB row	SA DB/KB shoulder press	SA cable pull down
	Press-up	SA cable pull	Jammer press	SA high-to-low cable pull
	Block BB bench press	DA cable row		
	BB floor press			
	DB/KB floor press			
Easy	Cable horizontal press			

BB, Barbell; *DA*, double arm; *DB*, dumbbell; *KB*, kettlebell; *SA*, single arm.

option, keeping resistance through full range, while giving the player the ability to alter arm position for comfort. As a regression, a CKC exercise would be a good option due to reduced stability demands required, such as a weighted press-up, again hand position and width can be manipulated for comfort. In our athletes, a bodyweight press-up normally equates to 55–60% of bodyweight, so this value can be used as a guide to prescribing resistance loads safely. Additional weight can be added to the individual's back, and although it is a regression of bench press, it can still be loaded heavily through full shoulder range.

Some players will experience pain at the bottom position of bench press (see Fig. 22.9D). In these cases, reducing the range of their lift tends to work well. Initially we would advocate a block bench, approximately three-quarters range of full bench press. However, if further restriction was needed, a floor press is a good option (see Fig. 22.9E). In our experience, very few players, even those with acutely painful shoulders, are unable to tolerate a double arm (DA) floor press. DB and SA options are other viable options when manipulating the stimulus, as well as manipulation of sets and reps.

Horizontal pull

Pulling tends to be less problematic for acutely injured shoulders. In terms of horizontal pulling, ensuring a bilateral primary UB exercise with a unilateral accessory UB pull remains important (see Table 22.6).

A prone BB bench pull remains the main lift for most programmes. Unfortunately, due to the bench support bar placement, it is not possible to achieve full range. The use of kettlebells (KB) is a good alternative, due to an ability to pull to end-range, while a wider grip ensures comfort.

For athletes who have difficulty lying prone, such as those with sternoclavicular joint injuries, some anterior chest wall injuries or acromioclavicular (ACJ) sprains, a bent-over row can be used. We prefer using a fixed cable-based horizontal pull; again this can be utilized as DA/SA. It is also possible to vary the height of the cable resistance to incorporate a high-to-low row to target lower scapular retractors. A chest-height row or a low-to-high pull provides a similar stimulus to a bent-over row. Grip type and placement can be altered here for comfort.

Vertical push

Given the demands of professional rugby union, the positions above the horizontal line of the shoulder pose the highest risk for developing serious shoulder injuries (e.g., tackle position). Therefore, it is important to ensure that our athletes are strong overhead to withstand these forces. Additionally, given the risks involved with pressing overhead and the potential for compensatory strategies to occur causing stress on anatomical structures (e.g., lumbar spine) care must be taken to ensure that the lift is performed competently.

The most technically challenging vertical push we use is the military press (see Fig. 22.9F). This is difficult in terms of the risks mentioned above so we utilize a DA/SA DB vertical press as a readily available alternative. Instead of challenging the athlete with a heavier weight, a bottoms-up KB press will challenge shoulder control; this can be done in a standing or seated position. Similar to the horizontal movements, it is appropriate to alternate between DA and SA lifts.

Generally, we find that a jammer press is tolerated well by most athletes, and is suited to squad gym sessions, potentially due to its closed chain nature.

Vertical pull

Chin-ups remain the 'Gold Standard' for the development of vertical pulling strength. However, we note that a minority of the squad do not perform this exercise due to underlying structural limitations, previous injury history or technical fault.

Although the development of overhead pulling strength is a good option, it must be noted that the exercise is often performed poorly, to such an extent that individuals place additional stress on other anatomical structures (e.g., the lumbopelvic region) and drive muscle patterning issues that can lead to injuries in other areas. However, this is a great UB strength exercise when performed proficiently. When undertaking this exercise, ensure:

- 'shoelaces pulled up', i.e., ankle in dorsiflexion
- pelvic neutral (avoid anterior and posterior tilting)
- trunk engaged, i.e., ribs down, belt buckle up
- minimal thoracic extension
- cervical spine/skull maintaining neutral.

As a regression, SA cable pull-downs can be utilized, with DA variations employed as indicated. As mentioned previously, these can be manipulated in terms of lower body position (standing, seated, kneeling, half-kneeling) and grip position.

Rotator cuff reactive strength

Up to this point in the athlete's rehabilitation, the rotator cuff has been prioritized as a humeral rotator and a glenohumeral joint stabilizer. Rotator cuff reactive strength is trained in order to challenge the shoulder in a way that replicates the demands of the sport, specifically seen in play in a tackle situation, where the shoulder complex is required to absorb large forces.

It is important that the cuff is able to react quickly and appropriately, primarily in the absorption of these forces in order to maintain joint integrity while tackling and passing, which are primarily executed by the global prime movers of the shoulder complex.

Our focus when training cuff reactive strength is predominately focused on the anterior cuff, its role in decelerating external rotational forces about the humeral head, especially in abduction. This is because forced abduction and external rotation is one of the most common mechanisms of serious structural shoulder injuries (Hart and Funk, 2013). These exercises are progressed through ranges when appropriate, with the aim of improving rate of force development (RFD), thus allowing the cuff to absorb forces efficiently (Fig. 22.12).

Return to play

Sport- and position-specific skills

In much the same way as systematically overloading an athlete's rehabilitation programme, great care must be taken to gradually expose an athlete to the demands of the sport upon their return from injury (Fig. 22.13).

The rehabilitation process is in place to ensure primarily that the athlete has the underpinning physiological characteristics needed to participate in the game. However, without the graded exposure to game- and position-specific tasks, the athlete will not be able to increase their confidence nor will they be able to develop these skills further. In the early to midstages, these game-based skills can be mimicked in the gym setting to allow controlled exposure and provide a training stimulus (e.g., medicine ball lateral throws to replicate passing, or barbell shoulder pressing to replicate line-out lifting). Importantly, a player needs exposure to these skills as soon as medically possible. After all, during a medium to long-term rehabilitation there is ample time to develop aspects of their own game that is not high risk, such as passing, line-out throwing or kicking.

Reactive strength rotator cuff exercises		
0–30° Shoulder flexion	30–90° Shoulder flexion	90°+ Shoulder flexion
Exercise selection and progressions		
1. Ball slap to stop	1. Ball slap to stop	1. Ball slap to stop
2. Ball throw and catch	2. Elbow supported ball catch/reload/throw	2. Half kneeling catch/reload/throw
	3. Elbow unsupported weighted ball catch/reload/throw	3. Supine catch/reload/throw
Increase weight/resistance as appropriate		

Fig. 22.12 Reactive strength rotator cuff exercises.

Sport / position specific skills									
30–60° Shoulder flexion		60–90° Shoulder flexion		90–120° Shoulder flexion		120–150° Shoulder flexion		FROM Shoulder flexion	
Forwards	Backs	Forwards	Backs	Forwards	Backs	Forwards	Backs	Forwards	Backs
Video analysis		Introduction to passing with physiotherapist		May commence contact skills + progressions		Level 2 contact skills		Level 3 contact skills	
Review own game skills to highlight strengths/weaknesses		Passing with coaches		Scrum techinque with coaches	Continue to develop specific/relevant skills as needed	Intro to line-out lifting with physio controlled line-out lifting/catching	Continue to develop specific/relevant skills as needed	Line-out contesting	Continue to develop specific/relevant skills as needed
Review of skills with coaches		Introduction to kick/catch with physiotherapist		Maul techique				Full scrummaging	
Skill development planning with coaches Game skill visualization		Kick/catch with coaches		Noncontact skills sessions		Non contact modified rugby session Controlled mauls and scrums		Live mauls Full rugby sessions	

Fig. 22.13 Sport-/position-specific skills. FROM, Full range of motion.

Contact skills		
Level 1 contact	Level 2 contact	Level 3 contact
Falling/rolling technique Introduction to tackle technique Exposure to breakdown positions	Introduction to controlled contact senarios Commencing exposure to decision making/contact while fatigued	Live, uncontrolled contact senarios Replication of game contact senarios under fatigue
Contact with pads, tackle bags	Contact with pads, tackle bags	*'Bone to bone' contact* Targeting any highlighted tackle technique deficiencies
Building confidence and technical ability	Continue to develop confidence and technical ability	
Minimal intent and intensity	Increasing intent and intensity	Maximum intent and intensity
Scrum techinque with coaches	Controlled scrummaging (e.g., 1v1, 2v2)	Full scrummaging
Maul techique	Controlled mauls	Full mauls
Physiotherapist led, coach supervised	Coach led, physiotherapist supervised	Coach led, physiotherapist supervised

Fig. 22.14 Contact skills.

Return to contact skills

Care must be taken to expose the athlete to graded and controlled contact scenarios, progressing to controlled full contact before reintegration into team-based training. Most likely their original injury was a result of a contact scenario. Therefore this progressive exposure to the contact enables not only the development of the player's own confidence during contact but also the confidence that their rehabilitated shoulder can withstand the demands of the sport and allow them to dominate on the field of play again.

The exposure to a return to contact can commence early. However it is helpful to have skilled rugby coaches to discuss proper technique, review the player's mechanism of injury and assess video clips of their tackle or contact techniques over a period of time to highlight any issues, so that these can be addressed during rehabilitation. The use of visualization and cuing in the early stages assists with this early exposure and development of improved contact technique.

Once the athlete is able to recommence contact, a graded exposure can commence as highlighted in Fig. 22.14. This

should be largely based around ensuring that contact and tackle technique is developed from a remedial to a high level with a skilled rugby coach when available. The importance of improving technique should not be underestimated. Correct tackling technique should allow forces to be dissipated throughout the body rather than isolating the shoulder to absorb massive forces that will obviously increase the risk of reinjury.

Prior to the athlete being cleared to return to full contact training and especially before the athlete has been cleared to return to play, it can be useful to discuss openly with the athlete whether they feel there are any areas where they feel deficient. Highlighting this early allows time for these to be addressed. The result of such discussions may include increasing cuff or global shoulder strength, conditioning or confidence in contact situations.

Despite spending time creating a structured and objectively lead RTP criteria, there are instances where athletes will progress based on function rather than by meeting objective strength scores. This occurs when, due to the severity of the injury, it is unlikely that full shoulder function will return. In these cases, the RTP criteria are considered flexible and

Return to	Milestone	Contact	Other considerations
Static skills	Pain-free FROM	Low level, submaximal tackle technique sessions including falling/rolling. (technique focus only)	Contact visualization - explanation
	Achieving cuff endurance at 90°		Video reviews of preinjury tackle technique
	Achieving cuff strength at 45°		Video reviews of best practice tackle technique (individual/other)
	Achieving reactive cuff strength at 0°		Discussion with coaches
Return to Contact level 1	Cuff strength >80% (HHD)	Low-level tackle technique sessions inc. falling/rolling. (Technique focus with progression of forces and intent)	Continue visualization, video review and coach discussion
	DA UB strength >80% preinjury baseline		Introduction to noncontact skills sessions
	SA UB strength >80% of noninjured side		Video review of completed tackle technique sessions
Return to Contact level 2	Cuff strength >85% (HHD)	Continuing tackle technique sessions. (Competence focus, maximum forces and intent. Tackle pad/bag contacts only)	Noncontact position specific sessions (backs-/forwards-specific drills)
	DA UB strength >85% preinjury baseline		Noncontact team training
	SA UB strength >85% of noninjured side		
	Technically competent completion of RTC 1		
Return to Contact level 3	Cuff strength >85% (HHD)	Progression of tackle technique sessions. (Outcome focus, maximum forces and intent, controlled full contact scenarios progressing to live uncontrolled situations)	Noncontact units sessions (backs-/forwards-specific drills)
	DA UB strength >85% preinjury baseline		Noncontact team training
	SA UB strength >85% of noninjured side		Continue to build confidence with contact scenarios
	Technically competent completion of RTC 2		Can participate in controlled contact drills in training
Return to Train full	Cuff strength >85%	Continuing tackle technique sessions. Content selected based on player's weakness or needs	Full participation in training
	DA UB strength >85% preinjury baseline		Build confidence with live, uncontrolled contact scenarios
	SA UB strength >85% of noninjured side		Address any issues/concerns highlighted by athlete
	Technically competent completion of RTC 3		
Return to Play	Cuff strength >85%	Continuing tackle technique sessions. Content selected based on player's weakness or needs	On-feet loading considerations
	DA UB strength >85% preinjury baseline		Full team training without limitations
	SA UB strength >85% of noninjured side		Athlete feels ready to return to play
	Technically competent in live contact scenarios		
Return to Perform	Cuff strength >90%	Continuing tackle technique sessions. Content selected based on player's weakness or needs	Discussion and review with coaches
	DA UB strength >90% preinjury baseline		1:1 training with coaches on highlighted skill deficits
	SA UB strength >90% of noninjured side		Working to exceed previous baselines (UB, LB, conditioning, skills)
	Continue to address deficits		

Fig. 22.15 Reintegration table. *DA*, Double arm; *FROM*, full range of motion; *HHD*, handheld dynamometry; *LB*, lower body; *RTC*, return to contact; *SA*, single arm; *UB*, upper body.

decisions are largely based around function, performance and ability to tolerate the demands of the sport.

Reintegration and return to performance

Outcome measures

Key outcome markers are used to monitor progress during rehabilitation to give an objective measurement on specific key qualities and attributes. In practice, isolated rotator cuff strength and power testing together with global shoulder strength testing is used. These are key markers for progressions and scores; this will be compared to both baseline strength scores and comparisons between injured and noninjured sides (Fig. 22.15).

One method of isolated strength testing is handheld dynamometry (HHD). This does come with a caveat:

this method is very operator dependent. For this reason, protocols and procedures to ensure the tests remain standardized are important. We test strength in internal and external rotation in three ranges: 0 degrees, 45 degrees and 90 degrees of shoulder flexion/abduction, and towards the end of the pathway we also test strength in end-ranges of abduction/external rotation (90 degrees /90 degrees).

Postoperative shoulder injuries should also be tested with isokinetic dynamometry on the consultant's recommendation, comparing peak torque and maximum force production, alongside analysis of the athlete's force curve to highlight any deficits.

Alternatively, a sphygmometer can be employed as a simple method of monitoring strength scores in terms of pressure (mmHg). This may provide an option if HHDs are not readily available.

Strength testing is only one component of outcome measures and must be viewed in conjunction with all other pillars in the decision-making process. Care must be taken to ensure that RTP decisions are not solely based on these test results but also take into account a holistic view of the athlete (e.g., tackle technique competence).

Tackle technique sessions can be run as standalone sessions or integrated within rehabilitation sessions led by physiotherapists. Simple tasks such as controlled falling or rolling can be performed on soft mats; other tasks such as a fending, controlled tackling onto a tackle pad and exposure to other contact scenarios can be performed. These tasks are very useful to help build confidence and reduce fear avoidance – as most of these players will have been injured in tackle situations. During the mid-to-late stage of rehab and on return to play and return to perform, coach feedback and expertise is a valued component. When tackle technique is poor there is a huge potential for injury, especially when the shoulder is placed in 'at risk' positions such as those mentioned above. We feel that if the player uses their body effectively during rugby activities then the forces the shoulder is exposed to are dissipated throughout the body rather than being concentrated around the shoulder joint itself. This process is an integral part of the rehabilitation process. No amount of cuff endurance, cuff strength or shoulder strength will adequately protect the shoulder when tackle technique is inadequate.

Inseason management

When rugby sessions are part of an athlete's weekly schedule, the planning and implementation of rehabilitation becomes more difficult. Most challenging are the management of category 2 and 3 injuries during the inseason period, where the aim is to manage the player's symptoms and rehabilitation while making the player available for selection.

These cases are dealt with on an individual basis as not all injuries will be able to be 'managed' and may require time away from the demands of rugby to allow a focused rehabilitation process to occur.

A decision to attempt to manage an athlete's injury inseason should not be taken lightly. As the Medical Department works as a single cog in a much larger system, it is important to involve and collaborate with other departments in this process, specifically the Strength and Conditioning Department and the Coaching Team. This multidisciplinary input ensures that all involved parties, including the athlete, are aware of the injury, the prognosis and risks involved in managing an athlete inseason.

All parties should have input in the decision-making process and assist in creating a framework to attempt to allow the athlete to be managed inseason. All parties must be aware that when managing an athlete inseason, then the main rugby aim is ensuring availability for selection for games. Consequently, it should be understood that availability for rugby training will likely be modified. For example, a player will be unlikely to participate in full contact training drills, and their UB gym sessions will be modified to more suitable shoulder-friendly exercises with a large emphasis on shoulder rehabilitation exercises.

Outside of rugby games and training the biggest priority for the athlete is to rehabilitate their shoulder. As a result, this takes priority over all other aspects of training. This is not to say that the athlete does not perform any other training in this period, but rather any available window of opportunity to perform rehabilitation is taken. In practice there needs to be a fluid approach taken with rehabilitation; overall training content and exercises progressions, although well thought out and structured, often have to be modified to enable their completion during the busy training week. Outside of UB strength and rehabilitation sessions, microdosing of selected exercises can be beneficial. This is essentially a 'little and often' approach – for instance having the athlete perform 2–3 specific exercises aimed at addressing large deficits throughout the day or week, such as before mobility sessions, gym sessions or pitch-based sessions.

Ultimately, despite the aim being to 'manage' the athlete, it is important to review the process regularly. For instance, when attempting to manage the injury, if the player is unable to perform on the field due to the nature of their injury then a rehabilitation-only approach or liaison with orthopaedic surgeon for their medical opinion may be more suitable.

Conclusion

The framework presented here has been found to be useful in clinical practice. However, it is essential that each player's injury is fully assessed and understood to ensure that the rehabilitation pathway being followed is specific to them, their injury, their individual deficits, their sporting demands and the resources available. Clinical reasoning and a tailored approach are always key in managing any pathology; the framework we propose should not be seen as a universal panacea for all shoulder problems.

References

Boileau, P., Villalba, M., Hery, J., Balg, F., Ahrens, P., Neyton, L., 2006. Risk factors of shoulder instability after arthroscopic Bankart repair. Journal of Bone & Joint Surgery 88 (8), 1755–1763.

Brandenburg, J.P., Docherty, D., 2002. The effects of accentuated eccentric loading on strength, muscle hypertrophy, and neural adaptations in trained individuals. Journal of Strength and Conditioning Research 16 (1), 25–32.

De Mey, K., Danneels, L., Cagnie, B., Borms, D., T'Jonck, Z., Van Damme, E., et al., 2014. Shoulder muscle activation levels during four closed kinetic chain exercises with and without Redcord slings. Journal of Strength and Conditioning Research 28 (6), 1626–1635.

Escamilla, R.F., Yamashiro, K., Paulos, L., Andrews, J.R., 2009. Shoulder muscle activity and function in common shoulder rehabilitation exercises. Sports Medicine 39 (8), 663–685.

Hart, D., Funk, L., 2013. Serious shoulder injuries in professional soccer: return to participation after surgery. Knee Surgery, Sports Traumatology, Arthroscopy 23 (7), 2123–2129.

Hegedus, E.J., Goode, A., Campbell, S., Morin, A., Tamaddoni, M., Moorman, C.T., et al., 2007. Physical examination tests of the shoulder: a systematic review with meta-analysis of individual tests. British Journal of Sports Medicine 42 (2), 80–92.

Hendricks, S., Matthews, B., Roode, B., Lambert, M., 2014. Tackler characteristics associated with tackle performance in rugby union. European Journal of Sport Science 14, 753–762.

Herrington, L., Horslet, I., Whitaker, L., Rolf, C., 2008. Does a tackling task effect shoulder joint position sense in rugby players? Physical Therapy in Sport 9 (2), 67–71.

Hortobágyi, T., Devita, P., Money, J., Barrier, J., 2001. Effects of standard and eccentric overload strength training in young women. Med Sci Sports Exerc 33 (7), 1206–1212.

May, S., Chance-Larsen, K., Littlewood, C., Lomas, D., Saad, M., 2010. Reliability of physical examination tests used in the assessment of patients with shoulder problems: a systematic review. Physiotherapy 96 (3), 179–190.

McMullen, J., Uhl, T.L., 2000. A kinetic chain approach for shoulder rehabilitation. Journal of Athletic Training 35 (3), 329–337.

Morgan, R., Herrington, L., 2013. The effect of tackling on shoulder joint positioning sense in semi-professional rugby players. Physical Therapy in Sport 1–5.

Mullaney, M.J., Perkinson, C., Kremenic, I., Tyler, T.F., Orishimo, K., Johnson, C., 2017. EMG of shoulder muscles during reactive isometric elastic resistance exercises. The International Journal of Sports Physical Therapy 12 (3), 417–424.

Quarrie, K., Wilson, B., 2000. Force production in the rugby union scrum. Journal of Sports Sciences 18 (4), 237–246.

Reardon, C., Tobin, D.P., Tierney, P., Delahunt, E., 2017. Collision count in rugby union: A comparison of micro-technology and video analysis methods. Journal of Sports Sciences 35 (20), 2028–2034.

Reed, D., Cathers, I., Halaki, M., Ginn, K., 2018. Shoulder muscle activation patterns and levels differ between open and closed-chain abduction. Journal of Science and Medicine in Sport 21 (5), 462–466.

Sciascia, A., Cromwell, R., 2012. Kinetic chain rehabilitation; a theoretical framework. Rehabilitation Research and Practise 1–9.

Seminati, E., Cazzola, D., Preatoni, E., Trewartha, G., 2016. Specific tackling situations affect the biomechanical demands experienced by rugby union players. Journal of Sports Biomechanics 16 (1), 58–75.

Sporrong, H., Lamerud, G., Herberts, P., 1995. Influences on shoulder muscle activity. European Journal of Applied Physiology and Occupational Physiology 71 (6), 485–492.

Sporrong, H., Palmerud, G., Herberts, P., 1996. Hand grip increases shoulder muscle activity: an EMG analysis with static hand contractions in 9 subjects. Acta Orthopaedica Scandinavica 67 (5), 485–490.

Torrance, E., Clarek, C.J., Monga, P., Funk, L., Walton, M.J., 2018. Recurrence after arthroscopic labral repair for traumatic anterior instability in adolescent rugby and contact athletes. The American Journal of Sports Medicine 46 (12), 2969–2974.

Usman, J., McIntosh, A., Fréchède, B., 2014. An investigation of shoulder forces in active shoulder tackles in rugby union football. Journal of Science and Medicine in Sport 14 (6), 547–552.

Wattanaprakornkul, D., Cathers, I., Halaki, M., Ginn, K., 2011a. The rotator cuff muscles have a direction specific recruitment pattern during shoulder flexion and extension exercises. Journal of Science and Medicine in Sport 14 (5), 376–382.

Wattanaprakornkul, D., Halaki, M., Cathers, I., Ginn, K., 2011b. Direction-specific recruitment of rotator cuff muscles during bench press and row. Journal of Electromyography and Kinesiology 21 (6), 1041–1049.

Chapter | 23 |

Assessment of the sporting shoulder

Marcus Bateman

Principles

The diagnostic filter

As with any form of clinical assessment, there should be prior knowledge and understanding of what we are assessing. There are a wide range of pathologies that can affect the shoulder and our clinical assessment should be a means of narrowing down the possibilities in a reasoned and systematic way to finally conclude one single accurate diagnosis.

Early identification of serious pathology

The first priority of assessment should always be to exclude pathologies that have the potential for loss of life or limb such as infection, serious neurovascular trauma or malignancy. Whilst such presentations thankfully are rare, the life-changing consequences of missed or delayed diagnosis mean these pathologies should always be at the forefront of our minds. There are less serious but also very important pathologies specifically related to the shoulder girdle that should be considered as requiring urgent intervention, such as pectoralis major tendon ruptures and traumatic rotator cuff tears. Such injuries require early surgical repair to facilitate successful healing and give the greatest chance of return to play.

In the absence of trauma, acute septic arthritis (infection of a joint) is the first pathology to exclude. Patients typically present with a recent onset of severe pain even at rest and with slight movement of the shoulder, fever symptoms, general feeling of being unwell and objective signs of joint inflammation such as swelling, increased heat and redness of the skin surrounding the joint.

History

Age as a predictor of pathology

Age is a key factor in the clinical reasoning process when considering the likelihood of certain pathologies. Take for example frozen shoulder, which is typically seen in those aged 40 to 60 years. It occasionally presents in individuals in their 30s but this is usually associated with type 1 diabetes. It is never seen in those under 30; this is also true of primary osteoarthritis of the glenohumeral joint. Therefore young patients presenting with both shoulder stiffness and pain should have a high index of suspicion for more serious pathology such as inflammatory arthropathy, septic arthritis or malignancy. Whilst the incidence of most cancers increases with age, teenagers and adults in their early 20s have the highest incidence of osteosarcoma.

The most common symptom of shoulder pain is 'impingement' – the patient describes sharp mechanical catching pain during certain activities. These symptoms are usually a sign of degenerative rotator cuff pathology in patients over 40 but in the young should be considered a possible sign of 'subclinical' instability.

Mechanism of onset

Probably the most important part of the history is the mechanism of onset. The absence of significant trauma obviously rules out fractures, acromioclavicular (AC) joint dislocation and rotator cuff tears in patients aged under 40. With trauma it is important to determine the arm position on impact. For example, a direct blow to the acromion, such as falling sideways from a bicycle whilst still holding the handlebars or falling sideways to the ground whilst holding a rugby ball against the chest, raises the suspicion of clavicle fracture or AC joint dislocation. A direct blow or fall with the shoulder in an abducted externally rotated position raises suspicion of anterior shoulder dislocation. A sudden severe pain when lifting heavy weight raises suspicion of tendon rupture, for example the pectoralis major or biceps brachii.

Instability symptoms

It is important to understand that instability is different from laxity. Laxity is excessive movement in a joint compared to what is considered normal, whereas instability is when that laxity causes symptoms such as pain, uncontrolled subluxation or dislocation, and loss of function. Patients may present with 'impingement' symptoms of sharp catching pain in certain ranges of movement (usually overhead). This is common from middle age onwards as a symptom of rotator cuff degeneration. In the young, however, especially in those under 25 years, it is more likely to be an early symptom of instability and should be correlated with clinical examination findings of laxity or instability provocation. Conversely instability may be obvious subluxation or dislocation of a joint, which needs to be correlated with any previous trauma, as there is a high risk of structural injury to the capsule–ligamentous complex resulting in a high redislocation rate, especially in the young after trauma. Subjective questioning is very important in patients with significant instability as an absence of trauma guides the treatment pathway towards nonoperative management.

Occupation (sport) and potential sport-specific risk

Collision sports clearly carry greater risk of traumatic injury than noncollision sports, but there are other sport-specific issues to consider. Sports with high shoulder demand include those that involve throwing (e.g., javelin, cricket, baseball, handball), swimming, racquet sports and volleyball. Such sports practised repetitively for years can lead to acquired shoulder abnormalities through microtrauma or increased risk of certain injuries. Superior labrum anterior posterior (SLAP) tears, for example, are commonly seen in throwing sports with a key subjective factor of loss of throwing power/distance or pain when throwing. Another common adaptation in overhead sports is the gradual gain of shoulder external rotation with corresponding loss of internal rotation, called glenohumeral internal rotation deficit (GIRD). This may lead to higher risk of shoulder 'impingement' symptoms, but unlike those patients with underlying laxity, these patients have restriction to their range of movement either in internal rotation or in total range of rotation arc.

Pain location

Pain location can be useful in directing the clinical examination. Pain in the upper trapezius and medial scapula border regions is much more likely to be related to the cervical spine rather than the shoulder, so the first element of the objective examination should be to assess the neck. Sometimes the patient will localize the pain very accurately and this is typical of localized AC joint or biceps pathology, when the patient often points directly to the area with one finger. Most commonly though the pain is more diffuse: either in the region of the deltoid, which is common for rotator cuff related pain, or in the region of the deltoid insertion midway down the humerus, common for glenohumeral joint pain. If the patient describes a deep anterior pain that is not palpable, especially with clunking during movement or a vague sense that something feels out of place, then this should raise suspicions of SLAP tear.

Aggravating factors

Night pain is usually considered to be a red flag sign of serious pathology, but in relation to the shoulder is a common complaint. It is important therefore to clarify whether this is purely positional, i.e., waking when rolling over onto the affected shoulder, or whether it is persistent and unrelated to changes of position. The latter scenario is a very common feature of frozen shoulder but may also represent infection, tumour or inflammatory joint disease.

Neurological symptoms

It is rare for patients with local shoulder pathology to complain of neurological symptoms. Shooting pains or sensory deficits that extend below the elbow towards the hand are usually related to the cervical spine. An uncommon but significant pathology that can affect people of any age is brachial neuritis (also known as Parsonage–Turner syndrome), which can affect any or multiple nerves of the brachial plexus. This typically presents as severe neuralgic pain in the absence of trauma that may affect the shoulder girdle or the whole limb and is poorly controlled with analgesia. The cause is uncertain but often occurs during times of physiological stress on the body such as during illness, after surgery and childbirth. Initial pain is followed by muscle weakness and sensory disturbance of the nerves affected.

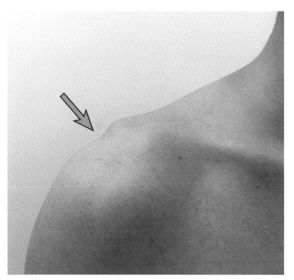

Fig. 23.1 Deformity of the acromioclavicular joint consistent with dislocation.

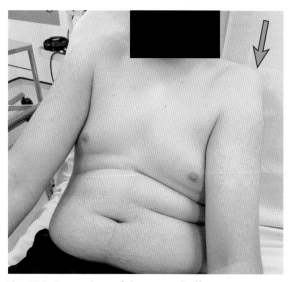

Fig. 23.2 Comparison of the squared-off appearance of an anteriorly dislocated shoulder (*arrow*) versus the rounder appearance of the unaffected side.

It is also important to ask about neurological symptoms after significant trauma, as these can be easily overlooked. This is particularly important after shoulder dislocation (axillary nerve), humeral shaft fractures (radial nerve), clavicle fracture and traction injuries to the arm (brachial plexus). If the patient complains of sensory deficit or weakness then the objective examination should focus on establishing the pattern of neurological deficit and whether this relates more to a cervical radiculopathy, peripheral nerve entrapment neuropathy or trauma, or a plexus-level pathology.

Clinical examination

On the field assessment

This should be as brief as possible to avoid disruption to the sport but always prioritizing the individual's health. Assessment should include observation of skin integrity or blood loss directed by the site of pain followed by assessment of deformity to the bony structure such as displacement of the clavicle or a squared-off appearance to the deltoid, which can indicate glenohumeral joint dislocation (Fig. 23.1). Any significant findings should result in the player leaving the field for further detailed assessment; likewise if there is significant pain with passive movement of the shoulder or significant pain on firm palpation of the clavicle, scapula or upper arm.

Off the field assessment

Observation

On the field, it is often not possible to expose the limb for a thorough visual assessment but this is imperative in any off the field examination. Look for:

Deformity. Does the shoulder contour look rounded like the contralateral shoulder or is there a squared-off appearance to indicate a possible glenohumeral joint dislocation? If squared-off, is there a prominence anteroinferior to the coracoid or posteriorly to indicate the direction of dislocation (Fig. 23.2)? Does the distal end of the clavicle appear significantly higher than the acromion and asymmetrical compared with the contralateral side to indicate an AC joint dislocation or distal end clavicle fracture? Does the clavicle look shortened or bulbous in the middle indicating a possible fracture? Is there significant winging of the scapula at rest to raise suspicion of long thoracic nerve pathology? Subtle asymmetry or pseudowinging, where just the inferior angle of the scapula is prominent, as opposed to true winging, where the whole of the medial scapula border is prominent (Fig. 23.3), is common and not a cause for concern. Is there a Popeye deformity of the bicep, either with a shift of the muscle belly proximally to indicate a distal tendon rupture, or a bulge of the muscle belly with hollowing near the axilla indicating a long head proximal tendon rupture?

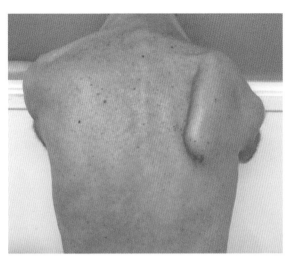

Fig. 23.3 Right scapula true winging pictured here with the patient leaning with both hands against a wall.

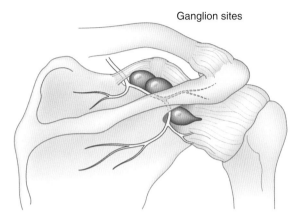

Ganglion sites

Fig. 23.4 Diagram showing how a ganglion may compress the suprascapular nerve at different sites along its course. (Adapted from Moore T. P., Hunter R. E., 1996. Suprascapular nerve entrapment. Operative Techniques in Sports Medicine 4 (1), 8–14.)

Bruising. Immediate significant bruising and discolouration after trauma is indicative of bony or vascular injury so should be regarded as an emergency. Typically bruising is seen 24–48 hours after injury and if extensive or present after an incident that did not involve direct trauma, for example when lifting a heavy weight, should be regarded as an indicator of a significant injury such as a fracture or tendon tear.

Wasting. Muscle wasting is rarely seen in those aged under 50 years so should be regarded as significant. It may represent the sequelae of pathology to the nerve supplying the affected muscle or tear of the tendon attachment. In the shoulder the deltoid should be inspected, especially after shoulder instability, as the axillary nerve is prone to injury. The supraspinatus and infraspinatus muscles of the rotator cuff can easily be examined visually by inspecting the muscle bulk above and below the scapula spine. Isolated infraspinatus wasting is rare and should not be mistaken for a sign of a rotator cuff tear, as cuff tears begin in the superior portion of the tendon attachment (i.e., supraspinatus portion) and extend posteriorly into the infraspinatus portion in larger tears. Isolated infraspinatus wasting therefore is not tear-related but usually a sign of compression of the inferior branch of the suprascapular nerve. Paralabral cysts may form after labral injury in the shoulder, such as after instability or with the repeated microtrauma of throwing sports, and these have the potential to compress the suprascapular nerve. This compression may be near the suprascapular notch, in which case both branches can be affected, resulting in wasting of both supraspinatus and infraspinatus, or near the spinoglenoid notch, in which case just the inferior branch is affected resulting in isolated wasting of the infraspinatus (Fig. 23.4) (Moore and Hunter, 1996). When wasting of both supraspinatus and infraspinatus is

present, then rotator cuff tear is most likely (dependent on the subjective history) but suprascapular nerve lesion or brachial neuritis should always be considered as differential diagnoses.

Swelling. Swelling in the shoulder is rare, and so when present should be viewed as a significant finding. After trauma this usually indicates a high likelihood of bone fracture. In the absence of trauma, swelling of the glenohumeral joint could be a sign of serious pathology such as infection or malignancy, except in the elderly when it is more likely to be related to degenerative rotator cuff tear arthropathy (arthritis as a result of superior migration of the humerus against the acromion due to massive rotator cuff tear). Likewise, obvious swelling of the AC joint without trauma should be considered concerning in younger patients, whereas it can be seen in more elderly patients as a consequence of rotator cuff tear arthropathy.

Redness. Redness is a key sign of active inflammation so when present over a joint should raise immediate suspicion of infection unless caused by trauma to the skin itself. Priority should be given to the exclusion of sepsis and should direct the assessment accordingly with detailed subjective questioning about red flags and appropriate imaging and laboratory tests.

Palpation

Bony tenderness. This should be assessed after trauma. Palpate the length of the clavicle, acromion and scapula spine whilst prompting the patient to report any significant tenderness that may indicate a fracture. Firm palpation through the muscles overlying the humerus may also raise suspicion of a fracture if significantly tender. If tenderness is present, try to assess if the bone is solid during active or passive movement of the limb. If movement can be felt, or crepitus, then radiographic imaging is required.

Joints. The sternoclavicular (SC) joint, AC joint and glenohumeral joint should be palpated for tenderness, excessive heat, swelling, crepitus during movement, and stability. The SC and AC joints are very superficial and so easy to palpate, whereas the glenohumeral joint may be difficult if there is significant overlying soft tissue. Significant pain provoked by even light touch over a joint, especially when associated with redness and heat, is a significant concern and should be considered as a septic joint until proven otherwise.

Range of movement

Firstly assess the active range of movement of external rotation compared with the unaffected side. If there is a deficit then reassess passively. A restriction of passive external rotation indicates stiffness of the glenohumeral joint such as from frozen shoulder, arthropathy, infection or a locked dislocation. In this event, expect all of the other shoulder movements to also be restricted. This may limit your ability to perform further clinical tests and the focus of the assessment should then shift to the cause of the restriction (see Imaging).

Restricted active external rotation but with full passive range suggests significant weakness of the posterior-superior rotator cuff (supraspinatus, teres major and infraspinatus) as seen in rotator cuff tears or suprascapular nerve lesions. In the presence of significant joint sepsis, it is important to note that even very small subtle movements such as rotation of the forearm away from the abdomen to less than neutral are severely painful. As well as assessing for range of movement deficits also assess for hypermobility. Most adults have external rotation range between 50 and 80 degrees. If the patient has 90 degrees or more, consider this to be hypermobile; it may be a predisposing factor for instability.

Next, assess functional movement behind the back by measuring how far the patient can reach their hand up their spine and compare to the unaffected side. A painful restriction may be as a result of one of a number of pathologies but a full range of pain-free motion excludes glenohumeral joint stiffness.

Assess shoulder flexion total range of both shoulders together whilst observing the dynamic movement of the scapulae. Significant winging or obvious asymmetry should be noted. If normal, ask the patient to repeat the movement 10–20 times whilst holding a 1-kg weight in each hand, to observe whether any dynamic scapular winging or symmetry is noticeable with loading or fatigue (i.e., scapula movement appears abnormal after 10–20 repetitions of the movement whereas it appeared normal initially).

Assess shoulder abduction through a full arc of movement prompting the patient to report any pain symptoms.

Pain in the middle arc, approximately 60–120 degrees, may indicate rotator cuff or bursa-related pain. Pain at the very extreme at full abduction may indicate pain from the AC joint. Again, assess for hypermobility of abduction – considered relevant if greater than 180 degrees is achieved (i.e., beyond the vertical, with the elbow behind the head).

In overhead athletes consider specific assessment of total range of movement deficit (TROMD) or GIRD. This is measured with the patient in supine lying to reduce scapular movement. The patient's arm is abducted to 90 degrees and the total range of movement is measured using a goniometer or inclinometer from extreme external rotation to extreme internal rotation. The measurement is then compared to the unaffected side. A 20-degree deficit (TROMD) has been reported to be clinically relevant (Kibler et al., 2012). GIRD is measured in a similar way with the patient supine but this time measuring the range of movement from vertical to extreme internal rotation before comparing to the other side (Fig. 23.5). A GIRD of 8 degrees has been reported to be clinically relevant (Kibler et al., 2012).

Clinical tests

Clinical tests should never be interpreted in isolation as none of the 'special' clinical tests of the shoulder have high specificity and sensitivity. Tests should always be an adjunct and the findings correlated to the subjective history.

The rotator cuff

The most significant finding of rotator cuff testing is weakness as this may indicate a structural defect such as a tendon tear or be as a result of neurological deficit. It is very common for pain to be provoked by these tests and such findings are not necessarily just attributable to the rotator cuff, so should be taken in context of the whole assessment.

The subscapularis can be tested in three ways (Pennock et al., 2011):

The belly press test. The patient places the hand on the belly with the elbow at 90 degrees and forward of midline. The tester tries to pull their hand away from the belly whilst the patient resists. If the forward elbow position is maintained then the test is normal. If the elbow drops back (i.e., the shoulder extends) then this highlights a possible tear of the subscapularis.

The bear hug test. The patient places their hand on their opposite shoulder with the elbow unsupported on the chest. The tester tries to pull their hand away from their shoulder. If the patient is unable to maintain the starting position then this suggests a possible subscapularis tear.

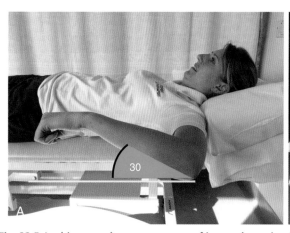
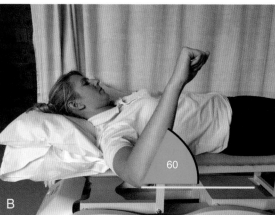

Fig. 23.5 In this example, measurement of internal rotation in supine reveals a 30-degree glenohumeral internal rotation deficit (GIRD) affecting the patient's right shoulder (B) in comparison to the left shoulder (A).

The lift-off test. The patient places their hand behind their back with the dorsum of the hand against the lumbar spine. The tester applies resistance whilst the patient tries to lift their hand away from the spine (posteriorly). Significant weakness suggests a possible subscapularis tear. This test may not be possible as patients in pain may not be able to even get their hand to the starting position.

The posterior-superior rotator cuff (supraspinatus, infraspinatus, teres minor) can be tested in many ways (Beaudreuil et al., 2009) including:

Isometric external rotation test. The patient stands with both elbows flexed to 90 degrees and the shoulders in neutral rotation. The patient is instructed to externally rotate the shoulders whilst the tester resists the movement with both hands. Strength can then be compared to the unaffected side.

External rotation lag sign. If there is considerable weakness of isometric external rotation then passively rotate the shoulder to full external rotation. Ask the patient to maintain this position before letting go of their arm. A positive sign is when the patient is unable to maintain the position and the arm swings back towards the neutral position. This suggests a massive cuff tear or significant suprascapular nerve lesion.

The full can test. The arm is abducted to 90 degrees in the plane of the scapula with the hand orientated so that the thumb points upwards. The tester applies a downward force to assess for pain and strength compared with the unaffected side. Some patients may not tolerate 90 degrees abduction so the test can be modified to a lower position. Pain and weakness may indicate a rotator cuff tear; however bursitis and calcific tendinitis may produce similar findings.

The empty can (Jobe's) test. This is similar to the full can test, however the hand is orientated so that the

thumb points towards the floor. Sometimes symptoms are provoked in this position when the full can test appears normal.

Acromioclavicular joint pain and instability (Yewlett et al., 2012)

Palpation. AC joint pain is very localized and the joint will be tender to firm palpation.

The scarf test. The patient flexes the shoulder to 90 degrees and adducts the hand towards the opposite shoulder. Overpressure is applied. A positive test reproduces pain locally over the AC joint.

Instability testing. If there is a dislocation of the AC joint the tester should offload the weight of the arm and assess whether the deformity reduces. If it does then the patient is less likely to require surgical intervention. Next, assess for any sagittal instability by applying an anteroposterior and posteroanterior force to the clavicle. If there is significant translation then the patient is more likely to require surgical stabilization as it suggests that all three of the stabilizing ligaments have ruptured.

Pectoralis major rupture

Bateman method. This method of testing the pectoralis major involves the tester standing face-to-face with the patient. First the patient places both hands on the tester's shoulders and applies a downward force (Fig. 23.6A). The tester then has two free hands to palpate the contour of the pectoral muscle belly and tendon attachment for asymmetry. This contracts the lower (sternal) fibres. Second, the patient places their hands on the lateral aspect of the tester's deltoids and applies an adduction force (i.e., trying to clap their hands together) (Fig. 23.6B). This includes both the upper (clavicular) and lower fibres. Again

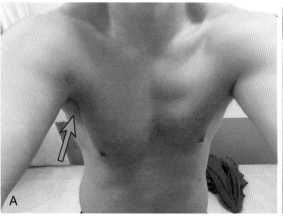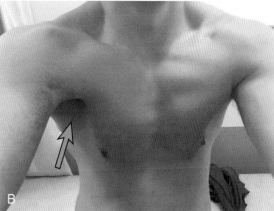

Fig. 23.6 The pectoral muscle contour of a patient with a right pectoralis major tendon rupture whilst the patient applies (A) a downward pressure on the assessor's shoulders, (B) an adduction pressure on the assessor's shoulders.

the tester palpates for symmetry of the muscle belly or tendon attachment. Any significant difference suggests a possible rupture and should be referred for imaging.

Bicep rupture

Ask the patient to tense their bicep and observe any deformity (as mentioned above). This is the most obvious diagnostic sign. If unsure, whilst the bicep remains tensed perform the hook test.

Hook test (O'Driscoll et al., 2007). This is performed by placing a hooked finger behind the distal tendon and pulling forward. An intact tendon can easily be felt as a solid structure whereas a ruptured tendon may not be palpable or offer no resistance.

Test the bicep further by resisting supination of the forearm for pain and weakness whilst noting any deformity of the muscle belly.

SLAP tear and proximal biceps tendinopathy

The subjective history of deep anterior pain, clunking, vague instability and a weak throw are the most important factors, but suspicions may be reinforced by clinical tests.

Palpation. The long head of bicep tendon may be tender proximally over the bicipital groove.

O'Brien's active compression test (O'Brien et al. 1998). The patient's arm is flexed to 90 degrees and adducted 30 degrees with the thumb pointing upwards. The tester applies a downward force that the patient is told to resist, and notes pain deep in the shoulder anteriorly. The thumb is then pointed downward and the same downward force applied. If the pain increases with the thumb pointing down then this may indicate a SLAP tear or proximal

biceps pathology. A positive test may also indicate AC joint pathology so the result must be taken in context of the history and other clinical tests.

Resisted throw (Taylor et al., 2017). To simulate the patient's symptom of a weak throw, ask the patient to place the arm in a throwing position whilst the tester then applies a force to resist the motion. Assess for pain or weakness that may indicate a SLAP tear or proximal biceps pathology.

Glenohumeral joint laxity and instability

Glenohumeral joint laxity is rather subjective with regard to the amount of translation that is significant and also relies on the patient being sufficiently relaxed to be tested fully.

The sulcus sign (Neer and Foster, 1980). The patient sits with the arm relaxed at their side. The tester applies a downward traction force to the humerus whilst observing inferior translation of the humeral head. This test may also induce apprehension of dislocation – a finding of instability.

The apprehension and relocation tests (Farber et al., 2006). With the patient sitting or supine lying the arm is abducted to 90 degrees with the elbow flexed to 90 degrees. The tester places one hand on the anterior shoulder and with the other passively externally rotates the shoulder. If the patient is apprehensive in this position of further shoulder subluxation this is a sign of anterior instability. This finding is reinforced if an anterior-to-posterior pressure is applied to the shoulder during a repeat test and the feeling of apprehension reduces.

The jerk test (Seung-Ho et al., 2004). With the patient sitting the shoulder is flexed to 90 degrees and adducted with internal rotation. The tester applies a force at the flexed elbow so that the humeral head is pushed posteriorly in the glenoid (Fig. 23.7). This may reproduce

299

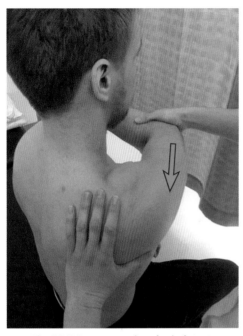

Fig. 23.7 Demonstrating the jerk test.

apprehension or a painful clunk within the shoulder indicating posterior instability.

Generalized laxity: Beighton score

In the presence of instability symptoms or pain without trauma in young athletes, screening of generalized joint mobility should be performed. The Beighton score assesses hypermobility, with 4 points or more considered relevant (Grahame, 2007):

- 1 point each for elbow hyperextension
- 1 point each for passive little finger extension of 90 degrees or more
- 1 point each for thumb parallel to forearm on passive wrist flexion
- 1 point each for knee hyperextension
- 1 point for touching palms to floor in standing with knees extended.

Differential tests for the neck and neurological screening

When sensory disturbance is present in the upper limb or when the pattern of pain includes the neck/upper trapezius region/medial scapula border region, then a cervical spine and neurological assessment is required (see Chapter 26).

Functional assessment

The closed kinetic chain upper extremity stability test (Goldbeck and Davies, 2000). This can be used as a functional assessment tool, especially if a preinjury baseline score has been documented for comparison. This high-level functional assessment can measure if an athlete has returned to preinjury fitness. Male patients adopt a full press-up starting position whereas as females adopt a kneeling press-up starting position. The hands are placed against markers that are spaced 36 inches apart. The patient is instructed to move one hand to touch the other and vice versa. The test measures the number of touches in a 15-s time period. The test is repeated three times and a mean score recorded. Reference scores have been reported; however, variety exists, so the test is best used against the individual patient's baseline normal scores.

Imaging

Imaging should be used to support the diagnosis based on the history and clinical presentation. Always be mindful that imaging findings are not 100% accurate and may yield false negative or false positive findings.

Plain film X-ray. Radiography of the shoulder has low radiation exposure and is a cheap, accessible form of imaging. Plain X-ray is recommended for patients with shoulder stiffness, those in significant pain and after trauma to exclude fracture, dislocation, osteoarthritis and calcific tendinitis. Plain X-ray may also show evidence of malignancy, infection or avascular necrosis. Two views in different planes are preferable over a single view.

Ultrasound scan. Ultrasound is often preferred to magnetic resonance imaging for suspected rotator cuff pathology as it has similar accuracy, is cheaper and better tolerated by patients. It may also be performed directly in the clinic. The added benefit is the ability to assess the soft tissue structures during movement to identify unusual pathologies such as long head of bicep tendon subluxation.

Computed tomography (CT). A cross-sectional imaging modality using a high dose of radiation mainly to assess bone. This is rarely used in the shoulder except following complex fractures, dislocations when a bony lesion is suspected, or in planning arthroplasty surgery.

Magnetic resonance imaging (MRI). High-resolution cross-sectional imaging is used to identify rotator cuff/bicep/pectoral tendon tears, paralabral cysts, osteoarthritis and tumours. It is, however, poorly tolerated by patients due to claustrophobia and the length of time for the scan to complete. The image quality may also be degraded by small movements or the presence of metallic implants in the area.

Magnetic resonance arthrogram (MRA). This is similar to MRI but with the addition of an injection of a liquid contrast agent into the glenohumeral joint prior to the scan. The contrast allows for clearer assessment of labral and capsule tears. This is the preferred modality for patients with instability symptoms.

Laboratory tests

Bloods and aspiration. If the patient presents with a recent onset of a severely painful, red, hot, swollen joint with systemic features of feeling unwell then a joint aspiration with microscopy, culture and sensitivity should be performed. In addition, urgent blood screening to assess for raised inflammatory markers (erythrocyte sedimentation rate and C-reactive protein) and white cell count should be undertaken. In less urgent cases where joint swelling and stiffness is present without severe pain or systemic features, an aspiration may not be required but bloods should first be screened for infection and inflammation along with routine liver function, electrolytes and possibly rheumatoid factor and anti–cyclic citrullinated

peptide (anti-CCP) antigens if inflammatory arthritis is suspected.

Neurophysiology. Peripheral nerve conduction testing and electromyography (EMG) testing of the shoulder girdle can be useful in differentiating between cervical radiculopathy and peripheral nerve lesions. In the shoulder it can be a useful test if brachial neuritis is suspected to assess which nerves are affected, or after shoulder dislocation to assess axillary nerve injury. If repeated after 3–6 months it can measure signs of recovery if clinically apparent progress is slow.

Conclusion

Accurate shoulder assessment fundamentally requires a foundation of knowledge of shoulder pathology, aetiology and epidemiology. Clinical assessment should use all available information – subjective and objective – to narrow down the wide array of possible diagnoses, ideally to one or a small number that can then be investigated further with imaging if appropriate. Reliance purely on objective clinical tests without sufficient understanding of pathology and correlation with subjective findings leads to misdiagnosis. Remember that the history is key.

References

Beaudreuil, J., Nizard, R., Thomas, T., Peyre, M., Liotard, J.P., Boileau, P., et al., 2009. Contribution of clinical tests to the diagnosis of rotator cuff disease: a systematic literature review. Joint Bone Spine 76, 15–19.

Farber, A.J., Castillo, R., Clough, M., Bahk, M., Mcfarland, E.G., 2006. Clinical assessment of three common tests for traumatic anterior shoulder instability. Journal of Bone and Joint Surgery 88, 1467–1474.

Goldbeck, T.G., Davies, G.J., 2000. Test-retest reliability of the Closed Kinetic Chain upper extemity stability test: a clinical field test. Journal of Sport Rehabilitation 9, 35–45.

Grahame, R., 2007. The need to take a fresh look at criteria for hypermobility. Journal of Rheumatology 34, 664–665.

Kibler, W.B., Sciascia, A., Thomas, S.J., 2012. Glenohumeral internal rotation deficit: pathogenesis and response to acute throwing. Sports Medicine and Arthroscopy Review 20, 34–38.

Moore, T.P., Hunter, R.E., 1996. Suprascapular nerve entrapment. Operative Techniques in Sports Medicine 4, 8–14.

Neer, C.S.,2nd, Foster, C.R., 1980. Inferior capsular shift for involuntary inferior and multidirectional instability of the shoulder. A preliminary report. Journal of Bone and Joint Surgery. American Volume 62, 897–908.

O'Brien, S.J., Pagnani, M.J., Fealy, S., Mcglynn, S.R., Wilson, J.B., 1998. The active compression test: a new and effective test for

diagnosing labral tears and acromioclavicular joint abnormality. The American Journal of Sports Medicine 26, 610–613.

O'Driscoll, S.W., Goncalves, L.B.J., Dietz, P., 2007. The hook test for distal biceps tendon avulsion. The American Journal of Sports Medicine 35, 1865–1869.

Pennock, A.T., Pennington, W.W., Torry, M.R., Decker, M.J., Vaishnav, S.B., Provencher, M.T., et al., 2011. The influence of arm and shoulder position on the bear-hug, belly-press, and lift-off tests: an electromyographic study. The American Journal of Sports Medicine 39, 2338–2346.

Seung-Ho, K., Jae-Chul, P., Jun-Sic, P., Irvin, O., 2004. Painful jerk test: a predictor of success in nonoperative treatment of posteroinferior instability of the shoulder. The American Journal of Sports Medicine 32, 1849–1855.

Taylor, S.A., Newman, A.M., Dawson, C., Gallagher, K.A., Bowers, A., Nguyen, J., et al., 2017. The "3-pack" examination is critical for comprehensive evaluation of the biceps–labrum complex and the bicipital tunnel: a prospective study. Arthroscopy 33, 28–38.

Yewlett, A., Dearden, P.M.C., Ferran, N.A., Evans, R.O., Kulkani, R., 2012. Acromioclavicular joint dislocation: diagnosis and management. Shoulder & Elbow 4, 81–86.

Chapter | **24** |

The sporting elbow

Daniel Williams, Shivan Jassim and Ali Noorani

The aim of this chapter is to present an overview of common conditions concerning the sporting elbow. Our objectives are:
- to present elbow joint anatomy, biomechanics of normal activity and throwing
- to present perspectives of acute and chronic elbow instability, tendinopathies and tendon ruptures
- to outline treatment plans for these conditions.

Introduction

The function of the elbow is to position the hand in space and act as the fulcrum for forearm activity to facilitate activities of daily living. The demands of athletes go beyond normal day-to-day function; therefore, minor limitations in range of movement or power can dramatically affect athletic performance.

The primary complaints of the elbow relate to pain, instability and stiffness. These symptoms are the result of both acute injuries and sequelae of chronic or repetitive minor trauma. Resolution of one of these symptoms may lead to a deterioration in another.

The throwing arm can be the main focus for chronic symptoms in an athlete. High strains are placed upon the elbow at the various stages of throwing, compounded by the multiple cycles that are undertaken in training and competitions. As such, careful coaching to optimize technique is vital for injury prevention and management. The best treatments for many conditions affecting the sporting elbow are still under debate. Therapy, minimally invasive treatments and surgery all have key roles in rehabilitation to regain a pain-free, stable elbow with a full range of motion.

Elbow anatomy

Osteology

The elbow joint comprises of three articulations (Fig. 24.1):
- the ulnohumeral joint, acting as a hinge for flexion and extension at the elbow
- the radiocapitellar joint, acting as a pivot for forearm pronation–supination
- the proximal radioulnar joint, also involved with forearm pronation–supination.

The ulnohumeral joint can be thought of as a uniaxial hinge except at the extremes of motion. The axis of rotation is at the centre of the arcs formed by the trochlear sulcus and the capitellum. The range of movement (ROM) is usually around 0–150 degrees of flexion/extension, although functional range for activities of daily living is less than this – approximately 30–130 degrees. The functional range for supination is 50 degrees at the radiocapitellar joint. The sports person may have and require a greater range of motion, such as hyperextension at the elbow in throwing athletes.

Ligaments

The ligaments of the elbow (Fig. 24.2) are important primary stabilizers. The medial (ulnar) collateral ligament (MCL) arises from the anteroinferior position of the medial epicondyle and inserts into the sublime tubercle of the medial coronoid. The MCL provides resistance to valgus forces through its three main components:
- anterior band (most important)
- transverse band
- posterior band, important in maximal elbow flexion.

The lateral collateral ligament (LCL) complex is composed of:

ELBOW

ELBOW

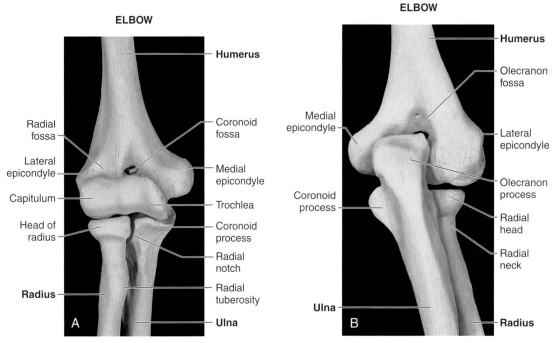

Fig. 24.1 The bones of the elbow. (A) Anterior view. (B) Posterior view.

- radial collateral ligaments (RCL)
- lateral ulnar collateral ligament (LUCL)
- accessory collateral ligament
- annular ligament, stabilizing the proximal radioulnar joint.

The LUCL is the primary stabilizer to varus and external rotation. It arises from the isometric point on the lateral epicondyle and attaches onto the supinator crest of the ulna.

Muscles

The muscles crossing the elbow joint have a role in its dynamic stability, as well as motor control of the forearm in the following ways:

- elbow extension by the triceps and, to a much lesser degree, anconeus
- elbow flexion by brachialis, brachioradialis and biceps brachii
- forearm supination by biceps brachii and supinator
- forearm pronation by pronator teres and pronator quadratus.

Biomechanics

The biomechanics of throwing have been widely studied, particularly that of baseball pitchers. Extraordinary forces are generated, making the elbow vulnerable to injury. The throw can be divided into five distinct phases:

Phase I (windup). In this preparatory phase the elbow flexes and the forearm is slightly pronated.

Phase II (cocking). The shoulder abducts and moves into maximal external rotation, the elbow flexes to between 90 degrees and 120 degrees and the forearm fully pronates.

Phase III (acceleration). A large forward-directed force in generated as the extremity moves into rapid elbow extension. Biomechanical studies demonstrate large medial shear forces, lateral compressive forces and valgus stress on the elbow. Most of the valgus stress is transmitted to the anterior bundle of the MCL. The remainder of the stress is dissipated by the secondary supporting structures namely the flexor–pronator musculature (Rossy and Oh, 2016).

Phase IV (deceleration). Eccentric contraction occurs in all muscles to slow the arm. High torque is generated during this phase, placing the shoulder and biceps at risk of injury.

Phase V (follow-through). In this final phase the forces are dissipated, and the body rebalances to stop forward motion.

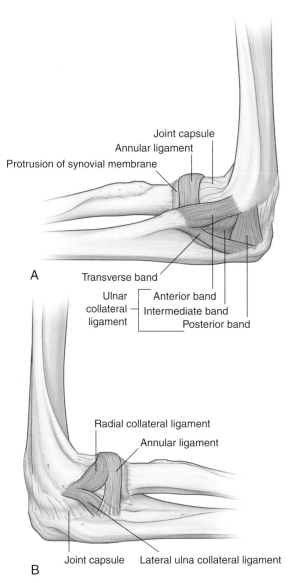

A

Joint capsule
Annular ligament
Protrusion of synovial membrane

Transverse band

Ulnar collateral ligament
Anterior band
Intermediate band
Posterior band

Radial collateral ligament
Annular ligament

B

Joint capsule   Lateral ulna collateral ligament

Fig. 24.2 Medial (A) and lateral (B) aspects of the left elbow showing the joint capsule and the radial and ulnar collateral ligaments.

Elbow instability

Elbow stability is vital for good, pain-free elbow function. Stability relies upon the relationship between the static stabilizers of the joint articulations and capsuloligamentous structures. Dynamic stability is conferred by the muscles crossing the joint. Instability follows fairly well-defined patterns and can be a result of a traumatic injury or secondary to chronic overuse syndromes.

In 2001, O'Driscoll et al. proposed the 'fortress of elbow stability', outlining primary and secondary stabilizers of the elbow (O'Driscoll et al., 2001). The primary stabilizers are the ulna humeral joint, preventing posterior translation of the ulna, the anterior band of the MCL, resisting valgus stress, and the LUCL, resisting external rotation and varus stress. The secondary stabilizers are radiohumeral joint and the common flexor and extensor origins. This system is commonly used today. However, it is worth acknowledging other structures important for stability, most notably the anterior capsule, and the dynamic stabilizers, notably biceps brachii, brachialis and triceps.

Acute instability

The elbow is the second most frequently dislocated joint. A simple elbow dislocation is defined as a dislocation where there are no concomitant fractures apart from small periarticular avulsions of 1 or 2 mm (Josefsson et al., 1984). It is not within the remit of this chapter to discuss more complex fracture dislocations. Most dislocations are posterior or posterolateral (Fig. 24.3). It has long been proposed that the mechanism of dislocation is valgus and external rotation. With the forearm fixed, this posterolateral rotation results in progressive subluxation and dislocation of the radial head (Osborne and Cotterill, 1966, O'Driscoll et al., 1992), resulting in a lateral-to-medial soft tissue injury described by O'Driscoll as the 'Horii circle' (O'Driscoll, 1999). More recent video analysis of recorded elbow dislocations suggests a mechanism of hyperphysiologic valgus in an extended elbow (Schreiber et al., 2013). This would result in the reverse pattern of injury starting with the anterior capsules and anterior band of the MCL and progressing laterally. This pattern of injury has been supported by magnetic resonance imaging (MRI) studies, which seem to suggest the medial structures are injured more commonly than the lateral structures – the latter being never injured in isolation (Rhyou and Kim, 2012; Schreiber et al., 2014). With this in mind, Robinson et al. (2017) proposed a ladder of instability starting with the medial ligament complex and progressing to the common flexor origin, anterior capsule, lateral ligament complex and finally the common extensor origin.

Investigation, immobilization and treatment algorithms vary considerably between surgeons and units. The risk of requiring surgery for recurrent instability following conservatively managed simple dislocations is 2.3% (Modi et al., 2015). As previously mentioned, MRI scans show ligamentous injuries in all patients (Schreiber et al., 2014), thus the risk of overtreatment following MRI is significant. The authors wonder if the same is true following examination under anaesthesia (EUA). In fact, Josefsson et al. (1987)

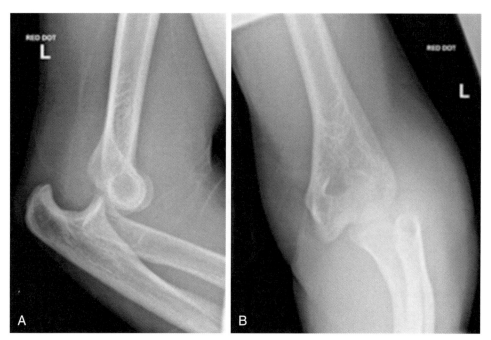

Fig. 24.3 Radiograph demonstrating a simple a posterolateral elbow dislocation. (A) Lateral radiograph. (B) Anteroposterior radiograph.

performed a randomized controlled trial (RCT) comparing operative and nonoperative management of 30 patients with acute dislocations. All patients underwent an EUA before randomization. Under anaesthetic, all the patients were found to have medial instability and 16 of the 30 had both medial and lateral instability. All patients at surgery had rupture or avulsion of both medial and lateral ligaments. However, the results showed no difference in outcome in terms of range of motion or recurrent instability at 1 year between those who underwent surgery versus conservative management.

An RCT of 100 patients comparing immobilization in a long arm cast for 3 weeks with early mobilization (within 2 days) show no difference in range of motion, outcome scores, heterotrophic ossification or recurrent instability after the first 6 weeks. However, in the first 6 weeks, patients in the early mobilization group performed better in all of these metrics (Iordens et al., 2015).

The senior author prefers an early mobilization and uses an overhead rehabilitation protocol. The patient begins early elbow range of motion (within a week) in a supine position with the shoulder flexed to 90 degrees. Controlled flexion and extension is performed with the hand and forearm held above the head with the forearm in pronation. This approach minimizes the effects of gravity and the angular forces. Forearm rotation is normally held in neutral when resting but can be adjusted in specific injury patterns.

For example, pronation stabilizes the LCL-deficient elbow and supination stabilizes a MCL-deficient elbow.

Although surgery for recurrent instability is rare following a simple elbow dislocation, the condition is not benign. In a study of 110 simple elbow dislocations at a mean of 88 months post injury, 8% of patients complained of subjective instability, 56% stiffness and 62% pain. Nineteen percent of the athletes in the cohort had to give up their sport or modify their technique (Anakwe et al., 2011).

Chronic instability
Posterolateral rotatory instability

Posterolateral rotatory instability (PLRI) is the most common form of symptomatic chronic elbow instability. It occurs because of failure in the LUCL. Disruption of the LUCL causes abnormal external rotation of the radius and ulna in relation to the distal humerus. This results in posterior displacement of the radial head relative to the capitellum. Most commonly this occurs following trauma but can be secondary to an iatrogenic insult such as arthroscopy, release of the lateral epicondyle or following steroid injections. With lateral elbow pain, locking and catching being the predominant presenting complaint, it is often initially misdiagnosed as tennis elbow, radial tunnel syndrome or radiocapitellar arthritis.

PLRI is a clinical diagnosis and can be easily missed if not suspected. A careful history and detailed examination is key. As described, the posterolateral subluxation of the radial head classically occurs when an axial load is applied to an arm positioned in supination and valgus such as pushing up from a wide-armed chair. The clinical examination and provocation tests are designed to simulate this position. Specific examinations for a patient with possible PLRI include the lateral pivot shift test (Fig. 24.4), the posterolateral draw test, the table-top relocation test, the chair sign and pain and instability in performing an active floor push-up.

Plain radiographs and MRI are useful in excluding other diagnoses such as radiocapitella joint arthritis and lateral epicondylitis but has little value confirming injury or damage to the LUCL. O'Driscoll et al. (1992) classified PLRI into distinct stages from 1 to 3 based on the degree of subluxation/dislocation and soft tissue injury. Fig. 24.5 is a

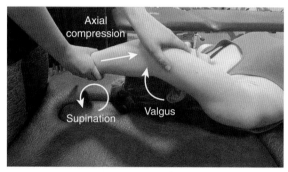

Fig. 24.4 The lateral pivot shift test. In a supine patient with the forearm hypersupinated, a valgus stress is applied along with axial load. The elbow starts in full extension and is slowly flexed. Instability usually occurs around 30–45 degrees.

radiograph of a patient with a grade 2 PLRI and a perched posterolateral dislocation.

Although activity modification and physiotherapy working on the dynamic elbow stabilizers can help, surgery is frequently indicated in patients with persistent, symptomatic instability. In this situation surgery is important, not only for symptomatic relief but also to prevent the arthritic change, which can occur rapidly in the unstable elbow. The avascular and hypocellular physiology of ligamentous tissue mean that direct repair is seldom indicated in chronic instability. The aim of surgery is therefore to secure a robust, stable and durable graft from the isometric point on the lateral epicondyle to supinator crest. Multiple autografts, allografts and synthetic ligaments have been used and secured in different ways. All of the series are too small and heterogeneous to make comment on the best possible technique.

Despite this, results of reconstruction are very good. A review by Anakwenze et al. (2014) found that 91% of patients had a good to excellent outcome following surgery with a range of motion from approximately 5 to 135 degrees. They reported an 11% complication rate and 8% rate of recurrence. Other studies have reported the rate of recurrent instability to be as high as 25% (Jones et al., 2012). Reuter et al. (2016) performed a retrospective review of seven studies containing 148 patients who had repair or reconstruction for PLRI. They found that there was no consensus on postoperative immobilization or rehabilitation. Most of the cases had a postoperative limit on extension set to 30 degrees, but this varied from between 1 day and 6 weeks. Overall, patients in their series regained high acceptable results following reconstruction.

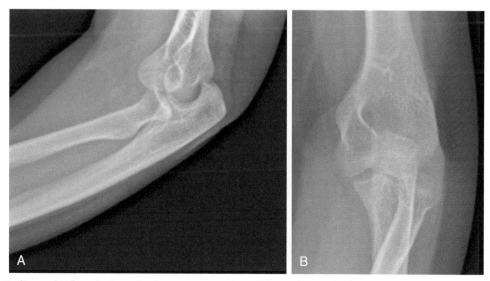

Fig. 24.5 Radiograph of grade 2 posterolateral rotatory instability and a perched posterolateral dislocation. (A) Lateral radiograph. (B) Anteroposterior radiograph.

Valgus instability

The anterior band of the MCL is the primary static restraint to valgus stress. The anterior band extends in a fan-like manner from the anteroinferior ridge of the medial epicondyle to its attachment on the sublime tubercle on the medial ulna. Injury can follow acute trauma, be secondary to repetitive valgus stress (microtrauama) or be iatrogenic, usually as a result of excessive release from the ulna.

Overhead athletes such as baseball pitchers and javelin throwers are not only most susceptible to this injury but also most likely to become symptomatic. Such athletes will often complain of medial elbow pain, and also loss of velocity or accuracy in throwing. Symptoms usually resolve with rest and activity modification. Chronic valgus extension overload can lead to posteromedial olecranon impingement, radiocapitellar compression and ulna nerve symptoms at the elbow.

In chronic cases there can be very little to see on examination. There may be tenderness of the MCL and a loss of extension secondary to medial olecranon spurring. Care should be taken to evaluate the ulna nerve function and stability. Valgus stability should be tested throughout the range of motion, but is most sensitive at 20–30 degrees. Specific tests for valgus instability include the milking manoeuvre and the moving valgus stress test.

Plain radiographs should be taken and, although these are usually unremarkable, they may reveal degenerative changes in chronic cases, particularly medial olecranon osteophytes. Stress radiographs show gapping or side-to-side asymmetry. Magnetic resonance arthrogram is the gold standard and can reveal partial-thickness or under-surface tears.

Chronic medial instability is uncommon in those who do not participate in overhead throwing sports. Conservative treatments should be attempted in most cases and these include a period of rest followed by flexor pronator strengthening and the development of a better throwing technique. Rettig et al. (2001) found that conservative treatment allowed only 42% of athletes to return to their previous level of sport and this took on average nearly 6 months. They found no way of predicting which patients would do well with nonoperative management (Rettig et al., 2001). This has led to an increase surgery for valgus instability. Multiple techniques, grafts and methods of fixation have been described. In 1974 successful reconstruction of the medial ulna collateral ligament on Tommy John, a Major League Baseball pitcher, was performed. Reconstruction of the MCL is still commonly referred to as the 'Tommy John procedure'. The technique was published in 1986 (Jobe et al., 1986) and involved a free tendon graft weaved in a figure of eight through bone tunnels in the ulna and medial epicondyle. This technique has been adapted and new docking techniques have led to a higher return to sport

and lower complication rates (Watson et al., 2014a). In this review of 1368 patients the overall complication rate was 12.9 %, most commonly an ulna nerve neuropraxia and the return to play rate was 78.9%.

Lateral epicondylitis

Lateral epicondylitis (LE) is an overuse injury that occurs as a consequence of overload at the common extensor origin, specifically the extensor carpi radialis brevis (ECRB). It most often affects the dominant arm and is more frequently seen in those performing prolonged and rapid activities such as typing, manual work and piano playing. Up to 50% of tennis players develop lateral epicondylitis during their careers and this has led to the condition commonly being referred to as 'tennis elbow'. The recurrent eccentric wrist extension and forearm pronation, especially during the backhand stroke, is thought to be responsible. This is exacerbated by poor technique, a heavy racquet and suboptimal grip size.

Despite the common belief, LE is not an inflammatory condition, Cook and Purdam (2009) proposed a continuum model, incorporating clinical, histological and imaging information. They describe a process of repeated microtrauma, tendon disrepair and finally degeneration. Microscopically, the appearance at the insertion site is that of angiofibroblastic hyperplasia and disorganized collagen, with an absence of inflammatory cells, i.e., a degenerative process rather than an inflammatory one.

The athlete will present with lateral elbow pain around the bony prominence which radiates down the forearm. This is usually associated and exacerbated by gripping and a repetitive contraction of the wrist extensors. Patients often complain of a subjective reduction in grip strength.

Examination reveals tenderness at the origin of ECRB in (or just distal to) the lateral epicondyle. There are a number of provocation tests to aid diagnosis, all aimed at stimulating pain at the lateral epicondyle. They involve resisted wrist extension (Cozens test; Fig. 24.6) or finger (primarily middle finger) extension (Maudsley test; Fig. 24.7). In addition, patients that have had previous treatment with injections of corticosteroid to the site may exhibit signs of lipoatrophy, such as depigmentation or thinning of skin around the lateral epicondyle.

Diagnosis is primarily clinical, based on the history and examination. Investigations can be useful to exclude other causes of lateral epicondyle pain. Common differential diagnoses include cervical radiculopathy, degenerative changes or radial tunnel syndrome, a compression neuropathy of the posterior interosseous nerve.

Plain radiographs are usually unremarkable, although occasionally reveal minor calcification in the common

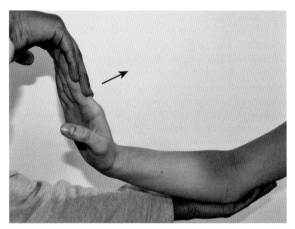

Fig. 24.6 The Cozens test. Stabilize the elbow in 90 degrees of flexion with one hand whilst palpating the lateral epicondyle. Position the patient's hand in radial deviation, forearm pronation and full wrist extension. The patient is asked to hold this position against manual flexion force applied to the hand and wrist providing resisted wrist extension. The test is considered positive if it produces pain in the area of the lateral epicondyle.

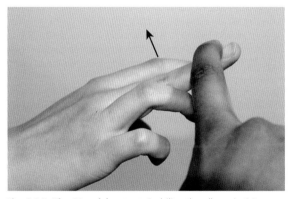

Fig. 24.7 The Maudsley test. Stabilize the elbow in 90 degrees of flexion with the wrist in neutral extension and palm parallel to the ground. Whilst palpating the lateral epicondyle ask to the patient to extend the middle finger against your counterforce. A positive test is indicated by pain over the lateral epicondyle.

extensor origin; they are useful to exclude radiocapitellar arthritis. Ultrasound can be useful in the hands of an experienced operator and can nicely demonstrate a thickened hypoechoic ECRB tendon. In addition, Doppler phases can detect neovascularization. MRI can demonstrate thickening or a tear of the ECRB origin with increased signal intensity on T2-weighted sequences. MRI may also identify an under-surface tear of the lateral collateral ligament. The senior author feels that when present, this results in

microinstability and a subsequent increase in the strain on common extensor origin (secondary stabilizer). This may contribute to refractory tennis elbow.

LE is usually self-limiting and resolves in 12–18 months. The aim of treatment is to control pain, preserve function and prevent deterioration whilst allowing the athlete to return to normal function. LE is a condition that tends to respond favourably to nonoperative methods. Consequently injections and surgery should be reserved for recalcitrant cases.

Resting and avoiding the aggravating behaviour can lead to symptom resolution, although in the elite athlete this is not a favourable strategy. Therefore, in addition to correction of technique, a number of therapies exist for the treatment of LE:

Physiotherapy

Physiotherapy is the mainstay of treatment for LE. Regimes are targeted at maintaining elbow range of movement in addition to eccentric strengthening of the common extensors. This has shown to be superior to rest alone, although no single regime has been demonstrated to be superior to another. In addition, stabilization of the scapula by recruiting the periscapular muscles is vital for elbow rehabilitation. Physiotherapy combining elbow manipulation and exercise has a superior benefit to 'wait and see' in the first 12 weeks. This benefit is no longer apparent by 26 weeks, both are superior to steroid injections (Bisset et al., 2006).

Antiinflammatory agents

Nonsteroidal antiinflammatory drugs and analgesia can help manage symptoms and enable therapy in the initial phase of the disease process. Steroid injections have been well studied in LE. The action of steroids is predominantly antiinflammatory and therefore their mechanism of action is poorly understood. There is now good evidence that steroid injections, despite providing good short-term pain relief, are detrimental in the medium and long term for pain, grip strength, symptom severity and duration compared to no treatment (Coombes et al., 2010; Olaussen et al., 2013). Despite this high-level evidence, there has been no impact on the widespread use of steroids to treat this condition (Fujihara et al., 2018).

Bracing

Counterforce braces broaden the area of applied stress on the ECRB muscle and reduce tension in the common extensor origin. Although the biggest biomechanical change in load on the ECRB tendon occurs when braces are placed over the muscle belly, the best clinical results occur when placed just distal to the epicondyle. They have been used with beneficial effect to reduce symptoms and have been shown to be better than wrist splintage. In fact, with immediate effect they can improve pain-free grip strength (Sadeghi-Demneh and Jafarian, 2013). Their effect in the intermediate and long term is less clear despite good tolerance and low risk profile.

Biological treatments

Numerous biological treatments are available and are being investigated for the treatment of LE, most notably platelet-rich plasma (PRP). Variation in the preparation, activation and control groups in randomized controlled trials (RCTs) have made it difficult to draw conclusions as to its efficacy in comparison with more traditional treatments. Multiple RCTs have shown efficacy of PRP over steroid injections, which we now know to be detrimental in tendinopathy (Lebiedziński et al., 2015; Peerbooms et al., 2010). Peerbooms et al. (2010) showed a 73% success rate at 52 weeks compared with 51% for steroid injections. PRP has also been shown to be superior to local anaesthetic injection at 8 weeks (Mishra and Pavelko, 2006). The evidence is however conflicting, with some studies showing no significant difference (de Vos et al., 2014). In the shoulder, biopsies of tendinopathic rotator cuff tendons following PRP have shown altered tissue characteristics including reduced cellularity, vascularity and increased levels of apoptosis (Carr et al., 2015). Although this had no deleterious clinical effects, for the first time the safety of PRP has been brought into question.

Other nonsurgical treatments have been described such as nitrate patches, radiofrequency thermal ablation, extracorporeal shockwave therapy, laser therapy and acupuncture. Whilst each of these modalities has some low-level evidence to support them, their role in the treatment algorithms of LE remains unclear. The existing literature does not provide conclusive evidence that there is one preferred method of nonsurgical treatment for this condition (Sims et al., 2014). Lateral epicondylitis is a condition that is usually self-limited in 95% of patients, resolving over a 12- to 18-month period. In fact, there is a paucity of evidence that in the long term any nonsurgical intervention is better than observation alone (Sayegh and Strauch, 2015).

Surgical treatment

A number of surgical techniques exist, all of which aim to debride and resect tendinopathic tissue from the ECRB tendon and decorticate the lateral epicondyle. All of the techniques, be it open, percutaneous or arthroscopic, can be performed as day case procedures and allow early rehabilitation.

Within each procedure, some variations of technique exist, such as whether or not to close the ECRB tendon or reattach the tendon to the common extensor origin. Arthroscopic techniques have the advantage of examining the rest of the elbow for alternative pathologies but arguably have longer surgical times and greater risks compared to open techniques. There are no studies that have demonstrated a clear advantage of one technique over another, including variations within open surgery. High satisfaction rates have been reported with each technique. Complications of surgery include infection, heterotopic ossification, nerve injury and iatrogenic LUCL injury.

Although limited by a small sample size, a study comparing sham surgery with a debridement of the diseased portion of the tendon, showed no differences in the outcome at 6 months and 2.5 years. Both groups showed significant improvement in symptoms (Kroslak and Murrell, 2018).

It is the senior author's opinion that surgery should be reserved for recalcitrant LE that has undergone a prolonged period of nonoperative management. MRI should be undertaken in secondary care to exclude a tear in the common extensor origin or LCL. In recalcitrant cases with no tear, it is also worth considering PRP prior to surgery as, despite the lack of consensus in the literature, it is minimally invasive and there is evidence that 89% of patients have improved pain and 82% return to work. Only 7% of patients in this series converted to surgical treatment (Ford et al., 2015). The senior author's algorithm for treating LE is shown in Fig. 24.8. We recommend referral to secondary care after failure of conservative treatment for 3 months. At this point 70% of patients have improved following physiotherapy (Olaussen et al., 2013). Although this rises to nearly 90% at 6 months, in order to avoid missing a more serious diagnosis and given the detrimental impact on patient quality of life, we believe that 3 months is reasonable.

Medial epicondylitis

Medial epicondylitis (ME) has many similar features to LE in that it is an overuse injury that affects the common flexor/pronator mass origin leading to degenerative tendinosis. It is associated with sports that have a repetitive forearm pronation and wrist flexion. It is less common than LE, harder to treat and has a less extensive evidence base for treatment.

Frequently ME is referred to as 'golfer's elbow', but is also prevalent in weightlifters, baseball pitchers, rowers and cricket bowlers, all of whom undergo repetitive wrist flexion/forearm pronation. In addition, ME may develop as a secondary response to a single large valgus force across

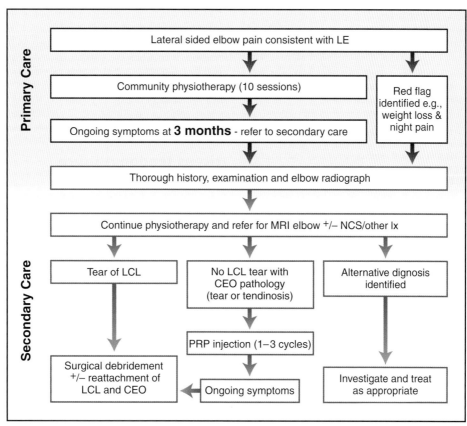

Fig. 24.8 Algorithm for the treatment of lateral epicondylitis. *CEO*, Common extensor origin; *Ix*, investigations; *LCL*, lateral collateral ligament; *LE*, lateral epicondylitis; *NCS*, nerve conduction studies; *PRP*, platelet-rich plasma.

the elbow often causing an avulsion of the common flexor pronator origin.

Tears were originally thought to predominantly affect the pronator teres and flexor carpi radialis tendon origins; however, more recent studies show that all muscles of the common flexor origin (with the exception of palmaris longus) are affected. Microscopically it is indistinguishable to LE, showing angiofibroblastic tendinosis.

Patients present with pain located at the medial epicondyle, worse with gripping. There is tenderness over the distal medial epicondyle and pain with resisted forearm pronation/wrist flexion. ME commonly coexists with an ulna neuritis and this is thought to be a consequence of traction, entrapment and compression. Careful examination to look for signs of valgus instability (MCL insufficiency) and ulnar nerve compression/neuropathy should be performed in order to avoid misdiagnosis.

As with LE, plain radiographs and MRI may show intra-tendinous calcification or traction spurs and can be useful in excluding alternative diagnoses, such as MCL tears or osteochondral injuries that may mimic ME.

The treatment modalities described for LE are all appropriate in the treatment of ME. However, as with LE the evidence base does not demonstrate superiority of one technique over another and in many cases only short-term benefits are demonstrated. In terms of surgical intervention, excision of pathological tissue at the common flexor origin is the main aim of treatment, with options for performing cubital tunnel release in cases of ulnar nerve compression. The complication profile includes injury to the ulnar or medial antebrachial cutaneous nerves and inadvertent release of the origin of the MCL. Results of surgery are, once again, good to excellent in around 90% of patients. Poorer outcomes are associated with ulnar nerve symptoms (Gabel and Morrey, 1995).

Tendon ruptures/avulsions

Distal biceps tendon rupture

Distal biceps tendon ruptures classically occur in middle-aged men, with only a few reports in the literature of distal biceps ruptures occurring in female patients. The classic history is of a significant extension force applied to the flexed elbow followed by an eccentric biceps contraction and a tearing sensation in the region of the antecubital fossa. The patient will often describe a 'pop' or giving way. The tear can occur as a result of an acute tear or in conjunction with chronic, often asymptomatic, degeneration.

The pathology of tendon rupture is not well understood and tends to occur at the insertion on the radial tuberosity. This may be due to the relative hypovascular nature of this area. It is also believed that mechanical impingement may lead to attrition when the forearm is pronated and the space between the ulna and the radial tuberosity is significantly reduced.

The clinical story and picture can make the diagnosis clear. Patients will often have significant anticubital fossa (ACF) echimosis, abnormal muscle contour with pain and weakness on supination and flexion. O'Driscoll et al. (2007) described the hook test for distal biceps ruptures that has a sensitivity and specificity of 100%, better than MRI. With the elbow held at 90 degrees of flexion, the forearm is supinated and the shoulder abducted to 90 degrees and internally rotated, the examiner can then hook the tip of his/her thumb around the lateral edge of biceps tendon in the ACF if the distal biceps is not ruptured.

Patients may have a partial tear or the examination may be confused by the presence of intact lacertus fibrosus. These patients should undergo further investigation. Plain radiographs are usually normal as the tendon rarely avulses off the tuberosity. The imaging modality of choice is MRI. The elbow should be scanned in the so-called FABS position (flexed elbow, abducted shoulder, forearm supinated). This creates tension in the tendon and minimizes its obliquity and rotation, resulting in a 'true' longitudinal view of the tendon (Chew and Giuffrè, 2005).

Although a nonoperative approach can be taken, a complete rupture is estimated to result in a 40% reduction in supination power and 30% flexion power. This is unacceptable to most athletes (Morrey et al., 1985).

Surgical technique to repair the tendon largely involves anatomical repair to the radial tuberosity. Controversy still exists regarding whether to use a one- or two-incision technique; the former is associated with higher rates of nerve injury and the latter with higher rates of heterotopic ossification. In addition, the use of different fixation techniques is the subject of much debate in orthopaedic literature. Options including fixation with suture anchors, bone tunnels, interference screws or suspensory cortical buttons have all had their methods described. Watson et al. (2014b) performed a review of fixation methods and techniques. They noted that the complication rate did not differ significantly between a one- and a two-incision approach. They found that the use of a bone tunnel and a cortical button had significantly lower complication rates compared with other fixation methods.

Ideally repairs are performed early before there is significant retraction, adhesion and degeneration of the tendon. However, good results have been obtained with delayed presentation. Even when the tension created by the contracted distal biceps tendon is high it may be reliably reattached to the anatomic insertion with up to 90 degrees of elbow flexion with excellent outcomes (Morrey et al., 2014). With progressively stronger fixation methods, rehabilitation protocols postoperatively can utilize earlier range of motion activities.

Triceps tendon rupture

Injury to the distal triceps is less common than the distal biceps, although the patient demographic and associated risk factors are similar. The mechanism of rupture is usually a forceful eccentric muscle contraction against a large load. Tears tend to occur at the triceps insertion onto the olecranon head rather than at the musculotendinous junction.

Patients complain of a painful pop at the elbow. They usually have full passive range of motion with an obvious extensor lag. Triceps power must be tested against gravity to avoid underestimating the degree of injury. Plain radiographs should be taken as they may show an avulsion fracture of the olecranon tip. MRI can occasionally be helpful if there is any diagnostic uncertainty and can pick up incomplete rupture.

Once again, nonoperative treatment has no role in the athlete, owing to reduced strength in elbow extension. Elbow immobilization is poorly tolerated and early surgical fixation should aim to be robust enough to allow early movement. Surgical repair is usually performed through a single, open posterior incision and may utilize suture anchors, bone tunnels or a combination.

Rehabilitation is aimed at allowing early passive motion and avoiding active elbow extension against gravity during the early phase of healing.

Key messages

- The elbow joint in the athlete can be affected by pain, stiffness and instability.
- The aim of all nonoperative and operative treatments is to permit early range of motion. Immobilization in plaster casts should be avoided.
- Tendinopathies around the elbow are common and usually self-limiting. There is much controversy regarding the best treatment. Early surgery should be avoided where possible.
- Instability can follow acute trauma or chronic attenuation. Meticulous work-up is required for accurate diagnosis and treatment planning.
- Nonoperative treatment has no role in acute tendon ruptures around the elbow in the athlete.

References

Anakwe, R.E., Middleton, S.D., Jenkins, P.J., McQueen, M.M., Court-Brown, C.M., 2011. Patient-reported outcomes after simple dislocation of the elbow. The Journal of Bone and Joint Surgery. American Volume 93 (13), 1220–1226.

Anakwenze, O.A., Kwon, D., O'Donnell, E., Levine, W.N., Ahmad, C.S., 2014. Surgical treatment of posterolateral rotatory instability of the elbow. Arthroscopy 30 (7), 866–871.

Bisset, L., Beller, E., Jull, G., Brooks, P., Darnell, R., Vicenzino, B., 2006. Mobilisation with movement and exercise, corticosteroid injection, or wait and see for tennis elbow: randomised trial. British Medical Journal 333, 939.

Carr, A.J., Murphy, R., Dakin, S.G., Rombach, I., Wheway, K., Watkins, B., et al., 2015. Platelet-rich plasma injection with arthroscopic Acromioplasty for chronic rotator cuff tendinopathy: a randomized controlled trial. The American Journal of Sports Medicine 43 (12), 2891–2897.

Chew, M.L., Giuffrè, B.M., 2005. Disorders of the distal biceps brachii tendon. RadioGraphics 25 (5), 1227–1237.

Cook, J.L., Purdam, C.R., 2009. Is tendon pathology a continuum? A pathology model to explain the clinical presentation of load-induced tendinopathy. British Journal of Sports Medicine 43, 409–416.

Coombes, B.K., Bisset, L., Vicenzino, B., 2010. Efficacy and safety of corticosteroid injections and other injections for management of tendinopathy: a systematic review of randomised controlled trials. Lancet 376, 1751–1767.

de Vos, R.J., Windt, J., Weir, A., 2014. Strong evidence against platelet-rich plasma injections for chronic lateral epicondylar tendinopathy: a systematic review. British Journal of Sports Medicine 48 (12), 952–956.

Ford, R.D., Schmitt, W.P., Lineberry, K., Luce, P., 2015. A retrospective comparison of the management of recalcitrant lateral elbow tendinosis: platelet-rich plasma injections versus surgery. Hand 10 (2), 285–291.

Fujihara, Y., Huetteman, H.E., Chung, T.T., Shauver, M.J., Chung, K.C., 2018. The effect of impactful articles on clinical practice in the United States: corticosteroid injection for patients with lateral epicondylitis. Plastic and Reconstructive Surgery 141 (5), 1183–1191.

Gabel, G.T., Morrey, B.F., 1995. Operative treatment of medial epicondylitis. Influence of concomitant ulnar neuropathy at the elbow. The Journal of Bone and Joint Surgery. American Volume 77 (7), 1065–1069.

Iordens, G.I., Van Lieshout, E.M., Schep, N.W., et al., 2015. Early mobilisation versus plaster immobilisation of simple elbow dislocations: results of the FuncSiE multicentre randomized clinical trial. British Journal of Sports Medicine 51 (6), 531–538.

Jobe, F.W., Stark, H., Lombardo, S.J., 1986. Reconstruction of the ulnar collateral ligament in athletes. The Journal of Bone and Joint Surgery. American Volume 68-A, 1158–1163.

Jones, K.J., Dodson, C.C., Osbahr, D.C., Parisien, R.L., Weiland, A.J., Altchek, D.W., et al., 2012. The docking technique for lateral ulnar collateral ligament reconstruction: surgical technique and clinical outcomes. Journal of Shoulder and Elbow Surgery 21 (3), 389–395.

Josefsson, P.O., Gentz, C.F., Johnell, O., Wendeberg, B., 1987. Surgical versus non-surgical treatment of ligamentous injuries

following dislocation of the elbow joint. A prospective randomized study. The Journal of Bone and Joint Surgery. American Volume 69, 605–608.

Josefsson, P.O., Johnell, O., Gentz, C.F., 1984. Long-term sequelae of simple dislocation of the elbow. The Journal of Bone and Joint Surgery. American Volume 66, 927–930.

Kroslak, M., Murrell, G.A.C., 2018. Surgical treatment of lateral epicondylitis: a prospective, randomized, double-blinded, placebo-controlled clinical trial. The American Journal of Sports Medicine 46 (5), 1106–1113.

Lebiedziński, R., Synder, M., Buchcic, P., Polguj, M., Grzegorzewski, A., Sibiński, M., 2015. A randomized study of autologous conditioned plasma and steroid injections in the treatment of lateral epicondylitis. International Orthopaedics 39 (11), 2199–2203.

Mishra, A., Pavelko, T., 2006. Treatment of chronic elbow tendinosis with buffered platelet-rich plasma. The American Journal of Sports Medicine 34 (11), 1774–1778.

Modi, C.S., Wasserstein, D., Mayne, I.P., Henry, P.D., Mahomed, N., Veillette, C.J., 2015. The frequency and risk factors for subsequent surgery after a simple elbow dislocation. Injury 46, 1156–1160.

Morrey, B.F., Askew, L.J., An, K.N., Dobyns, J.H., 1985. Rupture of the distal tendon of the biceps brachii. A biomechanical study. The Journal of Bone and Joint Surgery. American Volume 67 (3), 418–421.

Morrey, M.E., Abdel, M.P., Sanchez-Sotelo, J., Morrey, B.F., 2014. Primary repair of retracted distal biceps tendon ruptures in extreme flexion. Journal of Shoulder and Elbow Surgery 23 (5), 679–685.

O'Driscoll, S.W., Goncalves, L.B., Dietz, P., 2007. The hook test for distal biceps tendon avulsion. The American Journal of Sports Medicine 35 (11), 1865–1869.

O'Driscoll, S.W., Morrey, B.F., Korinek, S., An, K.N., 1992. Elbow subluxation and dislocation. A spectrum of instability. Clinical Orthopaedics and Related Research 280, 186–197.

O'Driscoll, S.W., 1999. Elbow instability. Acta Orthopaedica Belgica 65 (4), 404–415.

O'Driscoll, S.W., Jupiter, J.B., King, G.J., Hotchkiss, R.N., Morrey, B.F., 2001. The unstable elbow. Instructional Course Lectures 50, 89–102.

Olaussen, M., Holmedal, O., Lindbaek, M., Brage, S., Solvang, H., 2013. Treating lateral epicondylitis with corticosteroid injections or non-electrotherapeutical physiotherapy: a systematic review. British Medical Journal Open 3,e003564.

Osborne, G., Cotterill, P., 1966. Recurrent dislocation of the elbow. The Journal of Bone and Joint Surgery. American Volume 48, 340–346.

Peerbooms, J.C., Sluimer, J., Bruijn, D.J., Gosens, T., 2010. Positive effect of an autologous platelet concentrate in lateral epicondylitis in a double-blind randomized controlled trial: platelet-rich plasma versus corticosteroid injection with a 1-year follow-up. The American Journal of Sports Medicine 38 (2), 255–262.

Rettig, A.C., Sherrill, C., Snead, D.S., Mendler, J.C., Mieling, P., 2001. Nonoperative treatment of ulnar collateral ligament injuries in throwing athletes. The American Journal of Sports Medicine 29, 15–17.

Reuter, S., Proier, P., Imhoff, A., Lenich, A., 2016. Rehabilitation, clinical outcome and return to sporting activities after postero-lateral elbow instability: a systematic review. European Journal of Physical and Rehabilitation Medicine.

Rhyou, I.H., Kim, Y.S., 2012. New mechanism of the posterior elbow dislocation. Knee Surgery, Sports Traumatology, Arthroscopy 20 (12), 2535–2541.

Robinson, P.M., Griffiths, E., Watts, A.C., 2017. Simple elbow dislocation. Shoulder & Elbow 9 (3), 195–204.

Rossy, W.H., Oh, L.S., 2016. Pitcher's elbow: medial elbow pain in the overhead-throwing athlete. Current Reviews in Musculo-skeletal Medicine 9 (2), 207–214.

Sadeghi-Demneh, E., Jafarian, F., 2013. The immediate effects of orthoses on pain in people with lateral epicondylalgia. Pain Research and Treatment 2013, 353597.

Sayegh, E.T., Strauch, R.J., 2015. Does nonsurgical treatment improve longitudinal outcomes of lateral epicondylitis over no treatment? A meta-analysis. Clinical Orthopaedics and Related Research 473 (3), 1093–1107.

Schreiber, J.J., Potter, H.G., Warren, R.F., Hotchkiss, R.N., Daluiski, A., 2014. Magnetic resonance imaging findings in acute elbow dislocation: insight into mechanism. The Journal of Hand Surgery 39, 199–205.

Schreiber, J.J., Warren, R.F., Hotchkiss, R.N., Daluiski, A., 2013. An online video investigation into the mechanism of elbow dislocation. The Journal of Hand Surgery 38, 488–494.

Sims, S.E., Miller, K., Elfar, J.C., Hammert, W.C., 2014. Non-surgical treatment of lateral epicondylitis: a systematic review of randomized controlled trials. Hand (N Y) 9 (4), 419–446.

Watson, J.N., McQueen, P., Hutchinson, M.R., 2014a. A systematic review of ulnar collateral ligament reconstruction techniques. The American Journal of Sports Medicine 42 (10), 2510–2516.

Watson, J.N., Moretti, V.M., Schwindel, L., Hutchinson, M.R., 2014b. Repair techniques for acute distal biceps tendon ruptures: a systematic review. The Journal of Bone and Joint Surgery. American Volume 96 (24), 2086–2090.

Chapter | 25 |

Hand and wrist injuries: a focus on boxing

Ian Gatt

Introduction

The hand and wrist are the commonest sites of injury in boxing. The author has been working with the national GB squad over the last three Olympic cycles: London 2012, Rio 2016, and is currently planning for Tokyo 2020. After investing a considerable amount of time in understanding the main injuries occurring in this sport, several assessment approaches, therapeutic techniques and preventative strategies have been implemented through trial and error. Auditing indicates injury incidence in these areas has decreased, whilst overall training availability has increased. This chapter will provide an insight into the main injuries occurring at the hand and wrist in this sport.

To understand injuries occurring at the hand and wrist in boxing it is useful to appreciate a few technical aspects. Boxers can either adopt an *orthodox stance* (leading with left arm and left leg) or a *southpaw stance* (leading with right arm and right leg); on occasion you will also encounter *switchers*, who alternate between stances during a contest. An appreciation of diverse stances and dominance can impact on injury management. Linked with stance are the types of shots thrown in a contest. These are mainly divided into either straight or bent arm shots. The lead hand is predominately used for:

- *jabs* (straight arm shot)
- *hooks* (bent arm shots going from outward to inwards)
- *upper cuts* (bent arm shot going from downwards to up-wards).

The rear hand is used predominately for:

- *cross* (straight shot)
- *upper cuts.*

Hooks are not commonly thrown with the back hand due to its greater distance from the opponent when compared to the lead hand. Hooks, using the back hand, can however be used during *in-fighting* (i.e., when both boxers are in proximity).

During any contest, boxers can throw either of these shots depending on the tactics. Boxers can either throw single shots or multiple shots during any given phase of attack.

As with any sport, understanding the forces that are generated, and in turn absorbed, by an athlete are key to understanding the injuries. In boxing, single maximal punch speed has been measured at 8.16 m/s for amateurs (Walilko et al., 2005) and 8.9 m/s for professional boxers (Atha et al., 1985). Atha et al. (1985) reported that to replicate an equivalent punch force of 4096 N, as recorded in their study, a 6-kg padded wooden mallet would have to deliver a shot at 20 mph. The level of expertise will produce different punching forces. In elite, intermediate and novice groups the maximal punching forces for the rear hand have been recorded at 4800 N, 3722 N and 2381 N, respectively (Smith et al., 2000).

The type of shot will also produce different punching forces. Most studies assessing forces in boxing agree that the lead hook will produce more force than a lead jab, whilst a rear cross shot will produce a larger force than the lead hook (Lenetsky et al., 2013). It seems highly plausible that the forces produced are absorbed mainly by the knuckles, i.e., the metacarpophalangeal (MCP) joints, and this relates to the hand injuries that have been reported in several studies (Hame and Malone, 2000; Loosemore et al., 2017). This has also led to the term 'boxer's knuckle' becoming widely used (Gladden, 1957). Forces also travel into the rest of the hand and wrist, resulting in diverse injuries. Of note are carpometacarpal (CMC) joint injuries observed in elite amateur boxers, which can significantly impact on days lost from training (Loosemore et al., 2016).

Finally, boxers undergo different types of boxing training, ranging from no impact to the highest amount of impact at the hand–wrist region. These go in the order: shadow boxing, stick hitting, water bags, soft bags, heavy bags, pads, technical sparring, and open sparring. This information is useful when progressing a boxer from no impact to full return to boxing activities, with manipulation

315

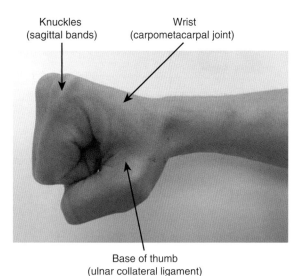

Knuckles
(sagittal bands)

Wrist
(carpometacarpal joint)

Base of thumb
(ulnar collateral ligament)

Fig. 25.1 Sites of main injuries incurred in boxing.

of variables of intensity (percentage of shot thrown) and volume (number of rounds, usually expressed in 3 min/round) possible. A practitioner should therefore have full knowledge of the diverse activities prior to designing a conservative or postoperative programme.

Main injuries occurring at the hand and wrist in boxing

Boxers incur injuries to all parts of their bodies, which is linked to specific sport mechanics and other general conditioning strategies, like running. Hand and wrist injuries, however, remain the bread and butter of this sport. At Olympic national level, between 2005 and 2009, hand–wrist injuries accounted for approximately 35% of all injuries in training and competition for the GB squad (Loosemore et al., 2017). Further, total days lost to training and overall duration were significantly greater for these areas than any other body part. Hand and wrist injuries are also a burden in the professional ranks, with many boxers requiring time off from training and competition. This chapter will therefore focus on understanding and managing the main injuries sustained in this sport that affect training availability (Fig. 25.1), which are:

- sagittal band ('extensor hood') injuries at the knuckles (MCP joints)
- CMC instability at the wrist
- ulnar collateral ligament (UCL) injuries at the base of the thumb.

The knuckles: sagittal band injuries

Knuckles, which are also known as metacarpophalangeal joints, provide the highest incidence of any injury at the hand–wrist region, although training with this injury is mostly possible, even when symptoms are present. Acutely, injuries occur due to hitting a bony anatomical region on an opponent in sparring or competition; shots to the opponent's forehead with a lead hand or back hand jab, or to the elbow when throwing an uppercut. This can result in tears of one of the sagittal bands (also called 'extensor hood') of the knuckle (Figs 25.1 and 25.2). It is postulated that, together with direct contact, there is also a shearing force occurring at the knuckle when impacting an opponent. This would create a lengthening force on one side of the knuckle with a shortening force occurring on the other, explaining why only one of the two anchoring sagittal bands are commonly injured. This shearing is further reinforced by clinical findings when assessing knuckle joint mobility posttrauma: increased transverse accessory glide in one direction (commonly ulnar direction), with decreased mobility in the opposite direction (radial direction). These joint mobility findings at the knuckle are similarly observed when clinically assessing a 'jarred' thumb, whereby commonly the UCL (one of the collaterals) is injured resulting from a shearing force occurring in an abduction (valgus or radial) direction.

Symptoms at the knuckles also occur insidiously, mainly linked to repeated hitting of training equipment, like a boxing bag. The knuckles most commonly injured are the first and second (i.e., index and middle finger). This is due to contact on impact occurring predominantly at these areas, as observed by pressure film impact testing performed in GB Boxing. Occasionally the fourth knuckle (i.e., little finger) is injured, usually as a result of an acute injury. The ring finger knuckle is rarely injured.

Presentation/testing for sagittal band injuries

Presentation and testing for sagittal band injuries is shown in Box 25.1.

Objective measures

Objective measures for any sporting injury are important as they link the subjective information to the severity of an injury. The information gathered will assist clinical decisions and training availability. In boxing, objective measures for hand and wrist injuries have been instrumental in providing the required level of care in this sport, safeguarding these athletes. This also applies to the other injuries discussed in this chapter.

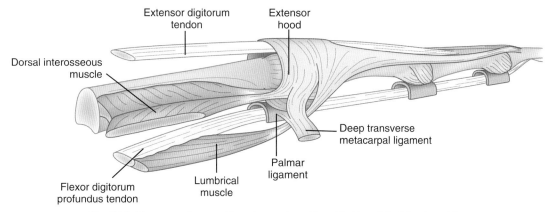

Fig. 25.2 Finger anatomy with extensor hood (sagittal bands) of the knuckle.

Box 25.1 **Sagittal band injuries**

Mechanism

- Direct impact
- Often due to poor bandaging or glove quality

Examination

- Swelling over the knuckle is common
- Pain on palpation over either side of the extensor hood (one side more than the other)
- A defect may be felt (feels like a hole with no tissue resistance), indicating a potential tear of the sagittal bands or of the capsule
- Occasional pain on the volar (palm) aspect of the metacarpophalangeal (MCP) joint
- Stiff joint end-feel on passive flexion of the MCP joint – can sometimes be *boggy* (inflammatory) or *empty* (no resistance felt on passive flexion – feels quite hypermobile)
- Extensor tendon subluxation on flexion – not always and can also occur in normal individuals – can be confirmed with dynamic ultrasound imaging

---

Range of motion

Making a fist can be painful in both acute and chronic conditions with a reduced visible or measured range of motion (ROM). Joint ROM is best tested using a metal finger goniometer placed directly over the knuckle (Fig. 25.3A). The wrist should initially be placed in full extension to eliminate the extensor musculature. The wrist can then be placed in full flexion to test muscle flexibility (finger extensors). Identifying which structures (muscle vs. joint) may be reducing knuckle ROM can assist in choosing appropriate strategies. From the screening performed in GB Boxing pre-injury, it is expected that the first knuckle usually has less ROM than the second, and the second less ROM than the third and fourth. This is possibly due to micro- or macro-trauma occurring over the years in these areas. Obviously, comparison between sides is recommended.

Strength (hand function)

The ability to make a fist in boxing is important, especially in the terminal phase of the punch. Impairment in this crucial phase of the punch may result in potential energy loss from soft tissue motion when tensing muscles at contact (Richards, 1997). In addition to reduced power output, the inability to make a fist creates a less stable wrist at contact which places the hand-wrist structures at risk of injury or further injury.

The hand has three main prehensile patterns; power grip, pinch grip and key grip. The recommended test for power grip in knuckle injuries uses the hand grip dynamometer (Fig. 25.3B) and the procedure discussed by Gatt et al. (2018): in standing, arm by side with full elbow extension, with all measurements performed alternatively three times with no rest. For each measurement, the dynamometer is squeezed for 3 s with the peak value of strength recorded.

Diagnostic work-up (investigations)

The subjective information, objective assessment and reaction to initial treatment should guide the practitioner as how best to proceed. If symptoms are quite persistent, or based on clinical rationale, an ultrasound scan should be considered. An ultrasound scan can identify structural damage to the joint, pick up a chronic synovitis or identify a subluxation of the extensor tendon occurring over the dorsal aspect of the knuckle (dynamic ultrasound most appropriate), which in most cases can be observed with the naked eye during flexion of the knuckle. The results may assist in supporting the current treatment approach or indicate the need for more invasive approaches like injection

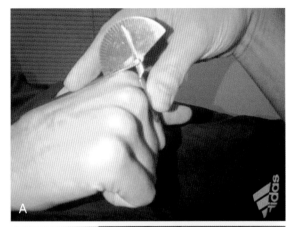

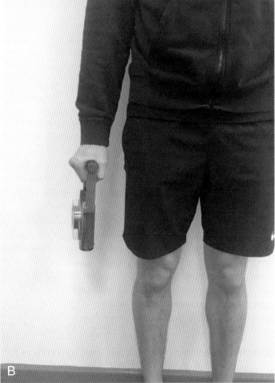

Fig. 25.3 Objective measures for the knuckles. (A) Finger goniometer for range of motion. (B) Hand grip dynamometer for power grip assessment.

therapy or surgical interventions. The information from an ultrasound scan should not be used to dictate whether surgery should ensue but rather add to the knowledge utilized to manage the boxer. More detailed investigation using magnetic resonance imaging (MRI) can be useful, especially in identifying the integrity of the capsule.

Conservative management
Protective strategies

Most boxers can manage full training status with an injured knuckle if relatively pain-free on impact. Sometimes these knuckles can be pain-free for a period, and then exacerbate based on competition or training requirements. It has been observed that reducing the forces acting on the knuckle can maintain full availability status whilst allowing the area to heal during the initial stages of an injury; equally it can help reduce the likelihood of recurrence or chronicity. Strategies to consider are predominantly gloves and bandaging techniques. Quality and size of gloves should be addressed as most boxers use gloves that are either too small, have poor padding or simply have been worn out. Boxers should consider acquiring at least two pairs of gloves: one for sparring and another for bags/pads. Protecting the knuckles starts with wrapping the hand–wrist before applying the gloves, with consideration for appropriate offloading strategies. These include using:

- better quality foam covering the four knuckles
- foam 'donuts' on any effected knuckle to offload areas of tenderness (Fig. 25.4A)
- buddy taping with the adjacent finger to reduce valgus forces (Fig. 25.4B)
- figure-of-eight bandaging at the knuckle to reduce flexion of the knuckle (Fig. 25.4C)
- a 'bar' on the palm of the hand with the wraps (Fig. 25.4D)
- considering the use of softer bags (e.g., water bags)

Ice and compression

In the acute phase, cold should be considered using crushed ice, if available, with traditional ice bags (with cling film to keep bag firmly in place). This should be followed by compression, using a 2.5-cm cohesive bandage around the knuckle (figure-of-eight approach as shown in Fig. 25.4C). Nowadays there is also electric or battery-powered equipment that can be used to provide cold and compression to the area. This has the added advantage of using continuous versus sequential compressive approaches. Subsequently it should be used to assist pain management after any impact sessions during early return to training. If it is an area that can flare up occasionally then using ice regularly will assist long-term management. As a preventative strategy, hands can be immersed, postsession, in an ice and water bucket (suggested is 20 s in and 40 s out × 5).

Manual therapy (joint mobilizations)

Manual therapy assessment and treatment is advisable in the initial stages of any hand and wrist injury. Flexion

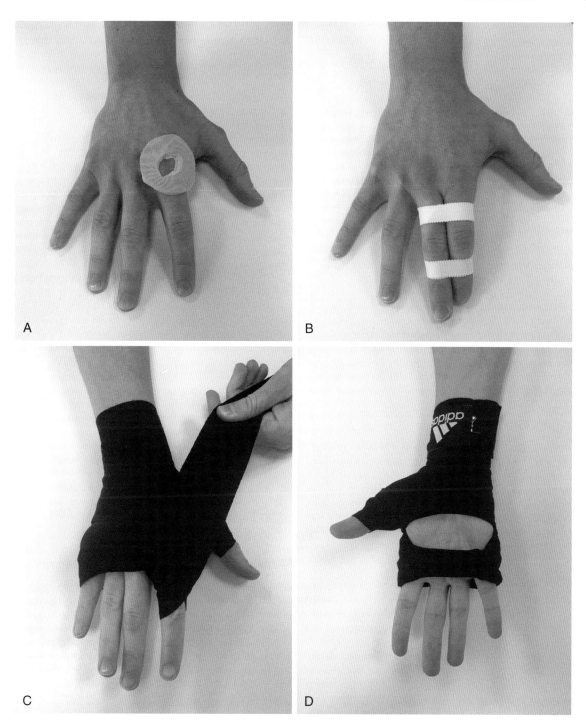

Fig. 25.4 Offloading strategies for the knuckles. (A) Foam 'donut' being used for the first knuckle. (B) Buddy taping of the index and middle finger. (C) Figure-of-eight technique at the index finger. (D) A 'bar' created using bandaging.

ROM is commonly lost due to joint jarring. Assessment of posteroanterior (PA) joint glide is recommended and any dysfunction restored to improve flexion ROM and the end feel. Abduction and adduction is another movement available at the knuckles occurring in a sagittal plane. As discussed earlier, the knuckles can be jarred in a more ulnar direction. This can impair the amount of sagittal plane movement occurring. Assessment of transverse joint glide is recommended as, even when flexion ROM is restored, if there is a transverse glide dysfunction it can prolong symptoms. Apart from local dysfunction it is important to assess the rest of the hand, wrist and forearm, as joint limitations in these areas can indirectly affect symptoms at the knuckle.

Electrotherapy modalities

Electrotherapy modalities like laser, which from clinical practice appear to yield positive results in terms of pain, can be included as part of the therapeutic approach. Class IIIb lasers have been the most commonly used models suited for therapeutic use. In recent years, class IV lasers have been introduced for Hand-Wrist injuries, with anecdotal evidence indicating that they supersede class IIIb lasers due to the higher intensity generated. Further evidence is required, a discussion of which is beyond the scope of this chapter; however, the author has used class IIIb for several years with positive feedback in these areas.

Acupuncture

Acupuncture has a beneficial role in symptom management and should be considered with care when utilized around training requirements (i.e., hypersensitization posttreatment is common). When considering knuckle injury, it is worth considering the interosseous muscles, as well as extrinsic muscles in the forearm, which can provide referred pain into the hand and mimic knuckle symptoms.

Soft tissue mobilization

Mobilization of soft tissue structures should be considered using positive or negative pressure techniques (i.e., pushing into the skin or lifting the skin). Positive pressure can be achieved using traditional massage techniques or with the assistance of instrument-assisted soft tissue massage (IASTM) techniques. Negative pressure can be achieved using connective tissue techniques, cupping or electrical equipment providing suction. All these techniques may be considered for soft tissue structures at the hand–wrist and forearm. Specifically, for the knuckles, IASTM tools can be used over the injured region for pain management. These techniques have been found to be effective when performed prior to commencing training due to their ability to

desensitize (numb) the area. Boxers can be thought how to self IASTM to maximize long-term impact of this strategy.

Rehabilitation (exercise therapy)

Rehabilitation forms the mainstay of managing any injury at the hand–wrist in boxing. The main aims of exercises at the knuckle are to maintain good flexion range of motion around this joint, condition the muscles/tendons around this joint, and desensitize pain. It has been observed that by performing a few key exercises (Fig. 25.5) prior to initiating the hand-wrapping process, hand and wrist injuries can be managed more effectively. These strategies have also been observed to reduce the risk of injuries by creating a more direct warm-up of the hand–wrist region. Exercises should also be performed posttraining, ideally after icing the knuckles if there is an active injury, to maximize the management of these conditions.

Use of resistance bands, resistance bars and spike balls should be considered for most stages of injury in this region (Fig. 25.5). Resistance bands (Fig. 25.5A) are used to develop strength/endurance of the hand extensors, resistance bars (Fig. 25.5B) are used to develop strength/endurance of the wrist flexors-extensors and forearm pronators-supinators, and the spike ball or reflex ball (Fig. 25.5C) aims at desensitizing the knuckle through vigorous massage over the symptomatic region. This technique can also be used for other hand–wrist injuries, complementing IASTM techniques aimed at pain management.

Stretching of the finger extensors is also important, as maintaining a closed fist allows less stress over the knuckle by reducing the stretch of the central extensor tendon on the sagittal bands. Therefore, stretching a closed fist (especially ensuring that the index and middle knuckles remain closed) into flexion, with elbow in full extension is a very useful strategy.

Antiinflammatories and injection therapy

Antiinflammatories are best avoided, especially in the first 72 hours of any acute injury, as they can disrupt the healing process, impacting on quality collagen layout and making the repair weaker. When a joint is predominantly inflammatory rather than mechanical, and is not responding well to the treatment strategies described so far, a course of antiinflammatories as guided by a physician could assist symptom progression. This should be combined with appropriate offloading strategies to maximize outcome.

When there is a chronic inflammatory component to the pathology, and no change in symptoms in response to treatment, consider a steroid injection in this area followed by an initial offload for up to 72 hours before subsequent

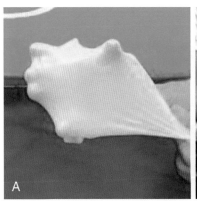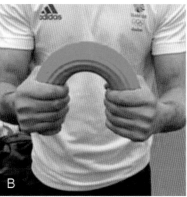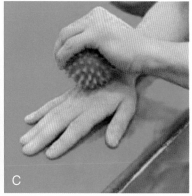

Fig. 25.5 Rehabilitation for the knuckles. (A) Resistance band openers for extensor tendon and knuckle joint conditioning. (B) Resistance bar wrist flexion-extension and forearm pronation-supination regime. (C) Spike ball massage for pain desensitization.

Box 25.2 **Postoperative protocol for extensor hood repairs**

1. *Immobility phase (0–4 weeks):* Athlete in removable splint to prevent excessive combined knuckle and wrist flexion
2. *Initial loading phase (4–6 weeks):* ROM/initial conditioning with no extensor tendon loading
3. *Progressive loading phase (6–8 weeks):* Increase in conditioning with extensor tendon loading
4. *Return to boxing phase (8–14 weeks):* Graduated return to boxing
5. *Full training phase (14–16 weeks):* Monitoring of boxer in full training status

---

return to training strategies. Injections are not a first-line of treatment and the other strategies described previously should be appropriately considered first.

Surgical intervention

The subjective and objective information combined with the reaction to initial treatment should guide the practitioner on how best to proceed. Boxers with severe acute injuries with torn sagittal bands can be maintained in training and competition as symptoms allow. Short- versus long-term performance gain should be considered. If symptoms are persistent, affecting training availability or competition performance, a surgical intervention might be warranted.

Surgical procedures are successful in most cases and a tailored rehabilitation protocol postoperation can augment the outcome of surgery (Box 25.2). Most boxers will require a period of 4 months before returning to full training status. Depending on the surgeon and type of surgery, the initial stages may vary. However, optimal loading during the entirety of the rehabilitation phase is important for a safe and timely return to training and competition.

Carpometacarpal joint injuries

The incidence of CMC joint injuries in GB Boxing is less than that of knuckle injuries; however, the severity and impact on training availability is greater. The common mechanism of injury is forced flexion of the wrist on impact against the opponent during which the hand is held in a considerably closed fist, which forces the CMC joint(s) into flexion. Like the knuckles, the second and/or third CMC joints are most commonly injured due to the contact on impact occurring over their respective knuckles. Unlike their ulnar counterparts (fourth and fifth CMC joints), the second and third CMC joints offer no joint mobility, which also puts them at risk when forcefully flexed.

The rear hand is more commonly injured during a cross shot when hitting the opponent at the top of the head. During the terminal part of the shot, the opponent has been observed on retrospective video analysis to forward flex their neck as a protective mechanism, augmenting the flexion torque at the wrist. Although correct bandaging techniques and gloves can reduce the incidence, injuries can still occur and require appropriate management.

Presentation/testing

CMC joint injury presentation is shown in Fig. 25.6 and Box 25.3 provides a summary of presentation and testing for these injuries.

Objective measures
Range of motion

ROM can be measured using an inclinometer or a smartphone with the appropriate application. The forearm should be placed on a flat surface with the elbow bent

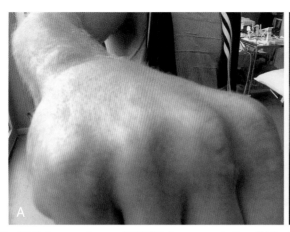
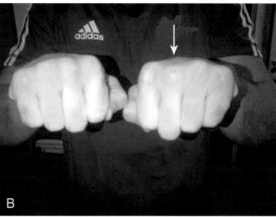

Fig. 25.6 Carpometacarpal (CMC) injury presentation. (A) Swelling over the back of the hand and (B) piano key effect occurring at the third or middle finger CMC in the left hand (middle finger knuckle seen to drop in relation to other knuckles in the hand).

Box 25.3 **Carpometacarpal joint injuries**

Mechanism

- A hit to the top of the opponent's head or body resulting in forced flexion at the wrist

Examination

- Swelling over the back of the hand is common (see Fig. 25.6A)
- Piano key effect if there is laxity occurring at the carpometacarpal (CMC) joint (see Fig. 25.6B)
- Carpal bossing (bony lump on back of hand) at the CMC joint (late sign)
- Tender on palpation of the CMC joint
- Pain on making a fist with potential laxity of second and/or third CMC joints
- Pain on axial loading (e.g., placing force through knuckle with a press-up)
- Inability to complete a barbell or dumbbell *reverse* biceps curl (i.e., palm facing down)
- Can often have >20% loss of grip strength when tested with hand grip dynamometer in comparison to baseline (Gatt et al., 2018)

From Gatt, I., Smith-Moore, S., Steggles, C., Loosemore, M., 2018. The Takei handheld dynamometer: an effective clinical outcome measure too for hand and wrist function in boxing. Hand (N Y) 13 (3), 319–324.

---

and hand hanging off the table with the palm facing down (Fig. 25.7A). For flexion and extension, the measuring device should be placed just proximal to the third knuckle over the metacarpal bone. Flexion with a closed fist and extension with an open hand measure the extensor and flexor musculature, respectively. Flexion with

an open fist and extension with a closed fist measure the joint ROM at the wrist. These motions should be measured and compared to the opposite side. It is also advisable to measure radial and ulnar deviation, as these movements are important for wrist biomechanics. For these measurements, the same position and method for flexion and extension is adopted; however, the forearm should be turned to a midprone (between full supination and pronation) position. The hand is maintained in a fist. The measuring device should be placed along an imaginary line between the proximal interphalangeal (PIP) joint of the index finger and web space between the thumb and the index (Fig. 25.7B). The amount of ROM and symptoms between sides can assist in understanding the severity of the injury.

Strength (hand function)

When presenting with a CMC joint injury, hand grip dynamometer testing should be considered as one of the first tests as the information obtained will guide clinical examination and decision making. As with knuckle injuries, using a hand grip dynamometer will assist in understanding the functional ability of making a fist at such a stage (Gatt et al., 2018). From clinical experience, a 0–20% hand grip deficiency with a midrange pain measure on gripping is considered a mild to moderate injury, with conservative management possible. More than 20% hand grip deficiency combined with a high pain measure indicates a poor prognosis and surgery should be considered. Hand grip measurements should be a key component of assisting progression during the loading stages of this injury. When available, isokinetic testing is useful in this situation. It can enhance both assessment and therapeutic strategies.

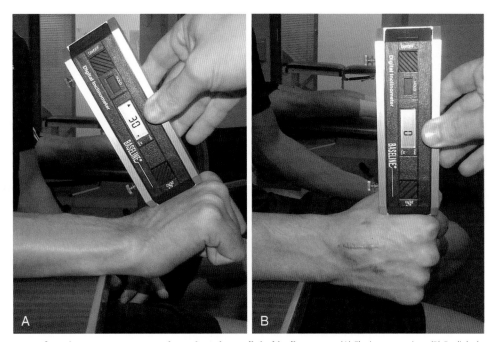

Fig. 25.7 Range of motion measurement at the wrist using a digital inclinometer. (A) Flexion-extension. (B) Radial-ulnar deviation.

Diagnostic work-up (investigations)

Based on clinical rationale, a dynamic ultrasound scan to assess ligamentous laxity at this joint should be considered. This is best supported using an MRI (3T MRI is suggested), which can provide more detailed information about the structures. In some cases, avulsion of the extensor carpi radialis brevis (ECRB) at the base of the third metacarpal (MC) and/or extensor carpi radialis longus (ECRL) at the second MC can be observed, with the former more commonly occurring. This information, together with the other objective measures of hand grip strength, ROM and functional abilities, combined with symptoms in and outside boxing will help guide management. A plain X-ray should be considered to rule out potential bone injury. Fractures do not commonly occur in the long shaft of the second and third MC bone, however, avulsion fractures involving the insertion of the ECRL and ECRB tendons can occur at the base of the MC bone. In contrast, more fractures have been recorded at the long shaft of the fifth MC bone. This is possibly due to more movement available at the fifth CMC joint, when compared to the second and third CMC joints, affecting torsion occurring in the long shaft of the MC bone.

Conservative management

Protective strategies

To prevent injuries from occurring, it is important to reduce the risk of forced flexion occurring at the wrist. 'Criss-Cross' techniques (Fig. 25.8A) using sports tape over the back of the hand–wrist region have been found to be effective. In the professional ranks this approach can be continued in competition. In the amateur ranks, as tape is traditionally not allowed albeit rule changes in recent years for elite competitors, it is important to use a portion of the bandage to create these criss-cross effects. More info can be found on YouTube (BOX Instructor tutorial – Hand wrapping). Unlike the knuckles, continued training with an injury at the CMCs can be difficult.

Mild injuries can potentially be maintained in full training using criss-cross taping placed underneath the bandage (i.e., directly on the skin) as an adjunct to an off-the-shelf protective splint (Fig. 25.8B). This form of orthotic has been found to be highly successful in reducing the strain at the CMC joints by decreasing flexion occurring at the wrist. Moderate injuries should be managed with an immediate period of rest. A minimum of 3 weeks of total rest in the area, wearing the splint throughout the whole day (and night if tolerated) is suggested. Hand grip dynamometry testing should be performed once a week to assess progression. If improvement is noted then prognosis may potentially be favourable, otherwise surgery should be considered. Severe injuries should be considered for early surgical intervention as otherwise outcome may not be successful. During the initial stages of return to training of moderate injuries, continued wearing of the splint during training becomes an integral strategy to prevent reinjury. This is also very useful during the early stages of return to impact postoperatively.

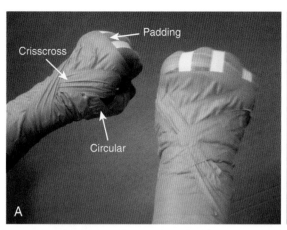 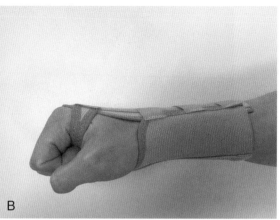

Fig. 25.8 Carpometacarpal protection aimed at preventing excessive wrist flexion. (A) Use of circular and crisscross taping techniques, and (B) off-the-shelf wrist splint.

Ice and compression

As with a knuckle injury, cold and compression should be considered in the acute stage of this type of injury. Subsequently it should be used to assist pain management after any impact sessions during early return to training.

Manual therapy

Although there is hardly any movement at the second and third CMC joints, joint play (specifically AP glide) can still be affected, influencing the symptoms. As this joint will be jarred into flexion, mobilizing using an AP glide can restore the accessory mobility of this joint helping to relieve symptoms. Proximally, it is also important to assess the carpal joints, which may have been affected by the initial trauma. Furthermore, like the knuckles it is important to assess for forearm motion (supination and pronation), as restrictions could affect the position of the wrist on impact. In clinical practice, assuring good mobility of all these areas has enhanced outcomes.

Electrotherapy

Like knuckle injuries, laser can be a useful adjunct to the healing process. In addition, the use of low-intensity pulsed ultrasound (LIPUS) directly over the area has yielded good clinical results, easing symptoms. This can be performed as 20 min of continuous treatment, once a day, 3–4 × week, for a period of 3–4 weeks.

Acupuncture

As for knuckle injuries, acupuncture can be useful in symptom management for mild to moderate CMC injuries where no ligament laxity is noted. Care should be taken as initially it may make the area more sensitive before yielding any results. This may affect training availability; therefore timing and type of approach requires attentive consideration.

Soft tissue mobilization

Intrinsically, desensitization using IASTM tools locally, reinforced by spike ball is a good strategy for pain management. Extrinsically, it is important to maintain the musculature of the dorsal forearm (extensors) as these can influence myofascial movement and ROM at the wrist. A regime of autostretching and self-release of the extensor musculature using, for example, a vibrating 'peanut' or rolling the forearm directly on a barbell on a rack can improve symptoms.

Rehabilitation (exercise therapy)

Rehabilitation is an integral part of safely returning to training or maintaining training with this injury. With this injury, it is important not to have any pain during impact or equally during rehabilitation, as it can negatively affect progression. For mild injuries, the author suggests the adoption of similar exercises described in the knuckle injuries section for both pre- and posttraining: resistance bands, resistance bars and spike balls (see Fig. 25.5A–C). In addition, the posttraining use of forearm resistance rotations (Fig. 25.9A) should be considered to improve forearm mobility through wrist control.

Vibration therapy plays a significant role in pain resolution. The use of vibration platforms (Fig. 25.9B) and hitting tyres with a metal bar (Fig. 25.9C) can provide increased stability at the wrist through proprioceptive feedback. Other exercises that are highly effective in wrist

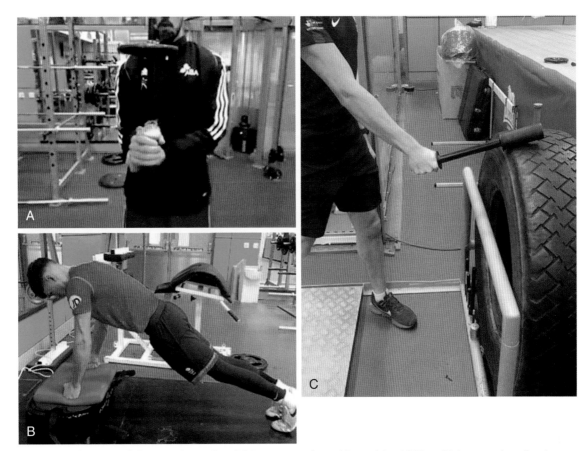

Fig. 25.9 Hand-Wrist stability exercises using; (A) Forearm rotations with a weighted 'T' bar. (B) A power plate vibration platform. (**C**) Tyre hits with a metal bar.

stability are dumbbell or barbell reverse biceps curls (palms facing down), which should be performed with the cue on keeping the wrist fixed during the entire motion. In moderate injuries these exercises can be introduced if the area is relatively symptom-free. Postoperatively these exercises will assist in appropriate progression throughout the stages. If available, isokinetic machines should be considered for rehabilitation, especially when strength deficits are present.

Antiinflammatories and injection therapy

Ideally, antiinflammatories are avoided, as they potentially make the area laxer and therefore more unstable. With mild injuries these drugs may not impact too negatively, and may be clinically justified. For moderate injuries, sclerotherapy (also called prolotherapy) should be considered when the splint is being worn during the rest phase period. Clinically this approach has yielded favourable results and, if undertaken, repeat injection is suggested after 2 weeks for a

more desirable outcome. For severe injuries, none of these strategies should be considered. Antiinflammatories may negatively affect the outcome of the operation. Sclerotherapy will not adversely affect the outcome of an operation and might be considered if attempting to progress a boxer to full impact due an upcoming major bout or competition before the surgery.

Surgical management

In most cases these injuries result in surgery due to loss of functionality at the hand–wrist region and inability of a boxer to return to impact activities. Optimal results are dependent on correct surgical technique, appropriate rehabilitation and progression to loading strategies (Box 25.4 and Fig. 25.10). Loading progression should include the use of a splint, as discussed previously, and measurement using the hand grip dynamometer forms an integral part of safe return to boxing.

Ulnar collateral ligament injury at the base of the thumb (MCP joint)

UCL injuries are not as common as knuckle and CMC injuries, and boxers are generally able to continue boxing training with this type of injury. The mechanism of injury is a valgus (abducted) force occurring at the MCP of the thumb causing a degree of ligamentous injury. In boxing the design of the glove and 'tucking the thumb' towards the fist (i.e., maintaining the thumb closer to the fist) using correct bandaging techniques contribute to injury reduction strategies in this region.

Presentation/testing

Presentation and testing is shown in Box 25.5.

Objective measures

Range of motion

Like the knuckles, joint ROM is best tested using a metal finger goniometer placed directly over the MCP joint. Flexion is generally more affected than extension, this mainly because, together with an abduction force, the thumb is also forced into extension. Forced flexion will be stiff and painful with most injuries.

Strength (hand function)

Like both knuckle and CMC joint injuries, strength measurements will assist with the clinical reasoning and management of this injury. In contrast to knuckle and CMC joint injuries however, hand grip dynamometry does not appear to be a valid tool for UCL injuries. Three tools have been found to be useful: handheld dynamometer (HHD), pinch grip

dynamometer, and weighted plates. The preferred choice, although most expensive device, is the HHD (Fig. 25.11A) as it maintains the thumb in an abducted position, thus biasing the UCL ligament providing improved functional testing for this type of injury. The suggested methodology is like the hand grip dynamometry discussed for the knuckles and CMCs. The pinch grip dynamometer (Fig. 25.11B), like the HHD, is useful to clinically assess UCL injuries; however, as the thumb is maintained in more adduction, results could be erroneous (i.e., they might indicate symptoms but not show the true severity of the injury). Further, this device is more suited to test a key grip, which although does not appear as relevant for a UCL injury, can be useful in other sports that require this type of hold (e.g., archery). In the absence of these devices, weighted plates may be considered (Fig. 25.11C). For example, ask the athlete to hold 10-kg plates in both hands using a pinch grip hold (i.e., opposing the thumb pulp towards the pulp of the fingers) and time to failure up to a maximum of 2 min. The main difference between plate holds and the HHD is that the former will more likely test endurance, whilst the latter is aimed at testing strength. Equally, however, they provide a measure of difference between the two sides, combined with a pain measure, which can help reveal the severity of an injury.

Diagnostic work-up (investigations)

Based on clinical rationale, a dynamic ultrasound scan to assess ligamentous laxity at this joint should be considered. This will be based predominantly on the symptoms reported, objective measures of strength and clinically on the amount of laxity encountered. The main reason for a scan is to assess whether a Stener lesion is present. This occurs when the aponeurosis of the adductor pollicis muscle becomes interposed between the ruptured UCL and its site of insertion at the base of the proximal phalanx. A Stener lesion does not allow appropriate healing and therefore an operative procedure is warranted. If no Stenor lesion is present, clinical findings and ability to continue training should guide the decision-making process.

Conservative management
Protective strategies

To prevent injuries from occurring, it is important to reduce the risk of extension-abduction occurring at the thumb by flexing-adducting the thumb whilst bandaging. This can be reinforced with tape by using a circular bandage technique going medial-to-lateral from dorsal-to-volar, in a way that encapsulates the base of the thumb and continues more proximally up the arm (Fig. 25.8A). This technique is also useful for CMC injuries by creating more static stability at the wrist. For further protection at the thumb 'figure-of-eight' techniques using

Progressive impact plan
Name: xxxxxxxxxxxxxxxxxxxx
Phase: Progressive loading
Dates: 11.12.17–07.01.18
Aims: Return to full training–from 8.1.18

GB BOXING

Week 1	11.12.2017	12.12.2017	13.12.2017	14.12.2017	15.12.2017	16.12.2017	17.12.2017
	Monday	Tuesday	Wednesday	Thursday	Friday	Saturday	Sunday
	60–80% water bags (4 rounds)	60–80% water bags (4 rounds)	Rest	80–100% water bags (2 rounds) 40–60% bags (4 rounds)	80–100% water bags (2 rounds) 40–60% bags (4 rounds)	Rest	Rest
Splint	On	Off		On	Off		
Week 2	18.12.2017	19.12.2017	20.12.2017	21.12.2017	22.12.2017	23.12.2017	24.12.2017
	Monday	Tuesday	Wednesday	Thursday	Friday	Saturday	Sunday
	60–80% bags (6 rounds)	60–80% bags (6 rounds)	Rest	80–100% bags (6–8 rounds)	80–100% bags (6–8 rounds)	80–100% bags (3 rounds) 60–80% pads (3 rounds)	Rest
Splint	On	Off		On	Off	On	
Week 3	25.12.2017	26.12.2017	27.12.2017	28.12.2017	29.12.2017	30.12.2017	31.12.2017
	Monday	Tuesday	Wednesday	Thursday	Friday	Saturday	Sunday
	Rest	80–100% bags (3 rounds) 60–80% pads (3 rounds)	Tech spar (4 rounds) 80–100% pads (4 rounds)	Rest	Tech spar (4 rounds) 80–100% pads (4 rounds)	80–100% bags/pads only (6 rounds)	Rest
Splint		Off	On		On	Off	
Week 4	01.01.18	02.01.18	03.01.18	04.01.18	05.01.18	06.01.18	07.01.18
	Monday	Tuesday	Wednesday	Thursday	Friday	Saturday	Sunday
	Rest	80–100% bags only (6 rounds)	Open spar (4 rounds) bags/pads only (4 rounds)	Rest	Open spar (4 rounds) Bags/pads only (4 rounds)	80–100% bags only (6 rounds)	Rest
Splint		Off	On		On	Off	

Full training from 08.01.18 with use of splint as guided by medical team

Fig. 25.10 Progressive impact plan for carpometacarpal joint postoperative procedures.

sport tape (Fig. 25.12A), which are commonly used in most sporting UCL injuries, can be considered prior to bandaging the hand. In competition this strategy is also useful when wrapping professional boxers, as well as in the amateur style of competition, obviously within the rules of the specific competition. For more moderate injuries, a bespoke thermoplastic splint (Fig. 25.12B) should be considered, which can allow continued healing of an injury while maintaining appropriate training availability.

Ice and compression

As with previous injuries discussed, cold and compression should be considered in the acute stage of an injury. Subsequently it should be used for pain management after any impact sessions during early return to training.

Manual therapy

In the same way as for knuckle injuries, manual therapy is a useful adjunct in the acute phase of UCL injuries to assess

327

and manage the injury. Flexion mobilizations will assist in restoring full ROM, whilst transverse ulnar glides should be aimed at restoring dysfunction created from the abduction force. A common finding posttreatment can be that the laxity felt when doing a valgus test has been reduced; equally, the reduced mobility felt during a varus test has been improved. It is the opinion of the author that manual therapy performed in the acute stage can impact positively on outcomes in mild-to-moderate injuries.

Electrotherapy

As for knuckle injuries, laser can be a useful adjunct to the healing process. This should not be utilized during the initial bleeding phase of a UCL injury; it is best considered after 24 hours.

Acupuncture

Similarly to knuckle and CMC injuries, acupuncture can be useful in symptom management for mild-to-moderate UCL injuries where no gross ligament laxity is noted. This modality is particularly useful for trigger points of the intrinsic musculature of the thumb (thenar eminence and dorsal first interosseous).

Soft tissue mobilization

The same rationale as for knuckle and CMC injuries applies to UCL injuries. Since ligaments are the effected structures, desensitization using IASTM tools locally reinforced by spike ball is a good strategy for pain management. Extrinsically, it is important to maintain the musculature of the thumb (both dorsal and volar aspect). Stretching can also assist symptoms. This is best performed with a straight elbow, thumb held inside a closed fist, and the wrist moved towards ulnar deviation.

Rehabilitation (exercise therapy)

For mild injuries, the exercises described for knuckle injuries (Fig. 25.5) are suitable for both pre- and posttraining: resistance bands, resistance bars and spike balls. In addition, the posttraining use of pinch plate holds (Fig. 25.11C) can be used. These can be progressed with dynamic plate passes (i.e., passing a weighted plate from one hand to another using the shoulders as pendulum) and dynamic plate drops (i.e., letting a weighted plate drop and catching it with the other hand). Both exercises should be performed using a pinch hold approach. Finger push-offs (Fig. 25.13), where the aim is to push off the wall and land onto the same hand only with pulps of all fingers and thumb touching the wall, is a good exercise for loading the thumb as well as other structures at the hand. This exercise can be progressed by alternating from one hand to another. The use of vibration, as discussed at the CMC joints, should also be considered to provide stability at the thumb with the hand position possibly changing from weight-bearing on the knuckles on the power plate to weight-bearing on the pulp of the fingers and thumb.

Antiinflammatories and injection therapy

Antiinflammatories should ideally be avoided; however from clinical experience, UCL injuries often yield better results with these medications compared to knuckle and CMC joint injuries. When applicable due to a chronic inflammatory component of the pathology, and due to no change in symptoms, a steroid injection in this area followed by an initial offload for up to 72 hours and subsequent return to training strategies can be considered. Injections tend to be less commonly used with these injuries compared to knuckle injuries, and more frequently used when compared to CMC injuries (where they should be avoided). As previously mentioned, injections are not a first-line treatment and the other strategies described previously should be appropriately considered first.

Surgical management

In most cases these injuries can be managed conservatively, unless a Stenor lesion is detected from diagnostic work-up. Optimal surgical outcome is dependent on correct surgical technique, appropriate rehabilitation and progression to loading (Box 25.6). Unlike the knuckles and CMCs, the thumb does not bear impact on every shot and therefore progression to loading is not as straightforward. Therefore, if symptoms have been minimal when performing bags, it is important to initially consider the use of a bespoke thermoplastic splint (Fig. 25.12B) with progression to figure-of-eight taping (Fig. 25.12A) during pads and sparring activities to avoid reinjury. Strength at the thumb is important and therefore the use of an HHD for activity progression is suggested.

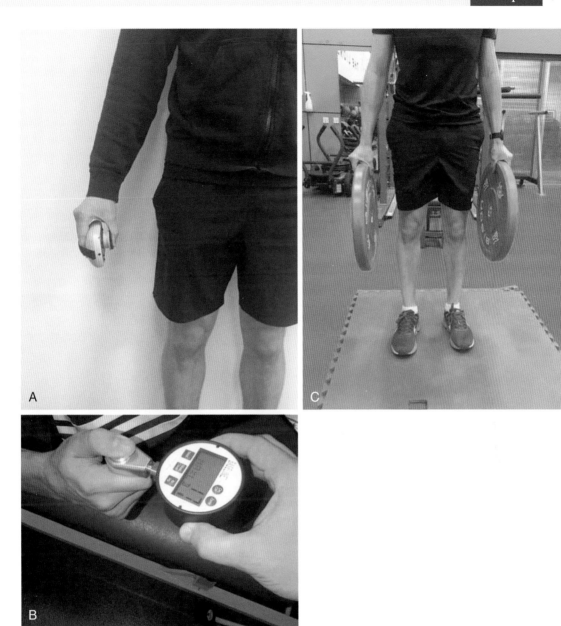

Fig. 25.11 Objectives measures for ulnar collateral ligament (UCL) injuries. (A) Pinch grip using a handheld dynamometer. (B) Key grip using a pinch grip dynamometer. (C) Pinch grip using weighted plate holds (10 kg is suggested using holds of 60–120 s for most athletes).

Conclusion

The knuckle, wrist and thumb are the most at-risk anatomical regions in boxing. Regardless of whether the boxer is an amateur or professional athlete, these injuries can equally occur. Wrapping the hands properly and using the right glove are the most important factors to help reduce the risk of injury. Following this, maintaining good flexibility, especially for the wrist extensors, together with conditioning exercises, are important. Presessions are advisable to perform some specific hand–wrist exercises prior to bandaging as part of a correct warm-up routine. Postsessions, it is also

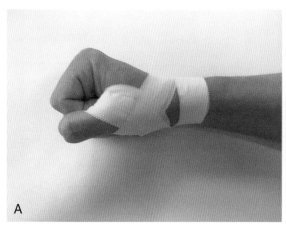

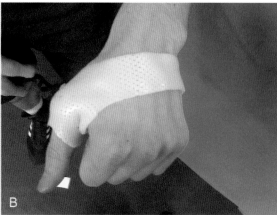

Fig. 25.12 Ulnar collateral ligament protection techniques. (A) Figure-of-eight strapping with sports tape and (B) bespoke thermoplastic splinting.

Box 25.6 **Postoperative protocol for ulnar collateral ligament injuries of the thumb (MCP)**

1. *Immobility phase (0–4 weeks):* Athlete in cast/removable splint
2. *Initial loading phase (4–6 weeks):* ROM/initial conditioning with no extensor tendon loading. Use of removable splint (mainly to avoid 'catching it')/night splint
3. *Progressive loading phase (6–8 weeks):* Increase in conditioning activities
4. *Return to boxing phase (8–12 weeks):* Graduated return to boxing (use of bespoke thermoplastic splint for pads/sparring activities)
5. *Full training phase (12–14 weeks):* monitoring of boxer in full training status (no splint)

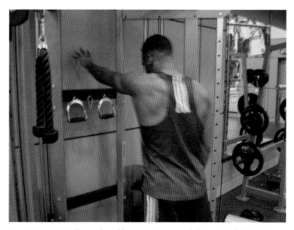

Fig. 25.13 Wall push-off exercise used for rehabilitation of knuckles, carpometacarpal joint and ulnar collateral ligament injuries by loading these structures in a controlled manner. This engages the kinetic chain: elbow, shoulder, shoulder blade and trunk.

advisable to routinely ice the hand–wrist region to prevent accumulation of microtrauma, which can lead to injury.

Conservative management of these injuries follows the order: UCL, knuckle and CMC joint (Fig. 25.13). It is therefore important to have a methodological approach to clinical examination to decide between a conservative or operative approach. Appropriate initial management of these injuries, particularly CMCs, can impact on resolution of symptoms. Therefore education should form part of injury-reduction strategies. Further, as the hand and wrist regions predominantly incur joint sprains rather than muscle strains, understanding the complex joint mechanics will enhance symptom outcome. Any form of treatment modality or exercise regime should also follow a bespoke and clinical evidence-based approach, with a clear justification.

Finally, if symptoms do not resolve in a timely fashion or if you suspect the athlete may have sustained a serious injury, it is important to consider imaging or referral to a surgeon. Subjective measures of pain linked to functional activities in boxing (i.e., hitting a bag or an opponent in sparring), together with objective measures (mainly strength and mobility linked with pain on execution) should guide the choice of any management and progression.

References

Atha, J., Yeadon, M.R., Sandover, J., et al., 1985. The damaging punch. British Medical Journal (Clinical Research Edition) 291 (6511), 1756–1757.

Gatt, I., Smith-Moore, S., Steggles, C., Loosemore, M., 2018. The Takei handheld dynamometer: an effective clinical outcome measure too for hand and wrist function in boxing. Hand (N Y) 13 (3), 319–324.

Gladden, J.R., 1957. Boxer's knuckle; a preliminary report. The American Journal of Surgery 93 (3), 388–397.

Hame, S.L., Melone, C.P., 2000. Boxer's knuckle in the professional athlete. The American Journal of Sports Medicine 28 (6), 879–882.

Lenetsky, S., Harris, N., Brughelli, M., 2013. Assessment contributors of punching forces in combat sports athletes: implications for strength and conditioning. Strength & Conditioning Journal 35 (2), 1–7.

Loosemore, M., Lightfoot, J., Gatt, I., et al., 2016. Hand and wrist injuries in elite boxing: a longitudinal prospective study (2005–2012) of the Great Britain Olympic boxing squad. American Association of Hand Surgery 1–7.

Loosemore, M., Lightfoot, J., Palmergreen, D., et al., 2017. Boxing injury epidemiology in the great britain team: a 5-year surveillance study of medically diagnosed injury incidence and outcome. British Journal of Sports Medicine 49, 1100–1107.

Richards, L., 1997. Posture effects on grip strength. Archives of Physical Medicine and Rehabilitation 78 (10), 1154–1156.

Smith, M.S., Dyson, R.J., Hale, T., et al., 2000. Development of a boxing dynamometer and its punch force discrimination efficacy. Journal of Sports Science and Medicine 18 (6), 445–450.

Walilko, T.J., Viano, D.C., Bir, C.A., 2005. Biomechanics of the head for olympic boxer punches to the face. British Journal of Sports Medicine 39 (10), 710–719.

Chapter | 26 |

The cervical spine: risk assessment and rehabilitation

Alan J. Taylor and Roger Kerry

Introduction

The neck is often the forgotten area of the body in terms of assessment and management (Fig. 26.1). In other anatomical regions, therapists focus on returning patients to preinjury levels. Rehabilitation strategies target identified muscle strength and endurance deficits in comprehensive training programmes that take patients through a range of exercises, from isometrics through to plyometrics, whilst concomitantly identifying and enabling psychological strategies. Every element is incorporated into the rehabilitation programmes, as patients go through a complex return-to-fitness schedule, which conditions them for the demands of their sport, pastime or physical activity. In the craniocervical region, however, therapists have historically offered little more than range of motion exercises and isometric deep neck flexor exercises, perhaps coupled with elements of manual therapy and advice, before encouraging their charges to get back into action. This strategy often has limited success and many go on to suffer chronicity (Lamb et al., 2012). This chapter explores the underlying reasons for this apparent mismatch and offers direction for therapists who rehabilitate the cervical spine in sport or any environment.

Risk assessment of the cervical spine in a sporting context

The incidence of catastrophic neck injury and concussion has decreased significantly over the last 30 years, as changes to the rules of various sports have resulted in fewer direct collisions that to neck or head trauma. Despite this, well over half of catastrophic injuries in sport are neck injuries. This type of injury is reported in a range of contact sports such as rugby, football, boxing and American football, and extends to a wide range of noncontact sports such as skiing, cycling, equestrian, lacrosse (Petschauer et al., 2010), scuba diving (Brajkovic et al., 2013) and surfing. Injuries are reported at all levels, from school (Olympia et al., 2007) and recreational through to professional level (Rihn et al., 2009). This chapter confines itself to the more common minor cervical spine or concussion injuries that occur secondary to sporting injuries or direct collisions between players. This type of injury may cause acceleration–deceleration trauma (Langer et al., 2008) to the head or neck, and result in complex presentations of dizziness, neck pain and headaches, which are both difficult to assess and manage effectively.

Headache and dizziness: danger or direction for treatment?

For any clinician, the posttrauma patient who presents with a combination of neck pain, headache and dizziness or other associated symptoms is challenging. It may well be that the spectre of possible serious pathology, such as fracture or associated cervical artery dysfunction (CAD), may be a factor in why clinicians appear reluctant to rehabilitate the cervical spine.

How should clinicians proceed?

In the event of sporting trauma and the evidenced absence of cervical spine fracture via the Canadian C-spine Rule pathway (Stiell et al., 2001), there are two primary key considerations for the clinician:
- cervical arterial dysfunction (CAD)
- traumatic brain injury (TBI).

Cervical arterial dysfunction

The International Framework for Examination of the Cervical Region for Potential of Cervical Arterial Dysfunction (IFOMPT;

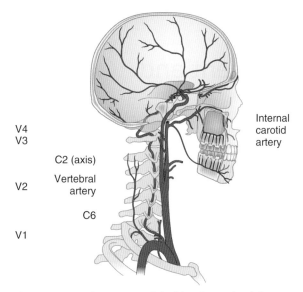

V4
V3

C2 (axis)

Vertebral
artery

V2

C6

V1

Internal
carotid
artery

Fig. 26.1 Normal anatomy of the blood vessels of the head and neck. (Reproduced with permission from McCarthy, C. 2010. Combined Movement Theory. Churchill Livingstone, Edinburgh.)

Rushton et al., 2014) offers direction to clinicians for safe risk assessment via sound clinical reasoning. CAD is an umbrella term that covers a range of vascular pathologies from atherosclerosis through to arterial dissection (Table 26.1).

In a sporting situation, based on the age and health of the athlete, underlying vascular disease would be considered less likely, whilst traumatic arterial dissection, although rare, would be a potential hypothesis. Dissection is known to occur as a result of blunt trauma to vessels due to direct impact on vessels (Degen et al., 2017) and/or as a result of unknown mechanisms linked to a range of activities such as rugby tackles or scrums and noncontact activities such as jogging (Fragaso et al., 2016; Suzuki et al., 2018).

Internal carotid artery dissection

As far back as 1974, Crissey hypothesized and described four mechanisms that may lead to injury of the carotid artery (Crissey et al., 1974):
- neck hyperextension associated with rotation
- direct blow to neck
- blunt intraoral trauma
- basilar skull fracture involving the carotid canal.

Clinical presentation

Commonly the presentation of carotid artery dissection involves headache of acute onset, which makes early differentiation between it and concussion difficult. Fig. 26.2 illustrates the common pain sites. It is suggested that ipsilateral pain may

Table 26.1 Range of arterial pathologies covered by the term cervical artery dysfunction (CAD)

Structure/site	Pathology	Symptoms/presentation
Carotid artery	Atherosclerosis • stenotic • thrombotic • aneurysmal	Commonly silent, possible carotidynia, possible transient ischaemic attack (TIA), stroke
Carotid artery	Hypoplasia	Commonly silent
Carotid artery	Dissection	Pain, TIA, cranial nerve palsies, Horner's syndrome
Vertebral artery	Atherosclerosis	Rare. Commonly silent, possible TIA, stroke
Vertebral artery	Hypoplasia	Commonly silent
Vertebral artery	Dissection	Pain, TIA, cranial nerve palsy
Temporal artery	Giant cell arteritis	Temporal pain (headache), scalp tenderness, jaw and tongue claudication, visual symptoms (diplopia or vision loss – may be permanent)
Cerebral vessels	Reversible cerebral vasoconstriction syndrome	Severe 'thunderclap' headaches
Any cervicocranial vessel	Vascular anomaly or malformation	Possible headache/neck pain, i.e., unruptured carotid aneurysm

affect neck, face, jaw region and head simultaneously. Detection may be easier in the 50% or more who have gone on to develop Horner's syndrome. This occurs due to either compression, stretch or hypoperfusion of the sympathetic fibres within the wall of the carotid artery. An acute onset Horner's syndrome (decreased pupil size, drooping eyelid and decreased sweating on the affected side of the face) associated with neck pain and headache is almost pathognomonic of carotid artery dissection. Around 10% of patients may suffer cranial nerve palsies, usually affecting levels IX–XII. Additionally some patients report pulsatile tinnitus, thought to be associated with the murmur of the dissection and resulting stenosis.

Any combination of the above symptoms or examination findings should raise the clinician's index of suspicion of carotid dissection and the patient should be referred on for immediate investigation without further delay. Orthopaedic or manual therapy examination is not indicated and should not be carried out as routine in such cases. Further examination for a suspected lesion is usually carried out via magnetic resonance angiography (MRA) or computerized tomography angiography (CTA). Duplex ultrasound is used in some centres as a preliminary investigation.

Management

At the time of publication there are no evidence-based guidelines for management of carotid dissection. Most are managed on a case-by-case basis with patients being treated conservatively with antithrombotic treatment or antiplatelet therapy or both (Rao et al., 2011). In selected cases, endovascular stent placement has been suggested as a safe and effective option to restore vessel lumen integrity and prevent stroke (Martinelli et al., 2017).

Vertebral artery dissection

Vertebral artery dissection (VAD) has been reported as one of the most common identifiable causes of stroke in those aged 18–45 (Kristensen et al., 1997). It is recognized that VAD is a potentially treatable cause of transient ischemic attack (TIA) and stroke (Beletsky et al., 2003). As the greatest risk of stroke in craniocervical dissections seems to occur in the first few weeks after dissection (Biousse et al., 1995), prompt diagnosis is essential. VAD should be considered within the clinical reasoning and diagnostic assessment of patients presenting with dizziness or craniocervical pain following sporting trauma.

Clinical presentation

Crucially, clinicians should be aware that VAD may present in the early stages as neck pain or headache. Gottesman et al. (2012) in a systematic review reported that 76% of studied individuals presented with neck pain or headache 'at some point during their presentation' (Fig. 26.3). Dizziness or vertigo was reported in ~58% of VAD patients. Sports identified specifically in this study were jogging, horse riding, skiing, surfing and tennis. Although rare, there is a strong suggestion that VAD should be considered as a differential diagnosis in patients with neck pain, headache and dizziness; this would seem particularly pertinent in trauma cases. The authors state that 'This is particularly important for younger patients where the combination of dizziness with craniofacial or cervical pain might otherwise be mistaken for a benign diagnosis such as vestibular migraine'.

The neurological consequences of VAD are linked to postinjury cerebral ischaemia linked to thromboembolism, hypoperfusion, haemorrhage or a combination of these.

Management

Traumatic VAD can have devastating complications, with reports of a 24% stroke rate and 8% death rate (Sanelli et al.,

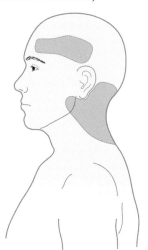

Fig. 26.2 Typical somatic pain distribution related to pathology and trauma of the internal carotid artery. (Reproduced with permission from McCarthy C, 2010 Combined Movement Theory, Churchill Livingstone, Edinburgh.).

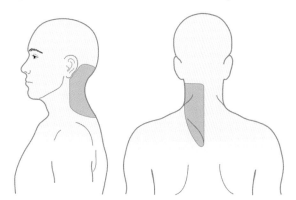

Fig. 26.3 Typical somatic pain distribution related to pathology and trauma of the vertebrobasilar arterial system. (Reproduced with permission form McCarthy C, 2010, Combined Movement Theory, Churchill Livingstone, Edinburgh.)

2002). Early recognition of this as a medical emergency is key. Patients who are diagnosed with VAD who have not developed ischaemic symptoms are managed with anticoagulation or antiplatelet therapy, depending on potential bleeding risk, location of lesion and extent of injury (Simon and Mohseni, 2017). Operative repair and endovascular therapy are used with high-grade lesions and those with contraindications to anticoagulation or antiplatelet therapy that are at elevated risk for progression. Currently, there is no evidence to support any one management option, and diagnosed patients seem to be dealt with on a case-by-case basis. Similarly, there appears to be no evidenced route back to sport for those who have been affected by cervicocranial vascular injury.

Ongoing dizziness

In the absence of evidenced fracture or traumatic CAD, clinicians still need to manage the posttraumatic cases where neck pain and dizziness remains a feature. There are three key considerations:
- traumatic brain injury
- cervicogenic dizziness
- sensorimotor dysfunction.

Traumatic brain injury

The reader is also referred to Chapter 27, which discusses the management of head injuries. The 2017 Concussion in Sport Group (CISG) (McCrory et al., 2017) consensus statement suggested that sports-related concussion (SRC) is 'often defined as representing the immediate and transient symptoms of TBI'. TBI is often used interchangeably with concussion and the Berlin expert panel who put this consensus document together modified the previous CISG definition as follows:
- SRC is a TBI induced by biomechanical forces.
- Several common features may be utilized to clinically define the nature of a concussive head injury:
  - SRC may be caused either by a direct blow to the head, face, neck or elsewhere on the body with an impulsive force transmitted to the head.
  - SRC typically results in the rapid onset of short-lived impairment of neurological function that resolves spontaneously. However, in some cases, signs and symptoms evolve over several minutes to hours.
  - SRC may result in neuropathological changes, but the acute clinical signs and symptoms largely reflect a functional disturbance rather than a structural injury and, as such, no abnormality is seen on standard structural neuroimaging studies.
  - SRC results in a range of clinical signs and symptoms that may or may not involve loss of consciousness. Resolution of the clinical and cognitive features

typically follows a sequential course. However, in some cases symptoms may be prolonged.

The consensus statement described six specific clinical domains that can be incorporated into a specific diagnosis of SRC as follows:
1. symptoms: somatic (e.g., headache), cognitive (e.g., feeling like in a fog) and/or emotional symptoms (e.g., lability)
2. physical signs (e.g., loss of consciousness, amnesia, neurological deficit)
3. balance impairment (e.g., gait unsteadiness)
4. behavioural changes (e.g., irritability)
5. cognitive impairment (e.g., slowed reaction times)
6. sleep/wake disturbance (e.g., somnolence, drowsiness).

It was suggested that, 'If symptoms or signs in any one or more of the clinical domains are present, an SRC should be suspected and the appropriate management strategy instituted'.

Advanced clinical reasoning is the hallmark of good decision making in such cases. It is recommended that, 'all athletes should have a clinical neurological assessment (including evaluation of mental status/cognition, oculomotor function, gross sensorimotor, coordination, gait, vestibular function and balance) as part of their overall management' (McCrory et al., 2017). Therapy clinicians should triage onto a physician or neuropsychologist if SRC is suspected.

Persistent symptoms

It is known that SRC symptoms may become persistent in some cases. The standard definition for persistent symptoms is, 'symptoms that persist beyond expected time frames (i.e., >10–14 days in adults and >4 weeks in children)' (McCrory et al., 2017). The Berlin expert consensus suggests that 'at a minimum, the assessment should include a comprehensive history, focused physical examination, and special tests where indicated (e.g., graded aerobic exercise test)'. They go on to recommend that 'treatment should be individualized and target specific medical, physical and psychosocial factors identified on assessment'.

Management

There is preliminary evidence supporting the use of:
1. an individualized symptom-limited aerobic exercise programme in patients with persistent postconcussive symptoms associated with autonomic instability which induces abnormalities in organ systems and may contribute to cardiovascular dysregulation
2. a targeted physical therapy programme in patients with cervical spine or vestibular dysfunction
3. a collaborative approach including cognitive behavioural therapy to deal with any persistent mood or behavioural issues.

Clinicians should be aware that there is a growing body of literature indicating that psychological factors may play a significant role in symptom recovery and contribute to risk of persistent symptoms in some cases. The assessment and management of such cases requires a careful and comprehensive history taking and an advanced level of clinical reasoning and decision making.

Cervicogenic dizziness

Cervicogenic dizziness (CGD) presents in a very similar way to CAD and elements of TBI. CGD is characterized by neck pain with or without headache, but with associated descriptions of imbalance, unsteadiness, disorientation and reduced range of neck motion (Reiley et al., 2017). CGD is currently a diagnosis of exclusion and there is a lack of consensus in the literature regarding the testing and resultant diagnosis. Reiley et al. (2017) proposed a stepwise process for diagnosing CGD, which is detailed in Fig. 26.4.

Reiley et al. (2017) state that 'Cervicogenic dizziness should NOT be considered if the patient does not have neck pain', suggesting that, 'neck pain can occur at rest, with movement, or with palpation. Symptoms caused by CGD should be exacerbated by movements that elicit neck pain and should subside with interventions that alleviate neck pain'. However, these statements appear largely unsupported by studies or research findings.

The word 'dizzy' describes a range of sensations. The clinician's priority is to elucidate the exact nature of a patient's report of 'dizziness' or 'vertigo', as the two may be erroneously used interchangeably. One method is to ask the patient to describe the feeling(s) without using the word 'dizzy'. Four subjective types of dizziness have been identified: vertigo, disequilibrium, presyncope and lightheadedness (Reilly, 1990). Clinicians must be able to distinguish different kinds of dizziness, since a differential diagnosis is peculiar to each type.

Definitions

Vertigo refers to the illusion of environmental motion, classically described as 'spinning' or 'whirling'. The sense of motion is usually rotatory, 'like getting off a merry-go-round' or 'the ground tilts up and down, like being on a boat at sea' (Reilly, 1990). *Dorland's Illustrated Medical Dictionary* (Dorland, 2012) splits it into two types.

- objective vertigo – a sensation as if the external world were revolving around the individual
- subjective vertigo – a sensation as if the individual were revolving in space.

True vertigo is generally thought to reflect a dysfunction at some level of the vestibular system. Vertigo is not thought to be a symptom arising from the cervical spine, but is more likely linked to peripheral vestibular disorders or lesions within the vestibular pathways of the central nervous system (CNS).

Disequilibrium is a disturbance in balance or coordination that impairs ambulation. Classically patients suggest that 'the problem is in my legs', but others feel 'dizzy in the head, too'. As ambulation makes the problem worse, gait analysis and neurologic examination are essential.

Presyncope means that the patient senses *impending* loss of consciousness. In cases where the patient has not ever actually lost consciousness, the complaint 'I feel like I will pass out' could be due to a range of explanations. However, a consideration of possible ischaemia, which may lead onto full syncope, should be investigated accordingly.

Lightheadedness refers to a sensation 'in the head' that is clearly not vertiginous or presyncopal, and that is *not* invariably related to ambulation. Some describe 'floating' or feeling 'like my head is not attached to my body', being 'high' or 'giddy'.

Patients may describe some elements of each of the above categories, which makes the assessment of postsporting trauma very challenging (Reiley et al., 2017).

Sensorimotor dysfunction

In sporting trauma with protracted unexplained dizziness, a full neurological screen is indicated involving assessment of radicular symptoms, myotomes, dermatomes, deep-tendon reflexes, upper motor neuron signs and cranial nerve function. Appropriate triage should made in the presence of abnormal neurological findings. In the absence of fracture, cervical instability, CAD or neurological dysfunction, it is logical to consider sensorimotor assessment.

Sensorimotor considerations

The term 'sensorimotor' is used to describe the complexity of the afferent, efferent and central processing components that provide and maintain stability in the postural control system (Kristjansson et al., 2009). Sensorimotor deficits (Yu et al., 2011) are thought to be a feature of traumatic neck injury such as whiplash-associated disorder (WAD); so it follows that there may be sensorimotor considerations in the case of sporting trauma to the cervicocranial region. Indeed, preliminary findings post-concussion in 54 elite rugby union players suggest minor altered balance strategies and altered trunk muscle control (Hides et al., 2017).

Disturbances to the afferent input from the neck are postulated as causes of dizziness, unsteadiness, visual disturbances, altered postural stability and cervical proprioception, which may be linked to head and eye movement control (Kristjansson et al., 2009). Fig. 26.5 illustrates the systems involved in this complex interaction. It is beyond the scope of this chapter to go into detailed pathophysiological descriptions of this system. However, it is suggested that the following areas are considered as part of assessment:

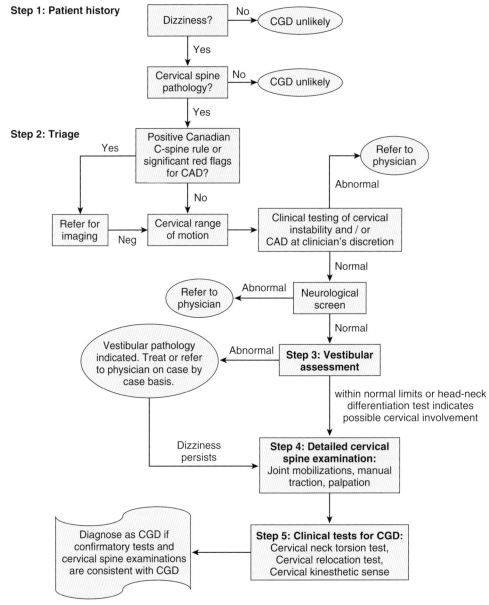

Step 1: Patient history

Step 2: Triage

Fig. 26.4 Stepwise algorithm for the diagnosis of cervicogenic dizziness (CGD). *CAD,* Cervical artery dysfunction. (Reproduced with permission from Reiley, A.S., Vickory, F.M., Funderburg, S.E., Cesario, R.A., Clendaniel, RA., 2017. How to diagnose cervicogenic dizziness. Archives of Physiotherapy 7, 12.)

- head–neck awareness
- neck movement control
- postural ability: dizziness and/or unsteadiness
- oculomotor disturbances.

The cervical spine contributes to somatosensory awareness via a range of mechanisms.

Mechanoreceptors, reflexes and the sympathetic nervous system

It is known that there is a high density of mechanoreceptors in the muscle spindles, joints and ligaments of the upper cervical spine. These cervical afferents are thought to provide proprioceptive sense and information to the CNS (Kristjansson

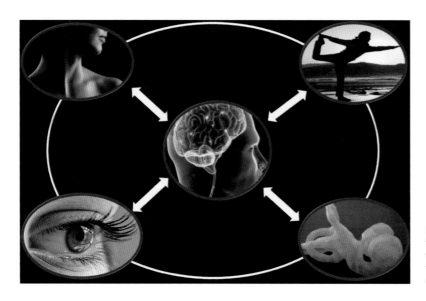

Fig. 26.5 The inputs and outputs from neck proprioception, visual, vestibular, and balance systems that are involved in sensorimotor dysfunction.

et al., 2009). These messages travel via sensory pathways to the thalamus, cerebellum and somatosensory cortex. Cervical afferents also mediate information and reflexes from the vestibular and visual systems and communicate with the sympathetic nervous system (SNS) via bidirectional beta-receptors in the muscle tissues. This complex system of communication plays a role in neck reflex activity, which interlinks head orientation, eye movement and postural stability (Treleaven, 2008).

Possible mechanisms

Disruption in sensorimotor control may result in a sensation of *disequilibrium* or reports of *dizziness* though the following mechanisms:

- because of direct trauma or from alterations in afferent feedback due to altered muscular function
- due to chemical neural irritation from local inflammatory responses in the surrounding tissues
- as part of a direct effect from centrally driven mediators
- the SNS may exert an effect on muscle spindle activity, resulting in alterations in muscular function.

Clinical examination

Assessment of oculomotor function can be conducted by examining the quality of eye movements and control. The clinician should also consider any reproduction of symptoms during testing.

Assessment of oculomotor control

1. **Smooth pursuit eye movement (in neutral).** Examination of oculomotor control includes observation of the eyes following a moving target (smooth pursuit) while keeping the head still. The eyes should move smoothly without nystagmus.

2. **Saccadic eye movement.** The patient is asked to quickly move the eyes to fix his/her gaze between several targets. Targets are placed in several different movement directions. Inability to fixate on target, overshooting the target, or taking more than two eye movements to reach the target might indicate a poor performance. In this case, the eyes will move in a jerky or jumpy style, which is normal.

3. **Smooth pursuit neck torsion test (SPNT).** The same as test 1 but with the trunk rotated to achieve 45 degrees of cervical rotation (head remains still). Impaired performance in torsion compared to neutral is suggestive of a cervical afferent influence. This manoeuvre stimulates the cervical but not the vestibular receptors and has shown potential to identify abnormal cervical afferent input, as an underlying cause of sensorimotor disturbance (Tjell and Rosenhall, 1998; Williams et al., 2017; Yu et al., 2011).

If reproduction of dizziness and or blurred vision occurs during tests 1 and 2, the clinician is immediately reassured that the spectre of CAD is much lower on the index of suspicion, as the vascular system has NOT been stressed during either of these manoeuvres. In other words, symptoms were reproduced by eye movements alone.

Test 3 should be performed after an initial check for dizziness in the first instance (following the 45-degree torsion position), followed by smooth pursuit eye movement. Reproduction of dizziness following eye movements would again implicate oculomotor dysfunction related to sensorimotor disturbance.

Further testing

Once the clinician is reassured that CAD is unlikely, further testing of the sensorimotor system can take place via assessment of gaze stability and eye–head coordination.

4. **Gaze stability.** The patient is asked to maintain visual focus on a target as he/she actively moves the head slowly into variations of rotation/flexion/extension. The clinician should observe for the ability to maintain focus, smoothness of movement and/or reproduction of symptoms. Impaired function may provide a direction for rehabilitation.

5. **Eye–head coordination.** The patient initiates eye movement to a point to focus and then, while maintaining focus, moves the head to that point. This can be performed to the left and right, and up and down. The clinician should observe for the inability of the patient to keep their head still while their eyes move, loss of focus during the head movements and/or reproduction of symptoms. These findings would support a sensorimotor hypothesis (Kristjansson and Treleaven, 2009) and provide a direction for rehabilitation.

6. **Optokinetic assessment.** The patient is positioned 90 cm away from a wall with a laser pointer attached to his/her head; the patient is asked to rotate left, right or into extension and relocate to a 'normal head position'. The measurement of the end position compared to the starting position is taken in millimetres, either negative or positive, to indicate over- or undershooting, respectively. The clinician should observe for any reproduction of dizziness, jerky movements or a large discrepancy in joint position error (de Vries et al., 2015) when testing with eyes open compared to eyes closed. A finding of impaired proprioception may provide a direction for rehabilitation.

7. **Head–body disassociation.** The patient is asked to maintain a stable head position, using laser as feedback if necessary, whilst moving their torso in a range of activities.

8. **Postural control system.** This includes all the sensorimotor and musculoskeletal elements involved in the control of postural orientation and equilibrium. The tonic neck reflex (TNR) is activated by muscles in the cervical spine and activates muscles in the body to create a base of support for balance and stable posture. The function of the system can be assessed indirectly via tests such as the Romberg's test or the Balance Error Scoring System (BESS) (Iverson and Koehle, 2013) to evaluate vestibular, visual and proprioceptive contributions to balance. Impaired balance, as compared to normative data, may be a direction for rehabilitation of affected patients.

Motor function

The neck musculature is responsible for maintenance of cervicocranial posture and for directing motion of the head. As such, it has been used as an indicator of neck dysfunction. However, uncertainty remains about the effectiveness of exercise for neck pain (Gross et al., 2015). A systematic review in 2015 suggested that, despite a paucity of high-quality evidence, 'Using specific strengthening exercises as part of routine practice for chronic neck pain, cervicogenic headache and radiculopathy may be beneficial' (Gross et al., 2015). The Neck Pain Guidelines: Revision 2017, incorporated exercise as part of multimodal treatment for acute and chronic neck pain. Controversy remains as to the optimal dosage, type and frequency of exercise (Gross et al., 2015). Notwithstanding the uncertainty, there is some encouraging preliminary research that suggests that neck strengthening may have a role in decreasing neck injury rates (Naish et al., 2013) and may indeed be a protective factor for reducing concussion. Neck muscles are accessory for breathing (Axen et al., 1992) and the cervical extensors maintain head position via an endurance role (Taylor et al., 2006), which is minimal during normal activity but may be tested maximally in sporting environments.

Clinical management and rehabilitation strategies

Isometric training

Isometric training has long been advocated in the management of cervical spine pain and dysfunction (Jull et al., 2008). The use of craniocervical flexion test (CCFT) as an assessment for deep neck flexor (DNF) function and endurance has been a feature of physiotherapy practice for decades. DNF exercises have been prescribed as a remedy for patients with neck pain and dysfunction. However, the authors propose that this apparent overfocus on isometric deep neck flexors is akin to offering static quadriceps exercises to a patient with acute or chronic knee dysfunction in the vain hope that they will recover full function. Clinicians should consider isometric exercise as merely a starting point in the rehabilitation process and incorporate progressive resistance programmes that include all cervical muscle groups. That said, recruitment of deep neck flexors is supported broadly by the literature (Jull et al., 2009) and may be considered to be a reasonable starting point for neuromuscular rehabilitation following sports injury. This, however, should be rapidly followed by an exercise regime that targets a variety of muscle groups, as preliminary investigations have found isometric neck strength and training were directly related to neck injury and concussion risk in sport (Hrysomallis, 2016).

Global strength training

Neck strengthening has been associated with reduced injury rates in rugby (Naish et al., 2013) and postulated to be a protective factor reducing risk for concussion in high school sports (Collins et al., 2014). Strength deficits can be identified either by manual muscle testing, handheld

Table 26.2 Exercises used in the neck strengthening intervention programme for a men's professional rugby union team

Name of exercise	Description of exercise
Isometric cable hold – neck flexion	In standing, a head harness is placed around the forehead with the cable at the level of the occiput. Player faces away from the weight stack and retracts the neck by 'tucking in' the chin. Player takes the weight then steps and leans forward to lift the weight stack using the neck flexors. Weight is held for 5 s
Isometric cable hold – neck extension	In standing, a head harness is placed around the forehead with cable at the level of the forehead. Player faces toward the weight stack and retracts the neck by 'tucking in' the chin. Player takes the weight then steps and leans backward to lift the weight stack using the neck extensors. Weight is held for 5 s
Isometric cable hold – right and left lateral flexion	In standing, a head harness is placed around the forehead so the cable is just above the left/right ear. Player faces side-on to where the weight stack is located. Player then takes a sideways step away from the weight stack and leans laterally using the lateral neck muscles. Weight is held for 5 s
Isometric cable hold – 45-degree neck flexion left and right	In standing, place the head harness so it is located between the occiput and the left/right ear. Player steps away from the weight stack on an angle so that the resistance is pulling the neck into extension on one side (left or right) at a 45 degree angle. Weight is held for 5s
Isometric cable hold – bent-over neck extension	In a crouched position, hips and knees are flexed at approximately 120 degrees. Player faces towards the weight stack and retracts the neck by 'tucking in' the chin, then takes the weight. The cable is directed towards the floor. The player then pulls backward using neck extensors. Weight is held for 5 s
Isometric cable hold – bent-over lateral flexion	In a crouched position, hips and knees are flexed at approximately 120 degrees. Player crouches side-on to the weight stack and places the head harness around the head so the cable is positioned just above the left/right ear. Player takes a sideways step away from the weight stack and leans sideways using the lateral neck muscles. Weight is held for 5 s
Tight head prop isometric cable hold – bent-over right lateral neck flexion with shoulder/pectoral fly	Exercise is performed in a cable fly machine. In a crouched position, hips and knees are flexed at approximately 120 degrees. Head harness is placed around the forehead so the cable is at the level of the left ear. Player positions themselves side-on to the weight stack then takes a sideways step to the right away from the weight stack and leans laterally using the right lateral neck muscles. At the same time, the player uses their arm right to pull the other cable positioned on the floor into the chest. Weight is held for 5 s
Loose head prop isometric cable hold – bent-over lateral neck flexion with shoulder latissimus dorsi pull-down	Exercise is performed in cable fly machine. In a couched position, hips and knees are flexed at approximately 120 degrees. Head harness is placed around the forehead so the cable is just above the level of the left ear. Player positions themselves side-on to the weight stack and takes a sideways step to the right away from the weight stack and leans laterally using the right lateral neck muscles. At the same time, the player uses their left arm to pull the other cable positioned on the floor to perform a horizontal latissimus dorsi pull-down. Weight is held for 5 s
Scrum truck simulation – lateral neck flexors and extensors	Exercise is performed in the scrum-simulating machine. While loading the pads with leg drive, the player's neck muscles resist a load applied to the head by the physiotherapist or strength and conditioner. This exercise can be performed at all angles with feedback provided by a sphygmomanometer placed between the hands of the person creating the load and the player's head. The isometric load is created for 5 s

Source: Naish, R., Burnett, A., Burrows, S., Andrews, W., Appleby, B., 2013. Can a specific neck strengthening program decrease cervical spine injuries in a men's professional rugby union team? A retrospective analysis. Journal of Sports Science and Medicine 12 (3), 542–550, with permission.

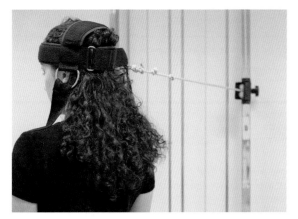

Fig. 26.6 Isometric cable hold for side flexion.

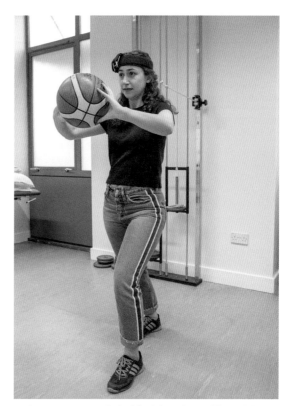

Fig. 26.8 Isometric hold with task specific activity.

Table 26.2 describes a range of isometric progressions specific to rugby. Figs 26.6–26.8 also illustrate progressions from isometric holds through to function-specific strength training. The training approach should adopt the principle of progressive resistance training, where the resistance is incrementally increased when the prescribed number of repetitions is attained (Minshull and Gleeson 2017).

Endurance training

To date, two papers have shown that both strength and endurance training were effective for treating neck pain (Nikander 2006; Ylinen et al., 2007). However, these studies were on chronic neck pain patients and it remains unknown whether this can be extrapolated to a sporting population who are likely to be at a much higher starting point from a strength and endurance perspective. At this point, it is reasonable to include endurance training in a balanced programme for return to sport.

Plyometric training

The effectiveness of plyometric training and perturbation training on head acceleration, cervical stiffness and injury risk

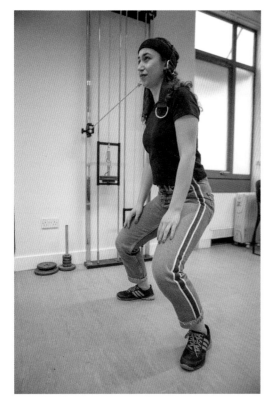

Fig. 26.7 Isometric hold of neck during squat performance.

dynamometer (Versteegh et al., 2015) or more sophisticated methods such as the GS Gatherer (Barrett et al., 2015). Preliminary research suggests neck strength, range of motion and susceptibility to fatigue can be influenced by focused neck training regimes (Hrysomallis, 2016).

A range of testing and rehabilitation exercises are accessible to patients and clinicians with basic gym equipment.

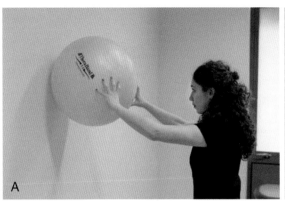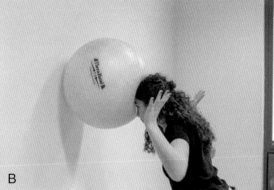

Fig. 26.9 Simple neck specific plyometric targeting and impact. (A) Preparation stage, hold ball at suitable height for a target for head, (B) letting go of ball with hands and moving head onto ball before ball falls.

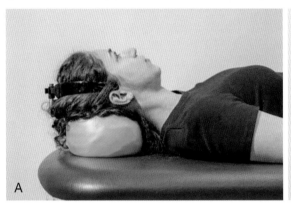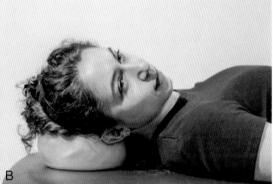

Fig. 26.10 Early stage sensorimotor activity with laser. From a neutral position (A), patient is instructed to move laser within a small target area whilst head is on deflated ball (B).

remain unclear. Whilst these techniques are used as part of training programmes anecdotally in top-level sport including Formula 1 motor racing, martial arts, boxing and rugby, few studies have evaluated their efficacy. Fig. 26.9 demonstrates and example of simple, neck-specific plyometric exercises.

Sensorimotor system training

Proprioceptive neck training as part of a sensorimotor training programme has been proposed as another area for development, but may be restricted because of the perceived need for sophisticated and expensive equipment (Alricsson et al., 2004). Identified deficits in cervical spine joint position sense (proprioception) can be retrained simply using laser pointers mounted on headbands as described above (Figs 26.10–26.12). Similarly identified deficits in oculomotor control can be divided into exercises performed with the head stationary and while the head is moving. This mimics common sports activities. Athletes need to progress to functional, dynamic tasks, progressing from walking to running with head turns to the left and right or up and down, whilst

retaining direction and velocity (Fig. 26.13). Introducing ball work is particularly relevant to this area of training to add increasing complexity. Therapists should strive to introduce key functional elements of the sport into all the training tasks, in order to maintain interest and facilitate return to play.

Mental health perspectives

It is well recognized that physical and psychological readiness to return to sport after injury do not always coincide (Clement et al., 2015; Podlog and Eklund, 2010). Andersen (2001) argues that returning an injured athlete to full activity is a complicated and multifaceted process. The process is influenced by a plethora of factors, including the characteristics of the injury along with biological, psychological and social variables. These factors have been listed as: the characteristics of the injury, sociodemographic factors, biological, psychological and social/contextual factors (Brewer et al., 2002).

343

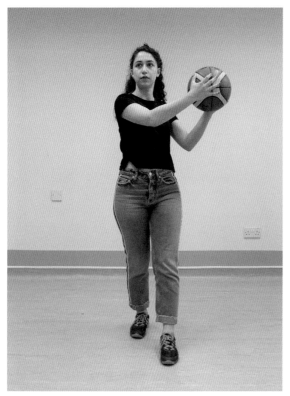

Fig. 26.11 Early stage sensorimotor activity with laser. Patient rotates head to hit various laser targets with head and deflated ball.

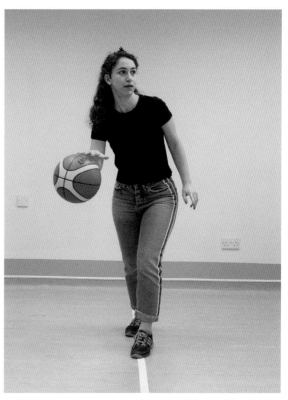

Fig. 26.13 Late stage sensorimotor activity. Training task specific head–body–limb coordination and control.

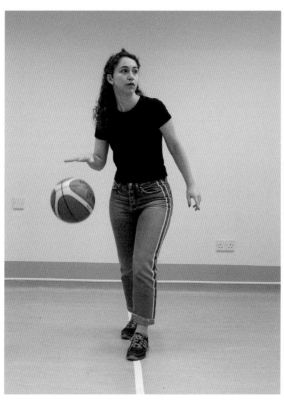

Fig. 26.12 Midstage sensorimotor activity. Task-specific head–body disassociation with laser feedback.

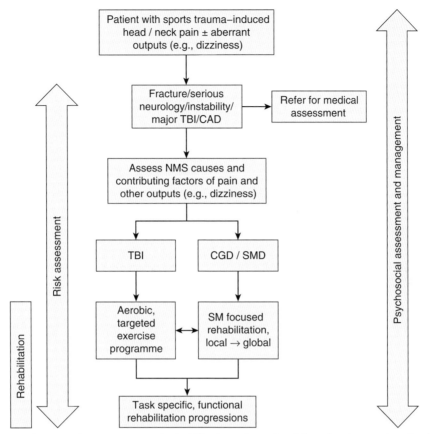

Fig. 26.14 Algorithm for the risk assessment and rehabilitation of people with neck pain associated with sports trauma. *CAD,* Cervical artery dysfunction; *CGD,* cervicogenic dizziness; *NMS,* neuromuscular system; *SMD,* sensorimotor dysfunction; *TBI,* traumatic brain injury.

The cervical spine is often considered a vulnerable part of human anatomy by athletes and clinicians. Commonly athletes may not fully disclose their injury-related emotions; equally, some clinicians may be reluctant to progress rehabilitation due to perceived risk. Studies have suggested that in any injury there should be a consideration of strategies to improve an athlete's emotional integrity and regularly monitor psychosocial factors throughout rehabilitation (Forsdyke et al., 2016). Considerations of the athlete's self-confidence and emotions of anxiety/fear is thought to increase the likelihood of a successful rehabilitation. The injury experience can be framed as an opportunity for growth and development. Wherever possible, clinicians should enable athletes to perceive an injury experience as positive, as this is known to be related to positive outcomes. Physical and psychosocial recovery from injury seldom occurs within the same timeframe. It is essential to ensure that injured athletes are physically, psychologically, socially, tactically and technically ready to return to sport (Forsdyke et al., 2016). Similarly, clinicians should be knowledgeable and skilled at delivering the pragmatic management options that are supported by the current evidence in an anatomical region that is sadly neglected.

Summary

- The cervical spine is often an underrehabilitated area of the body.
- Clinicians must have a systematic approach to risk assessment that considers potential fracture, instability and/or cervical arterial dysfunction in cases of sports trauma.
- Dizziness and associated symptoms may be linked to benign dysfunction of the cervical spine or postconcussive syndromes, which may have links to the sensorimotor system, all of which can be successfully identified and rehabilitated.
- Rehabilitation should take a multifaceted approach, incorporating motor, sensory and psychosocial dimensions.
- A risk assessment and rehabilitation strategy is summarized in Fig. 26.14.

References

Alricsson, M., Harms-Ringdahl, K., Larsson, B., Linder, J., Werner, S., 2004. Neck muscle strength and endurance in fighter pilots: effects of a supervised training program. Aviation, Space, and Environmental Medicine. 75 (1), 23–28.

Andersen, M.B., Van Raalte, J.L., Brewer, B.W., 2001. Sport psychology service delivery: staying ethical while keeping loose. Psychology: Research and Practice. 32 (1), 12–18.

Axen, K., Haas, F., Schicchi, J., Merrick, J., 1992. Progressive resistance neck exercises using a compressible ball coupled with an air pressure gauge. Journal of Orthopaedic & Sports Physical Therapy. 16 (6), 275–280.

Barrett, M.D., McLoughlin, T.F., Gallagher, K.R., Gatherer, D., Parratt, M.T., Perera, J.R., et al., 2015. Effectiveness of a tailored neck training program on neck strength, movement, and fatigue in under-19 male rugby players: a randomized controlled pilot study. Open Access Journal of Sports Medicine. 6, 137–147.

Beletsky, V., Nadareishvili, Z., Lynch, J., Shuaib, A., Woolfenden, A., Norris, J.W., Canadian Stroke Consortium, 2003. Cervical arterial dissection: time for a therapeutic trial? Stroke 34 (12), 2856–2860.

Biousse, V., D'Anglejan-Chatillon, J., Touboul, P.J., Amarenco, P., Bousser, M.G., 1995. Time course of symptoms in extracranial carotid artery dissections. A series of 80 patients. Stroke 26 (2), 235–239.

Brajkovic, S., Riboldi, G., Govoni, A., Corti, S., Bresolin, N., Comi, G.P., 2013. Growing evidence about the relationship between vessel dissection and scuba diving. Case Reports in Neurology 5 (3), 155–161.

Brewer, B.W., Andersen, M.B., Van Raalte, J.L., 2002. Psychological aspects of sport injury rehabilitation: toward a biopsychosocial approach. In: Mostofsky, D.L., Zaichkowsky, L.D. (Eds.), Medical and Psychological Aspects of Sport and Exercise. Fitness Information Technology, Morgantown, WV, pp. 41–54.

Cantu, R.C., 2014. Neck strength: a protective factor reducing risk for concussion in high school sports. Journal of Primary Prevention. 35 (5), 309–319.

Clement, D., Arvinen-Barrow, M., Fetty, T., 2015. Psychosocial responses during different phases of sport-injury rehabilitation: a qualitative study. Journal of Athletic Training 50 (1), 95–104.

Collins CL, Fletcher EN, Fields SK, Kluchurosky L, Rohrkemper MK, Comstock RD, Crissey, M.M., Bernstein, E.F., 1974. Delayed presentation of carotid intimal tear following blunt craniocervical trauma. Surgery 75 (4), 543–549.

de Vries, J., Ischebeck, B.K., Voogt, L.P., van der Geest, J.N., Janssen, M., Frens, M.A., et al., 2015. Joint position sense error in people with neck pain: a systematic review. Manual Therapy 20 (6), 736–744.

Degen, R.M., Fink, M.E., Callahan, L., Fibel, K., Ramsay, J., Kelly, B.T., 2017. Internal carotid artery dissection after indirect blunt cervical trauma in an ice hockey goaltender. American Journal of Orthopedics 46 (3), E139–E143.

Dorland W.A.N. 2012. Dorland's Illustrated Medical Dictionary, thirty second ed. Saunders/Elsevier, Philadelphia, PA.

Forsdyke, D., Smith, A., Jones, M., Gledhill, A., 2016. Psychosocial factors associated with outcomes of sports injury rehabilitation in competitive athletes: a mixed studies systematic review. British Journal of Sports Medicine 50 (9), 537–544.

Fragoso, Y.D., Adoni, T., do Amaral, L.L., Braga, F.T., Brooks, J.B., Campos, C.S., et al., 2016. Cerebrum-cervical arterial dissection in adults during sports and recreation. Arquivos de Neuro-Psiquiatria 74 (4), 275–279.

Gottesman, R.F., Sharma, P., Robinson, K.A., Arnan, M., Tsui, M., Ladha, K., et al., 2012. Clinical characteristics of symptomatic vertebral artery dissection: a systematic review. Neurologist 18 (5), 245–254.

Gross, A., Kay, TM., Paquin, JP., Blanchette, S., Lalonde, P., Christie, T., et al. Cervical Overview Group. Exercises for mechanical neck disorders.

Hides, J.A., Franettovich Smith, M.M., Mendis, M.D., Smith, N.A., Cooper, A.J., Treleaven, J., et al., 2017. A prospective investigation of changes in the sensorimotor system following sports concussion. An exploratory study. Musculoskeletal Science & Practice 29, 7–19.

Hrysomallis, C., 2016. Neck muscular strength, training, performance and sport injury risk: a review. Sports Medicine 46 (8), 1111–1124.

Iverson, G.L., Koehle, M.S., 2013. Normative data for the balance error scoring system in adults. Rehabilitation Research and Practice 2013, 846418.

Jull, G.A., Falla, D., Vicenzino, B., Hodges, P.W., 2009. The effect of therapeutic exercise on activation of the deep cervical flexor muscles in people with chronic neck pain. Manual Therapy 14 (6), 696–701.

Jull, G.A., O'Leary, S.P., Falla, D.L., 2008. Clinical assessment of the deep cervical flexor muscles: the craniocervical flexion test. Journal of Manipulative and Physiological Therapeutics 31 (7), 525–533.

Kristensen, B., Malm, J., Carlberg, B., Stegmayr, B., Backman, C., Fagerlund, M., et al., 1997. Epidemiology and etiology of ischemic stroke in young adults aged 18 to 44 years in northern Sweden. Stroke 28 (9), 1702–1709.

Kristjansson, E., Treleaven, J., 2009. Sensorimotor function and dizziness in neck pain: implications for assessment and management. Journal of Orthopaedic & Sports Physical Therapy 39 (5), 364–377. .

Lamb, S.E., Williams, M.A., Williamson, E.M., Gates, S., Withers, E.J., Mt-Isa, S., et al., 2012. Managing Injuries of the Neck Trial (MINT): a randomised controlled trial of treatments for whiplash injuries. Health Technology Assessment 16 (49), iii-iv, 1–141.

Langer, P.R., Fadale, P.D., Palumbo, M.A., 2008. Catastrophic neck injuries in the collision sport athlete. Sports Medicine and Arthroscopy Review 16 (1), 7–15.

Martinelli, O., Venosi, S., BenHamida, J., Malaj, A., Belli, C., Irace, F.G., et al., 2017. Therapeutic options in the management of carotid dissection. Vascular Surgery 41, 69–76.

McCrory, P., Meeuwisse, W., Dvořák, J., Aubry, M., Bailes, J., Broglio, S., et al., 2017. Consensus statement on concussion in sport – the 5th international conference on concussion in sport held in Berlin, October. British Journal of Sports Medicine 51 (11), 838–847.

Minshull, C., Gleeson, N., 2017. Considerations of the principles of resistance training in exercise studies for the management of knee osteoarthritis: a systematic review. Archives of Physical Medicine and Rehabilitation 98 (9), 1842–1851.

Naish, R., Burnett, A., Burrows, S., Andrews, W., Appleby, B., 2013. Can a specific neck strengthening program decrease cervical spine injuries in a men's professional rugby union team? a retrospective analysis. Journal of Sports Science and Medicine 12 (3), 542–550.

Neck pain guidelines: revision 2017: using the evidence to guide physical therapist practice. Journal of Orthopaedic & Sports Physical Therapy. 47 (7), 2017, 511–512.

Nikander, R., Mälkiä, E., Parkkari, J., Heinonen, A., Starck, H., Ylinen, J., 2006. Dose-response relationship of specific training to reduce chronic neck pain and disability. Medicine & Science in Sports & Exercise. 38 (12), 2068–2074.

Olympia, R.P., Dixon, T., Brady, J., Avner, J.R., 2007. Emergency planning in school-based athletics: a national survey of athletic trainers. Pediatric Emergency Care 23 (10), 703–708.

Petschauer, M.A., Schmitz, R., Gill, D.L., 2010. Helmet fit and cervical spine motion in collegiate men's lacrosse athletes secured to a spine board. Journal of Athletic Training 45 (3), 215–221.

Podlog, L., Eklund, R.C., 2010. Returning to competition after a serious injury: the role of self-determination. Journal of Sports Sciences. 28 (8), 819–831.

Rao, A.S., Makaroun, M.S., Marone, L.K., Cho, J.S., Rhee, R., Chaer, R.A., 2011. Long-term outcomes of internal carotid artery dissection. Journal of Vascular Surgery 54 (2), 370.

Reiley, A.S., Vickory, F.M., Funderburg, S.E., Cesario, R.A., Clendaniel, R.A., 2017. How to diagnose cervicogenic dizziness. Archives of Physiotherapy 7, 12. ; PubMed Central PMCID: PMC5759906..

Reilly, B.M., 1990. Dizziness. In: Walker, H.K., Hall, W.D., Hurst, J.W. (Eds.), Clinical Methods: The History, Physical, and Laboratory Examinations, third ed. Butterworths, Boston. Chapter 212.

Rihn, J.A., Anderson, D.T., Lamb, K., Deluca, P.F., Bata, A., Marchetto, P.A., et al., 2009. Cervical spine injuries in american football. Sports Medicine 39 (9), 697–708.

Rushton, A., Rivett, D., Carlesso, L., Flynn, T., Hing, W., Kerry, R., 2014. International framework for examination of the cervical region for potential of cervical arterial dysfunction prior to orthopaedic manual therapy intervention. Manual Therapy 19 (3), 222–228.

Sanelli, P.C., Tong, S., Gonzalez, R.G., Eskey, C.J., 2002. Normal variation of vertebral artery on CT angiography and its implications for diagnosis of acquired pathology. Journal of Computer Assisted Tomography. 26 (3), 462–470.

Simon, L.V., Mohseni, M., 2017. Vertebral Artery Injury. StatPearls Publishing, Treasure Island (FL).

Stiell, I.G., Wells, G.A., Vandemheen, K.L., Clement, C.M., Lesiuk, H., De Maio, V.J., et al., 2001. The Canadian C-spine rule for radiography in alert and stable trauma patients. JAMA 286 (15), 1841–1848.

Suzuki, S., Tsuchimochi, R., Abe, G., Yu, I., Inoue, T., Ishibashi, H., 2018. Traumatic vertebral artery dissection in high school rugby players: a report of two cases. Journal of Clinical Neuroscience 47, 137–139.

Taylor, M.K., Hodgdon, J.A., Griswold, L., Miller, A., Roberts, D.E., Escamilla, R.F., 2006. Cervical resistance training: effects on isometric and dynamic strength. Aviation, Space, and Environmental Medicine. 77 (11), 1131–1135.

Tjell, C., Rosenhall, U., 1998. Smooth pursuit neck torsion test: a specific test for cervical dizziness. American Journal of Otolaryngology 19 (1), 76–81.

Treleaven, J., 2008. Sensorimotor disturbances in neck disorders affecting postural stability, head and eye movement control. Manual Therapy 13 (1), 2–11.

Versteegh, T., Beaudet, D., Greenbaum, M., Hellyer, L., Tritton, A., Walton, D., 2015. Evaluating the reliability of a novel neck-strength assessment protocol for healthy adults using self-generated resistance with a hand-held dynamometer. Journal of Physiotherapy 67 (1), 58–64.

Williams, K., Tarmizi, A., Treleaven, J., 2017. Use of neck torsion as a specific test of neck related postural instability. Musculoskeletal Science & Practice 29, 115–119.

Ylinen, J., Häkkinen, A., Nykänen, M., Kautiainen, H., Takala, E.P., 2007. Neck muscle training in the treatment of chronic neck pain: a three-year follow-up study. Europa Medicophysica 43 (2), 161–169.

Yu, L.J., Stokell, R., Treleaven, J., 2011. The effect of neck torsion on postural stability in subjects with persistent whiplash. Manual Therapy 16 (4), 339–343.

Chapter 27

Management of head injuries

Etienne Laverse, Akbar de Medici, Richard Sylvester, Simon Kemp and Ademola Adejuwon

Introduction

Concussion, also known as mild traumatic brain injury (mTBI), describes a clinical syndrome that follows head trauma. It accounts for >80% of the estimated 1.4 million TBI cases seen in hospitals in England and Wales annually and affects 1.6 to 3.8 million individuals in the US each year (Cancelliere et al., 2014; Levin and Diaz-Arrastia, 2015). Contact and collision sports have various degrees of risk for causing head trauma. Examples of higher risk sports include hockey, horse racing, rugby, soccer, football, basketball, cricket, snowboarding and skiing (Giza et al., 2013).

Although classified as 'mild', repeated mTBI can result in significant neurocognitive sequelae. Rarely, in the short term (hours to weeks), it may result in a potentially fatal 'second impact syndrome' where a player with mTBI has returned to play and then suffers catastrophic consequences following a second impact that is associated with cerebral autodysregulation and oedema (Khong et al., 2016; Khurana and Kaye, 2012). The long-term sequelae may consist of progressive cognitive impairment. It is therefore essential all individuals involved in sports, including coaches, trainers, parents and athletes, to have a practical understanding of the recognition and management of head injuries of their athletes.

Symptoms

The syndrome of mTBI comprises a constellation of symptoms following the biomechanical injury to the brain. Commonly reported symptoms include headache, visual disturbance, memory impairment, disorientation and loss of consciousness. Brain injury occurs as a consequence of either a force applied directly to the head, face or neck from contact with an opponent, the ground or another object, or from a force applied elsewhere to the body, with the impulsive force transferred to the head.

Diagnosis and management

Management guidelines in sport have been prepared largely from recognized consensus processes, e.g., the 2017 Concussion Sport Group (CISG) consensus statement (McCrory et al., 2016), with the aim of preventing further injury and limiting cumulative impact of repeated head injuries. Certain factors are thought to contribute to the risk of sustaining an mTBI. For example, it has been reported that female athletes may be more at risk in sports such as soccer or basketball. The type of sport played will also have an impact on the risk of head contact/collision frequency and intensity varies (Giza et al., 2013).

The first step in the management of mTBI is the prompt recognition of a potential mTBI. Suspected cases should be assessed by a member of the medical team or healthcare professional appropriately trained in how to carry out such assessments. Standard on-field immediate trauma care should be initiated, including the appropriate management of potential cervical spine injuries. The Sport Concussion Assessment Tool – 5th edition (SCAT5) (2017) should be used to support the initial assessment by healthcare professionals. It is also important in the early phase to identify signs and symptoms that may reflect more significant injury, e.g., persisting focal deficit or low Glasgow Coma Scale (GCS) score. These indicators suggest moderate to severe brain injuries requiring further investigations and management. This should lower the threshold for brain imaging such as computed tomography (CT) or magnetic resonance imaging (MRI).

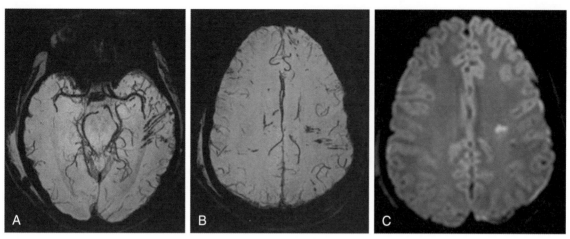

Fig. 27.1 MRI of diffuse axonal injury. Susceptibility-weighted imaging (SWI) and diffusion-weighted imaging (DWI) showing microbleeds and shearing injuries respectively.

Any athlete with suspected concussion should be removed from play, medically assessed and monitored for deterioration. No athlete diagnosed with concussion should return to play on the day of injury.

Subsequent steps in the management of mTBI comprise a graduated return to study, work and play that includes regular assessments for symptoms and graded physical activity, in order to allow for full recovery, optimal fitness and safety for future sporting activities.

mTBI involves complex pathophysiological processes affecting the brain following mechanical impact. Angular, rotational or linear acceleration of the brain can result in neuronal shearing and dysfunction. Only 10% of these cases have an associated loss of consciousness; this is thought to be a result of transient interruption in the reticular activating system (Khurana and Kaye, 2012). It is believed that a complex time-dependent evolution of pathologies (a neurometabolic cascade) occurs postinjury – this is substantiated in animal models. Disruption of ion channels on neural membranes allows for an efflux of K^+ and an influx of Ca^{2+}, and an activation of Na^+/K^+ pumps in an attempt to restore ionic balance. This process is highly energy consuming. Inflammatory cytokines are also considered to underlie the molecular cascade of events that follow mTBI and inflammation may play a central pathophysiological role (Khurana and Kaye, 2012).

The diagnosis and management of mTBI is largely based on the detection and monitoring of signs and symptoms. It is acknowledged that objective markers to diagnose, grade and prognosticate are lacking; research is underway to explore molecular and brain imaging markers to assist in the process. Optimal management is crucial as there may also be scholastic and financial implications, particularly for younger athletes (Hobbs et al., 2016).

All current diagnostic schema require that the athlete experiences an external force to the head followed by some alteration in brain function. The guidelines mandate that in all suspected cases of mTBI the individual should be removed from play and assessed by a licensed healthcare provider. mTBI education targeted at athletes and coaches is therefore important to encourage symptom reporting and prompt recognition of mTBI.

Frequently observed features following mTBI include a vacant stare, confusion, delayed motor and verbal responses, disorientation, memory deficits and incoordination. The majority of single-episode noncomplicated adult mTBI patients recover spontaneously within the first few days to weeks postinjury, with 80–95% of athletes having returned to baseline neurocognitive measures between 3 and 6 months postinjury. Cognitive dysfunction can persist for a longer period and diffuse axonal injury (DAI) in the brain (Figs 27.1 and 27.2) is thought to be the primary pathology (Kawata et al., 2016; Siman et al., 2015).

Immediate pitch-side recognition of mTBI

The current consensus is that anyone with a suspected mTBI should immediately be removed from the field of play. mTBI should be suspected following a head injury event if any of the signs or symptoms in Box 27.1 are observed or reported.

Several professional sports have introduced off-field screens for athletes with suspected and possible mTBI. These screening protocols are designed to determine whether a player who has sustained a head injury event where the consequences of the head impact are unclear needs to be definitively removed from play; they are not used to make or refute a diagnosis of concussion, unless

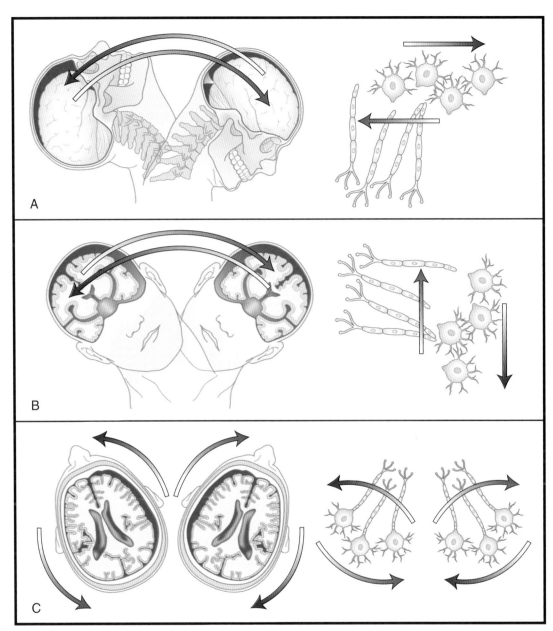

Fig. 27.2 Traumatic brain injury: axonal and sheer injury. Angular or linear acceleration of the brain can result in neuronal shearing and dysfunction.

observable signs at the time of the head impact are seen. These protocols are only used in elite adult sports where trained and experienced doctors are present. In all other settings, 'recognize and remove' should be used.

The key elements of the 10-minute off-field World Rugby Head Injury Assessment (HIA 1) are: review of game footage for presence of observable signs, memory assessment

questions, tests of immediate and delayed memory, ability to reverse strings of numbers, tandem gait/walking test of balance, concussion symptom check, review by doctor for other signs of concussion (Fig. 27.3) and second review of game footage for presence of observable signs.

If observable signs are seen on the video, or if the player makes errors in the assessment, or if in the doctor's

Box 27.1 Observable signs and symptoms of mild traumatic brain injury

Signs

- Loss of consciousness
- Lying motionless on the ground
- Slow to rise/unsteady/balance problems
- Grabbing/clutching head
- Dazed/blank look

Symptoms

- Headache
- Dizziness
- Fatigue/drowsiness
- Nausea/vomiting
- Feeling or demonstrating slowed down/mental clouding, emotional change or sadness
- Blurred vision

judgement the player is showing any signs of concussion, then the player does not return to play. This approach was first pioneered during the Rugby World Cup 2015 and has seen the number of players not removed at the time of their concussion reduce from 50% to less than 10%.

The addition of sideline and medical room real-time video review offers improved identification and evaluation of head impacts and allows for a more comprehensive review of the whole process.

Red flags

A *red flag* is a potential indicator of serious pathology. Although mTBI usually runs a benign course, the possibility of more severe injury should be considered as part of the assessment process as these may require additional management steps. Signs and symptoms that may indicate more significant injury, and therefore prompt further investigations such as brain imaging (Figs 27.4 and 27.5), are shown in Box 27.2.

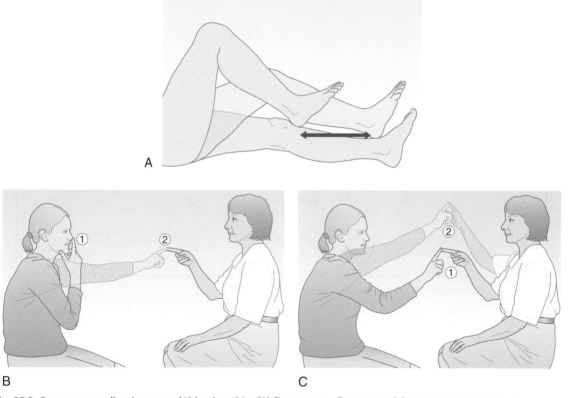

Fig. 27.3 Common coordination tests: (A) heel to shin; (B) finger–nose–finger test; (C) examiner moving the target finger. (1) Elbow flexed; (2) elbow extended.

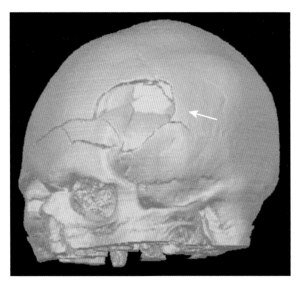

Fig. 27.4 Depressed skull fracture.

- symptom evaluation (e.g., headache, nausea, dizziness, feeling as if 'in a fog', sensitivity to light/noise)
- memory tests
- concentration tests
- neurological screen
- coordination tests
- balance tests.

The use of mTBI SCAT5 symptom scales help with the documenting of symptom progression as a function of time. Greater symptom burden at initial presentation is associated with poorer recovery. Headache is the most common symptom, followed by dizziness.

If a concussive event is witnessed or suspected and if any one of the above domains is deemed to be abnormal, then mTBI should be suspected and the appropriate management instituted. Where more serious injury is suspected, e.g., with the identification of red flag symptoms or signs, athletes should be transferred to the nearest emergency/trauma centre for more acute care.

Investigations

mTBI is a clinical diagnosis and investigations are used when more severe injury is suspected. These include standard CT brain imaging and/or MRI. Standard brain scan sequences are usually normal in mTBI. CT scans can detect acute bleeding (e.g., subdural haemorrhage) and cranial fractures. However, certain MRI sequences, such as susceptibility-weighted imaging (SWI) (see Fig. 27.1), may reveal microvascular changes associated with mTBI in the form of microbleeds, and diffusion tensor imaging

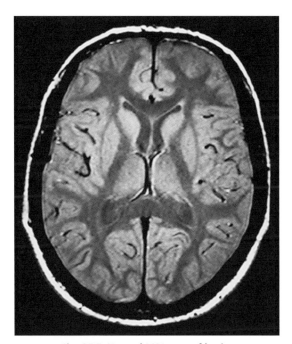

Fig. 27.5 Normal MRI scan of brain.

Clinical assessment

Athletes suspected of an mTBI should initially be assessed by healthcare providers using the SCAT5. The diagnostic process comprises an assessment of multiple domains, including:

can provide information on diffuse axonal and vascular injuries that standard scans may not detect (Sharp et al., 2011; Sharp and Jenkins, 2015). The clinical significance of these findings is not fully understood. Nonetheless, subtle vascular changes or other brain changes may not be revealed by the usual standard scans and therefore radiological correlates are not routinely observed.

Acute management

The athlete with suspected mTBI should be immediately removed from play and be medically evaluated on-site using standard emergency prehospital care. Particular attention should be given to excluding cervical spine injury. If this cannot be excluded, the athlete must be immobilized, leaving in place any sports equipment not interfering with clinical management, such as a helmet, and transferred to hospital for further evaluation and imaging.

Following the initial assessment and exclusion of significant traumatic injuries, a more focused assessment of domains affected by mTBI should be examined using standardized assessment tools such as the SCAT5.

mTBI is an evolving injury in the acute phase and the athlete should be observed over the initial few hours following injury for any deterioration (e.g., decreasing GCS score). Follow-up serial evaluation is advised as symptoms may evolve or have a delayed onset; a symptom check list is useful to track recovery.

It is important to appreciate that symptoms may develop over several hours and the extent of injury may not be immediately apparent. Therefore athletes should not be allowed to return to play on the day of injury. An expanding epidural haematoma can be the cause of neurological deterioration following a period of apparent improvement and in a minority of cases; cerebral contusion and subdural haematomas may also account for a lucid interval.

Treatment of mTBI

The key objective is to limit further injury. Cognitive and physical activities should be adjusted according to symptoms. The amount of exercise and rest following an injury should be proportional and complete prolonged rest is not considered to be the best approach. However, activities that require concentration, i.e., cognitively demanding tasks (e.g., playing video games) may exacerbate symptoms and premature physical exercise might intensify postconcussion symptoms and should be avoided for 24–48 hours. After an initial period of rest the athlete should look to return to activities of normal daily living. If symptoms are still present, these activities should be below the level that exacerbates symptoms (symptom-limited activity or relative rest). There is limited evidence to support the use of pharmacotherapy in the acute phase of mTBI management.

Following complete resolution of symptoms and after the minimum rest period stipulated by sport (14 days for rugby union and association football), the athlete can commence a stepwise return to play, ideally under medical supervision. A number of sport-specific protocols exist. These typically comprise distinct levels (Table 27.1). Adult athletes may progress each day to the next level if they are able to complete the current level without provocation of symptoms (Hobbs et al., 2016; McCrory et al., 2016); however, those aged 19 years and under are recommended to take 48 hours rather than 24 hours to complete each stage. Thus the adult athlete can complete the full protocol within a week if they remain asymptomatic throughout. If symptoms should recur, then it is advised that the athlete return to the previous level and attempt the physical activity again after a 24-hour period of rest. Medical review prior to resuming full contact training is recommended. Neuropsychological tests may help with providing objective measures of cognitive function and reduce a reliance on subjective symptom reporting by the athlete when advising on return to play. Recovery of cognitive performance to preseason level is part of the criteria used to decide when the athlete can return to play. However, this approach is itself not infallible and there is a definite need for more objective markers to aid in the assessment.

Chronic/persistent symptoms

Athletes generally recover within days to weeks. Risk factors for delayed recovery include:
- young age (<16 years)
- acute onset of migraine-type headaches
- memory deficit
- a recent history of mTBI.

The strongest predictor of slower recovery from mTBI is the severity of a person's initial symptoms in the first few days after injury. Notably, a low level of symptoms in the first day after injury is a favourable prognostic indicator. Studies have indicated that a preinjury neuropsychiatric disorder is related to persistence of symptoms for 3 months or longer after mTBI. Where symptoms extend beyond the usual 10–14 days in adults (>4 weeks in children), more specialist input can be helpful, such as from neurologists or sports physicians with expertise in managing mTBI. This can be in the setting of a dedicated concussion clinic (e.g., Institute of Sport and Exercise Health, London, UK) where additional investigations such as more detailed neuropsychological tests and advanced neuroimaging (e.g.,

Table 27.1 Graduated return to play protocol in athletes with mild traumatic brain injury

Rehabilitation stage	Functional exercise at each stage of rehabilitation	Objective for each stage
1. No activity	Physical and cognitive rest	Recovery
2a. If symptoms persist at 24 hours: symptom-limited activity	Initially activities of daily living that do not provoke symptoms. Consider time off or adaptation of work or study	Return to normal activities (as symptoms permit)
2b. Light aerobic exercise	Walking, swimming or stationary cycling, keeping intensity <70% of maximum predicted heart rate; no resistance training	Increase heart rate
3. Sport-specific exercise	Skating drills in ice hockey, running drills in soccer. No head impact activities	Add movement
4. Noncontact training drills	Progression to more complex training drills, e.g., passing drills in football and ice hockey; may start progressive resistance	Exercise, coordination and cognitive load
5. Full contact practice	Following medical clearance participate in normal training activities	Restore confidence and assess functional skills by coaching staff
4. Return to play	Normal game play	

SWI, fluid-attenuated inversion recovery or T2*-weighted sequences) can be considered in a multidisciplinary setting.

Symptoms such as dizziness and difficulty with balance may be a result of vestibular abnormalities and specialist input in the management of these can be addressed in such specialist clinics. Interventions including psychological, cervical and vestibular rehabilitation may be of benefit. Pharmacological treatment of headache (particularly with migrainous features) can be helpful if these symptoms persist beyond the first month after mild TBI.

The illustrative case in Box 27.3 highlights the potential complexities of mTBI and underscores the benefit of seeking specialist input for complex cases.

There has been increasing interest in the long-term effects of head injury in sports, primarily the neurocognitive abnormalities that can have a significant impact on players' (and retired players') wellbeing, with important psychosocial consequences. This has all led to increasing public concern about the effects of head injury in contact sports. It is thought that repetitive head injury, including subconcussive hits to the head, may be associated with a neurodegenerative tauopathy – chronic traumatic encephalopathy (CTE) with accumulation of tau protein in perivascular spaces in deep cortical sulci – in athletes (Ling et al., 2017).

Thus, seemingly innocuous mTBI may be associated with significant functional brain pathology. As a consequence of this increased recognition, sporting bodies have taken steps to minimize and, where possible, prevent the risk of mTBI. For example, stricter rule enforcement of red cards for high elbows in heading duels in professional soccer is supported by evidence of lower risk of head contacts and mTBI with such enforcements.

A history of mTBI is known to increase the risk of future injuries and baseline symptoms, as well as long-term cognitive and psychiatric dysregulation in athletes. It is also difficult to predict which athletes will suffer in the long-term as symptom resolution does not automatically indicate full recovery from the traumatic event.

The current approach to diagnosing mTBI relies on patient-reported symptoms and a neurological exam to assess the extent of injury. However athletes are known to underreport symptoms and this can negatively affect the diagnostic process. Neuropsychological tests are helpful and brain imaging in certain cases may provide added useful clinical information. Nonetheless the clinical evaluation remains limited as the extent of injury to the brain, particularly the microstructural changes that result from mTBI, remains largely unknown. The graduated return-to-play protocol is a useful guide to allow safe return to play – yet it is not effective for every case. Defining recovery by being symptom-free potentially risks premature return to play, putting athletes at risk of further trauma.

Research is underway to assess the validity of fluid biomarkers in the evaluation of mTBI in order to add further objective measures to the current assessment. However, these are not yet incorporated into clinical practice (Mercier et al., 2013). The majority of mTBI biomarker studies are generally hypothesis driven. It is hypothesized that damage to the neurovascular unit, consisting of brain microvascular

Box 27.3 **Case study**

Persistent symptoms following mild traumatic brain injury (mTBI)

A 21-year-old male university rugby player presents at 4-months postinjury, sustained playing rugby. He has no markers of severe TBI acutely and a normal CT head scan.

Persistent symptoms

The patient is unable to return to studies or physical activity due to severe headaches with migrainous features, he is using analgesia daily, experiences imbalance and dizziness, visual vertigo, fatigue, poor concentration and subjective memory impairment, low mood and anxiety.

Examination findings

Normal neurological and vestibular examination.

Investigation findings

MRI brain scan with susceptibility-weighted imaging sequences are normal with no evidence of diffuse axonal injury. Vestibular assessment shows evidence of unilateral peripheral vestibular dysfunction. Neuropsychology – mild global impairment largely due to attentional difficulties felt to reflect influence of low mood rather than impaired brain function.

Management approach

Posttraumatic migraine complicated by analgesia overuse is managed by reducing analgesia intake to <2 days/week and starting amitriptyline 10 mg (dose gradually increasing to 40 mg). Vestibular dysfunction managed with vestibular rehabilitation directed by a specialist physiotherapist. Mood disorder managed with cognitive behavioural therapy.

Outcome

Gradual symptom resolution over 3 months allowing return to academic studies and full physical activity.

endothelial cells and neurons, may permit some molecules to cross the blood–brain barrier (Kawata et al., 2016). Developing methods to detect these markers may help to diagnose mTBI promptly and accurately and, in turn, help to mitigate the long-term neurological effects. The need for diagnostic biomarkers as a more objective means to assess mTBI in athletes and to aid in prognosis is also highlighted in the recent consensus statement from the 5th International Conference on Concussion in Sport held in Berlin in 2016 (McCrory et al., 2017).

Electroencephalogram (EEG), advanced neuroimaging techniques, genetic testing and fluid biomarkers are some of the modalities that are currently being studied in the research setting and may add further objective components to our investigative and management steps of mTBI in the future.

It is envisaged that fluid biomarkers, including blood neuronal proteins, that reliably reflect the extent of neuronal injury could diagnose and predict clinical recovery and/or determine risk of potential cumulative impairments after injury. Neurofilament light polypeptide (NFL), found in large-caliber myelinated axons, is an example of a biomarker that has been found to be elevated in serum and cerebrospinal fluid (CSF) after TBI. Studies of boxers showed a positive correlation between head blows and CSF NFL levels as well as with symptom burden and recovery (Roy, 2017).

Although no gold standard exists for the diagnosis of mTBI, it is hoped that molecular and imaging markers may in the future improve the accuracy of assessing the severity of injury and help with prognosis and guidance for return to play. At present, it is important that established guidelines are adhered to, so that improved recognition of the syndrome can allow for optimal management to be instituted early in order to mitigate the long-term consequences of repeated mTBI.

Key points and take-home message

- Athletes with suspected concussion should be immediately removed from the field of play.
- Standard trauma care should be applied acutely, including examining for cervical spine injury.
- The process for diagnosing concussion acutely involves a clinical exam supported by the SCAT5 assessment tool.
- The mainstay of treatment is symptomatic management followed by a graded programme of exercise prior to full return to play.
- Modifications may need to be made to scholastic or work programmes.
- Athletes aged 19 years and below should be treated more conservatively.
- Athletes with persistent symptoms should be referred for specialist assessments by neurologists or sports physicians, e.g., in a concussion clinic setting.
- Repeated or single episodes of mTBI may be associated with long-term neurocognitive impairment and chronic traumatic encephalopathy.
- Radiological and molecular biomarker research is underway and may contribute further objective tools to aid in the overall management of mTBI.

References

Cancelliere, C., Hincapié, C.A., Keightley, M., Godbolt, A.K., Côté, P., Kristman, V.L., et al., 2014. Systematic review of prognosis and return to play after sport concussion: results of the international collaboration on mild traumatic brain injury prognosis. Archives of Physical Medicine and Rehabilitation 95, S210–S229.

Giza, C.C., Kutcher, J.S., Ashwal, S., Barth, J., Getchius, T.S.D., Gioia, G.A., et al., 2013. Summary of evidence-based guideline update: evaluation and management of concussion in sports: report of the Guideline Development Subcommittee of the American Academy of Neurology. Neurology 80, 2250–2257.

Hobbs, J.G., Young, J.S., Bailes, J.E., 2016. Sports-related concussions: diagnosis, complications, and current management strategies. Neurosurgery Focus 40, E5.

Kawata, K., Liu, C.Y., Merkel, S.F., Ramirez, S.H., Tierney, R.T., Langford, D., 2016. Blood biomarkers for brain injury: what are we measuring? Neuroscience and Biobehavioral Reviews. 68, 460–473.

Khong, E., Odenwald, N., Hashim, E., Cusimano, M.D., 2016. Diffusion tensor imaging findings in post-concussion syndrome patients after mild traumatic brain injury: a systematic review. Front Neurology 7, 156.

Khurana, V.G., Kaye, A.H., 2012. An overview of concussion in sport. Journal of Clinical Neuroscience 19, 1–11.

Levin, H.S., Diaz-Arrastia, R.R., 2015. Diagnosis, prognosis , and clinical management of mild traumatic brain injury. The Lancet Global Health 4422, 1–12.

Ling, H., Morris, H.R., Neal, J.W., Lees, A.J., Hardy, J., Holton, J.L., et al., 2017. Mixed pathologies including chronic traumatic encephalopathy account for dementia in retired association football (soccer) players. Acta Neuropathology 133, 337–352.

McCrory, P., Meeuwisse, W., Dvorak, J., Aubry, M., Bailes, J., Broglio, S., et al., 2017. Consensus statement on concussion in sport—the 5 th international conference on concussion in sport held in Berlin, October 2016. British Journal of Sports Medicine 51 (11), 838–847.

Mercier, E., Boutin, A., Lauzier, F., Fergusson, D.A., Simard, J.-F., Zarychanski, R., et al., 2013. Predictive value of S-100β protein for prognosis in patients with moderate and severe traumatic brain injury: systematic review and meta-analysis. British Medical Journal 346, 1–16, f1757.

Roy, P., 2017. A blood test for concussion? Neurology 1780–1781.

Sharp, D.J., Jenkins, P.O., 2015. Concussion is confusing us all. Practical Neurology 15, 172–186.

Sharp, D.J., Beckmann, C.F., Greenwood, R., Kinnunen, K.M., Bonnelle, V., De Boissezon, X., et al., 2011. Default mode network functional and structural connectivity after traumatic brain injury. Brain 134, 2233–2247.

Siman, R., Shahim, P., Tegner, Y., Blennow, K., Zetterberg, H., Smith, D.H., 2015. Serum SNTF increases in concussed professional ice hockey players and relates to the severity of postconcussion symptoms. Journal of Neurotrauma. 32, 1294–1300

Sport concussion assessment tool, 2017. Fifth ed. British Journal of Sports Medicine 51, 851–858. .

Chapter | 28 |

A high-performance approach to optimizing a major league soccer preseason

David McKay

Introduction

Preceding any team's competitive season, it is highly advisable to have a productive preparatory period. This preparation is known as the *preseason*, is commonly 3–12 weeks in duration and prepares the players, physically and tactically, for the demands of *inseason* competition. A variety of nonmodifiable aspects should be considered, including multiple games with short turn-around times, extensive travel, unique environmental factors, and the demands of the head coach's philosophy and desired style of play. The majority of time spent will be dedicated to building the players' fitness levels beyond previous inseason levels, along with teaching very specific tactical concepts in training and within a scheduled preseason games progression.

The preseason is when physical standards are established and reinforced. These standards set the expectations for the entire season. Arguably one of the two greatest objectives of the performance staff, in conjunction with the coaching staff, is to improve the players' soccer-specific athleticism. The other is having all players within the squad available for selection and ready to compete in the first game of the competitive season.

Professional soccer is continually becoming faster and more physically demanding; therefore the importance of the preseason for preparing players to meet the demands of this explosive sport has amplified considerably (Bush et al., 2015). In relation to this, players are now expected to return to preseason training with a respectable foundation of physical conditioning and strength to reduce their risk of injury and maximize performance improvements (Gabbett et al., 2016). Thus, implementation of an individualized offseason programme can optimize preseason readiness.

Below we outline how to arrive at, plan and deliver an optimal preseason to prepare for the grind of a soccer season.

The foundation: offseason

The offseason period often varies from 3 to 12 weeks in professional soccer. Implementing a low-volume offseason programme has shown to significantly increase the risk of injury upon returning to competitive training (Blanch and Gabbett, 2015). Ensuring a balance between passive/active recovery and offseason training is vital. The initial part of the offseason presents an opportunity for complete and active (crosstraining, tennis, etc.) recovery in an attempt to physically and mentally recover from the wear and tear of inseason competition (Malone et al., 2015). Following this period of prescribed recovery, an individualized, sport-specific programme is implemented, focusing on key performance indicators such as:
1. strength/power development
2. running volumes and intensities
3. soccer-specific conditioning.

Strength/power development

Having the appropriate amount of strength and power has been shown to build an individual's resilience to the competitive demands of the game and reduce the likelihood for injury; in addition, it can improve key physical components such as sprint speed, jump height and running efficiency (Suchomel et al., 2016). Developing these qualities during the preseason and inseason can be challenging, due to congested fixture lists and the high volume of prioritized on-field training sessions. Therefore it is essential to develop these qualities within the offseason training programme. Table 28.1 gives an overview of the offseason programme template.

The purpose of this strength and power training is to stress the muscles and tendons to allow them to adapt in preparation for the upcoming season. Hamstrings play a major role in high-speed movements, which are becoming more frequent in the modern game. Eccentric hamstring strength has received a lot of interest because of its suggested protective effect on hamstring strain injuries (Opar et al., 2015). An eccentric strength training protocol (such as the Nordic hamstring lower) can produce significant delayed onset muscle soreness (DOMS) and without progressive exposure to this it may negatively affect performance and increase risk of injury.

Including a larger volume of Nordic hamstring lowers during the offseason will allow for a minimal effective maintenance dose (Presland et al., 2018) in the preseason and inseason to avoid DOMS whilst minimizing hamstring injury risk (Bourne et al., 2016).

Table 28.2 sets out our offseason eccentric hamstring programme. This protocol is only one piece of a hamstring-strengthening programme; it is also essential to include unilateral and bilateral hip- and knee-dominant hamstring exercises (Bourne et al., 2016) to mitigate injury risk. Another key factor is high-speed running exposure of over 90% of a player's maximum velocity (Malone et al., 2017).

Running volumes and intensities

After a significant amount of time off, the player's base fitness accumulated over time through a chronic training load will be considerably reduced. For field-based sports that are predominantly running based, like soccer, it is vital to rebuild this chronic training load in the offseason in order to increase tissue tolerance and cardiovascular endurance for the start of the preseason (Kelly and Coutts, 2007). This is also done with a progressive training plan that increases running volumes and intensities.

The offseason weekly plan consists of two session classifications: linear and multidirectional work. Session classifications consist of alternating variables, including volume and intensity. There are 4 days within the weekly programme: linear volume, multidirectional intensity, linear intensity, and multidirectional volume. The volumes and intensities of the sessions will progressively increase until the final week of the offseason. During the final week of the offseason, the players will only complete three sessions in an attempt to taper for the first week of preseason training.

Manipulating intensities and volumes can be achieved in many ways. Some common modifiable variables include total distance covered, distance covered at high speeds, percentage of maximal velocity reached, numbers of

Table 28.1 Offseason training programme

Week	Focus	Sets/reps	Frequency
1	Base strength introduction	3 × 8	2 upper body 2 lower body
2	Base strength + introduce eccentric loading	3–4 × 5–6	2 upper body 2 lower body
3	Submaximal strength + eccentric loading + introduce power	3–4 × 5–6	2 upper body 2 lower body
4	Maximal strength/ power + eccentric overload	3–4 × 5–6	1 upper body 1 lower body 1 total body
5	Maximal strength/ power	3–5 × 4–5	1 upper body 1 lower body 1 total body
6	Maximal strength/ power (taper)	3 × 4–5	1 upper body 1 lower body 1 total body

Table 28.2 Offseason eccentric hamstring programme

Week	Exercise	Sets/reps	Tempo	Frequency
1	Glute bridge with eccentric hamstring slide	3 × 5	5-s eccentric	2 sessions
2	Band-assisted Nordic hamstring lower	3 × 4		2 sessions
3	Band assisted/unassisted Nordic hamstring lower	3 × 3/1 reps (3 assisted/ 1 unassisted)		2 sessions
4	Band assisted/unassisted Nordic hamstring lower	3 × 2/2 reps (2 assisted/ 2 unassisted)		2 sessions
5	Nordic hamstring lower	3 × 3		2 sessions
6	Nordic hamstring lower	3 × 4		1 session

accelerations and decelerations and numbers of controlled and random changes in direction (Russell et al., 2016). Monitoring and progressing high-speed running exposures ranging from 60% to over 90% of an individual's maximum speed is also vital, as it appears to significantly stress the posterior chain musculature and mitigate risk of injury (Malone et al., 2017). Therefore, it is recommended to build these speeds from early in the offseason, with the exposures to maximal velocity coming in the last 1–2 weeks in preparation for the start of preseason. The inclusion of high-velocity running is especially important for athletes who will participate in speed testing upon their arrival at preseason camp. By exposing the players to high velocities prior to preseason, it allows the coaching staff more freedom to plan training sessions with regards to the size of the playing areas.

Soccer-specific conditioning

The final piece of our offseason programme is the integration of soccer-specific training, which is often neglected, as it is not directly under the performance staff's scope of practice. This may be achieved through collaboration with the coaching staff. By integrating the soccer-specific work with the physical work, the players can accomplish technical and physical development. For example, a wide player may work on the technical aspects of crossing a ball followed by a high-intensity recovery run on the linear-quality running day. Similarly, that same wide player could work on the technical aspects of defending in a 1v1 situation on the multidirectional-quantity day. Soccer-specific conditioning not only refines technique but also progressively exposes a player to 'high-risk' technical demands such as ball-striking, which may increase the risk of injury if overloaded incorrectly (Charnock et al., 2009).These sessions also expose the athletes to specific movement patterns, cognitive processes, footwear and ground surfaces they will be exposed to during preseason training.

Box 28.1 outlines the strategies we use to connect all three components of the offseason.

The structure: preseason

The main objectives for our high-performance staff in preseason training are as follows:
1. Assess the initial fitness status of the players upon arrival.
2. Work in collaboration with the technical staff to plan, progress and monitor training loads to improve the squad's fitness levels.
3. Strength/power development.

> ### Box 28.1 **Strategies to connect components of offseason training**
>
> - Sessions always start with general prep (warm-up) specific to the upcoming demands.
> - On-field conditioning and soccer specific training precede lower body strength/power sessions to minimize risk of injury.
> - Linear running days are paired with lower body strength/power sessions to keep the posterior chain stresses on the same day to minimize accumulation of fatigue throughout the week.
> - Either 1 or 2 days off follow the days focusing on linear running and lower body strength/power.
> - The first days back in the gym after an off-day consist of upper body strength and power work.

Testing

Our testing battery is divided into three phases. Phase 1 begins prior to the first training session. A full physical and blood panel is administered by the team's doctors in addition to the seven-site skinfold body composition test conducted by our performance nutritionist. The purpose of the full physical is to ensure that no issues have occurred over the offseason and that all new signings are medically cleared to train without restriction. The main areas of focus in relation to the blood panel are vitamin D and iron levels. The findings of this test allow the performance nutritionist to prescribe supplementation and individualized dietary plans. The body composition results are one of our standards for physical professionalism. All out-field players are required to return to the start of preseason at 10% body fat or below and goalkeepers at 13% body fat or below (these standards are on the higher end and could vary at different levels of play). If these standards are not met, then the players in question will have additional training sessions and nutritional interventions to improve their body composition.

Phase 2 is gym based and measures lower limb strength/power, endurance and asymmetries. Every player is prescribed an isokinetic muscle testing protocol on the Biodex machine and a one-repetition test on the Nordbord. We consider an imbalance of 15% or greater to place a player at significantly higher risk of injury and that individual will be required to perform additional strength work within their strength/power programme (van Dyk et al., 2016). In reference to the Nordbord, a score of 337 N or below indicates poor eccentric knee flexor strength and these players require additional strength work within their weekly sessions (Timmins et al., 2015).

The third and final phase of our testing battery occurs in the first week of preseason and is made up of the on-field performance tests. These tests are designed to focus on heart rate recovery, maximal aerobic capacity and maximum linear velocity. Our first day back to training involves a generic warm-up followed by 4 minutes of the yo-yo intermittent recovery test level 2 (submax yo-yo) followed by 3 minutes of standing still. The goal of this test is to attain approximately 80–85% of a player's maximum heart rate and then assess how well they can recover in the following 3-minute time period. Heart rate recovery (efficiency) has been shown to correlate with the status of the player's aerobic fitness and therefore quantifies the aerobic condition in which the players are returning to training (Veugelers et al., 2016). On our second day of training, the players complete a generic warm-up with a greater focus on change of direction and cutting movements. The yo-yo endurance test level 2 follows this and is used to assess both aerobic capacity ($\dot{V}O_{2max}$) and maximum heart rate. A secondary aim of this maximal field test is to create a competitive environment between individuals. Our standards for this test are as follows (goalkeepers do not participate):

- level 14.9 and above: fit to train without restriction
- level 13.6–14.8: fit to train but required to complete additional fitness training
- level 13.5 and below: not fit to train and required to train separate to the team until required improvement is made.

The final test of this phase, maximal linear velocity, takes place towards the end of the first week of preseason. On this day the warm-up contains multiple linear speed preparation activities. For example, marching, skipping and bounding variations progressing to partner harness–resisted marching/skipping/running followed by acceleration repeats and finishing with 20/30/40/50 yard 'build-ups' at increasing intensities. Following a complete rest (>3 minutes) the players are required to perform two 50-yard build-ups ending at 100% intensity.

The build-ups consist of:
- 0–8 yards at 50% maximum speed
- 8–20 yards at 50–80% maximum speed
- 20–50 yards at 80–100% maximum speed.

The results from this test are captured with our global positioning system (GPS) and presented in metres per second (m s^{-1}). This test captures the player's maximum speeds in order to monitor their weekly high-speed and sprint-speed exposures throughout the season. The timing of this test is very important, as exposing players to maximal velocity within the first couple of days may place them at increased risk of injury (Higashihara et al., 2018). This is a specific worry for new signings who may not have completed our offseason programme and arrive on day 1 underprepared. Therefore, we programme this test towards the end of the first week of training, which allows for players to be gradually exposed to increasing velocities within the training sessions.

At the beginning of preseason, these tests help to paint a picture of the physical status of the squad. The next step is to retest throughout preseason and the inseason in order to quantify improvement. Table 28.3 outlines our approach to retesting.

Table 28.3 Approach to retesting physical fitness

Test protocol	Frequency	Notes
Body composition	Every 4–6 weeks on same week day at the same time	
Blood work	Preseason/midseason	
Biodex		Only retested within a return to play protocol for an injured player
Nordbord	Weekly or biweekly within our lower body strength/power training sessions	
Submax yo-yo test	Every 4–6 weeks on multidirectional + 3 within the warm-up	
Yo-yo ETL2	Only retested within a return to play protocol for an injured player	
Linear maximum speed	Tracked weekly throughout the season for new maximum speeds but not retested	

ETL2, Yo-yo Endurance test level 2

Table 28.4 Example of building players' weekly training loads offseason

Week	Total distance (km)	Total high-speed running (m)
1	16 km	700 m
2	18 km	800 m
3	20 km	950 m
4	23 km	1100 m
5	25 km	1300 m
6	30 km	1500 m

Planning and progressing training loads

Offseason-to-preseason transition

A major objective of the performance staff, in conjunction with the coaching staff, is to have all players within a squad available and ready for selection for the first game of the competitive season. To achieve maximal availability there must be a safe and progressive plan in place whilst also overloading the players to improve their physical capacity. But doing so too rapidly or aggressively can be detrimental to a squad. To minimize the risk of injury during preseason, the training load all players were exposed to during the off-season must be understood and then used to avoid large spikes of volume and/or intensity (Hulin et al., 2013).

Table 28.4 shows an example of how we build the players' weekly (acute) training loads in the offseason from a volume (total distance covered in kilometres) and intensity (high-speed running distance covered in metres) standpoint (Blanch and Gabbett, 2015; Bowen et al., 2016). Note that we use these two metrics in order to simplify the prescription and monitoring process.

Once an initial distance is set, in this case 16 km of total distance covered and 700 m of high-speed running, it is recommended to stay below a 15% increase in load when progressing the following week (Blanch and Gabbett, 2015; Gabbett, 2016). Therefore, the priority of the offseason is to progress smoothly into the preseason. For example, if the goal of the first week of preseason is to achieve 35 km of total distance, then our goal of the last week in the offseason is to cover approximately 30–32 km (or 10–15% of 35 km). It is important to note that this 10–15% increase in training load serves as a guide and not a hard rule. Whilst using this percentage range as a guide, it is important to consider the compliance of each individual during the offseason. Due to a number of factors, such as access to

facilities, weather conditions and personal commitments, the load achieved may vary within a squad. Therefore, the battery of testing gives a key insight into the physical condition of the squad on day 1 of preseason.

Preseason: planning the big picture

Our preseason is split into three main phases and begins with a training overload phase, which consists of weeks 1, 2 and 3. Phase 2 is classed as the game overload phase and occurs during weeks 4 and 5. Phase 1 and 2 are followed by phase 3, a 1-week underload phase or taper.

Phase 1: training overload phase

Phase 1 aims to physically overload the players through technical and physical training sessions. The target training loads are determined from the offseason plan, although we aim to achieve weekly loads excessive of the average inseason week (25–30 km) to generate training adaptations and build up load tolerance. Week 1 is used to overload players without specifying one physical quality. Using moderate-sized teams (5v5–7v7) and moderate-sized playing dimensions (32 yards wide × 40 yards long to 50 yards wide × 60 yards long) we limit the opportunities to achieve high-speed running and can expect moderate amounts of accelerations and decelerations. During this week, high-speed running efforts are controlled within running drills separate to the soccer-specific sessions (for example, a box-to-box run in 12 s followed by 24 s of active recovery for 2 sets of 6 repetitions). The final part of week 1 is a 30-min friendly match (2 × 15 min) to build up tolerance to match play. During weeks 2 and 3 we continue to overload the players through technical and tactical sessions with the emphasis alternating between multidirectional loading and velocity loading along with recovery sessions. Multidirectional loading is achieved through high numbers of accelerations and decelerations with multiplanar changes of directions. The majority of these are achieved in drills utilizing 1v1–5v5 teams on a small to moderate playing area (15 yards wide × 20 yards long to 32 yards wide × 40 yards long). During multidirectional loading sessions the quadriceps, adductors and glutes are the muscle groups that are predominantly stressed. The coaching staff can use these drills to introduce tactical themes such as pressing, defensive organization and high-tempo transitions. Velocity loading is then achieved through exposure to linear high speeds (>5.5 m s^{-1}) for moderate volumes (400–600 m) and sprint speeds (>7 m s^{-1}) for low volumes (100–200 m). These occur during 9v9- to 11v11-sized team games using large areas (75 yards wide × 85 yards long to 75 yards wide × 120 yards long). The coaching staff can use these drills to introduce tactical styles such as counterattacks and defensive recovery. During velocity loading sessions the hamstrings are the muscle group predominantly stressed. Week 2 ends with the first friendly game where all players play for 45 minutes. Week 3 ends with a 60-minute friendly game.

Phase 2: game overload phase

Phase 2 involves overloading our players through competitive match play as opposed to tactical training sessions. However, the total distance volume is decreased by up to 20%. This phase is the most demanding of all preseason. Week 4 consists of two 75-minute match exposures separated by a 3-day turnaround. The days prior to and following games consist of recovery-based training sessions involving low-intensity tactical drills. This schedule exposes the players to multiple games with a quick turnaround time. Week 5 involves a week of tactical training with one 90-minute friendly game in preparation for the competitive season. We aim to reduce the load of week 4 by 5% for week 5.

Phase 3: underload or taper phase

The final phase is an underload phase. Week 6 is the last week of training leading into the first competitive inseason game. We aim to reduce the training load by 10% of week 5. This is accomplished through reducing training times and limiting additional sessions. If done correctly the players will be physically and mentally refreshed leading into the all-important first game of the season.

Game progression within 'big picture' planning

Having all players physically, mentally and tactically prepared for the first game of the competitive season requires all players be exposed to multiple games within the preseason. Preseason games provide the intensities, competitive environments and pressures that are seemingly impossible to replicate from training alone. The number of games played will typically depend on the length of the preseason, but with our preseason lasting 6 weeks teams commonly play 4–6 games. Our preseason games are progressed by the number of minutes played and our aim is to achieve roughly 375 minutes of competitive soccer per player using a 30/45/60/75/75/90-minute progression model. Our preseason game minutes progression aims to gradually increase tolerance to the competitive game demands. In order for each player to achieve an equal exposure to game minutes played, the coaching staff should be creative with their scheduling. We often schedule the first game as an intrasquad game made up of either 2 or 3 × 15-minute periods (number dependent) and ensure all players get 30 minutes

of game time. Following the intrasquad, a regular 90-minute game is scheduled and the squad makes up two different 11-man line-ups for each 45-minute period. For the 60- and 75-minute exposures we have implemented two separate fixtures on the same day. One team prioritizes the coaching staff's anticipated starting 11. The other squad is made up of reserve players. The final game is a 90-minute game. This game is scheduled one week before the season commences and typically takes place in a stadium. With this in mind a further reserve fixture is organized the next day to ensure the nonstarters accumulate the relevant playing time.

Monitoring

Implementing a quality objective and subjective monitoring system is vital to maximize the efficiency of the planning and manipulation of training loads. Our performance staff use real-time GPS for every session and game to quantify the volume and intensity of individual drills and sessions. From the live GPS feedback we can add or reduce training load to achieve daily and weekly targets. The key metrics we prioritize during preseason are: total distance, high-speed running (HSR) distance (55–70% of max velocity), sprint (SPR) distance (>70% max velocity), maximum velocity ($m\ s^{-1}$) and combined total of accelerations and decelerations (number of efforts >3.0 $m\ s^{-2}$).

Total distance is a gauge of absolute volume a player is exposed to. Total distance when divided by duration of session can also be used to display metres per min ($m\ min^{-1}$) and is a gauge of drill or session intensity. Metres per minute may show positional differences in certain drills, which can then be considered for future planning.

The following metrics are used to monitor velocity loading. HSR, SPR and peak speed are measured through metres per second. HSR can be individualized through achieving >55% of an individual's maximum velocity (attained during testing) or an absolute value of >5.5 $m\ s^{-1}$ held for at least 1 s. SPR is then classified as >70% of an individual's maximum velocity or an absolute value of >7 $m\ s^{-1}$ held for at least 1 s. HSR and SPR distance are both displayed as an accumulation of distance within a drill or session. Velocity metrics are monitored to ensure we progressively expose the players to greater volumes without creating an unnecessary spike. Velocity metrics can also be used to identify underloaded players, which has shown to be associated with increased injury risk (Hulin et al., 2015; Hulin et al., 2016).

We closely monitor intensity measures, including relative running speeds, to ensure our players achieve >90% of their maximum velocity on velocity loading days. It is vital that players are exposed to >90% of their maximum velocity within a 7- to 10-day period. Peak speed is also monitored to ensure overexposure does not occur (Malone et al., 2017).

The final metric that requires attention assesses multidirectional loading and is the total number of accelerations and decelerations (m s^{-2}) executed. It is important to monitor multidirectional loading metrics to avoid training monotony and potential overuse issues. Our goal is to taper exposures of high accelerations and deceleration (m s^{-2}) actions on the two days prior to game day, due to the biomechanical stress of the movement (Higashihara et al., 2018; Varley and Aughey, 2013).

As a performance staff, we monitor the above-mentioned metrics on a daily, weekly and rolling 4-weekly basis. We utilize the acute:chronic workload model to create a picture of the external physical loads being placed on the individual players (Hulin et al., 2013; Hulin et al., 2015). The acute:chronic workload model is used as an objective guide to monitor potential spikes or dips in training load, as both have an association with increased injury risk (Gabbett et al., 2016). The main limitation with using the acute:chronic ratio is the timeframe necessary to develop the denominator, making the ratio invalid throughout the first month of preseason.

To ensure our training prescriptions are aligning with the bigger picture of preseason, we feel it essential to receive subjective information from players on physical preparedness prior to training and rate of perceived exertion (RPE) following training (Borg, 1970; Hooper et al., 1995).

On the morning of each training day, players score their sleep quality, muscle soreness and overall fatigue on a scale of 1 to 5 (Hooper et al., 1995). This subjective information gives the performance staff an insight into how they have responded to the previous session. This information can also act as an alert system to highlight any unexpected responses that may require additional attention. It may also allow small adjustments to a session such as implementing a floater who has no defensive responsibility, which will limit their training load. In addition to these three areas of enquiry, we gain subjective feedback from the squad on a 1–10 RPE scale following every training session (Borg, 1970). The player's feedback allows us to assess the success of our training prescription and can also be used to show how players are responding to training intensity prescriptions. Both methods of receiving player feedback require an understanding of the scales used and honesty from the players to ensure they do not exaggerate or dilute the information we, as performance staff, require for efficient monitoring.

As previously mentioned, we also utilize heart rate monitors to test heart rate recovery status every 4–6 weeks. Daily heart rate tracking can be used to quantify the internal response to training. Monitoring heart rate responses is important to gain insight into the demands that different activities place on the players. Knowing the specific demands that varying activities place on the players is vital in the big picture planning and progression of a preseason.

Strength/power development

During the offseason, a player overloads their strength and power qualities which should be continued into the preseason as these qualities are fundamental to key performance aspects in soccer and injury risk mitigation (Stølen et al., 2005). The planning of strength/power sessions can be difficult, due to the high volume of tactical sessions and fixtures. Strength/power sessions are scheduled on the day before a recovery or off-day to allow additional recovery before the next on-field session. Strength/power sessions are not scheduled within 72 hours of a competitive fixture as it may induce detrimental levels of fatigue. In early stages of preseason, we often implement strength/power sessions immediately after the 30- and 45-minute match exposures as these games usually occur prior to an off/recovery day. Strength/power sessions mainly take place in the gym; however, we sometimes conduct them on-field when facilities and circumstances allow.

To ensure appropriate loading of strength/power work we often split the squad into three groups. The first group consists of the players who have completed the full off-season programme, increasing the likelihood of sustaining a sufficient foundation of strength. The second group consists of those that may not have completed the full offseason plan but do have over 5 years of strength/power training experience. Finally, the third group consists of new signings who have also not completed an offseason training schedule and have less than 5 years of strength/power training experience. The content of each group alters slightly in order to apply appropriate exercises. The repetitions and sets are also prescribed dependent on group and sessions goals. Table 28.5 demonstrates how we group a basic lower body strength/power session for the squad.

There are also opportunities within the on-field training sessions to train strength or power qualities. On appropriate training days, implementing a mini power session (microdosing) within the warm-up may provide the perfect opportunity to develop explosive qualities through the use of hurdle jumping variations and horizontal broad jumps. The focus within these mini power sessions is not on volume but rather intensity and rate of force development. These types of power exercises are not only used in warm-ups but also within competitive drills such as 1v1s or 2v2s. For example, an exercise starts with a specified number of hurdle jumps followed by a sprint to a ball, which the coach plays in from the sideline, followed by an attack on goal. Another opportunity to do on-field strength or power sessions comes when the players are divided into three teams within the session. In this scenario, two teams are playing small-sided games (SSGs) whilst the other team is resting. The team that is resting can use the time off for a mini strength or power session. This mini strength and power session could include body weight or loaded strength exercises, jumping variations, medicine ball throws and weighted sled drags.

Table 28.5 Grouping basic lower body strength/power session

Block	Exercise	Sets/reps
Group 1	Focus: maximum strength/reactive power	
A1	Hex bar deadlift	3 × 5
A2	Depth jump	3 × 3
B1	Nordic hamstring lower	3 × 3
B2	TRX anti-extension core	3 × 8
Group 2	Focus: base strength/power	
A1	Kettlebell deadlift	3 × 6
A2	Countermovement jump	3 × 4
B1	Nordic hamstring lower	3 × 2/2
B2	TRX anti-extension core (kneeling)	3 × 8
Group 3	Focus: base strength fundamentals/power development	
A1	Bodyweight hinge pattern	3 × 8–10
A2	Non-countermovement jump	3 × 5
B1	Eccentric hamstring slide (5 second eccentric)	3 × 5
B2	Plank position body saw	3 × 8–10

Summary

A team's preseason is used to build a solid physical platform that leads into the competitive season. This physical platform not only begins when the players return to training. A plan should be in place from the final day of the previous season. This plan is a specific offseason plan that focuses primarily on recovery before overloading strength and power qualities and progressively increasing running distance and intensities. These running volumes and intensities should ensure a foundation of exposures to HSR before the players return to training, mitigating the risk of injury associated with large spikes in training load. The preseason should then continue to progressively build tolerance to the demands of soccer training and competitive match play. Through careful planning, the performance and coaching staff can provide windows of opportunity for tactical, strength, power, aerobic and anaerobic development sessions in addition to competitive fixtures and recovery. Continual monitoring throughout the preseason allows for adjustments to be made to minimize unnecessary spikes or dips in training load. Preseason will not only determine the robustness of the playing squad but can also be vital in establishing physical standards to maintain throughout the season.

References

Blanch, P., Gabbett, T.J., 2015. Has the athlete trained enough to return to play safely? The acute: chronic workload ratio permits clinicians to quantify a player's risk of subsequent injury. British Journal of Sports Medicine 50 (8), 471–475.

Borg, G., 1970. Perceived exertion as an indicator of somatic stress. Scandinavian Journal of Rehabilitation Medicine 2, 92–98.

Bourne, M.N., Duhig, S.J., Timmins, R.G., Williams, M.D., Opar, D.A., Al Najjar, A., et al., 2016. Impact of the Nordic hamstring and hip extension exercises on hamstring architecture and morphology: implications for injury prevention. British Journal of Sports Medicine 51 (5), 469–477.

Bowen, L., Gross, A.S., Gimpel, M., Li, F.-X., 2016. Accumulated workloads and the acute: chronic workload ratio relate to injury risk in elite youth football players. British Journal of Sports Medicine 51 (5), 452–459.

Bush, M., Barnes, C., Archer, D.T., Hogg, B., Bradley, P.S., 2015. Evolution of match performance parameters for various playing positions in the English Premier League. Human Movement Science 39, 1–11.

Charnock, B.L., Lewis, C.L., Garrett Jr., W.E., Queen, R.M., 2009. Adductor longus mechanics during the maximal effort soccer kick. Sports Biomechanics 8, 223–234.

Gabbett, T.J., Hulin, B.T., Blanch, P., Whiteley, R., 2016. High training workloads alone do not cause sports injuries: how you get there is the real issue. British Journal of Sports Medicine 50 (8), 444–445.

Gabbett, T.J., 2016. The training-injury prevention paradox: should athletes be training smarter and harder? British Journal of Sports Medicine 50 (5), 273–280.

Higashihara, A., Nagano, Y., Ono, T., Fukubayashi, T., 2018. Differences in hamstring activation characteristics between the acceleration and maximum-speed phases of sprinting. Journal of Sports Sciences 36, 1313–1318.

Hooper, S.L., Mackinnon, L.T., Howard, A., Gordon, R.D., Bachmann, A.W., 1995. Markers for monitoring overtraining and recovery. Medicine & Science in Sports & Exercise 27, 106.

Hulin, B.T., Gabbett, T.J., Blanch, P., Chapman, P., Bailey, D., Orchard, J.W., 2013. Spikes in acute workload are associated with increased injury risk in elite cricket fast bowlers. British Journal of Sports Medicine 48 (8), 708–712.

Hulin, B.T., Gabbett, T.J., Caputi, P., Lawson, D.W., Sampson, J.A., 2016. Low chronic workload and the acute: chronic workload ratio are more predictive of injury than between-match recovery time: a two-season prospective cohort study in elite rugby league players. British Journal of Sports Medicine 50 (16), 1008–1012.

Hulin, B.T., Gabbett, T.J., Lawson, D.W., Caputi, P., Sampson, J.A., 2015. The acute: chronic workload ratio predicts injury: high chronic workload may decrease injury risk in elite rugby league players. British Journal of Sports Medicine 50 (4), 231–236.

Kelly, V.G., Coutts, A.J., 2007. Planning and monitoring training loads during the competition phase in team sports. Strength and Conditioning Journal 29, 32.

Malone, J.J., Di Michele, R., Morgans, R., Burgess, D., Morton, J.P., Drust, B., 2015. Seasonal training-load quantification in elite English premier league soccer players. International Journal of Sports Physiology and Performance 10, 489–497.

Malone, S., Roe, M., Doran, D.A., Gabbett, T.J., Collins, K., 2017. High chronic training loads and exposure to bouts of maximal velocity running reduce injury risk in elite Gaelic football. Journal of Science and Medicine in Sport 20, 250–254.

Opar, A.D., Williams, D.M., Timmins, G.R., Hickey, J.J., Duhig, J.S., Shield, J.A., 2015. Eccentric hamstring strength and hamstring injury risk in Australian Footballers. Medicine & Science in Sports & Exercise 47, 857–865.

Presland, J.D., Timmins, R.G., Bourne, M.N., Williams, M.D., Opar, D.A., 2018. The effect of Nordic hamstring exercise training volume on biceps femoris long head architectural adaptation. Scandinavian Journal of Medicine & Science in Sports.

Russell, M., Sparkes, W., Northeast, J., Cook, C.J., Love, T.D., Bracken, R.M., et al., 2016. Changes in acceleration and deceleration capacity throughout professional soccer match-play. The Journal of Strength & Conditioning Research 30, 2839–2844.

Stølen, T., Chamari, K., Castagna, C., Wisløff, U., 2005. Physiology of soccer. Sports Medicine 35, 501–536.

Suchomel, T.J., Nimphius, S., Stone, M.H., 2016. The importance of muscular strength in athletic performance. Sports Medicine 46, 1419–1449.

Timmins, R.G., Bourne, M.N., Shield, A.J., Williams, M.D., Lorenzen, C., Opar, D.A., 2015. Short biceps femoris fascicles and eccentric knee flexor weakness increase the risk of hamstring injury in elite football (soccer): a prospective cohort study. British Journal of Sports Medicine 50 (24), 1524–1535.

van Dyk, N., Bahr, R., Whiteley, R., Tol, J.L., Kumar, B.D., Hamilton, B., et al., 2016. Hamstring and quadriceps isokinetic strength deficits are weak risk factors for hamstring strain injuries: a 4-year cohort study. The American Journal of Sports Medicine 44, 1789–1795.

Varley, M.C., Aughey, R.J., 2013. Acceleration profiles in elite Australian soccer. International Journal of Sports Medicine 34, 34–39.

Veugelers, K.R., Naughton, G.A., Duncan, C.S., Burgess, D.J., Graham, S.R., 2016. Validity and reliability of a submaximal intermittent running test in elite Australian football players. The Journal of Strength & Conditioning Research 30, 3347–3353.

Chapter 29

An introduction to working in an elite football academy

Diane Ryding

Introduction

This chapter introduces general concepts around working with the developing athlete in an elite football academy. The athlete-centred approach and interdisciplinary working is presented along with aspects unique to working with children, especially those linked to growth and maturation. Many physiotherapists commence their sporting careers working with youth teams or academies; there are inherent differences to work practices when working with children and adolescents when compared to adults.

The interdisciplinary team and the athlete-centred approach

Football academies employ staff from multiple professions to be involved in developing the youth footballer (Fig. 29.1), with the ultimate aim of producing players who are at a standard to play for the professional team of that club.

A modern football academy adopts an athlete-centred approach, where the development needs of the player is the primary concern and there is a collaborative, interdisciplinary approach to developing that player. When working with the youth athlete, the parent is also a key member of this team. This athlete-centred approach empowers the player to be engaged in their own development and encourages the player to take ownership of their development journey. The player is provided with opportunities for self-evaluation, reflection and goal setting. The interdisciplinary team (IDT) facilitates the player to develop problem-solving and decision-making skills, which aims to enhance their individual performance and that of the team. Ultimately, the

athlete-centred approach involves planning for long term, even if it that means accepting short-term setbacks (Kidman et al., 2010).

The role of the IDT is to support the evolving needs of the player during each stage of their development and help them reach their maximal potential, although ultimately this 'potential' will vary between players. During regular IDT meetings, areas for player improvement and enrichment will be identified and planned interventions, goals and a timescale for reevaluation will be documented. The IDT will select the most appropriate members to work with the player, as not all professions will be required at all stages of the development process. It is important that any discussions of a sensitive or confidential nature only take place with appropriate persons present; medical confidentiality still applies in a sports setting.

Each member of the IDT must have a defined role but also have an appreciation of when the knowledge and skills of other professionals may be utilized, with interdisciplinary referral pathways identified. Within the wider IDT there will also be 'subteams' who work together such as the sports science and medicine team (Fig. 29.2). Intradepartmental integration, awareness of what other members of the IDT can offer, along with clear channels of communication between departments is crucial to ensuring that appropriate and timely input occurs. In order to develop the academy player to their maximum potential, the IDT must itself become an effective team.

Developing people, not just footballers

Childhood is a fleeting period in someone's lifetime. Those who work with children are privileged to be part of this defining and memorable time, but this comes with responsibility.

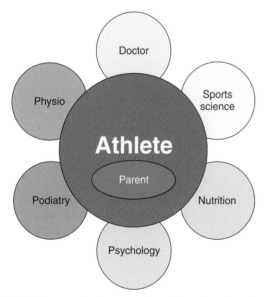

Fig. 29.1 The interdisciplinary team may include a number of professions.

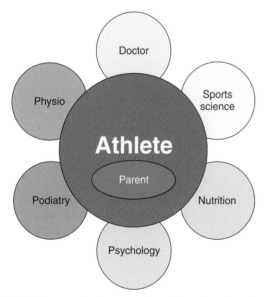

Fig. 29.2 The sports science and medicine department. Within the interdisciplinary team there will be smaller subteams that will need to work effectively together such as the medical team or sports science and medicine team.

A high percentage of children involved in academies will not progress to the professional ranks; it is therefore the responsibility of all academy staff to ensure the time spent is value-added regarding developing life skills alongside football. The IDT will ensure that personal and social development of

the child occurs. Aspects of development include teamwork, organization and time-management skills, problem solving, resiliency, respect, fair play and the importance of working hard. In relation to the football principles, the emphasis at the younger age groups is on player development and 'learning to train', whereas at the older age groups the emphasis is about 'learning to compete'.

Custodians of club culture and values

All members of the IDT will be custodians of the club culture and values and will have a key role in maintaining expectations and standards set by the club. Because some academy players do not start from the same baseline understanding of what constitutes socially acceptable behaviour, it is important that the club has a clear philosophy that sets the expected standards and values. Players and staff must ensure that values are upheld when representing the club, both on and off the field of play. Players are taught club philosophies such as respecting others, being gracious in victory and to show respect in defeat.

Clinical assessment and treatment planning in the young footballer

Environment

An appropriate, child-friendly environment is crucial to alleviate stress in the young player. Motivational quotes and positive messages may be displayed, along with advice from other IDT members or senior professional players. Prior to a clinical assessment, the child's parent or an appropriate adult should be present as a chaperone. The assessment procedure should be clearly explained throughout and anatomical posters and models will help to illustrate the diagnoses.

Subjective assessment

If an adult is asked to explain the history of an injury during an assessment, they may provide information on the initial mechanism of injury along with the duration and current presentation of symptoms. Children may not volunteer the information as easily. Questioning of the paediatric player may need to be more probing, in order to uncover pertinent information. The therapist may also need to consider external factors and any nonfootballing activities. For example, does the child have a new computer game that they have spent hours playing? If it has been snowing outside, have they been sledging? Has the player been injured playing another sport or while playing for another team that they may be reluctant to disclose? Children and adolescents may be apprehensive about offering certain information for fear they will get into trouble; reassure them that as children they are expected to take part in other activities.

Pain scales

When assessing pain in the paediatric player, several subjective scales are available. Both the Wong–Baker FACES Pain Rating Scale (Wong and Baker, 1988) and the Faces Pain scale revised (FPS-R) (Hicks et al., 2001) use six graphically or cartoon-depicted faces with varying facial expressions. They are well established and recommended for use with children 5–12 years and 3–18 years of age, respectively, with evidence of validity, reliability and the ability to detect change (Stinson et al., 2006). The Numerical Pain Rating Scale (NPRS) uses a range of numbers, either 0 to 10 or 0 to 100, in either spoken or graphic format. The lowest number represents no pain and the highest number represents the most pain possible and has been deemed reliable in children over 8 years for acute pain (Pagé et al., 2012). The Visual Analogue Scale (VAS) is recommended for children over 8 years of age (Stinson et al., 2006).

Objective, observational and behavioural assessment

During the objective assessment, observe the young player as they walk into the room and when they are not consciously aware of being observed. Tell-tale signs such as muddy knees may indicate that the player has been participating in sports at school or playing out with friends.

The clinician must determine if the subjective and objective assessment correlates (see Safeguarding).

Following the clinical assessment and explanation of the diagnosis and treatment plan, ask the player to repeat what has been discussed. This will provide the assessing clinician with a good indication of their understanding.

A thorough clinical assessment will determine if further investigations are appropriate and or necessary. Even clinicians in a well-resourced club must use their clinical reasoning skills and ensure that additional diagnostic tools (such as magnetic resonance imaging), are used only when clinically indicated. Unnecessary referral for further investigations simply because they are easily accessible resources for the football club is inappropriate. Overuse of these diagnostic modalities could negatively affect the young player from a psychological perspective, creating false expectations of how injuries are assessed and diagnosed. This has the potential to increase expectations or create anxiety during the assessment phase of future injuries if the player is not referred for further diagnostic tests.

Rehabilitation planning

Concepts of the athlete-centred approach should be incorporated throughout the rehabilitation process. The aim is for the player to take ownership of their recovery and to feel empowered throughout the process. The physiotherapist should help the player to learn about their own body and always encourage questions (Fig. 29.3). To engage the player in their own goal setting, a 'problem list' can be reimagined as a 'challenge sheet', to provoke a greater appeal to paediatric athletes.

Rehabilitation is frequently planned as a criteria-based (rather than a timescale) model, where the goal is to

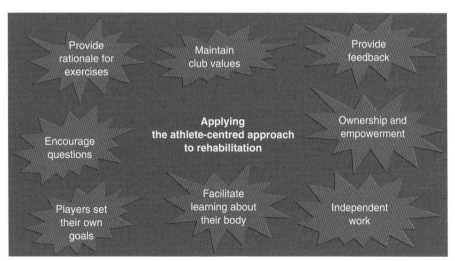

Fig. 29.3 Applying the athlete-centred approach to rehabilitation.

achieve the desired, documented criteria before progressing to the next phase. To maintain motivation, the player must be provided with rationale for the exercises/phases. They must have a good understanding of the rehabilitation process and goals to be attained prior to returning to football. Throughout the rehabilitation process, the physiotherapist will provide the player with opportunities for independent work and will ensure age-appropriate exercises, which should not be beyond a child's capabilities to appear more exciting. Regular feedback should be provided with the player being involved in reviewing their progress and reevaluating their goals.

Throughout rehabilitation, it is imperative to consider the young player in their entirety rather than just the injured joint or limb. Time must be used effectively to develop other aspects of the footballer such as cardiovascular fitness or strength and power gains. The rehabilitation phase is the perfect opportunity for the player to have additional input from other members of the IDT. The physiotherapist may coordinate gym or field-based sessions with the sports scientist. Referral pathways to the club nutritionist or psychologist should be activated once a player has sustained a long-term injury. Encourage the player to understand that maintaining a positive attitude during the rehabilitation phase is fundamental to their success. Ultimately, they cannot change what has happened to them, but they can control their attitude.

Avoiding over medicalization

When treating children and adolescent footballers, the emphasis is on education and an exercise-based approach to treatment. Joint mobilizations or soft tissue techniques may still be used but it is important to avoid creating dependency or overreliance involving manual techniques, taping or even treatment by one staff member. The aim is to encourage the right treatment environment where the young player learns about their own body and how to take care of it.

Taping

One controversial treatment in the adolescent player is the use of sports tape. Tape is applied to control oedema, to support an injured joint or to limit movement in a specific direction in order to protect a healing or previously injured joint/ligamentous structure. A rigid tape is used to restrict joint movement and elastic adhesive tape or elastic cohesive tape (which sticks to itself and not to the skin) is used for compression and to support joints or muscles.

Prior to tape application there must be a clear understanding of the aim of taping, the most appropriate tape to be used and the application technique. A consistent approach between club physiotherapists regarding the indication for use and tape application will help to maintain continuity. Adult players may at times receive a greater

amount of psychological rather than physical support from taping techniques. When working with paediatrics, avoid creating unnecessary dependency on tape.

Long-term athletic development

When working with senior professional athletes, there is frequently pressure to return from injury from external sources such as coaching staff, peer pressure or even for financial reasons. There may also be internal pressure from the athletes themselves. When working with paediatric footballers, the medical team must ensure that the long-term development of the player takes precedence over any external or internal pressures and short-term gains.

Growth and maturation

Growth and maturation are terms frequently used synonymously. Growth predominantly occurs during the first two decades of life and is an increase in the size of the body as a whole or of specific parts. Maturation is the process of progressing towards maturity or the adult stature (Malina, et al., 2004a). Maturation is considered in terms of stage and tempo, i.e., rate of maturation and timing (Cumming et al., 2018). To distinguish further, 'maturation is a process and maturity is a state', (Malina et al., 2004a, p. 302). An example of these differences is that children can be of equal height but of varying stages of skeletal maturity in relation to the percentage of attained end-height stature (i.e., adult height).

The adolescent growth spurt in females commences around 9 or 10 years of age, peaks at approximately 12 years of age and finishes at about 16 years. In males, the acceleration begins at 10 or 11 years, peaks at around 14 years and stops around 18 years of age (Malina et al., 2004a). Peak height velocity (PHV) is the period where maximum growth rate occurs and predicted maturity offset is defined as the amount of time before or after PHV (Kozieł and Malina, 2018).

What 'age' is the player?

A child is defined as being 'a human being below the age of 18 years' (UN General Assembly, 1989), although this definition can vary between countries. A child can, however, be of various 'ages' simultaneously when considering their chronological, biological and psychological age.

Chronological age

Chronological age is the age of a person measured in years, months, and days from their date of birth.

Biological or skeletal 'age'

The biological or skeletal 'age' or maturation status of the child is a dynamic rather than a static concept and can differ from that person's chronological age. Maturation status can be estimated by methods that compare the individual's maturation status against normative population data with regard to chronological age (Johnson et al., 2017). The maturity status indicates the progress the individual is making towards the attainment of biological maturity (Malina, 1971) and maturity can be defined by the difference between chronological age and skeletal age (Johnson et al., 2009). There are invasive and noninvasive techniques available to estimate maturation.

Assessing biological maturity: invasive methods

Wrist–hand X-rays. Skeletal age is considered the most accurate method of assessing biological maturity, with radiographs of the left hand and wrist being considered the gold standard (Engebretsen et al., 2010). This method aims to evaluate changes and provide an objective record of the maturity status of the developing skeleton at a single point in time. This is possible because the epiphyseal ossification and fusion of individual bones occurs at various times during the maturation process.

The three most frequently used methods to assess skeletal maturity according to Engebretsen et al. (2010) are the Greulich–Pyle method (Greulich and Pyle, 1959), the Tanner–Whitehouse method (Tanner et al., 1962, 1983, 2001) and the Fels method (Roach et al., 1988). The Gruelich–Pyle method compares the hand–wrist X-rays to pictures in an atlas and the Tanner–Whitehouse method (now on its third edition; TW3) assigns a numerical score based on the assessment of 20 bones depending on the appearance of maturity indicators. Finally, the Fels method takes into account a greater number of maturity indicators than the TW3 method and includes assessment of each carpal bone, the epiphyses and diaphysis of the radius, ulna and of the metacarpals and phalanges of the first, third and fifth digits (Malina et al., 2004a). By using these methods, children are classified as being either 'on time', late or early maturers by subtracting the skeletal age from the chronological age. Children are classed as early maturers or late maturers if their skeletal age is 1 year older or younger, respectively, than their chronological age. Normal maturers have a skeletal age that is within 1 year of their chronological age (Johnson et al., 2009; Malina et al., 2004b). Caution should be used when interpreting the wrist-hand X-ray data as there is a wide variation in biological maturity within players who are of similar chronological ages. Johnson et al. (2009) demonstrated that a third of players were shown to be outside of the 'normal' maturity category. There are also different maturity rates in different ethnic backgrounds (Malina et al., 2004a) and earlier osseous maturity in female adolescents (Engebretsen et al., 2010). This has implications when considering that there is likely to be a wide range of biological ages within children who are grouped together for sport using chronological age brackets.

The use of hand–wrist radiographs for determining skeletal age may not be ethical in the sporting environment (Dvorak et al., 2007a) and X-rays for the purpose of age determination in healthy children and adolescents may not be endorsed by ethical committees in many countries (Engebretsen et al., 2010).

Assessment of genital/pubic hair development. The Tanner's Sexual Maturity Scale was devised to assess physical development in children, adolescents and adults and has been used to determine maturation status (Marshall and Tanner, 1969, 1970). This requires either clinical assessment by a medical professional or a self-assessment of secondary sex characteristics to determine the stage of breast, genital or testicular maturation. During self-assessment, adolescents are provided with figure drawings representing Tanner's Sexual Maturity Scale and are asked to select the drawing/stage that best indicates their own stage of development. Schlossberger et al. (1992) found that there was a tendency for subjects to overestimate their development during the early stages of maturation and underestimate their development at later stages. The researchers also found that an impending examination could induce the teenager to be more accurate about self-assessment.

This technique is considered invasive in regards to the individual's personal space and is not routinely used in football. If employed, this technique would be limited to use within the pubertal years (Malina et al., 2012).

Assessing biological maturity: noninvasive methods

Methods using anthropometric measurements. Methods that use anthropometric data rather than skeletal assessment are deemed noninvasive indicators of adolescent biological maturation and are frequently used in football academies.

The Khamis and Roche (1994) and Mirwald et al. (2002) methods use prediction equations to determine the final adult stature (height) of the child. The chronological age, current standing height (stretch stature) and weight of the child are included in the equations for both prediction models. In addition to these parameters, the Khamis and Roche (1994) method also includes self-reported midparental height in the calculations and Mirwald et al. (2002) method takes sitting height into account. Both of these methods aim to predict when a child will go through PHV, allowing the clinician to assess how far a child is away from PHV and to predict the maturity offset value. The maturity offset value is calculated by subtracting chronological age at prediction from the predicted time at which PHV occurs. This can be a negative value if the child is prior to PHV, a zero value if they are circa PHV or a positive value if the child has passed PHV.

These anthropometric techniques are time efficient, require inexpensive equipment and require no extensive training to undertake. Consequently they are commonly used in football. There are, however, limitations to these prediction models. Malina and Kozieł (2014) found that predicted 'age at PHV' (APHV) has applicability among average maturing boys 12–16 years in contrast to late and early maturing boys. The Mirwald equation was found to underestimate the actual APHV at younger ages and in early maturers, and overestimate it at older ages and in late maturers. Kozieł and Malina (2018) found that the equations were not useful for early and late maturing girls, with a window for the assessment of average maturing girls not being apparent. The use of self-determined mid-parental height in the Khamis and Roche (1994) method is a limitation due to the risk of incorrect information being provided. Many of these studies are also based on Caucasian participants from middle-class socioeconomic backgrounds, whereas within football these models are applied to multiethnicities from various socioeconomic backgrounds.

Magnetic resonance imaging. The use of MRI offers the possibility of estimating biological/chronological maturity without the need for ionizing radiation but has yet to replace the use of hand–wrist radiographs.

Dvorak et al. (2007a,b) attempted to use left wrist MRIs for chronological age determination in an attempt to ensure appropriate chronological age participation in male footballers. Based on these two investigations, Engebretsen et al. (2010) concluded that MRI was a viable tool for screening male players in the U16 and U17 groups, but at the time there was no evidence to support the use of wrist MRI for age determination in male athletes below 14 years and above 17 years of age. In 2016, Tscholl et al. determined that due to earlier osseous maturity in female adolescents, the grade of fusion of the distal radial epiphysis on MRI is not recommended for pretournament age determination in female participants of U17 and younger. During this study, complete fusion of the distal radial epiphysis was observed in 14- and 15-year-old females.

More recently, an atlas of MRI studies of the knee spanning the paediatric and adolescent years was created and validated by Pennock et al. (2018). They found a strong correlation between chronological age and bone age with excellent interobserver and intraobserver reliability demonstrated. Smaller scale studies have looked at the feasibility of assessing skeletal age from left hand MRIs, with Hojreh et al. (2018) and Serinelli et al. (2015) finding good correlation to estimated chronological age. Future studies are required to evaluate these wrist study results in larger sample sizes that include individuals from a range of ethnicities and socioeconomic backgrounds.

In those over 18 years, the clavicle is used for the assessment of maturity as it is the last bone in the human body to complete fusion (Buckley and Clark, 2017). A pilot study by Schmidt et al. (2015) investigated the use of MRI to verify the age of players in U20 football tournaments and found that the presence of a fully ossified clavicular epiphyseal plate appears to provide evidence of completion of the 20th year of life. However, this also requires further study including a greater number of participants.

Psychological age

The term 'psychological age' refers to the emotional/cognitive/psychological development of a child. The correlation between the physical and psychological age of a child is not necessarily linear. A player may reach the height of an adult during the mid-teenage years but this does not mean that they have the emotional and cognitive maturity of an adult. The cognitive and emotional maturity status of the child must be considered when assessing and treating the player. For example, a 14-year-old player may be 6 ft/182 cm in height and physically look like an adult but this does not mean that their mind is able to process information like an adult.

The relative age effect and bio-banding

The *relative age effect* is a phenomenon that suggests there are asymmetries in the distributions of birth dates in senior professional and youth soccer players (Vaeyens et al., 2005). Players born early in the selection year are favoured and those born later in the year are discriminated against (Helsen et al., 2012). This is often due to maturation-associated selection.

In the UK the academic and academy calendar runs from 1 September through to 31 August and groups children together based on chronological age. Consequently, UK children born in the months of September to December may be at a selection advantage in comparison to younger players born later that selection year. These dates for chronological age banding can vary internationally, with many countries using 1 January to 31 December to group children chronologically. Consequently, in these countries children born between January to March may have the selection advantage. Musch and Hay (1999) determined that the relative age effect was shown to be present independent of variation in cut-off date.

With regard to academy player selection, Johnson et al. (2017) suggest that skeletal maturation status is more strongly associated with academy selection than birth quarter. This study suggests that academies tend to favour those born earlier in the selection year to a relatively small degree; in contrast, they favour earlier maturing athletes to a much greater extent. As discussed by Musch and Hay (1999), discrimination against the smaller, skeletally less mature players may limit their opportunities and they may drop out of sport earlier rather than continue until they reach maturity when the age disadvantage is overcome. Indeed, if skilled players are proportionately dispersed across the population, then it is a flawed strategy to select players from the early maturers group only, as potential talent in the late and normal maturers group will be excluded or missed (Johnson et al. 2017). Differences in maturation statuses also have the potential to work adversely against early maturers as they may use their physicality during the game rather than developing their technical abilities in the early teenage years. This can have negative consequences when the other players achieve the same maturation status and are said to 'catch up'.

To counteract the relative age effect, football coaches often take the date of birth of the player into consideration in regard to talent identification and player selection. However, benchmarking players against others of similar chronological ages does not account for maturation differences; consequently, bio-banding has been suggested. Bio-banding is the process of grouping athletes on the basis of attributes associated with growth or maturation, rather than chronological age (Cumming et al., 2017) in an attempt to 'level the playing field'.

Practical aspects of academy working

Safeguarding

Safeguarding is the process of protecting children and adults at risk. Many academies will have a designated safeguarding officer, but all members of the IDT have a responsibility for adhering to safeguarding policies in order to protect the children they work with and themselves. Always default to the code of conduct and ethics of your profession and work within the employer's safeguarding guidelines.

It is important to note that a child may use the physiotherapy or treatment room as an escape from the football pitch. Use clinical reasoning skills to determine the following:

- Does the mechanism of injury fit the presentation?
- Do the subjective history and objective assessment findings correlate?
- Has the player presented to the physiotherapist repeatedly for relatively minor incidents/injuries?
- When discussing the player returning to training, does the player appear apprehensive?

- Are there any bruises that cause concern or are in anatomical areas that are not commonly caused by the sport, e.g., chest/thorax/upper arm/shoulder with football.
- Have any concerns been brought to the attention of the medical team previously?

If concerns arise following the assessment, consider whether any of the following factors may be influencing the presentation of the player:

- Is the player being bullied? This may be by another player, a staff member or even by his or her parent after training.
- Is the player struggling within the group and finding the training difficult? Any minor injury may be catastrophized by a child who is not enjoying their football.
- Does the player appear anxious or display fear of failure?
- Is there evidence of overexpectation from the parent?
- Is the player being subjected to peer group pressure?

Creating a safe environment

Consider the appropriate safeguarding measures within the changing working environment, whether in the physiotherapy room, gym, swimming pool area or hotel. Best practice would be that staff members are not left unsupervised in confined areas with academy children. This promotes a safe environment for both the child and the staff member. Refer any inappropriate practice or behaviours immediately according to employer's guidelines. Always ensure that cultural and religious factors are considered when treating any patient.

If your club or employer does not have a safeguarding policy then you can find more information from the English Football Association's website in the document, *Keeping Football Safe and Enjoyable* (The Football Association, 2017).

Travelling with academy-age children
Pretour preparation

For all tours and tournaments, the club must complete pretour risk assessments. These risk assessments will include information on the players and the venues, including the hotel and stadia. It is important to be familiar with this and always work within the organizations' policies and procedures.

Transport

If the main medical kit is stowed in the hold of the aircraft or coach, a small medical bag can be carried as hand luggage to deal with minor injuries or incidents en route. Consider what would be required to deal with a child having a nosebleed or being travelsick. Ensure that players take any key medication in their hand luggage.

Back to basics

Encourage a balanced diet and try to keep dietary advice consistent, simple and understandable with young players. During competition, the food is often high in carbohydrate content and is consumed at least 2 hours prior to the commencement of games. A club nutritionist may lead the dietary strategy, but at academy level, the coaching and medical staff on the tour will often oversee the dietary requirements of the players.

Ensure players and staff wash their hands with soap or use alcohol gel regularly to mitigate the risk of spreading infectious disease within the team.

Consider environmental factors

- Hydration: Can the players drink the tap water? How much will they need to drink given the duration and frequency of matches and environmental factors such as temperature, humidity or altitude?
- What equipment and clothing are required for the climate? Will suncream be required?
- Take into consideration that many children may never have travelled outside of their local area.
- Homesickness can be a contributing factor to how a player presents.

Multiple roles of IDT members

Only a selection of the full complement of the IDT will travel with an academy team; consequently, for the welfare of the players, members frequently take on aspects of roles usually fulfilled by other professions. All staff will be *in loco parentis* and will take on a pastoral care role for children; they will look after the nutritional and hydration needs and ensure safeguarding procedures are adhered to.

First aid

Physiotherapists working in sport are frequently required to provide pitch-side emergency care during matches. It is important that any person accepting this responsibility has undertaken an appropriate sports first aid course and that these skills be practised regularly to maintain competence. Emergency action plans must be in place for all training and match venues.

Summary

The role of a physiotherapist in sport is multifaceted and goes beyond working solely in a treatment room. Any physiotherapist or sports therapist working within an academy system must be clear of their roles and responsibilities, both when working at home or overseas. They must be able to adapt their assessment and treatment strategies to the paediatric population and understand aspects around growth and maturation.

References

Buckley, M.B., Clark, K.R., 2017. Forensic age estimation using the medial clavicular epiphysis: a study review. Radiologic Technology 88 (5), 482–498.

Cumming, S.P., Lloyd, R.S., Oliver, J.L., Eisenmann, J.C., Malina, R.M., 2017. Bio-banding in sport: applications to competition, talent identification, and strength and conditioning of youth athletes. Strength and Conditioning Journal 39 (2), 34–47.

Cumming, S.P., Brown, D.J., Mitchell, S., Bunce, J., Hunt, D., Hedges, C., et al., 2018. Premier League academy soccer players' experiences of competing in a tournament bio-banded for biological maturation. Journal of Sports Sciences 36 (7), 757–765.

Dvorak, J., George, J., Junge, A., Hodler, J., 2007a. Age determination by magnetic resonance imaging of the wrist in adolescent male football players. British Journal of Sports Medicine. 41 (1), 45–52.

Dvorak, J., George, J., Junge, A., Hodler, J., 2007b. Application of MRI of the wrist for age determination in international U-17 soccer competitions. British Journal of Sports Medicine 41 (8), 497–500.

Engebretsen, L., Steffen, K., Bahr, R., Broderick, C., Dvorak, J., Janarv, P.-M., et al., 2010. The International Olympic Committee Consensus Statement on age determination in high-level young athletes. British Journal of Sports Medicine 44 (7), 476–484.

Greulich, W.W., Pyle, S.I., 1959. Radiographic atlas of skeletal development of the hand and wrist. The American Journal of the Medical Sciences 238 (3), 393.

Helsen, W.F., Baker, J., Michiels, S., Schorer, J., Van Winckel, J., Williams, A.M., 2012. The relative age effect in European professional soccer: did ten years of research make any difference? Journal of Sports Sciences 30 (15), 1665–1671.

Hicks, C., Baeyer, C., Spafford, P., van Korlaar, I., Goodenough, B., 2001. The Faces Pain Scale-Revised: toward a common metric in pediatric pain measurement. Pain 93 (2), 173–183.

Hojreh, A., Gamper, J., Schmook, M.T., Weber, M., Prayer, D., Herold, C.J., et al., 2018. Hand MRI and the Greulich-Pyle atlas in skeletal age estimation in adolescents. Skeletal Radiology 47, 963–971.

Johnson, A., Doherty, P.J., Freemont, A., 2009. Investigation of growth, development, and factors associated with injury in elite schoolboy footballers: prospective study. The British Medical Journal 338, b490.

Johnson, A., Farooq, A., Whiteley, R., 2017. Skeletal maturation status is more strongly associated with academy selection than birth quarter. Science and Medicine in Football 1 (2), 157–163.

Khamis, H.J., Roche, A.F., 1994. Predicting adult stature without using skeletal age: the Khamis-Roche method. Pediatrics 94 (4), 504–507.

Kidman, L., Lombardo, B.J., 2010. Athlete-centred Coaching: Developing Decision Makers, second ed. IPC Print Resources, Worcester, UK.

Kozieł, S.M., Malina, R.M., 2018. Modified maturity offset prediction equations: validation in independent longitudinal samples of boys and girls. Sports Medicine 48, 221–236.

Malina, R.M., 1971. A consideration of factors underlying the selection of methods in the assessment of skeletal maturity. American Journal of Physical Anthropology 35 (3), 341–346.

Malina, R.M., Kozieł, S.M., 2014. Validation of maturity offset in a longitudinal sample of Polish boys. Journal of Sports Sciences 32 (5), 424–437.

Malina, R., Eisenmann, J., Cumming, S., Ribeiro, B., Aroso, J., 2004b. Maturity-associated variation in the growth and functional capacities of youth football (soccer) players 13–15 years. European Journal of Applied Physiology 91 (5–6), 555–562.

Malina, R.M., Coelho, E., Silva, M.J., Figueiredo, A.J., Carling, C., Beunen, G.P., 2012. Interrelationships among invasive and non-invasive indicators of biological maturation in adolescent male soccer players. Journal of Sports Sciences 30 (15), 1705–1717.

Malina, R.M., Bouchard, C., Bar-Or, O., 2004a. Growth, Maturation, and Physical Activity. Human Kinetics, Champaign, IL.

Marshall, W.A., Tanner, J.M., 1969. Variations in pattern of pubertal changes in girls. Archives of Disease in Childhood 44 (235), 291–303.

Marshall, W.A., Tanner, J.M., 1970. Variations in the pattern of pubertal changes in boys. Archives of Disease in Childhood 45 (239), 13–23.

Mirwald, R.L., Baxter-Jones, A.D., Bailey, D.A., Beunen, G.P., 2002. An assessment of maturity from anthropometric measurements. Medicine & Science in Sports & Exercise 34 (4), 689–694.

Musch, J., Hay, R., 1999. The relative age effect in soccer: cross-cultural evidence for a systematic discrimination against children born late in the competition year. Sociology of Sport Journal 16 (1), 54–64.

Pagé, M.G., Katz, J., Stinson, J., Isaac, L., Martin-Pichora, A.L., Campbell, F., 2012. Validation of the numerical rating scale for pain intensity and unpleasantness in pediatric acute post-operative pain: sensitivity to change over time. The Journal of Pain 13 (4), 359–369.

Pennock, A.T., Bomar, J.D., Manning, J.D., 2018. The creation and validation of a knee bone age atlas utilizing MRI. The Journal of Bone and Joint Surgery 100 (4), e20.

Roche, A.F., Chumlea, W.C., Thissen, D., 1988. Assessing the skeletal maturity of the hand-wrist: FELS Method. Charles C. Thomas; Springfield, IL.

Schlossberger, N.M., Turner, R.A., Irwin, C.E., 1992. Validity of self-report of pubertal maturation in early adolescents. Journal of Adolescent Health 13 (2), 109–113.

Schmidt, S., Vieth, V., Timme, M., Dvorak, J., Schmeling, A., 2015. Examination of ossification of the distal radial epiphysis using magnetic resonance imaging. New insights for age estimation in young footballers in FIFA tournaments. Science & Justice 55, 139–144.

Serinelli, S., Panebianco, V., Martino, M., Battisti, S., Rodacki, K., Marinelli, E., et al., 2015. Accuracy of MRI skeletal age estimation for subjects 12–19. Potential use for subjects of unknown age. International Journal of Legal Medicine 129 (3), 609–617.

Stinson, J.N., Kavanagh, T., Yamada, J., Gill, N., Stevens, B., 2006. Systematic review of the psychometric properties, interpretability and feasibility of self-report pain intensity measures for use in clinical trials in children and adolescents. Pain 125 (1–2), 143–157.

Tanner, J.M., Whitehouse, R.H., Cameron, N., Marshall, W.A., Healy, M.J.R., Goldstein, H., 1983. Assessment of Skeletal Maturity and Prediction of Adult Height (TW2 Method), second ed. Academic Press, London, UK.

Tanner, J.M., Healy, M.J.R., Goldstein, H., Cameron, N., 2001. Assessment of Skeletal Maturity and Prediction of Adult Height (TW3 Method), third ed. Saunders, London.

Tanner, J.M., Whitehouse, R.H., 1962. Growth at Adolescence, second ed. Blackwell Scientific Publications, Springfield, Illinois, USA.

The Football Association, 2017. Keeping Football Safe and Enjoyable. Available from: Keeping Football Safe and Enjoyable (2017). Available at: http://www.thefa.com/-/media/thefacom-new/files/about-the-fa/2017/keeping-football-safe-en-joyable.ashx?la=en.

Tscholl, P.M., Junge, A., Dvorak, J., Zubler, V., 2016. MRI of the wrist is not recommended for age determination in female football players of U-16/U-17 competitions. Scandinavian Journal of Medicine & Science in Sports 26 (3), 324–328.

UN General Assembly, 20 November 1989. Convention on the Rights of the Child, vol. 1577. United Nations, Treaty Series, p. 3, available at: http://www.refworld.org/docid/3ae6b38f0.html. [Accessed January 2018].

Vaeyens, R., Philippaerts, R.M., Malina, R.M., 2005. The relative age effect in soccer: a match-related perspective. Journal of Sports Sciences 23 (7), 747–756.

Wong, D.L., Baker, C.M., 1988. Pain in children: comparison of assessment scales. Pediatric Nursing 14 (1), 9–17.

Chapter | **30** |

Growing bones: anatomy and fractures

Diane Ryding

Introduction

In paediatric medicine and rehabilitation, the assertion that 'children are not mini adults' frequently emerges, but what does this mean? How do injuries differ in the skeletally immature athlete? In order to understand paediatric musculoskeletal injuries, clinicians must be aware of anatomical variants between mature and immature skeletons, which lead to a unique set of injuries within the paediatric population. Specifically, the epiphyses, epiphyseal (growth) plates and the apophyses of a developing skeleton are all at risk from injuries.

This chapter will discuss paediatric long bone anatomy, bone growth and fractures that may occur in the developing skeleton. It is beyond the scope of this chapter to discuss all paediatric fractures, but those that may be seen within an elite football academy environment are included along with an overview of their management.

Paediatric long bone anatomy

Based on Malina et al. (2004):
* The *diaphysis* is the shaft of the bone. This contains the primary ossification centre, which is the site of bone deposition in the cartilage model, changing cartilage to bone. In long bones, this is located in the midportion of the bone.
* The *periosteum* is a membrane that covers the outer surface of the diaphysis. This layer has the ability to produce osteoblasts.
* The *epiphysis* is the rounded end of long bones that contributes to a joint. It develops from a secondary ossification centre formed in the cartilage at the end of the diaphysis. Long bones of the arms and legs have ossification centres at both ends. Short bones of the hand and foot only have secondary ossification centres at one end.

* The *physis/epiphyseal plate* is the name given to the epiphyseal cartilage/growth plate.
* The *metaphysis* is the region where ossification occurs. It is the narrow portion of a long bone between the epiphysis and the diaphysis which contains the growth plate.
* The *apophysis* is a normal bony outgrowth which is the secondary ossification centre. The musculotendinous unit attaches to the apophysis and the apophysis fuses with the bone over time.

> **Key point**
>
> The epiphysis contributes to a joint and apophysis to a teno-osseous attachment.

Bone growth

Prenatally, children begin with a skeleton of cartilage which is gradually replaced by bone as the child grows. At the end of each bone there is an ossification centre (epiphysis) with an adherent physis (growth plate), which is perpendicular to the long axis of the bone (Engebretsen et al., 2010). The bone grows in length in the direction of the epiphysis by the proliferation of cartilage cells and intercellular matrix at the metaphysis (Malina et al., 2004). The cartilage cells of the physis multiply and transform with mineralization and new bone is produced; this contributes to diaphysial growth (Engebretsen et al., 2010). In other words, the cartilage eventually calcifies and is replaced by bone (Fig. 30.1). The bone grows in width by laying down bone on the outer or subperiosteal surface. Bone on the inner (endosteal) surface is reabsorbed (Malina et al., 2004).

Bones cease to grow when the proliferation of cartilage cells slows and ossification proceeds at a faster pace. Eventually, there is epiphyseal union where the epiphysis and metaphysis fuse; at this time, skeletal maturity has occurred

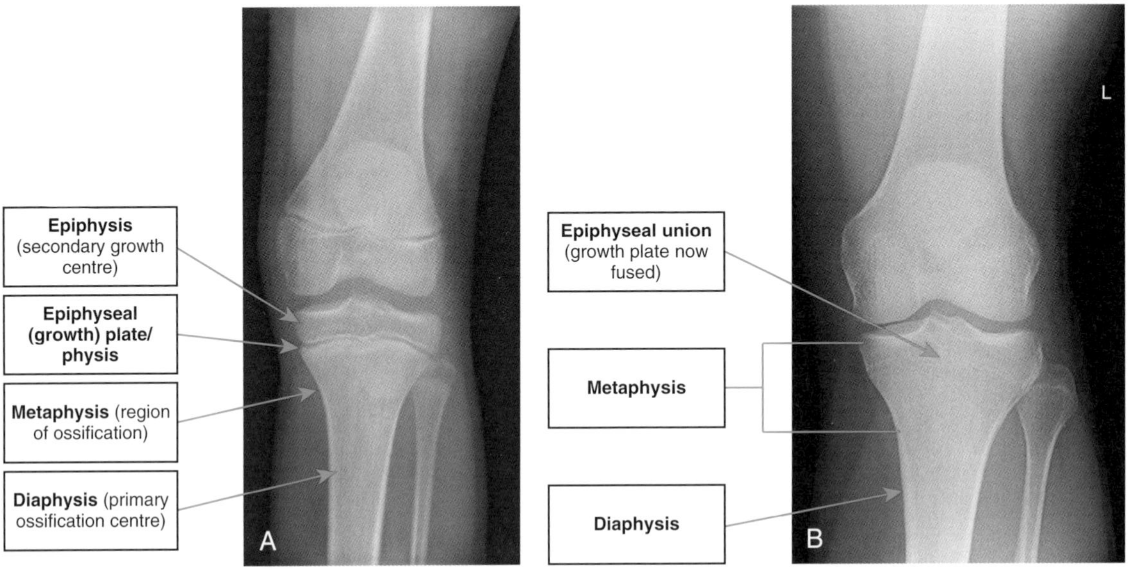

Fig. 30.1 Anatomical differences: child versus adult knee radiograph. (A) Paediatric left knee: immature/developing skeleton. (B) Adult left knee: mature/developed skeleton.

and the physis (growth plate) disappears. Females on average complete the ossification process of the secondary centres sooner than males (Malina et al., 2004).

Salter–Harris classification of physeal fractures

Due to the anatomical variants in growing bones, fractures can occur which affect the physis (growth plate). These fracture types are commonly described using the Salter–Harris classification I–IV (Salter and Harris, 1963) (Box 30.1) and can be remembered using the mnemonic 'Salter' (Fig. 30.2).

Signs and symptoms

Physeal fractures, like other fractures, may present with pain, swelling, deformity, limited movement, bony tenderness or reduced ability to weight bear in the lower limb.

Diagnosis and treatment

Physeal fractures can result in growth disturbances; therefore, in order to avoid potential long-term adverse consequences it is imperative that any paediatric player with a suspected fracture is referred for a radiograph. Any significant physeal fracture will commonly be followed up

---

Box 30.1 Salter–Harris classification of physeal features

- A type I fracture is a separation through the physis. It is more common in younger patients with a thicker physis.
- A type II fracture enters through the plane of the physis and exits through the metaphysis. The separate metaphyseal fragment is known as a Thurston Holland fragment. Type II accounts for 74% of physeal fractures.
- A type III fracture enters in the plane of the physis and exits through the epiphysis. This is a less common fracture type, but has the additional risk of posttraumatic arthritis and growth arrest.
- A type IV fracture crosses the physis, extending from the metaphysis to the epiphysis. This fracture type has an element of longitudinal instability. There is a risk of complete physeal arrest or asymmetric growth or deformity.
- A type V is a crush injury resulting in injury to the physis often due to compressive forces.

Based on Cepela, D.J., Tartaglione, J.P., Dooley, T.P., Patel, P.N., 2016. Classifications in brief: Salter-Harris classification of pediatric physeal fractures. Clinical Orthopaedics and Related Research 474 (11), 2531–2537.

---

for around 1 year postinjury in the orthopaedic outpatient department in order to monitor for any growth complications.

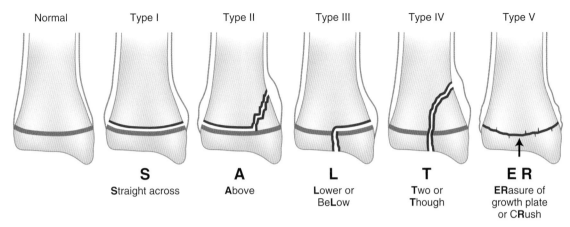

Fig. 30.2 Salter–Harris classification of physeal features. The mnemonic 'Salter' can be useful in remembering the different types.

Key points

A commonly held belief is that emergency department clinicians 'just tape' minor finger fractures and some parents are reluctant to spend hours waiting with their child for this, but the risk of incorrect management of a finger physeal fracture could have long-term implications for hand function.

Take care with the paediatric athlete who presents with a traumatic joint deformity. The deformity may not be due to a joint dislocation, but rather be an intraarticular physeal fracture. For example, an apparent 'patella dislocation' may actually be a physeal fracture of the distal femur.

Incomplete fractures

The bones of children have a greater degree of elasticity when compared to adult bones, leaving them susceptible to incomplete fractures. There are three common types:

Greenstick fractures

Greenstick fractures are transverse fractures through the cortex, where one side of the bone is broken and the other only bent and the break does not disrupt the opposite cortex, i.e., the bone bends and breaks much like a green twig. Ting et al. (2016) found them to occur in the 2–15 year-old age range, with a mean age of 6.9 years.

Torus (buckle) fracture

Torus (buckle) fractures are incomplete fractures of the shaft of a long bone characterized by bulging of the cortex, often involving the metaphyseal and diaphyseal junction (Fig. 30.3).

They occur during an axial loading force and often occur in the distal radius. Torus fractures of the distal radius are often managed in a splint rather than a cast; this is an inherently stable type of fracture with a low risk of displacement (Williams et al., 2013). They commonly occur in the preadolescents, but Ling and Cleary (2018) found them to occur in the 0–16 year-old age group, with a mean age of 9 years.

Clinical tip

In football, these fractures often present in a young goalkeeper who complains of wrist pain after stopping a shot (often reported as wrist hyperextension). They may also occur following a fall on an outstretched hand.

Bow fracture

Bow fractures affect long bones, most commonly the radius and ulna followed by the fibula. The bone bends or bows along its longitudinal axis following a loading force, but there is no distinct cortex disruption. In a small-scale review Vorlat and De Boeck (2003) found the mean age of radial bow fractures to be 7 years 5 months.

Fracture clinical decision tools

Clinical decision tools used in the assessment of lower limb injuries serve as guidelines for the requirement of radiographic examination, with the aim of avoiding unnecessary radiography in emergency departments (Fig. 30.4). These tools can be helpful for health professionals working in the acute sport setting.

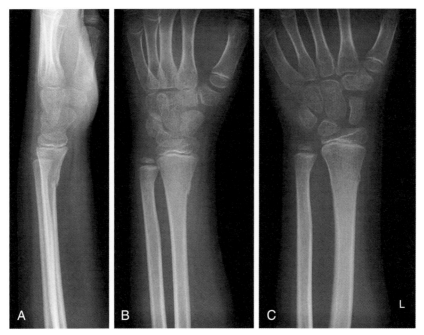

Fig. 30.3 **Buckle fracture.** (A) Lateral view, (B) oblique view, (C) PA view.

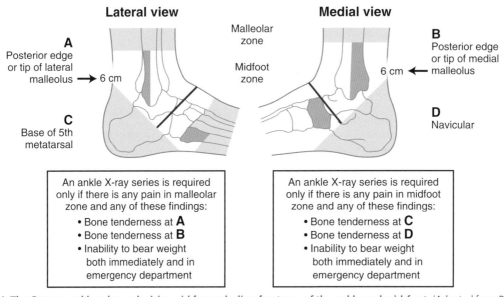

Fig. 30.4 **The Ottawa ankle rules, a decision aid for excluding fractures of the ankle and mid-foot.** (Adapted from Bachman et al. (2003).)

The Ottawa foot and ankle rules

A meta-analysis by Dowling et al. (2009) suggests that these rules appear to be a reliable tool to exclude fractures in children over 5 years of age when presenting with ankle and midfoot injuries. The pooled sensitivity was 98.5% (95% CI 97.3–99.2%) meaning that 1.5% of fractures might be missed using the rules.

The Ottawa knee rules

In 2003, Bulloch et al. validated the Ottawa knee rules for use in children over 5 years, determining that use of these rules can safely reduce the necessity for knee radiographs. Clinicians should, however, have a high index of suspicion and low threshold for further investigations (magnetic resonance imaging; MRI) if a paediatric player presents with a large knee effusion as Pennock et al. (2017) suggest that intraarticular fractures may not been seen on the plain radiographs of skeletally immature athletes.

Fracture treatment

The academy medical team should follow the orthopaedic advice on fracture immobilization in the immediate postfracture phase. If the fracture is stable and it is safe to do so, the medical team will work with the player on other body areas whilst protecting the healing structure during the immobilization phase. Once the fracture has healed, rehabilitation will consist of regaining range of movement, functional strength, proprioception and plyometric ability, along with building cardiovascular endurance and progressing back to position-specific end-stage activity. A phased return to training with load management will be utilized as required. The physiotherapist will ensure that the player is comfortable and confident in training before returning them to competitive games.

Chronic fractures affecting the growth plate

As well as acute physeal injuries, Caine et al. (2006) suggest that chronic physeal injuries can occur if sport training is of sufficient duration and intensity. In extreme cases, this may lead to bone growth disturbance.

Apophyseal avulsion fractures

The apophysis, as the secondary ossification centre, appears during puberty and it does not fuse until late adolescence

(Gidwani et al., 2004). During this time, it is the weakest part of the musculotendinous junction, which is why an apophyseal avulsion occurs rather than a muscle injury (Lozano-Berges et al., 2017; Schiller et al., 2017). In other words, the apophysis is the weakest link in the chain of muscle, tendon and bone (Gidwani et al., 2004).

During an apophyseal avulsion fracture, a fragment of bone is pulled away from the main bony mass as a result of a sudden tensile force applied due to a powerful muscle contraction (Porr et al., 2011). Apopyseal avulsion fractures commonly occur at the apophyseal attachments of large musculotendinous units but can also occur at the attachments of ligaments, e.g., at the origin of the anterior talofibular ligament.

In late adolescence, the growing cartilage ossifies and the connection between the apophysis and the body of the bone strengthens. At this point, the musculotendinous unit becomes the weakest structure in transferring the force between muscle and bone (Porr et al., 2011), explaining why the injuries change when working with skeletally mature athletes.

Pelvic apophyseal avulsion fractures

There are a number of sites in the adolescent pelvis that can sustain an avulsion injury (Fig. 30.5). Table 30.1 demonstrates this type of avulsion fracture, the corresponding muscle creating the traction and the potential muscle action during the mechanism of injury. Table 30.2 shows the findings of two studies on pelvic apophyseal fractures.

Signs and symptoms. Signs and symptoms of pelvic apophyseal avulsion fractures include the following:
- Acute, sudden onset of pain preceded by a forceful muscular contraction. A popping sensation is frequently reported.
- Difficulty ambulating and activity-limiting pain.
- Swelling and/or bruising may be observed.
- Pain and weakness on assessment of the corresponding muscle group.
- Localized pain, tenderness on palpation of the avulsion site.
  Clinically, an athlete with an anterior inferior iliac spine (AIIS) avulsion may be unable to straight leg raise whereas an ischial tuberosity avulsion may cause pain during sitting.

Diagnostics/imaging. In an elite academy environment, MRI is the first choice of investigation to identify an apophyseal avulsion. A plain radiograph or a computed tomography (CT) scan can also be used, although the ionizing radiation dosage must be taken into consideration. A CT scan may be necessary if surgery is required; surgery is mainly reserved for large fractures or when the fracture is considerably displaced (>20 mm).

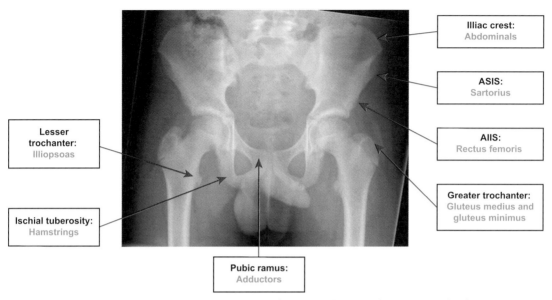

Fig. 30.5 Paediatric pelvic radiograph demonstrating sites of pelvic avulsions and muscles involved. *AIIS*, Anterior inferior iliac spine; *ASIS*, anterior superior iliac spine.

Table 30.1 Avulsion fractures

Pelvic avulsion type	Muscle	Potential action during avulsion
Anterior inferior iliac spine (AIIS) avulsion	Origin of rectus femoris	Can result after contraction of the rectus femoris. 50% of AIIS avulsions are caused by kicking (Schuett et al., 2015)
Anterior superior iliac spine (ASIS) avulsion	Origin of sartorius	Occurs during sudden contraction of the sartorius muscle when the hip is extended with the knee flexed (Schuett et al., 2015)
Ischial tuberosity	Origin of hamstrings	Commonly caused by a sudden eccentric load to the proximal hamstrings, as occurs in kicking (Schuett et al., 2015). Can be misdiagnosed as a hamstring strain and poor management can lead to complications with nonunion (Gidwani et al., 2004)
Iliac crest	Insertion of abdominals	Occurs with the forceful muscle contraction of internal/external obliques and transverse abdominis muscle. May occur with sudden rotational or change of direction activities and may include activities that include arm swing and opposing contraction of the gluteus medius and tensor fascia lata
Lesser trochanter	Insertion of iliopsoas	Sudden contraction of the hip flexors
Pubic ramus	Origin of adductors	Sudden contraction of the adductors. This may include a sudden change of direction
Greater trochanter	Insertion of gluteus medius and gluteus minimus	Rare in paediatrics, but can occur with a sudden contraction of lateral rotators, e.g., gluteus medius/minimus

Sources: Gidwani, S., Jagiello, J., Bircher, M., 2004. Avulsion fracture of the ischial tuberosity in adolescents–an easily missed diagnosis, British Medical Journal 329 (7457), 99–100. Schuett, D.J., Bomar, J.D., Pennock, A.T., 2015. Pelvic apophyseal avulsion fractures: a retrospective review of 228 cases. Journal of Pediatric Orthopaedics 35 (6), 617–623.

Table 30.2 The findings of two large-scale studies on pelvic apophyseal fractures

Schuett et al., 2015	Rossi and Dragoni, 2001
228 cases of pelvic apophyseal fractures in 225 patients	203 cases of pelvic apophyseal fractures in 198 adolescent athletes (multisports)
Age range: 10.7–18.2 years	Age range: 11–17 years
Mean age: 14.5 years ±1.4 years in males;14 years ±1.2 years in females	Mean age: 13.8 years
Males > females (76% male vs. 24% female)	Males > females (68.5% male vs. 31.5% females)
Apophyseal avulsions in frequency order	
AIIS (49%) ASIS (30%) Ischial tuberosity (11%) Iliac crest (10%)	Ischial tuberosity (109 cases; 54%*) AIIS (45 cases; 22%*) ASIS (39 cases; 19%*) Superior corner of pubic symphysis (7 cases; 3%*) Iliac crest (3 cases; 1.5%*)
The most common mechanism of injury was sprinting/running (39%) followed by kicking (29%)	
Surgery was indicated in only 3% of cases, fracture displacement >20 mm increased the risk of nonunion by 26 times	

*Percentages have been added to allow the reader to easily compare between studies.
AIIS, Anterior inferior iliac spine; *ASIS*, anterior superior iliac spine.
Sources: Rossi, F., Dragoni, S., 2001. Acute avulsion fractures of the pelvis in adolescent competitive athletes: prevalence, location and sports distribution of 203 cases collected. Skeletal Radiology 30 (3), 127– 131; Schuett, D.J., Bomar, J.D., Pennock, A.T., 2015. Pelvic apophyseal avulsion fractures: a retrospective review of 228 cases. Journal of Pediatric Orthopaedics 35 (6), 617–623.

Treatment.
- Initial treatment includes protecting and unloading the injured area, with the weight-bearing status being partial or non-weight-bearing with elbow crutches, depending on the index of suspicion and the injury presentation.

- Ice can be applied regularly for the first 2–3 days to ease pain and inflammation. Ice should be applied for a minimum of 10 minutes but not longer than 20–30 minutes. The optimal time between applications must be guided by pain and discomfort (ACPSEM, 2010).
- During this early offloading period, the range of movement in unaffected joints is maintained and general conditioning activities are continued whilst not compromising/stressing the site of the avulsion.
- Following the initial fracture healing phase, a gradual loading programme is commenced with consideration of the stresses placed on the affected tissues.
- A graduated rehabilitation programme will aim to regain full range of movement of the affected joint and those around (e.g., lumbar spine). The player must recover good strength, power and muscular flexibility of the limb as a whole, as well as regaining neural length, cardiovascular capacity and plyometric ability before progressing to sport-specific activities.
- A phased return to play is utilized (see Return to training and return to play below).

General advice for extended absence from football due to injury.
- Setting short- and long-term 'challenges' and targets will help engage the young player in their rehabilitation.
- Including the parent/guardian in the management plan helps them to support the child. Other members of the interdisciplinary team such as psychologists and coaching staff can help to maintain player motivation during extended injury periods. The player may also find it beneficial to speak to others who have been through similar experiences.
- Nutrition advice may be useful during this time whilst they are not as active.
- Parents may report that the player is demonstrating behavioural issues/mood swings at home during an extended injury period. Reassure the player that frustration is a common response following a significant injury but explain that although they cannot control what has happened to them, they can maintain a positive attitude and appropriate behaviour.

Return to training and return to play.
Amendments may be made to the training intensity, duration or frequency when a player is returning following an extended absence due to an injury. The player may take part in a phased return to play, with half-sessions or light technical work being completed initially, in order to reduce the exposure time and load when returning to training.

Paediatric athletes should return to training and be completing sessions fully without issues prior to being exposed to the intensity and load of a match situation when 'returning to play'.

Avulsion of the tibial spine (tibial eminence fractures)

This is a bony avulsion of the anterior cruciate ligament (ACL) from its insertion on the intercondylar eminence. It is relatively rare and is the functional equivalent to a rupture of the ACL in an adolescent or adult athlete. Scrimshire et al. (2018) found the mean age to be 11.8 years.

Signs and symptoms

Fractures of the tibial eminence may clinically mimic an ACL injury, with the player presenting with a painful knee, haemarthrosis, decreased range of motion and difficulty bearing weight.

Treatment

Further investigation and an orthopaedic review is required. The fracture type will determine whether a conservative or surgical approach is appropriate.

Tibial tubercle avulsion

The tibial tubercle develops from a secondary ossification centre in the proximal tibia and develops due to traction (Frey et al., 2009). Avulsion fractures are relatively rare occurrences and the avulsion commonly occurs during sprinting or jumping activities. Frey et al. (2009) state that the mechanically vulnerable period in males is approximately 13–16 years of age; mean age 13.7 years (range 11 years 5 months to 17 years 6 months). Pretell-Mazzini et al. (2016) found the mean age at time of surgery was 14.6 years; they state that due to the proximal tibial physis closing from posterior to anterior, the fracture pattern depends on the amount of physeal closure when the injury occurs. These fractures can be classified using the Watson-Jones (Watson-Jones, 1955) or Ogden (Ogden et al., 1980) classifications.

Frey et al. (2009) found a strong predominance of males with this injury and suggest that higher traction stresses are placed on the tibial tubercle due to males generally being physically larger with stronger quadriceps. The tibial physis also close later in males than in females.

No definitive correlation has been found between Osgood–Schlatter disease (OSD) and tibial avulsion fractures but Pretell-Mazzini et al. (2016) reported a prior history of OSD to be associated with tibial avulsion fractures in 23% of cases within the articles they reviewed. However, they state that it is still unclear as to what percentage of patients with OSD will go on to develop a fracture.

Signs and symptoms

- Sudden onset of pain in the tibial tubercle region during jumping or sprinting activities.
- The player presents with knee swelling/haemarthrosis, reduced range of movement, an extensor lag and high-riding patella with more significant avulsions. Palpation of tibial tubercle is painful and there may be a bony fragment or deformity identifiable.
- Compartment syndrome is a potentially severe complication that must be considered on initial presentation of this injury (Frey et al., 2009).

Diagnostics/imaging

Plain radiography or MRI is used for imaging and diagnosis.

Treatment

The fracture management depends of the degree of the avulsion. These cases can be managed conservatively with cast immobilization or treated surgically with either open or arthroscopic reduction and internal fixation/percutaneous screw fixation.

Calcaneum avulsion fractures

Avulsions of the Achilles tendon are rare paediatric injuries, but Yu and Yu (2015) describe chronic loads resulting in stress fractures which are misdiagnosed as Sever's disease.

Diagrammatic overview

A diagrammatic overview of paediatric fractures and other paediatric musculoskeletal conditions that can affect young athletes can be found in Chapter 31 (see Fig. 31.1).

Summary

It is important for those working with skeletally immature athletes to be fully aware of the skeletal differences between adults and children and the corresponding fracture types. Clinicians should have a low threshold for onwards orthopaedic referral if there is any suspicion of a fracture. This could aid early diagnosis or indeed avoid missing an epiphyseal plate fracture or a tendon/ligament avulsion. These conditions have the potential to lead to growth disturbances and can have long-term functional implications if mismanaged.

References

ACPSEM, 2010. Acute Management of Soft Tissue Injuries. ACPSEM, Sheffield, UK.

Bachmann, L.M., Kolb, E., Koller, M.T., Steurer, J., ter Riet, G., 2003. Accuracy of Ottawa ankle rules to exclude fractures of the ankle and mid-foot: systematic review. British Medical Journal 326, 417.

Bulloch, B., Neto, G., Plint, A., Lim, R., Lidman, P., Reed, M., et al., 2003. Validation of the Ottawa knee rule in children: a multicenter study. Annals of Emergency Medicine 42 (1), 48–55.

Caine, D., DiFiori, J., Maffulli, N., 2006. Physeal injuries in children's and youth sports: reasons for concern? British Journal of Sports Medicine 40 (9), 749–760.

Cepela, D.J., Tartaglione, J.P., Dooley, T.P., Patel, P.N., 2016. Classifications in brief: Salter-Harris classification of pediatric physeal fractures. Clinical Orthopaedics and Related Research 474 (11), 2531–2537.

Dowling, S., Spooner, C.H., Liang, Y., Dryden, D.M., Friesen, C., Klassen, T.P., et al., 2009. Accuracy of Ottawa Ankle Rules to exclude fractures of the ankle and midfoot in children: a meta-analysis. Academic Emergency Medicine 16 (4), 277–287.

Engebretsen, L., Steffen, K., Bahr, R., Broderick, C., Dvorak, J., Janarv, P.-M., et al., 2010. The International Olympic Committee Consensus Statement on age determination in high-level young athletes. British Journal of Sports Medicine 44 (7), 476–484.

Frey, S., Hosalkar, H., Cameron, D.B., Heath, A., Horn, B.D., Ganley, T.J., 2009. Tibial tuberosity fractures in adolescents. Journal of Children's Orthopaedics 2 (6), 469–474.

Gidwani, S., Jagiello, J., Bircher, M., 2004. Avulsion fracture of the ischial tuberosity in adolescents--an easily missed diagnosis. British Medical Journal 329 (7457), 99–100.

Ling, S.-N.J., Cleary, A.J., 2018. Are unnecessary serial radiographs being ordered in children with distal radius buckle fractures? Radiology Research and Practice 2018, 5143639.

Lozano-Berges, G., Matute-Llorente, Á., González-Agüero, A., Gómez-Bruton, A., Gómez-Cabello, A., Vicente-Rodríguez, G., et al., 2017. Soccer helps build strong bones during growth: a systematic review and meta-analysis. European Journal of Pediatrics 177, 295–310.

Malina, R.M., Bouchard, C., Bar-Or, O., 2004. Growth, Maturation, and Physical Activity. Human Kinetics, Champaign, IL.

Ogden, J.A., Tross, R.B., Murphy, M.J., 1980. Fractures of the tibial tuberosity in adolescents. The Journal of Bone and Joint Surgery. American Volume 62 (2), 205–215.

Pennock, A.T., Ellis, H.B., Willimon, S.C., Wyatt, C., Broida, S.E., Dennis, M.M., et al., 2017. Intra-articular physeal fractures of the distal femur: a frequently missed diagnosis in adolescent athletes. Orthopaedic Journal of Sports Medicine 5 (10), 2325967117731567.

Porr, J., Lucaciu, C., Birkett, S., 2011. Avulsion fractures of the pelvis - a qualitative systematic review of the literature. Journal of the Canadian Chiropractic Association 55 (4), 247–255.

Pretell-Mazzini, J., Kelly, D.M., Sawyer, J.R., Esteban, E.M.A., Spence, D.D., Warner, W.C., et al., 2016. Outcomes and complications of tibial tubercle fractures in pediatric patients: a systematic review of the literature. Journal of Pediatric Orthopedics 36 (5), 440–446.

Rossi, F., Dragoni, S., 2001. Acute avulsion fractures of the pelvis in adolescent competitive athletes: prevalence, location and sports distribution of 203 cases collected. Skeletal Radiology 30 (3), 127–131.

Salter, R.B., Harris, W.R., 1963. Injuries involving the epiphyseal plate. Journal of Bone and Joint Surgery 45 (3), 587–622.

Schiller, J., DeFroda, S., Blood, T., 2017. Lower Extremity avulsion fractures in the Pediatric and adolescent athlete. Journal of the American Academy of Orthopaedic Surgeons 25 (4), 251–259.

Schuett, D.J., Bomar, J.D., Pennock, A.T., 2015. Pelvic apophyseal avulsion fractures: a retrospective review of 228 cases. Journal of Pediatric Orthopedics 35 (6), 617–623.

Scrimshire, A.B., Gawad, M., Davies, R., George, H., 2018. Management and outcomes of isolated paediatric tibial spine fractures. Injury 49 (2), 437–442.

Ting, B.L., Kalish, L.A., Waters, P.M., Bae, D.S., 2016. Reducing cost and radiation exposure during the treatment of pediatric greenstick fractures of the forearm. Journal of Pediatric Orthopedics 36 (8), 816–820.

Vorlat, P., De Boeck, H., 2003. Bowing fractures of the forearm in children. Clinical Orthopaedics and Related Research 413, 233–237.

Watson-Jones, R., 1955. Fractures and Joint Injuries, vol. 2, fourth ed. Lippincott Williams & Wilkins, Baltimore.

Williams, K.G., Smith, G., Luhmann, S.J., Mao, J., Gunn 3rd, J.D., Luhmann, J.D., 2013. A randomized controlled trial of cast versus splint for distal radial buckle fracture. Pediatric Emergency Care 29 (5), 555–559.

Yu, S.M., Yu, J.S., 2015. Calcaneal avulsion fractures: an often forgotten diagnosis. American Journal of Roentgenology 205 (5), 1061–1067.

Chapter 31

Growing bones: osteochondroses and serious paediatric conditions

Diane Ryding

Introduction

This chapter presents an overview of both nonarticular and articular osteochondroses along with their management principles pertaining to an elite football academy environment. It also discusses serious and sinister 'not to be missed' conditions and disease processes such as bone or joint infections and tumours.

At the end of the chapter, a summary section provides an overview of the age range occurrences of conditions covered by both this and the prior chapter.

Osteochondroses

Osteochondroses is the term used to describe a group of self-limiting disorders that affect the growing skeleton. They are classed as *nonarticular* or *traction apophysitis* if they affect the secondary ossification centres, *intraarticular* if they affect a joint (commonly causing necrosis), or *physeal* as in Sheuermann's disease. They result from a period of growth, injury or overuse of the developing growth plate and surrounding ossification centres (Atanda et al., 2011).

Nonarticular osteochondroses: traction apophysitis

- Apophysitis of the tibial tubercle (Osgood–Schlatter disease; OSD).
- Apophysitis of the pole of the patella (Sinding-Larsen Johansson syndrome).
- Calcaneal apophysitis (Sever's disease).
- Apophysitis of the fifth metatarsal head (Iselin's disease).

Apophysitis treatment and management principles

Nonarticular apophysitis is commonly referred to as 'growing pains', is symptom driven, self-limiting in nature and will resolve with the closing of the physis. Explanation of the condition will reduce both player and parental concerns and will reassure them that the pain is not down to any sinister or serious pathology.

Assessment
Assess and address any tightness in lower limb musculature including iliopsoas, quadriceps, hamstrings, gastrocnemius and soleus muscles, which may demonstrate tightness following periods of rapid growth. Similarly, assess for any weakness in lower limb musculature, (including gluteal muscles). Identify any biomechanical abnormalities and refer to podiatry as appropriate.

Activity modification
Load management can be adopted to manage symptoms and to allow pain levels to remain within acceptable limits for the player. Amendments may be made to the intensity, duration or frequency of training, with the use of half-sessions or light technical work in order to reduce load. Consider the combined load of other activities or sports that the child participates in outside of football.

Self-management strategies
Ice application after training can provide pain relief.

Rehabilitation
If the player is struggling to cope with modified training load, then a period of rehabilitation may be required. During this time, other aspects of the physical development of the player can also be targeted, e.g., upper/lower body functional strength, neuromuscular control and flexibility. The

player may work to maintain their cardiovascular capacity by low-load but high-intensity cardiovascular activities. If the player is unable to complete even rehabilitation exercises due to pain, then a short period of rest may be beneficial.

Graduated return to play
If a player has not been playing due to symptoms, a graduated return to play can be adopted with the use of half-sessions or load management by modification of the duration or intensity of sessions.

Tibial tubercle traction apophysitis (Osgood–Schlatter disease)

OSD is a traction apophysitis of the tibial tubercle caused by repetitive strain on the quadriceps tendon (Circi et al., 2017). It presents in growing children (boys, 12–15 years; girls, 8–12 years), is due to repetitive strain on the secondary ossification centre of the tibial tubercle and symptoms are often exacerbated by running or jumping activities or by direct contact such as kneeling (Gholve et al., 2007). Radiographic changes include irregularity of the apophysis with separation from the tibial tubercle in the early stages due to microavulsions occurring at the chondrofibro-osseous tibial tubercle; fragmentation may occur in later stages (Circi et al., 2017; Gholve et al., 2007). The condition may reoccur for 12–18 months before the player reaches skeletal maturity in this region and there is closure of the apophysis (Circi et al., 2017).

Signs and symptoms
- May present unilaterally or bilaterally.
- Pain increases during or following sporting activity (running/jumping).
- Pain is often exacerbated by resisted quadriceps testing.
- There is likely to be lower limb tightness, specifically (but not exclusively) involving the quadriceps. The player often demonstrates a reduced heel-to-buttock measurement on prone knee bend due to a growth spurt.
- Pain is reported at the tibial tubercle on resisted quadriceps or when squatting or lunging.
- There is pain on palpation of the tibial tubercle.
- Assess for altered biomechanics, overpronation/rear foot varus.
- Long-term, the player may develop a permanent, painless bony prominence over the tibial tubercle.

Diagnosis. Commonly the diagnosis is made by clinical assessment, but the changes can be observed on plain radiographs, by ultrasonography or magnetic resonance imaging (MRI).

Treatment and management plan. See Apophysitis treatment and management principles, with specific attention to quadriceps stretches.

Inferior pole of the patella apophysitis (Sinding-Larsen Johansson syndrome)

This form of apophysitis affects the proximal patella tendon at its insertion into the inferior pole of the patella. It is a self-limiting condition, occurring between 10 and 14 years (Carr et al., 2001).

Signs and symptoms
- May present unilaterally or bilaterally.
- Pain increases during or following sporting activity.
- Pain is often exacerbated by resisted quadriceps testing.
- There is pain and point tenderness on palpation of the pole of the patella with possible soft tissue swelling.
- There is lower limb tightness/weakness specifically involving quadriceps as per OSD.

Diagnosis, treatment and management plan. Sinding-Larsen Johansson disease is often a clinical diagnosis, but changes can be observed via ultrasonography, radiographs or MRI. Management is similar to that given in Apophysitis treatment and management principles, with specific attention to quadriceps stretches.

Calcaneal apophysitis (Sever's disease)

Calcaneal apophysitis elicits heel pain relating to the calcaneal apophyseal growth plate. It occurs between the ages of 8 and 15 years (James et al., 2013), with the mean age at presentation being 10–10.8 years (Davison et al., 2016; Rachel et al., 2011). Its aetiology is unknown, but increased tension on the Achilles tendon due to the rapid growth may create traction on the calcaneal apophysis growth plate. Biomechanical abnormalities may also contribute to heel pain.

Signs and symptoms. Based on Scharfbillig et al. (2008) calcaneal apophysitis presents as follows:
- It may be unilateral or bilateral and present after a period of rapid growth.
- There is no history of trauma.
- Pain worse during/after sporting activity but improves with rest and is better in the mornings.
- There is pain and tenderness over calcaneal insertion of Achilles tendon or the pain may extend around the sides of the calcaneus or underneath.
- There is a positive squeeze test, where medial-lateral compression of the apophyseal area of the calcaneum elicits pain in the absence of serious trauma.
- It elicits pain on standing on tiptoes or on passive dorsiflexion.
- Tightness in gastrocnemius/soleus is frequently present.

Diagnostics/imaging. This is a clinical diagnosis; imaging is not normally necessary unless an avulsion is suspected.

Treatment and management plan. The treatment approach is based around a combination of physiotherapy (with specific attention to gastrocnemius and soleus stretches), a biomechanical assessment, use of a heel raise and load modification. See also Apophysitis treatment and management principles.

The biomechanical considerations (James et al., 2013) can be summarized as follows:

- A rear foot valgus position may affect the windlass mechanism and change the force required at the tendo-Achilles (TA).
- If repetitive impact forces are considered to be traumatizing the apophysitis, then the use of an orthotic with a heel cup or heel raise with shock-absorbing properties may be useful for cushioning and pain relief of the calcaneal soft tissues.
- An early heel raise or leg length discrepancy may increase TA loading. A heel raise may be used to correct these issues, but it must be inserted into every change of shoe.

Wiegerinck et al. (2016) compared a wait-and-see approach to wearing a heel raise or eccentric exercise at a 6-week and 3-month timescale; each resulted in a clinically relevant and statistically significant reduction of heel pain due to calcaneal apophysitis. From a child-reported perspective, at the 6-week stage the heel raise group improved more than the wait-and-see group, and from a parental perspective, eccentric exercises improved more than the wait-and-see group. The author concludes that patients and parents should be consulted about their preferred treatment option.

James et al. (2016) found a relative advantage in the use of heel raises over prefabricated orthoses at the 1- and 2-month timescale. However, at the 6- and 12-month stage, they found no relative advantage of either treatment approaches. This suggests that heel raises at the initial stages of therapy may aid children with Sever's disease to remain physically active.

Clinical tips

Review the footwear the child is wearing (school shoes/trainers); discourage them from wearing flat pump-like trainers without sufficient heel cushioning or midfoot support. Advise the player to wear trainers in the home rather than bare feet if they are struggling with symptoms. If a heel raise is provided as part of the management plan, explain to the child the increased importance of stretching gastrocnemius and soleus muscles.

Apophysitis of the fifth metatarsal base (Iselin's disease)

Iselin's disease is an osteochondrosis or traction apophysitis at the base of the fifth metatarsal (MT). Radiography may show a fragmented appearance to the apophysis with bony overgrowth (Gillespie, 2010). Iselin's disease is caused by repetitive minor trauma due to the force of the peroneus brevis tendon. It affects both males and females and first appears on radiographs at approximately 8–11 years in boys and 11–14 years in girls (Forrester et al., 2017). Fusion of the apophysis is usually complete by 17–18 years (Gillespie, 2010).

Signs and symptoms

- There may be nontraumatic (insidious onset) or traumatic (ankle inversion injury) cause.
- Pain and tenderness is found on palpation to the fifth MT base at the insertion of peroneus brevis.
- There may be swelling observable on the lateral aspect of the foot and the player may be limping due to pain.

Diagnostics/imaging. This is a clinical diagnosis, but X-ray imaging may be required to rule out a fracture or an os vesalianum accessory bone, which can cause pain.

Treatment and management plan. See Apophysitis treatment and management principles. A period of immobilization may be required in more severe cases and occasional surgical excision or fixation is required if there is ongoing pain or nonunion.

Articular osteochondrosis

This group includes the following:

- Legg–Calvé–Perthes disease (LCPD)
- Osteochondritis dissecans (OCD)
- Köhler's disease
- Freiberg's disease.

Legg–Calvé–Perthes disease

Legg–Calvé–Perthes disease is an idiopathic avascular necrosis of the proximal femoral epiphysis. It is commonly seen in children between the ages of 4 and 8 years, with a male bias (male to female ratio 4:1); it is bilateral in 10–13% of cases (Ramachandran and Reed, 2016).

LCPD is thought to be a multifactorial pathogenic process. Leroux et al. (2017) state that LCPD develops after at least two episodes of ischaemia (double insult), but the possible involvement of microtrauma, environmental insults, prenatal conditions, genetic factors, or hypercoagulability remains controversial.

Signs and symptoms

- The child presents with a limp. Groin, thigh or referred knee pain may be present without any history of trauma. However, pain may not be severe and the limp may be the significant finding.
- Reduced abduction and internal rotation of the hip on examination.

Diagnosis and treatment. Plain radiography and/or MRI scans are used to confirm diagnosis. Although not indicated in all cases, a surgical approach (commonly osteotomy), aims to prevent loss of joint congruency by restoring the epiphysis to its central position within the acetabular cup. This consequently guides the remodelling process (Leroux et al., 2017). Postoperative rehabilitation will be surgery dependent. In the younger age range, rest and antiinflammatories may be advised as a nonoperative approach.

Osteochondritis dissecans (OCD)

Osteochondritis dissecans (OCD) is a focal, idiopathic alteration of subchondral bone with risk for instability and disruption of the adjacent articular cartilage that may result in premature osteoarthritis (Edmonds and Shea, 2013). The aetiology is not completely understood but acute trauma, repetitive microtrauma, local vascular insufficiency and genetic factors have all been proposed as potential causes. Launay (2015) suggests a male bias with a male:female ratio of 4:1, and a prevalence between the ages of 10 and 13 years. The Research on Osteochondritis Dissecans of the Knee (ROCK) Study Group suggests 12- to 19-year-olds are most frequently affected (ROCK, 2018).

Signs and symptoms. History and clinical findings can be vague and diagnosis may rely on plain radiographs or MRI diagnosis (Bauer and Polousky, 2017). The following are typical at presentation:
- Activity-exacerbated nonspecific joint pain
- Vague, poorly localized pain
- Mechanical symptoms such as locking may indicate the presence of a loose body
- Joint effusion
- Limited joint range of movement
- Point tenderness over the affected femoral condyle
- Quadriceps atrophy may be a late finding.

Diagnosis and treatment. Plain radiographs may be of use, but MRI is recommended for staging (i.e., determining the lesion stability) (DiFiori et al., 2014), often by using the International Cartilage Repair Society (ICRS) Cartilage Lesion Classification System. Factors determining whether surgical intervention is indicated include physeal status, fragment stability, presence of a loose body, the patient's functional requirements along with the size, stage and depth of the lesion (Erickson et al., 2013).

Stable juvenile cyst-like lesions of <1.3 mm in length on MRI have the highest predictive validity for healing potential with nonoperative management (Krause et al., 2013). The aim of a conservative approach is to allow healing of the subchondral bone whilst ultimately gaining a functional pain-free joint. Rest and restriction of physical activities that cause excessive and repetitive compressive stress on the affected knee is often advised until symptoms have disappeared and the lesion is progressing toward healing (Andriolo et al., 2018). The lesion characteristics, location, articular cartilage involvement and stability, skeletal maturity and symptomology should all be considered when planning rehabilitation progressions (Paterno et al., 2014; Yang et al., 2014). Physiotherapy aims to protect the healing tissue whilst looking to reduce joint effusion, regain joint range of movement and strengthen lower limb musculature. Ultimately, a phased return to play and load modification is implemented. Krause et al. (2013), however, suggest that conservative management may fail in up to 50% of cases. Negative prognostic factors include larger lesion size, more severe lesion stages and greater skeletal maturity along with swelling or locking (Andriolo et al., 2018).

Köhler's disease

Köhler's disease is a rare idiopathic osteochondrosis of the tarsal navicular bone, with the National Organization for Rare Disorders (NORD, 2004) suggesting that it may be the result of stress-related compression at a critical time during the period of growth.

Signs and symptoms
- It is commonly unilateral in presentation.
- It presents in children aged 5–6 years but cases have been reported in 2- to 11-year-olds; it has a male bias (Sharp et al., 2003).
- Pain increases with weight-bearing, and the child walks on the lateral aspect of the foot. Midfoot and medial border pain and swelling are present on assessment (Gillespie, 2010).

Diagnosis and treatment. Plain radiographs may exclude a fracture but show fragmentation, sclerosis and narrowing or flattening of the tarsal navicular bone. Köhler's disease can also be an incidental radiographic finding with no pain and tenderness (Gillespie, 2010).

The condition itself is self-limiting in nature and is therefore managed symptomatically. Treatment can vary from a 'watchful wait' to a period of immobilization. Analgesics and foot orthoses may also help symptoms. Symptoms often resolve within 1 year, but may persist up to 2 years.

Freiberg's disease

Freiberg's disease is an osteochondrosis/osteonecrosis of the MT head. It commonly occurs in the second MT head (68%) but can occur in the other lesser metatarsals, most commonly the third (27%), and then the fourth (3%) (Carmont et al., 2009).

The aetiology is unknown but it is thought to be multifactorial. Trauma and circulatory issues (leading to avascular necrosis) play a major but not solitary role. The age at onset varies in the literature but it appears to occur at all ages after adolescence. In 10 female patients, Al-Ashhab et al. (2013) found the mean age to be 18.3 years (range 14–24 years). It has a female-to-male bias of 5:1 according to Katcherian (1994).

Signs and symptoms. Freiberg's disease typically presents with:

- Pain (and possibly swelling) at the head of the second MT (or lesser MT head)
- Antalgic gait or pain or stiffness on mobilizing
- Pain increasing with activity
- Pain increasing when increasing weight-bearing through forefoot as in calf raises/heeled footwear
- A small effusion may be palpable and a callus may be seen underneath the affected MT head (Lin and Liu, 2013).

Diagnosis and treatment. Radiographically, the second (or affected) MT head may appear flattened, with areas of increased sclerosis and fragmentation (Lin and Liu, 2013).

Conservative treatment focusing on offloading and relieving stress is uniformly accepted as the appropriate initial management (Cerrato, 2011). Activity reduction or modification is advised and Schade (2015) suggests nonsteroidal antiinflammatory medication, padding (under the MT head), orthotics or immobilization as conservative treatment options.

If conservative treatment fails, a wide variety of surgical procedures exist, but Schade (2015) suggests that the optimal procedure is unknown.

Physeal osteochondrosis

Scheuermann's disease

In Scheuermann's disease, there is abnormal development of the thoracic spine, where the anterior aspect of the vertebra does not develop as quickly as the posterior aspect; this produces a characteristic wedge-shaped deformity seen on radiographs and consequently causes the characteristic kyphosis. Other radiographic signs include Schmorl's nodes, anterior flattening of the vertebral endplate and anterior detachment of a ring apophysis. This osteochondrosis develops prior to puberty and becomes most prominent during the adolescent growth spurt (Fotiadis et al., 2008), with Gokce and Beyhan (2016) suggesting that typical onset of presentation is 13–16 years. It is not yet clear if there is a gender bias.

The aetiology of Scheuermann's kyphosis remains unclear; it is thought to be multifactorial with mechanical, metabolic and endocrine influences being postulated (Bezalel et al., 2014; Ristolainen et al., 2012). This is a self-limiting condition with disease progression ceasing once the individual reaches skeletal maturity.

Symptoms and diagnosis. This is predominantly a radiographic diagnosis, but initial presentation will include a structural thoracic kyphosis, which the patient cannot consciously correct. This kyphosis may appear more obvious in the forward flexed position. Spinal movement is reduced and there may be accompanying pain, although pain is not the predominant presentation. The generally accepted definition, published by Sørensen, is that at least three consecutive vertebral bodies with a minimum of 5 degreees of wedging must be present on X-ray to justify the diagnosis (Sørensen, 1964).

Treatment. High-quality evidence for the conservative management of Scheuermann's disease is lacking in the literature, with management being largely dependent on the degree of kyphosis. In 2010, the 7th Society on Scoliosis Orthopaedic and Rehabilitation Treatment (SOSORT) consensus paper was published on the conservative treatment of idiopathic and Scheuermann's kyphosis (de Mauroy et al., 2010). The consensus deemed that rigidity of the curve, anatomical location and local pain was key information before deciding on treatment methods. The consensus concurs with the usefulness of physiotherapy and rigid braces in aiming to correct thoracic hyperkyphosis during adolescence, with many choosing physiotherapy prior to bracing. The main therapeutic aims of physical exercise in patients at risk of requiring bracing are self-postural control, self-elongation and proprioception training. Muscular endurance, strengthening exercises, stretching (pectorals and hamstrings) and breathing techniques are also included, with 20 minutes of home exercises being the average. The main aim of bracing is to avoid hyperflexion on the anterior wall. Bracing aims to restore alignment of muscular forces, reduces continuous loading and provides the thoracolumbar discs space for proper development. Brace rigidity has been suggested as the main reason for unsuccessful treatment.

In terms of surgical options, Riouallon et al. (2018) suggest that both posterior-only and combined anterior/posterior (AP) primary fusion surgery for Scheuermann's kyphosis provides stable functional and radiological results; therefore AP fusion technique should be reserved for major deformations. The average age at the time of surgery was 23 years and the average kyphosis was 77 degrees. A long-term follow up showed that there was no correlation between the degree of kyphosis and self-reported quality of life or health or back pain (Ristolainen et al., 2012).

Other 'not to be missed' paediatric presentations

Slipped upper femoral epiphysis

A slipped upper (or capital) femoral epiphysis (SUFE/ SCFE) occurs when there is anatomic disruption through the proximal femoral physis and displacement of the femoral neck in relation to the femoral head. The femoral head remains anatomically positioned in the acetabulum while the metaphysis moves anteriorly and superiorly relative to the epiphysis. SUFE may present following minor trauma, but often its onset is insidious in nature. The exact cause of this condition is unknown but Alshryda et al. (2018) suggest that increased shear forces and weakness of the physis during adolescence may be contributory factors. Hormonal factors and the child being overweight have also been proposed.

Naseem et al. (2017) suggest an incidence of 1–10/100,000. Boles and El-Khoury (1997) suggest that males are more commonly affected than females, with the peak age of SUFE occurrence being slightly higher for boys (range 10–17 years; average 13–14 years) than for girls (range 8–15 years; average 11–12 years). Slips are often classified as stable if the patient is able to weight-bear (with or without crutches) or unstable if weight-bearing is not possible (Loder et al., 1993). However, Alshryda et al. (2018) suggest that researchers are now challenging this definition. Prompt identification of SUFE is crucial as suboptimal management can lead to substantial disability.

Signs and symptoms

Signs and symptoms of SUFE include:
- Pain in the hip/thigh and/or knee. This may be a sudden (nontraumatic) onset or gradual onset over a period of months. Hip pain can be referred to the knee via the medial obturator nerve; therefore, any child presenting with knee pain must also undergo a hip examination.
- Limping, antalgic or externally rotated gait with possible Trendelenburg signs.
- External rotation of the affected leg and a leg length discrepancy may be apparent.
- Reduced hip range of movement, especially internal rotation with pain and guarding.

Diagnosis and treatment. On suspicion of the player having a SUFE, provide them with crutches (non-weight-bearing) and arrange immediate referral to an emergency department for medical evaluation. A plain radiograph is often the primary diagnostic investigation.

A SUFE will require surgical pinning, which aims to hold the bones in place until the epiphyseal plate fuses. The type of fixation will depend on the distance that the head of the femur has slipped. Some surgeons may advocate pinning the unaffected side to prevent future slipping, as approximately 20% of patients have bilateral slips, but this is controversial. Long-term complications include osteoarthritis, chondrolysis and avascular necrosis (AVN), with a study by Loder et al. (1993) finding AVN developed in 47% of unstable slips (14 out of 30 hips) but none of the stable slips (0 out of 25). The rehabilitation process is guided by the orthopaedic surgeon.

Femoroacetabular impingement

The 2016 Warwick consensus defined femoroacetabular impingement (FAI) syndrome as 'a motion-related clinical disorder of the hip with a triad of symptoms, clinical signs and imaging findings. It represents symptomatic premature contact between the proximal femur and the acetabulum' (Griffin et al., 2016, p. 1170).

There are two types of FAI morphology, *cam* and *pincer*, both of which may occur independently or simultaneously. However, the presence of cam and/or pincer morphology does not always lead to FAI (van Klij et al., 2018).

Cam morphology. This is more prevalent in males than females (23.9% vs. 9.9%) ($P < 0.001$) (Li et al., 2017). It is also more prevalent in adults than adolescents but has been shown to gradually increase during skeletal growth (van Klij et al., 2018). Cam morphology has been observed from 10 years of age (Palmer et al., 2018).

Pincer morphology. This is equally common in males and females (29.7% vs. 35.1%) (Li et al., 2017), with pincer morphology being observed from 12 years of age (Li et al., 2017; Monazzam et al., 2013).

Ross et al. (2017) reviewed surgery for FAI in 39 skeletally immature patients and determined a mean age 15.8 years (range 12.8–19.3 years).

Symptoms and diagnosis

The following is based on the Warwick consensus by Griffin et al. (2016):

Symptoms, clinical signs and imaging findings must be present to diagnose FAI syndrome:
- Hip pain, clicking, catching, stiffness or giving way.
- Motion-related hip/groin pain; pain may also be reported in the back, buttock or thigh.
- Restricted hip range of motion (ROM), positive FADIR (flexion, adduction, and internal rotation) test – which is sensitive but not specific.

- Radiological findings of cam or pincer morphology. Computed tomography (CT), MRI or intra-articular hip injections may also aid diagnosis.

Treatment

The conservative approach includes patient education, activity modification and analgesia. Physiotherapy includes hip ROM, hip stability (gluteal activation), neuromuscular control and lumbopelvic dissociation.

The surgical approach aims to correct the hip morphology. Postoperative physiotherapy is generally a criterion-based approach led by the postoperative protocol (which is surgeon/surgery specific).

Lumbar spondylolysis and spondylolisthesis

Adolescent low back pain (ALBP) is common within the athletic population, but awareness of the presentation of spondylolysis and spondylolisthesis in the adolescent athlete is important for optimal outcomes to be achieved.

Spondylolysis

Spondylolysis is bony defect or stress fracture that develops through the pars interarticularis as the weakest part of the vertebra; it can occur unilaterally or bilaterally. A fracture is 'complete' if it passes through the pars or 'incomplete' if it appears on one side of the cortex and not the other (Gregory et al., 2004).

Spondylolysis may occur at any age or at any level, but the vast majority occur at L5 (85–95%), followed by L4 (5–15%), with the incidence appearing to be higher in the young athletic population (Standaert and Herring, 2000). In a study of cricketers and football players, Gregory et al. (2004) found the median age at onset of low back pain was 17.5 years (range 11.5–44.0 years) with most complete fractures being identified at L5 (66.7%), followed by L3 (15.7%), then L4 (6.9%). Incomplete fractures were more evenly distributed throughout the lower three lumbar levels, predominantly L5 (41.7%) followed by L4 (37.5%), then L3 (20.8%).

Spondylolysis is thought to be either developmental or acquired secondary to chronic low-grade trauma (Leone et al., 2011). Developmentally, the pars interarticularis ossification process occurs from posterior to anterior and congenital incompletion may predispose it to stress fractures (Lawrence et al., 2016; Purcell and Micheli, 2009). Spondylolysis or spondylolisthesis is believed to be acquired due to mechanical factors, as zero cases were detected in nonambulatory patients in comparison to the 5.8% incidence in the general population ($P < 0.001$) (Rosenberg et al., 1981).

Repeated hyperextension and rotation of the lumbar spine are proposed as predisposing factors (Gregory et al., 2004).

Spondylolisthesis

Spondylolisthesis can be defined as the anterior displacement of the vertebral body in reference to the bordering vertebral bodies (Gagnet et al., 2018). An aetiological classification of spondylolysis and spondylolisthesis was presented by Wiltse et al. in 1976 and includes five types: dysplastic (congenital defect), isthmic, (either pars fatigue following multiple healed stress fractures, pars elongation or an acute pars fracture), degenerative, traumatic or neoplastic. In young athletes, isthmic spondylolithesis is the predominant type identified, where there has been a bilateral pars fracture leading to slippage of the vertebra. This is frequently (but not exclusively) in a forwards direction and is commonly a slip of L5 on S1. In a long-term follow-up (45 years) Beutler et al. (2003) found that only patients who had a bilateral pars defect progressed to a spondylolisthesis.

A commonly adopted method of grading the severity of spondylolisthesis is the Meyerding classification (Meyerding, 1932), which grades the severity of the spondylolithesis based on the percentage that one vertebral body has slipped forward over the vertebral body below:

- grade 1: 0–25%
- grade 2: 26–50%
- grade 3: 51–75%
- grade 4: 76–99%
- grade 5: ≥100%.

Spondylolysis symptoms and diagnosis

No clinical test, either alone or in combination, can distinguish between spondylolysis and other forms of ALBP (Sundell et al., 2013), with Alqarni et al. (2015) suggesting that the commonly used one-legged hyperextension test (stork standing test) has virtually no value in diagnosing patients with spondylolysis. Consequently, Gregory et al. (2004) suggest that all athletes presenting with activity-related low back pain which increases with lumbar extension should be investigated for spondylolysis.

Spondylolysis can also be asymptomatic, but can be a cause of spine instability, back pain, and radiculopathy (Leone et al., 2011) with pain radiating to the buttock area or posterior thigh. Clinical findings may include tightness of the hip flexors and hamstrings, weakness of the abdominals and gluteals, and an excessive lordotic posture (Lawrence et al., 2016).

It is possible to diagnose spondylolysis via CT, MRI or by an oblique plain radiograph. Although CT scanning is more sensitive for visualizing the regional degenerative changes and sclerosis associated with pars defects, MRI is able to detect early bone marrow oedema, which can suggest a stress response without a visible fracture line (Leone et al., 2011). On an oblique radiograph, the 'Scottie dog sign' will identify a spondylolysis, where a defect/break in the pars interarticularis appears as a collar on the 'Scottie dog'. Compared to the other two methods, MRI does not emit ionizing radiation and is therefore the preferred primary investigation in adolescent athletes with suspected spondylolysis. It is important to note that spondylolysis can be an incidental finding on MRI in an asymptomatic patient.

Spondylolysis treatment

There is lack of large controlled clinical trials in the physiotherapeutic management of spondylolysis and treatment itself may depend on MRI findings. A criterion-based rehabilitation programme is designed around the degree of spondylolysis (unilateral/bilateral or high signal and visible fracture line), biological healing timescales and ultimately symptomology.

In the early phase, the player is provided with posture advice and will refrain from any sporting activities until symptoms settle/resolve, in order to allow bony healing. Within this healing phase, rehabilitation may include pain-free, low-load static core stability exercises in supported positions. Occasionally, surgeons advocate the use of spinal bracing during the healing phase. There is some evidence that low-intensity pulsed ultrasound (LIPU) may be beneficial in the treatment of early-stage lumbar spondylolysis for improving fracture healing timescales (Busse et al., 2002) and return to play (Tsukada et al., 2017), although further larger studies are required.

As symptoms reduce, exercises will be progressed to include stretches for hamstring, gluteal or hip flexor muscles as appropriate, along with lumbar/thoracic mobility exercises and progressive functional core stability work. Once the initial symptoms have resolved, there will be a progressive loading phase allowing for fracture healing timescales. The player will commence low load cardiovascular work, progressing back to jogging, sprinting, multidirectional work and sport specific training and a graduated return to play programme.

If lumbar pars injuries remain symptomatic after an extended period of conservative treatment, a surgical approach, such as spinal screw fixation, may be required

Spondylolisthesis symptoms and diagnosis

Patients with grade 1 or 2 slippage may not experience symptoms and therefore a conservative approach will be selected. A player with a lumbar spondylolisthesis causing nerve root compression may present with radiculopathy or report lower limb 'shooting pains' on lumbar extension.

They may adopt a kyphotic lumbar posture in order to reduce symptoms and relieve pressure from the nerve roots (Gagnet et al., 2018). A systematic review by Alqarni et al. (2015) suggests that there appears to be utility in palpating lumbar spinal processes for the diagnosis of lumbar spondylolisthesis. There may be a visible or palpable step at the level of the slip with associated soft tissue abnormalities. Imaging with MRI, X-ray or CT can confirm diagnosis.

Spondylolisthesis treatment

Lundine et al. (2014) found that nonoperative management of the minimally symptomatic or asymptomatic child with a high-grade spondylolisthesis does not lead to significant problems.

Those who do not respond to conservative treatment (pain relief, bracing and physiotherapy) or those with greater degrees of slippage (grade 3 and above) may require surgical fixation. Bouras and Korovessis (2015) suggest that if a player undergoes surgery (pars repair and short fusion), return to play will depend on the sport and varies from 6 to 12 months, with prohibition in collision sports.

Clinical tip

Although the classically described visible or palpable step may be present with someone with a high-grade spondylolisthesis, the ability to detect a lower-grade slip is dependent on the degree of the slippage and the surrounding soft tissues so it may not be perceptible. If it is suspected, it must be investigated!

Bone and joint infections: septic arthritis and acute osteomyelitis

Septic arthritis and osteomyelitis affect synovial joints and bone, respectively. Septic arthritis can occur in isolation or as a secondary process related to underlying osteomyelitis (Monsalve et al., 2015). Septic arthritis affects synovial joints and can be caused by bacterial, viral or fungi infiltration. Any joint may be affected but bacterial infections often affect the larger joints especially knees, ankles, shoulders, hips, elbows or wrists (NORD, 2009). Osteomyelitis is usually bacterial in origin and among children and teens, the long bones of the legs and arms are most frequently affected, especially the epiphysis (NORD, 2005). An infection can enter the joint through the bloodstream via a nearby wound or injury, with bacterial infections often progressing quickly.

Symptoms

A player with septic arthritis or osteomyelitis often presents with an acute onset of pain with an oedematous, warm,

Table 31.1 Sarcomas (bone and soft tissue cancers)

Sarcoma	Most common sites	Potential presentation
Osteosarcoma	Femur (42%, with 75% of these in distal femur) Tibia (19%, with 80% of these in proximal tibia) Humerus (10%, with 90% of these proximal) Skull or jaw (8%) Pelvis (8%)	Bimodal age distribution: first peak between 10–14 years, suggesting a relationship with the adolescent growth spurt; second peak in adults >65 Symptoms may include bone pain that gets worse at night or with activity. Swelling around the bone
Ewing sarcoma	Pelvic, femur and tibia along with the chest wall/scapula	Teenagers and young adults Symptoms as per osteosarcoma
Rhabdomyosarcoma	Skeletal muscle cells	Can occur in teens and adults, but commonly found in children under 10-years-old. Symptoms may include lumps (painful/nonpainful), swelling or bowel problems

From American Cancer Society, 2016. Types of cancers that develop in adolescents. Available at: https://www.cancer.org/cancer/cancer-in-adolescents/what-are-cancers-in-adolescents.html; Ottaviani, G., Jaffe, N., 2009. The epidemiology of osteosarcoma. Cancer Treatment and Research 152, 3–13. https://doi.org/10.1007/978-1-4419-0284-9_1.

tender joint/limb with restricted ROM and inability to weight-bear. The player may be pyrexial, systematically unwell or have a recent history of local infection or trauma (including simple abrasions).

Diagnosis and treatment

This is an orthopaedic emergency. Urgent referral to accident and emergency is required for further investigations which may include bloods (full blood count, C-reactive protein, erythrocyte sedimentation rate), sonography and joint aspiration or radiographs. Manz et al. (2018) advocate the use of MRI and systematic pathogen detection including nucleic acid testing to limit the use of broad-spectrum antibiotics along with the treatment duration. Septic joints may require arthrotomy and washout in theatre.

Clinical tip

If a player has been prescribed antibiotics for a recent infection, these may be masking septic arthritis and osteomyelitis symptoms and the presentation may be more subtle. Be aware of the 'red herring' reporting of an unclear injury in an aim to explain the presentation.

Tumours misdiagnosed as musculoskeletal injuries

The important message here is that the clinical presentation of a musculoskeletal tumour may mimic that of a sports-related

injury. A study by Muscolo et al. (2003) found that, 'poor quality radiographs and an unquestioned original diagnosis despite persistent symptoms were the most frequent causes of an erroneous diagnosis' (p. 1209). All medical staff working with paediatric players must remain conscious of potential red flags in the paediatric athlete including pain at rest, night pain or any symptoms that do not fit the normal pattern or that are worsening over time. Immediate medical referral must occur if the clinician has any suspicions.

Sarcomas are cancers that start in connective tissues such as muscles, bones or fat cells. Primary bone cancers can occur at any age but are often diagnosed in older children and teens (American Cancer Society, 2016) (Table 31.1).

Bone health, growth, maturation and injuries

Even with all the potential for bony injuries, a systematic review and meta-analysis by Lozano-Berges et al., 2017 suggests that beginning to play football at the prepubertal stage and continuing through puberty appears to be appropriate for improving bone health during these developmental and future stages.

While the relationship between maturation, growth and musculoskeletal conditions remains plausible, Swain et al. (2018) found that the current body of knowledge is at high risk of bias, impeding the ability to establish whether biological maturity and growth are independent risk factors for musculoskeletal conditions.

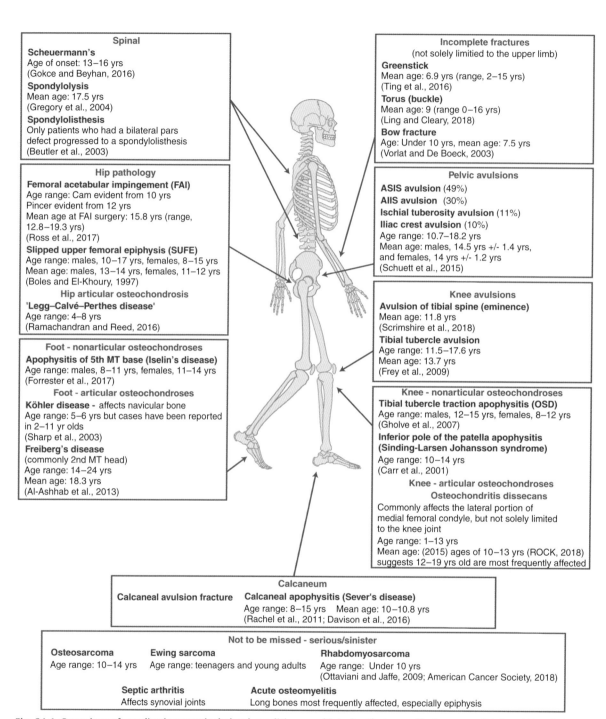

Spinal

Scheuermann's
Age of onset: 13–16 yrs
(Gokce and Beyhan, 2016)
Spondylolysis
Mean age: 17.5 yrs
(Gregory et al., 2004)
Spondylolisthesis
Only patients who had a bilateral pars
defect progressed to a spondylolisthesis
(Beutler et al., 2003)

Hip pathology
Femoral acetabular impingement (FAI)
Age range: Cam evident from 10 yrs
Pincer evident from 12 yrs
Mean age at FAI surgery: 15.8 yrs (range,
12.8–19.3 yrs)
(Ross et al., 2017)
Slipped upper femoral epiphysis (SUFE)
Age range: males, 10–17 yrs, females, 8–15 yrs
Mean age: males, 13–14 yrs, females, 11–12 yrs
(Boles and El-Khoury, 1997)
Hip articular osteochondrosis
'Legg–Calvé–Perthes disease'
Age range: 4–8 yrs
(Ramachandran and Reed, 2016)

Foot - nonarticular osteochondroses
Apophysitis of 5th MT base (Iselin's disease)
Age range: males, 8–11 yrs, females, 11–14 yrs
(Forrester et al., 2017)
Foot - articular osteochondroses
Köhler disease - affects navicular bone
Age range: 5–6 yrs but cases have been reported
in 2–11 yr olds
(Sharp et al., 2003)
Freiberg's disease
(commonly 2nd MT head)
Age range: 14–24 yrs
Mean age: 18.3 yrs
(Al-Ashhab et al., 2013)

Incomplete fractures
(not solely limitied to the upper limb)
Greenstick
Mean age: 6.9 yrs (range, 2–15 yrs)
(Ting et al., 2016)
Torus (buckle)
Mean age: 9 (range 0–16 yrs)
(Ling and Cleary, 2018)
Bow fracture
Age: Under 10 yrs, mean age: 7.5 yrs
(Vorlat and De Boeck, 2003)

Pelvic avulsions
ASIS avulsion (49%)
AIIS avulsion (30%)
Ischial tuberosity avulsion (11%)
Iliac crest avulsion (10%)
Age range: 10.7–18.2 yrs
Mean age: males, 14.5 yrs +/- 1.4 yrs,
and females, 14 yrs +/- 1.2 yrs
(Schuett et al., 2015)

Knee avulsions
Avulsion of tibial spine (eminence)
Mean age: 11.8 yrs
(Scrimshire et al., 2018)
Tibial tubercle avulsion
Age range: 11.5–17.6 yrs
Mean age: 13.7 yrs
(Frey et al., 2009)

Knee - nonarticular osteochondroses
Tibial tubercle traction apophysitis (OSD)
Age range: males, 12–15 yrs, females, 8–12 yrs
(Gholve et al., 2007)
**Inferior pole of the patella apophysitis
(Sinding-Larsen Johansson syndrome)**
Age range: 10–14 yrs
(Carr et al., 2001)
Knee - articular osteochondroses
Osteochondritis dissecans
Commonly affects the lateral portion of
medial femoral condyle, but not solely limited
to the knee joint
Age range: 1–13 yrs
Mean age: (2015) ages of 10–13 yrs (ROCK, 2018)
suggests 12–19 yrs old are most frequently affected

Calcaneum
Calcaneal avulsion fracture   **Calcaneal apophysitis (Sever's disease)**
Age range: 8–15 yrs   Mean age: 10–10.8 yrs
(Rachel et al., 2011; Davison et al., 2016)

Not to be missed - serious/sinister

Osteosarcoma   **Ewing sarcoma**   **Rhabdomyosarcoma**
Age range: 10–14 yrs   Age range: teenagers and young adults   Age range: Under 10 yrs
                                                                (Ottaviani and Jaffe, 2009; American Cancer Society, 2018)

Septic arthritis   **Acute osteomyelitis**
Affects synovial joints   Long bones most frequently affected, especially epiphysis

Fig. 31.1 Overview of paediatric musculoskeletal conditions and injuries that can affect young athletes. Abbreviations:
AIIS, Anterior inferior iliac spine; *ASIS*, anterior superior iliac spine; *MT*, metatarsal.

Summary

Any therapist working with paediatrics must be aware of the specific injuries and disease processes that may present in the developing skeleton, from the most common types of osteochondroses to serious and sinister pathology, where the risk of misdiagnosis could be detrimental to a young career or even the life of a young person (Fig. 31.1). Indeed the declaration that 'children are not mini adults' could not be more accurate.

References

Al-Ashhab, M.E.A., Kandel, W.A., Rizk, A.S., 2013. A simple surgical technique for treatment of Freiberg's disease. The Foot 23 (1), 29–33.

Alqarni, A.M., Schneiders, A.G., Cook, C.E., Hendrick, P.A., 2015. Clinical tests to diagnose lumbar spondylolysis and spondylolisthesis: a systematic review. Physical Therapy in Sport 16, 268–275.

Alshryda, S., Tsang, K., Chytas, A., Chaudhry, M., Sacchi, K., Ahmad, M., et al., 2018. Evidence based treatment for unstable slipped upper femoral epiphysis: systematic review and exploratory patient level analysis. Surgeon 16 (1), 46–54.

American Cancer Society, 2016. Types of cancers that develop in adolescents. Available at: https://www.cancer.org/cancer/cancer-in-adolescents/what-are-cancers-in-adolescents.html.

Andriolo, L., Candrian, C., Papio, T., Cavicchioli, A., Perdisa, F., Filardo, G., 2018. Osteochondritis dissecans of the knee - conservative treatment strategies: a systematic review. Cartilage 10 (3), 267–277.

Atanda Jr., A., Shah, S.A., O'Brien, K., 2011. Osteochondrosis: common causes of pain in growing bones. American Family Physician 83 (3), 285–291.

Bauer, K.L., Polousky, J.D., 2017. Management of osteochondritis dissecans lesions of the knee, Elbow and Ankle. Clinics in Sports Medicine 36 (3), 469–487.

Beutler, W., Fredrickson, B., Murtland, A., Sweeney, C., Grant, W., Baker, D., 2003. The natural history of spondylolysis and spondylolisthesis: 45-year follow-up evaluation. Spine 28 (10), 1027–1035. discussion 1035.

Bezalel, T., Carmeli, E., Been, E., Kalichman, L., 2014. Scheuermann's disease: current diagnosis and treatment approach. Journal of Back and Musculoskeletal Rehabilitation 27 (4), 383–390.

Boles, C., El-Khoury, G.Y., 1997. Slipped capital femoral epiphysis1. Radiographics 17 (4), 809–823. Available at: https://pubs.rsna.org/doi/pdf/10.1148/radiographics.17.4.9225384.

Bouras, T., Korovessis, P., 2015. Management of spondylolysis and low-grade spondylolisthesis in fine athletes. A comprehensive review. European Journal Of Orthopaedic Surgery & Traumatology : Orthopedie Traumatologie 25 (Suppl. 1(S1)), S167–S175.

Busse, J.W., Bhandari, M., Kulkarni, A.V., Tunks, E., 2002. The effect of low-intensity pulsed ultrasound therapy on time to fracture healing: a meta-analysis. CMAJ : Canadian Medical Association Journal 166 (4), 437–441. Available at: http://www.ncbi.nlm.nih.gov/pubmed/11873920. [Accessed 19 June 2018].

Carmont, M.R., Rees, R.J., Blundell, C.M., 2009. Current concepts review: Freiberg's disease. Foot & Ankle International 30 (2), 167–176.

Carr, J.C., Hanly, S., Griffin, J., Gibney, R., 2001. Sonography of the patellar tendon and adjacent structures in pediatric and adult patients. American Journal of Roentgenology 176 (6), 1535–1539.

Cerrato, R.A., 2011. Freiberg's disease. Foot and Ankle Clinics 16 (4), 647–658.

Circi, E., Atalay, Y., Beyzadeoglu, T., 2017. Treatment of Osgood–Schlatter disease: review of the literature. Musculoskeletal Surgery 101 (3), 195–200.

Davison, M.J., David-West, S.K., Duncan, R., 2016. Careful assessment the key to diagnosing adolescent heel pain. The Practitioner 260 (1793), 30–32. 3 Available at: http://www.ncbi.nlm.nih.gov/pubmed/27382917. [Accessed 26 May 2018].

de Mauroy, J., Weiss, H., Aulisa, A., Aulisa, L., Brox, J., Durmala, J., et al., 2010. 7th SOSORT consensus paper: conservative treatment of idiopathic Scheuermann's kyphosis. Scoliosis 5 (9), 1–15. Available at: http://www.scoliosisjournal.com/content/5/1/9. [Accessed 1 June 2018].

DiFiori, J.P., Benjamin, H.J., Brenner, J.S., Gregory, A., Jayanthi, N., Landry, G.L., et al., 2014. Overuse injuries and burnout in youth sports: a position statement from the American Medical Society for Sports Medicine. British Journal of Sports Medicine 48 (4), 287–288.

Edmonds, E.W., Shea, K.G., 2013. Osteochondritis dissecans: editorial comment. Clinical orthopaedics and related research. Association of Bone and Joint Surgeons 471 (4), 1105–1106.

Erickson, B.J., Chalmers, P.N., Yanke, A.B., Cole, B.J., 2013. Surgical management of osteochondritis dissecans of the knee. Current Reviews in Musculoskeletal Medicine 6, 102–114.

Forrester, R.A., Eyre-Brook, A.I., Mannan, K., 2017. Iselin's disease: a systematic review. Journal of Foot & Ankle Surgery 56 (5), 1065–1069. 2017/08/27.

Fotiadis, E., Kenanidis, E., Samoladas, E., Christodoulou, A., Akritopoulos, P., Akritopoulou, K., 2008. Scheuermann's disease: focus on weight and height role. European Spine Journal 17 (5), 673–678.

Frey, S., Hosalkar, H., Cameron, D.B., Heath, A., David Horn, B., Ganley, T.J., 2008. Tibial tuberosity fractures in adolescents. Journal of Paediatric Orthopaedics 2 (6), 469–474.

Gagnet, P., Kern, K., Andrews, K., Elgafy, H., Ebraheim, N., 2018. Spondylolysis and spondylolisthesis: a review of the literature. Journal of Orthopaedics 15 (2), 404–407.

Gholve, P.A., Scher, D.M., Khakharia, S., Widmann, R.F., Green, D.W., 2007. Osgood Schlatter syndrome. Current Opinion in Pediatrics 19 (1), 44–50.

Gillespie, H., 2010. Osteochondroses and apophyseal injuries of the foot in the young athlete. Current Sports Medicine Reports 9 (5), 265–268.

Gokce, E., Beyhan, M., 2016. Radiological imaging findings of scheuermann disease. World Journal of Radiology 8 (11), 895–901. Baishideng Publishing Group Inc.

Gregory, P.L., Batt, M.E., Kerslake, R.W., 2004. Comparing spondylolysis in cricketers and soccer players. British Journal of Sports Medicine 38, 737–742.

Griffin, D.R., Dickenson, E.J., O'Donnell, J., Agricola, R., Awan, T., Beck, M., et al., 2016. The Warwick Agreement on femoroacetabular impingement syndrome (FAI syndrome): an international consensus statement. British Journal of Sports Medicine 50 (19), 1169–1176. 2016/09/16.

James, A.M., Williams, C.M., Haines, T.P., 2013. Effectiveness of interventions in reducing pain and maintaining physical activity in children and adolescents with calcaneal apophysitis (Sever's disease): a systematic review. Journal of Foot and Ankle Research 6 (1), 16. 2013/05/07.

James, A.M., Williams, C.M., Haines, T.P., 2016. Effectiveness of footwear and foot orthoses for calcaneal apophysitis: a 12-month factorial randomised trial. British Journal of Sports Medicine 50 (20), 1268–1275. 2016/02/27.

Katcherian, D.A., 1994. Treatment of Freiberg's disease. The Orthopedic Clinics of North America 25 (1), 69–81. Available at: http://www.ncbi.nlm.nih.gov/pubmed/8290232. [Accessed 25 June 2018].

Krause, M., Hapfelmeier, A., Möller, M., Amling, M., Bohndorf, K., Meenen, N.M., 2013. Healing predictors of stable juvenile osteochondritis dissecans knee lesions after 6 and 12 months of nonoperative treatment. The American Journal of Sports Medicine, 41(10). SAGE PublicationsSage CA, Los Angeles, CA, pp. 2384–2391.

Launay, F., 2015. Sports-related overuse injuries in children. Orthopaedics & Traumatology: Surgery & Research 101 (1), S139–S147.

Lawrence, K.J., Elser, T., Stromberg, R., 2016. Lumbar spondylolysis in the adolescent athlete. Physical Therapy in Sport, 20. Elsevier, pp. 56–60.

Leone, A., Cianfoni, A., Cerase, A., Magarelli, N., Bonomo, L., 2011. Lumbar spondylolysis: a review. Skeletal Radiology, 40(6). Springer-Verlag, pp. 683–700.

Leroux, J., Abu Amara, S., Lechevallier, J., 2017. Legg-Calve-Perthes disease. Orthopaedics & Traumatology: Surgery Research. 2017/11/21.

Li, Y., Helvie, P., Mead, M., Gagnier, J., Hammer, M.R., Jong, N., 2017. Prevalence of femoroacetabular impingement morphology in asymptomatic adolescents. Journal of Pediatric Orthopedics 37 (2), 121–126.

Lin, H.-T., Liu, A.L.-J., 2013. Freiberg's infraction. Case Reports 2013 (jun18 1). p. bcr2013010121-bcr2013010121.

Ling, S.-N.J., Cleary, A.J., 2018. Are unnecessary serial radiographs being ordered in children with distal radius buckle fractures? Radiology Research and Practice 5143639.

Loder, R.T., Richards, B.S., Shapiro, P.S., Reznick, L.R., Aronson, D.D., 1993. Acute slipped capital femoral epiphysis: the importance of physeal stability. The Journal of Bone and Joint Surgery. American Volume 75 (8), 1134–1140. Available at: http://www.ncbi.nlm.nih.gov/pubmed/8354671. [Accessed 28 May 2018].

Lozano-Berges, G., Matute-Llorente, A., González-Agüero, A., Gómez-Bruton, A., Gómez-Cabello, A., Vicente-Rodríguez, G., et al. 2018. Soccer helps build strong bones during growth: a systematic review and meta-analysis. European Journal of Pediatrics 177, 295–310.

Lundine, K.M., Lewis, S.J., Al-Aubaidi, Z., Alman, B., Howard, A.W., 2014. Patient outcomes in the operative and nonoperative management of high-grade spondylolisthesis in children. Journal of Pediatric Orthopedics 34 (5), 483–489.

Manz, N., Krieg, A.H., Heininger, U., Ritz, N., 2018. Evaluation of the current use of imaging modalities and pathogen detection in children with acute osteomyelitis and septic arthritis. European Journal of Pediatrics 177 (7), 1071–1080.

Meyerding, H.W., 1932. 'Spondyloptosis. Surgery, Gynecology & Obstetrics 54, 371–377.

Monazzam, S., Bomar, J.D., Dwek, J.R., Hosalkar, H.S., Pennock, A.T., 2013. Development and prevalence of femoroacetabular impingement-associated morphology in a paediatric and adolescent population. The Bone & Joint Journal 95–B (5), 598–604.

Monsalve, J., Kan, J.H., Schallert, E.K., Bisset, G.S., Zhang, W., Rosenfeld, S.B., 2015. Septic arthritis in children: frequency of coexisting unsuspected osteomyelitis and implications on imaging work-up and management. American Journal of Roentgenology 204 (6), 1289–1295.

Muscolo, D.L., Ayerza, M.A., Makino, A., Costa-Paz, M., Aponte-Tinao, L.A., 2003. Tumors about the knee misdiagnosed as athletic injuries. The Journal of Bone and Joint Surgery. American Volume 85–A (7), 1209–1214. Available at: http://www.ncbi.nlm.nih.gov/pubmed/12851344. [Accessed 25 February 2018].

Naseem, H., Chatterji, S., Tsang, K., Hakimi, M., Chytas, A., Alshryda, S., 2017. Treatment of stable slipped capital femoral epiphysis: systematic review and exploratory patient level analysis. Journal of Orthopaedics and Traumatology 18 (4), 379–394.

NORD (National Organization for Rare Disorders), 2004. Köhler Disease [online] Available at: https://rarediseases.org/rare-diseases/kohler-disease/ [Accessed 8th April 2018].

NORD (National Organization for Rare Disorders), 2005. Osteomyelitis [online] Available at: https://rarediseases.org/rare-diseases/osteomyelitis/ [Accessed 10th April 2018].

NORD (National Organization for Rare Disorders), 2009. Arthritis, Infectious [online] Available at: https://rarediseases.org/rare-diseases/arthritis-infectious/ [Accessed 9th April 2018].

Ottaviani, G., Jaffe, N., 2009. The epidemiology of osteosarcoma. Cancer Treatment and Research 152, 3–13.

Palmer, A., et al., 2018. Physical activity during adolescence and the development of cam morphology: a cross-sectional cohort study of 210 individuals. British Journal of Sports Medicine 52, 601–610.

Paterno, M.V., Prokop, T.R., Schmitt, L.C., 2014. Physical therapy management of patients with osteochondritis dissecans: a comprehensive review. Clinics in Sports Medicine 33 (2), 353–374.

Purcell, L., Micheli, L., 2009. Low back pain in young athletes. Sports Health 1(3), 212–222.

Rachel, J.N., Williams, J.B., Sawyer, J.R., Warner, W.C., Kelly, D.M., 2011. Is radiographic evaluation necessary in children with a clinical diagnosis of calcaneal apophysitis (Sever disease)? Journal of Pediatric Orthopaedics 31 (5), 548–550.

Ramachandran, M., Reed, D.W., 2016. Legg-Calvé–perthes disease of the hip. Orthopaedics and Trauma 30 (6), 461–470.

Riouallon, G., Morin, C., Charles, Y.-P., Roussouly, P., Kreichati, G., Obeid, I., et al., 2018. Posterior-only versus combined anterior/posterior fusion in Scheuermann disease: a large retrospective study. European Spine Journal 27 (9), 2322–2330.

Ristolainen, L., Kettunen, J.A., Heliövaara, M., Kujala, U.M., Heinonen, A., Schlenzka, D., 2012. Untreated Scheuermann's disease: a 37-year follow-up study. European Spine Journal 21 (5), 819–824.

ROCK (Research in Osteochondritis of the Knee), 2018. Patient Education. [online] Available at: https://kneeocd.org/patient-education/#1492949877752-4d44c196-4604 [Accessed 5th March. 2018].

Rosenberg, N.J., Bargar, W.L., Friedman, B., 1981. The incidence of spondylolysis and spondylolisthesis in nonambulatory patients. Spine 6 (1), 35–38. Available at: http://www.ncbi.nlm.nih.gov/pubmed/7209672. [Accessed 19 June 2018].

Ross, J.R., Stone, R.M., Ramos, N.M., Bedi, A., Larson, C.M., 2017. Surgery for femoroacetabular impingement in skeletally immature patients: radiographic and clinical analysis. Orthopaedic Journal of Sports Medicine 5 (7_Suppl. 6). 2325967117S0025.

Schade, V.L., 2015. Surgical management of Freiberg's infraction. Foot & Ankle Specialist 8 (6), 498–519.

Scharfbillig, R.W., Jones, S., Scutter, S.D., 2008. Sever's disease: what does the literature really tell us? Journal of the American Podiatric Medical Association 98 (3), 212–223. Available at: http://www.ncbi.nlm.nih.gov/pubmed/18487595. [Accessed 26 May 2018].

Schuett, D.J., Bomar, J.D., Pennock, A.T., 2015. Pelvic apophyseal avulsion fractures: a retrospective review of 228 cases. Journal of Pediatric Orthopaedics 35 (6), 617–623.

Scrimshire, A.B., Gawad, M., Davies, R., George, H., 2018. Management and outcomes of isolated paediatric tibial spine fractures. Injury 49 (2), 437–442.

Sharp, R.J., Calder, J.D.F., Saxby, T.S., 2003. Osteochondritis of the navicular: a case report. Foot & Ankle International 24(6), 509–513.

Sørensen, K.H., 1964. Scheuermann's Juvenile Kyphosis: Clinical Appearances, Radiography, Aetiology, and Prognosis. Munksgaard, Copenhagen.

Standaert, C.J., Herring, S.A., 2000. Spondylolysis: a critical review. British Journal of Sports Medicine 34, 415–422.

Sundell, C.G., Jonsson, H., Ådin, L., Larsén, K.H., 2013. Clinical examination, spondylolysis and adolescent athletes. International Journal of Sports Medicine 34 (3), 263–267.

Swain, M., Kamper, S.J., Maher, C.G., Broderick, C., McKay, D., Henschke, N., 2018. Relationship between growth, maturation and musculoskeletal conditions in adolescents: a systematic review. British Journal of Sports Medicine 52, 1246–1252.

Ting, B.L., Kalish, L.A., Waters, P.M., Bae, D.S., 2016. Reducing cost and radiation exposure during the treatment of pediatric greenstick fractures of the forearm. Journal of Pediatric Orthopaedics 36 (8), 816–820.

Tsukada, M., Takiuchi, T., Watanabe, K., 2017. Low-intensity pulsed ultrasound for early-stage lumbar spondylolysis in young athletes. Clinical Journal of Sport Medicine 1.

van Klij, P., Heerey, J., Waarsing, J.H., Agricola, R., 2018. The prevalence of cam and pincer morphology and its association with development of hip osteoarthritis. Journal of Orthopaedic & Sports Physical Therapy 48 (4), 230–238.

Vorlat, P., De Boeck, H., 2003. Bowing fractures of the forearm in children. Clinical Orthopaedics and Related Research 413 (413), 233–237.

Wiegerinck, J.I., Zwiers, R., Sierevelt, I.N., van Weert, H.C., van Dijk, C.N., Struijs, P.A., 2016. Treatment of calcaneal apophysitis. Journal of Pediatric Orthopaedics 36 (2), 152–157.

Wiltse, L.L., Newman, P.H., Macnab, I., 1976. Classification of spondylolisis and spondylolisthesis. Clinical Orthopaedics and Related Research (117), 23–29. Available at: http://www.ncbi.nlm.nih.gov/pubmed/1277669. [Accessed 20 June 2018].

Yang, J.S., Bogunovic, L., Wright, R.W., 2014. Nonoperative treatment of osteochondritis dissecans of the knee. Clinics in Sports Medicine 33 (2), 295–304.

Chapter | 32 |

Cardiac event in the young athlete

Dean Chatterjee, Nikhil Ahluwalia and Aneil Malhotra

Introduction

Sudden cardiac death (SCD) in a young athlete is thankfully a rare event. Nevertheless, in sport it is vital to be aware of this devastating event and the consequences of it. Sudden cardiac death is defined as '… an event that is non-traumatic, non-violent, unexpected, and resulting from sudden cardiac arrest within six hours of previously witnessed normal health' (Sharma et al., 1997). Sudden cardiac death is the unexpected failure of heart function during exercise or sport or immediately after exercise without trauma. The heart stops pumping adequately and therefore the athlete loses consciousness, collapses and inevitably dies unless normal heart rhythm can be restored.

To understand the severity of the situation it is important to look at the overall figures in sudden cardiac death in athletes (Harmon et al., 2015a):
- incidence is approximately 1/50,000
- mean age at death in athletes is 23 years
- 40% of deaths in athletes are of those <18 years
- it is more common in males than females (9:1)
- 90% deaths occur during or immediately after exertion.
Looking at the figures, it is clear how vital it is to be aware of the condition. There are various causes of sudden cardiac death including congenital and anatomical abnormalities, cardiomyopathies, arrhythmias, undetermined and acquired causes. Clinical manifestations can range from chest pain, dyspnoea and palpitations to exertional dizziness and syncope. Athletes can also be asymptomatic.

The medical care of sports teams can be busy and hectic at the best of times. Both a clear screening policy for cardiac pathology, as discussed below, and thorough preparedness of interdisciplinary team for sudden cardiac arrest and SCD (Box 32.1) are key components to managing risk to athletes (Shah et al., 2018). The reader is also referred to Chapter 42 on emergency aid preparation.

Preparticipation cardiac screening (PPS) in athletes is premised on the detection of cardiac disorders associated with SCD. The juxtaposition of tragic pathology on a background of exemplary health status of young athletes has a significant emotional impact and presents a health concern that glares in the public eye. Consequently, the desire to identify those at highest risk through a screening process is understandable. However, the practical implementation of a robust, effective programme is complex. The contemporary controversies regarding PPS are around cost effectiveness, screening protocol and false positive cases in the context of exercise-induced cardiac remodelling.

Pathology associated with SCD can occasionally manifest forewarning symptoms leading to diagnosis via traditional healthcare pathways. However, many cases remain clinically indolent until a significant, often fatal, index event and electrocardiogram (ECG) analysis can dramatically improve sensitivity. Early detection through PPS can mitigate SCD risk through risk stratification, primary prevention and facilitate evidence-based activity recommendations (Corrado et al., 2006).

Sudden cardiac death in athletes

Estimates of SCD in the young population taken from death certificate-based data suggests at least 8 deaths per week in England and Wales (Papadakis et al., 2009). Overwhelming multisystem health benefits associated with regular exercise participation are seen at a population-level. However, the risk of SCD is almost 3 times as likely in athletes as compared to sedentary counterparts (Corrado et al., 2003). This is referred to as the 'paradox of exercise' and can be a highly visible tragedy as well as a significant loss of life years. SCD is the most common cause of death in young athletes in the UK, during activity but also off the field too (Wasfy et al.,

Box 32.1 **Match day preparation**

Match days are often chaotic for sports medicine departments and often compounded with player and managerial pressures. Staff availability may also vary in lower leagues, leading to multiple aspects of an emergency action protocol being performed by the same provider (e.g., the team physiotherapist or physician). Given that most sporting events are highly visible and publicized, the management of every incident is under scrutiny. Failures are often emphasized in the media, highlighting the need for emergencies to be dealt with systematically and efficiently.

It is crucial in this environment to be systematic and safe when approaching events such as sudden cardiac death. Sports clinicians do not deal with life-threatening injuries on a daily basis; therefore preparation is key. A medical team on match day should be prepared for any event possible and practicing scenarios is crucial. A summary of the key points are given here and a more detailed discussion of this topic is given by Shah et al. (2018).

While increased awareness of cardiac comorbidities in athletes through screening is helpful, time-critical interventions are crucial. In the event of a nontraumatic collapse, sudden cardiac arrest must be presumed. It is essential that all members of the match day team are ready and prepared for this. The team lead must remain calm at all times and each member must know their role and all strive to achieve the optimal outcome for the athlete. A systematic approach must be followed and reviewed throughout the event.

It is essential to be in regular contact with the management staff throughout the event. It will be worrying and upsetting for everyone involved. The casualty is not just another athlete but a team member and friend to many of the members of the team. Regular updates are vital to ensure everyone is updated on the condition of the player and everyone knows the next steps. The player's family members may be in the crowd and it is vital they are kept informed at all times.

From Shah, R., Chatterjee, A.D., Wilson, J., 2018. Creating a model of best practice: the match day emergency action protocol. British Journal of Sports Medicine 52, 1535–1536.

2016). The responsible pathophysiology is unclear, but the recurrent catecholamine exposure associated with chronic, intense exercise may induce the phenotypic manifestation of underlying cardiac disorders such as fatal arrhythmia.

The incidence of SCD in athletes is estimated at 0.3–8.0 per 100,000 athletes (Harmon et al., 2015a). The sports with the highest incidence of SCD in young athletes appear to be soccer and basketball (Harmon et al., 2011). This trend may be due to the popularity and high uptake of these sports, but also to the

sudden stop–start and dynamic movements involved that can cause adrenergic surges in athletes predisposed to SCD.

A much higher incidence is seen in male athletes compared to female athletes with a 9:1 bias; this ratio is as high as 19:1 among elite athletes (Harmon et al., 2011). Although this, in part, may be due to historically greater uptake of sport among men, it does not completely account for this bias. Furthermore, a higher incidence in black athletes than white athletes has been seen (Harmon et al., 2011).

It is important to clarify the distinction between SCD *during exercise* versus SCD *in the athlete who undertakes athletic volumes* of exercise. Population-level studies suggest that although SCD can occur during, or shortly after, exercise, the incidence of this in the general population is low (Papadakis et al., 2009). Preparticiptation screening is designed to address the latter cohort of SCD, occurring at anytime, in an athletic individual. SCD in young, competitive athletes can occur outside the context of exercise and even during sleep. This suggests an alternative, or indirect relationship between exercise-induced catecholamine surges and SCD.

Related cardiac conditions

Early athlete screening programmes were established to identify underlying cardiac disorders associated with fatal ventricular arrhythmias. It is important to focus a screening programme to target the most important underlying causes. In the context of SCD this requires consideration of age and athletic status, as aetiological distribution can vary according to these fixed variables. Whereas atherosclerotic disease and coronary artery anomalies are most prevalent causes in nonathletic populations and older athletes, inherited cardiomyopathies predominate in young athletes (Chugh and Weiss, 2015).

Overall, atherosclerotic coronary disease is the most common cause of SCD in all athletes. However, its pathogenesis does not lend itself well to existing screening technologies. Predicting atherosclerotic disease burden in asymptomatic individuals is not recommended due to cost, adverse effects of screening tools and historically high false positive rates. The focus of existing screening tools, particularly in athletic cohorts, is towards identifying the hereditary, structural and electrical cardiac disorders associated with SCD.

Targeted clinical evaluation of this cohort can highlight forewarning symptoms and have been reported in 30% of survivors (Vettor et al., 2015). These symptoms can include syncope, dizziness, chest pain, dyspnea and palpitations. These may be dismissed by the athlete or even traditional healthcare pathways. However, critical analysis of these symptoms is necessary to conserve value or risk significantly diluting positive predictive value.

Clinically quiescent cardiomyopathies frequently manifest as electrocardiographic abnormalities. Hypertrophic cardiomyopathy (HCM) is most commonly associated with SCD in contemporary American literature. The hallmark cardiac myocyte disarray that is the arrhythmogenic substrate in HCM, alongside ventricular hypertrophy, produces ECG abnormalities in 95% of cases. Arrhythmogenic right ventricular cardiomyopathy, now more accurately referred to as arrhythmogenic ventricular cardiomyopathy (AVC), is a more frequent culprit condition in some European studies. It presents with anterior T-wave changes in 80% of cases. Other cardiomyopathies, such as dilated cardiomyopathy, can also be detected, although their sensitivity by ECG is lower. Channelopathies such as congenital long QT syndrome, Brugada syndrome and Wolff–Parkinson–White syndrome (WPW) can also be demonstrated through characteristic abnormalities via this modality. However, penetrance of these conditions is incomplete and nonspecific and it is important to remember that screening is not a risk-stratification tool, rather a diagnostic test.

Evolution of the screening process has enabled expansion to detect additional cardiac disorders in a young population that, if subsequently diagnosed, may have a morbidity benefit from early intervention or surveillance, including for conditions such as valvular heart disease and aortopathies.

Congenital coronary abnormalities are another commonly cited cause of SCD, although the anatomical abnormality is difficult to predict without cardiac imaging tools such as echocardiography in the first instance and more detailed techniques such as cardiac computed tomography (CT).

Cardiac autopsy in deceased individuals has led to the recognition of a distinct aetiological contribution of sudden arrhythmic death syndrome (SADS) (Behr et al., 2007). The diagnosis of exclusion is made following sudden death in the context of a histopathologically normal heart at autopsy and unremarkable toxicology screen. The nature of this condition means it is not amenable to existing diagnostic tools and further study is required to characterize it. Further familial evaluation of first-degree relatives is also essential.

Who to screen

The study of SCD and the existing literature has tended to focus on young athletes. This is in part due to their physiological predisposition to elite athlete status and thus they are the greater focus of sporting regulation and sports science.

Earlier implementation of PPS enables the earlier detection of pathologies prior to symptoms and thus a greater population reduction in SCD. However, the phenotypic features that screening tools rely on for detection may not be present in youth and thus premature implementation may reduce sensitivity. ECG features that would be considered abnormal in adults may represent the developing 'juvenile ECG pattern', which resolve spontaneously and are benign (Basu et al., 2018). Premature ECG-based

screening may misinterpret these as disease and lead to anxiety and unnecessary downstream investigation. The juvenile ECG pattern tends to resolve by age 16 so it would be prudent to screen individuals older than this (Fig. 32.1).

In contrast, the emergence of recreational middle-aged athletes and veteran athletes should draw attention to a less-studied cohort that should not be ignored. The age-related distribution of SCD aetiologies means that in this group the pathological focus moves away from cardiomyopathy and towards atherosclerotic disease. Consequently, testing all-comers against the same criteria is not an option. A modified approach to this population may be required and the value of traditional screening pathways is less clear.

The implementation of a national policy of cardiovascular screening of athletes is explored in the Case study.

Case study

The Italian experience

Italy has recognized the role of the sports physician and the need for medical evaluation prior to sports participation since the 1950s. A nationally sponsored programme was established in 1982 to provide specialist medical attention and deliver preventative care to a population that was felt to have a greater need of medical care than provided to the general population. That the driver was clinical, as opposed to socioeconomic, enabled the institution of a mandatory preparticipation screening programme, including cardiac evaluation, for all competitive athletes.

Initial screening for all athletes comprises of an ECG, physical evaluation and history for the cost of €50. Of the amateur athletes screened, it has been found that 9% warrant further investigation based on physician's suspicion; 2% are found to have underling cardiac abnormalities – however not all require treatment or intervention. Olympic athletes are subjected to a more intensive screening programme including echocardiogram and exercise testing.

This programme has enabled the collection of more robust data. Time trend analysis over a 26-year period following the screening programme implementation demonstrated a sharp reduction in the annual incidence of SCD in screened athletes, falling from an initial peak value of 3.6 per 100,000 to 0.4 per 100,000 (Corrado et al., 2006). In contrast, the incidence in the nonathletic unscreened population remained at 0.7–0.8 per 100,000 over the same period. Thus the screening programme reduced the incidence of SCD in athletes to below that in the general population.

From Corrado, D., Basso, C., Pavei, A., Michieli, P., Schiavon, M., Thiene, G., 2006. Trends in sudden cardiovascular death in young competitive athletes after implementation of a preparticipation screening program. JAMA 296 (13), 1593–1601.

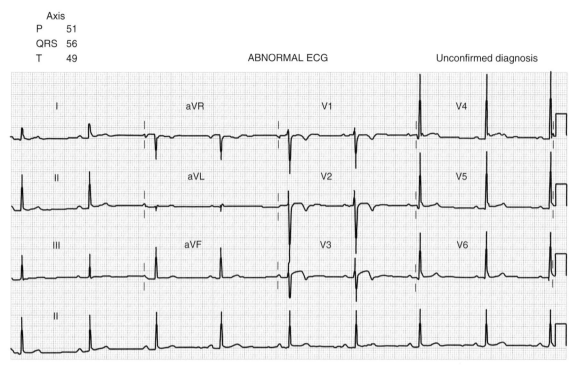

Fig. 32.1 An electrocardiogram (ECG) demonstrating a typical juvenile pattern in a 14-year-old athlete. Note the anterior T-wave inversion in V1–V2 and a biphasic T-wave in V3. Such findings are present in up to 10% of those under 15 years old and resolve in the vast majority of cases by the age of 16. Anterior T-wave inversion is associated with cardiomyopathy.

Screening programme design

The positive predictive value of a diagnostic test correlates to the pretest probability of the tested individual. A positive result in an unstratified, unselected cohort is more likely to represent a false positive. Therefore, the value of a screening test is to stratify and positively select those individuals with a high probability of underlying disease to undergo the subsequent diagnostic test.

A series of public health screening measures as the standard to audit proposed screening programmes against has been established by the World Health Organization (WHO). The Wilson and Jungner (1968) screening criteria dictate the screened condition should be: (1) a significant health problem, (2) that it can be detected sufficiently early, (3) to enable therapeutic intervention; there should be (4) a clear understanding of the pathophysiology, (5) the test itself should be economically justifiable and (6) it should be accepted by the general population.

With regard to cardiac screening in athletes, criteria (3) and (4) are well established and are directly related to the underlying disease. We have a good understanding of the most prevalent causes of SCD as a result of translational study and basic

research. Furthermore, effective medical and lifestyle interventions now exist to enable us to affect disease progression and reduce the risk of SCD. These are largely independent of the screening modality and thus do not depend on the screening tool. Criteria (2), (5) and (6) are dependent on the structure and components of the programme. Criterion (1) is ambiguous and although the great tragedy of SCD is universally recognized, the overall incidence of SCD is low and must be considered against the harm attributed to the screening of the population as well as the false positive cases subjected to cascade investigations and unnecessary anxiety. Indirectly, this is a reflection of the specificity of the screening tests. The most established tools for cardiac screening are:
• medical history and physical examination
• 12-lead resting ECG
• echocardiography.
A combination of these tend to form the basis of most PPS programmes.

Medical history and physical examination

The initial role of medical history is to determine the baseline prescreening probability of an individual. Screening is a risk-stratification tool and if an individual has a high probability of underlying cardiac disease, such as a family history of inherited cardiomyopathy, they should be redirected for appropriate specialist evaluation.

Direct patient assessment by history taking and examination should be undertaken with the intention of identifying suspicious symptoms in the athlete. However, the difficulty lies in ascribing value to nonspecific symptoms. The American Heart Association (AHA) strongly advocate the value of this assessment and delineate a high-yield, 12-point questionnaire to more effectively discriminate for significant features (Maron et al., 2007).

A pivotal cost issue is whether a front-line specialist physician is required to perform this questioning and examination. Retrospective comparisons of protocols with and without experienced specialists suggest the value inferred by an ability to appreciate true symptoms against unrelated symptoms such as isolated, atypical chest pain, translates into a significant decrease in the number of athletes referred for downstream testing and lower overall cost (Drezner et al., 2016).

However, stratification relies fully on preexisting symptoms in the athlete or recognizing the significance of features in their family. This has been shown to have poor sensitivity in order to detect cardiac disease (Harmon et al., 2015b). A thorough physical evaluation may enable the identification of valvular heart disease and aortopathies; however, this may not translate into a reduction in SCD.

Therefore, although a physician's assessment may satisfy criterion (6), the general population, the sensitivity is low and thus limits (2) early detection.

The role of the 12-lead resting ECG

The limitations of ECG screening to detect coronary artery disease are acknowledged and the focus of this modality is towards detecting inherited cardiomyopathies and ion channelopathies which manifest as ECG abnormalities. However, an appreciation of abnormality requires a deep understand of the normal resting 12-lead ECG and this is significantly more complicated in an athlete.

Long-term exercise can confer physiological, structural and electrocardiographic cardiac adaptations. These recognized features are referred to as 'athlete's heart' – a benign phenomenon (Baggish and Wood, 2011). Difficulty arises as some features can overlap with ECG and echocardiographic early findings of pathological cardiomyopathic processes, often referred to as 'grey zone' features. Attributing their aetiology in an athlete can be a challenging process.

Expert guidance has been issued to delineate the accepted limits of supraphysiological adaptations of exercise from those that may represent pathology and require further characterization. The most recent international consensus statement was published in 2017 to help guide the interpreting physician through the athlete's ECG (Fig. 32.2) (Drezner et al., 2017).

Retrospective analyses of screening protocols employing ECG screening alongside physician evaluation have recognized the superior sensitivity of the ECG in identifying those cases with underlying cardiomyopathies and channelopathies. The adjunctive clinical value of identification of WPW is also noted.

ECG screening is so widely recognized as fundamental that it has led experts in sports cardiology to call for a reconsideration and revision of those protocols that exclude the ECG to incorporate it (Harmon et al., 2015b).

Costs of infrastructure and training courses for preparticipation screening must also be taken into account in the calculation of the overall screening cost. Resources must also be accounted for when considering the role of echocardiogram; the potential to visualize the myocardium as well as valvular, congenital and septal defects improves the detection rate of certain pathologies but may appear normal when the primary defect is electrical.

ESC and AHA consensus for PPS in athletes

Contemporary recommendations by the European and American cardiology representative expert committees strongly advocate the uptake of PPS (Maron et al., 2007; Mont et al., 2017). These have been taken on board by regulatory bodies that oversee sports. The most prominent include the International Olympic Committee (IOC) and FIFA, who suggest a 12-lead ECG, medical history and physical examination as the basic standard. Within the UK, the English Football Association, Rugby Football Union (RFU) and Lawn Tennis Association have implemented programmes across the country in keeping with these recommendations too.

Although consensus management guidelines exist, the role of the multidisciplinary team is to provide the athlete with information and risk stratification to support autonomous decision making.

Ethical perspective

The preparticipation cardiac screening (PPCS) pathway is fraught with ethical issues. From the outset, subjecting an asymptomatic, healthy individual to a potentially life-changing test must be actively considered and counselled. Alongside the difficulties surrounding the management of athletes with quiescent cardiac disorders, the anxiety conferred by the uncertainty of the diagnostic process to all athletes subjected to adjunctive screening tests, as well as the potential for false positive

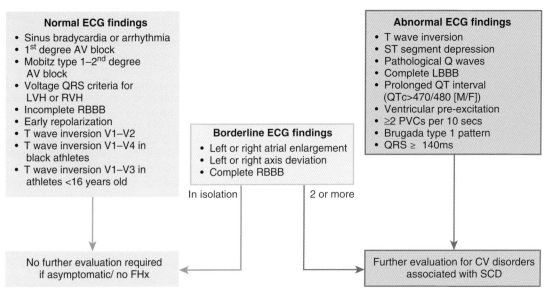

Normal ECG findings
- Sinus bradycardia or arrhythmia
- 1st degree AV block
- Mobitz type 1–2nd degree AV block
- Voltage QRS criteria for LVH or RVH
- Incomplete RBBB
- Early repolarization
- T wave inversion V1–V2
- T wave inversion V1–V4 in black athletes
- T wave inversion V1–V3 in athletes <16 years old

Borderline ECG findings
- Left or right atrial enlargement
- Left or right axis deviation
- Complete RBBB

Abnormal ECG findings
- T wave inversion
- ST segment depression
- Pathological Q waves
- Complete LBBB
- Prolonged QT interval (QTc>470/480 [M/F])
- Ventricular pre-excitation
- ≥2 PVCs per 10 secs
- Brugada type 1 pattern
- QRS ≥ 140ms

In isolation   2 or more

No further evaluation required if asymptomatic/ no FHx

Further evaluation for CV disorders associated with SCD

Fig. 32.2 The international recommendations for the interpretation of an athlete's electrocardiogram (ECG). *AV*, Atrioventricular; *CV*, cardiovascular; *FHx*, family history; *LBBB*, left bundle branch block; *LVH*, left ventricular hypertrophy; *PVCs*, premature ventricular contractions; *RBBB*, right bundle branch block; *RVH*, right ventricular hypertrophy; *SCD*, sudden cardiac death.

cases, must be considered. The incorporation of PPCS should be as part of a healthcare practitioner's duty of care through its aim of reducing the incidence of SCD. The provision of lifestyle and therapy advice may be further complicated by the uncertainty of diagnosis and the uncertainty of symptomatic penetrance of quiescent cardiomyopathy.

The consent process prior to screening should cover the components of the first-line test and also its implications, including informing the patient of the medical implications of a possible positive diagnosis as well as potential impact on competitive participation. This information must be sensitively conveyed to reflect the positive value of the test.

The intention of the screening test is to identify asymptomatic athletes with a significant underlying cardiac condition. However, the subsequent management of a healthy athlete is based on lifestyle and therapeutic recommendations in the absence of pathological symptoms. These concerns influence the test components and the need for clear management pathways for the various outcomes at each stage of the screening process. Integration with secondary sports cardiology support services, tests and specialists is the ideal.

As for all individuals receiving a diagnosis of cardiomyopathy or arrhythmogenic disorder, the highest risk individuals may require invasive preventative strategies such as implantable defibrillation or surgical intervention.

Conclusion

PPS is recommended by ESC and AHA and endorsed by a number of sporting bodies, including the IOC, the FA and RFU. No protocol will achieve 100% sensitivity due to the inherent incidence of SADS and difficulties identifying significant atherosclerotic coronary artery disease. However, cardiomyopathies are more common causes of SCD in young athletes and can be detected effectively with ECG screening.

Robust PPS of athletes with a medical history taking, clinical evaluation and resting 12-lead ECG is associated with a reduction in SCD prevalence. As the evaluation process becomes more efficient and standardized, the associated costs will reduce and further promote uptake.

References

Baggish, A.L., Wood, M.J., 2011. Athlete's heart and cardiovascular care of the athlete: scientific and clinical update. Circulation 123 (23), 2723–2735.

Basu, J., Malhotra, A., Styliandis, V., Miles, H.D., Parry-Williams, G., Tome, M., et al. 2018. 71 Prevalence and progression of the juvenile pattern in the electrocardiogram of adolescents. Heart 104, A63–A63.

Behr, E.R., Casey, A., Sheppard, M., Wright, M., Bowker, T.J., Davies, M.J., et al., 2007. Sudden arrhythmic death syndrome: a national survey of sudden unexplained cardiac death. Heart 93, 601–605.

Chugh, S.S., Weiss, J.B., 2015. Sudden cardiac death in the older athlete. Journal of the American College of Cardiology 65 (5), 493–502.

Corrado, D., Basso, C., Rizzoli, G., Schiavon, M., Thiene, G., 2003. Does sports activity enhance the risk of sudden death in adolescents and young adults? Journal of the American College of Cardiology 42 (11), 1959–1963.

Corrado, D., Basso, C., Pavei, A., Michieli, P., Schiavon, M., Thiene, G., 2006. Trends in sudden cardiovascular death in young competitive athletes after implementation of a preparticipation screening program. JAMA 296 (13), 1593–1601.

Drezner, J.A., Sharma, S., Baggish, A., Papadakis, M., Wilson, M.G., Prutkin, J.M., et al., 2017. International criteria for electrocardiographic interpretation in athletes: consensus statement. British Journal of Sports Medicine 51, 704–731.

Drezner, J.A., Harmon, K.G., Asif, I.M., Marek, J.C., 2016. Why cardiovascular screening in young athletes can save lives: a critical review. British Journal of Sports Medicine 50, 1376–1378.

Harmon, K.G., Asif, I.M., Klossner, D., Drezner, J.A., 2011. Incidence of sudden cardiac death in National Collegiate Athletic Association athletes. Circulation 123 (15), 1594–1600.

Harmon, K.G., Asif, I.M., Maleszewski, J.J., Owens, D.S., Prutkin, J.M., Salerno, J.C., et al., 2015a. Incidence, etiology, and comparative frequency of sudden cardiac death in National Collegiate Athletic Association athletes: a decade in review. Circulation 132, 10–19.

Harmon, K.G., Zigman, M., Drezner, J.A., 2015b. The effectiveness of screening history, physical exam, and ECG to detect potentially lethal cardiac disorders in athletes: a systematic review/meta-analysis. Journal of Electrocardiology 48 (3), 329–338.

Maron, B.J., Thompson, P.D., Ackerman, M.J., Balady, G., Berger, S., Cohen, D., et al., 2007. Recommendations and considerations related to preparticipation screening for cardiovascular abnormalities in competitive athletes: 2007 update: a scientific statement from the American Heart Association council on nutrition, physical activity, and metabolism: endorsed by the American College of Cardiology Foundation. Circulation 115 (12), 1643–1655.

Mont, L., Pelliccia, A., Sharma, S., Biffi, A., Borjesson, M., Terradellas, J.B., et al., 2017. Pre-participation cardiovascular evaluation for athletic participants to prevent sudden death: position paper from the EHRA and the EACPR, branches of the ESC. Endorsed by APHRS, HRS, and SOLAECE. Europace 19 (1), 139–163.

Papadakis, M., Sharma, S., Cox, S., Sheppard, M.N., Panoulas, V.F., Behr, E.R., 2009. The magnitude of sudden cardiac death in the young: a death certificate-based review in England and Wales. Europace 11 (10), 1353–1358.

Shah, R., Chatterjee, A.D., Wilson, J., 2018. Creating a model of best practice: the match day emergency action protocol. British Journal of Sports Medicine 52, 1535–1536.

Sharma, S., Whyte, G., McKenna, W.J., 1997. Sudden death from cardiovascular disease in young athletes: fact or fiction? British Journal of Sports Medicine 31 (4), 269–276.

Vettor, G., Zorzi, A., Basso, C., Thiene, G., Corrado, D., 2015. Syncope as a warning symptom of sudden cardiac death in athletes. Cardiology Clinics 33 (3), 423–432.

Wasfy, M.M., Hutter, A.M., Weiner, R.B., 2016. Sudden cardiac death in athletes. Methodist DeBakey Cardiovascular Journal 12 (2), 76–80.

Wilson, J.M., Jungner, Y.G., 1968. Principles and practice of mass screening for disease. Boletin de la Oficina Sanitaria Panamericana Pan American Sanitary Bureau 65 (4), 281–393.

Chapter | 33 |

Developing speed qualities in youth athletes

Johnny Wilson, Michael Sup, Mark Wilson, Marc-André Maillet and Said Mekary

Introduction

Speed is the distance travelled per unit of time (Elert, 2017). With higher speeds, an athlete is simply moving faster, regardless of direction. Pure sprint training drills, which focus on style and efficiency, are unidimensional and without sport-specific function and are outside the scope of this chapter. Instead, our interest is in the particular advantages of speed training for invasion sports (soccer, rugby, hockey, basketball, etc.) in young athletes. This chapter will focus on how to develop motor, cognitive and perceptual speed qualities in children between the ages of 5 and 16 years. Balyi and Hamilton (2004) separate maturation into three distinct stages: sampling years (ages 5–11 years), specialization years (ages 10–16 years) and investment years (ages 15–18 years). This group of authors will concentrate on the first two stages of accelerated trainability in this chapter.

Skilled speed training in youth athletes may be planned, reactive or both, but all should be in reference to dynamic movements, complex motor patterning, neuromuscular and proprioceptive efficiency (Mulvany and Wilson, 2018). In this chapter we will discuss:

- when children can begin to develop their functional speed ability
- the influences of nature (the inherent biological) and nurture (training and psychosocial effects)
- the accelerated windows of trainability and how to train speed ultraspecifically within these distinct but overlapping maturation stages (Ericsson, 2008).

When is it possible to develop speed qualities in children?

To build speed qualities in children, they need to be exposed to speed interventions routinely throughout their childhood. According to the American College of Sports Medicine (Faigenbaum and Chu, 2017) critical explosive movements can be introduced as early as 5 years of age. However, Avery Faigenbaum provides some stipulations, asserting that:

> *Although there is no minimum age requirement for participation in a youth training program, all participants should have the emotional maturity to accept and follow direction and should genuinely appreciate the potential benefits and risks associated with training.*

Faigenbaum, 2002, p. 32

Therefore, if a child has the emotional intelligence and is ready to participate in organized and structured sports such as cricket, soccer, rugby or basketball then they are generally ready to perform a supervised training programme.

Does a child have to possess the 'performance/speed gene'?

Any notion that a child is born fast or slow appears to be a fundamentally flawed argument. This mindset caters only for *nature* (that we are born a certain way and this cannot be changed) and excludes the huge potential that *nurture* can provide (the outcome of deliberate practice) (Ericsson, 1993). While we all have unique genetic makeups as human beings, the idea that a single 'speed/performance gene' or 'athlete gene', or even set of genes, exists is a myth (Tucker et al., 2012). Although it is true to say that we all have a genetic performance threshold, this threshold can only be realized through the process of deliberate and specific practice aimed at improving whatever aspect of performance we wish to, in this case speed (Ericsson, 1993). In other words, the view coaches might adopt is that it is the interaction between nature and nurture that determines the outcome of a child's ability to realize their physiological and psychological speed potential (Tucker et al., 2012; Vaeyens et al., 2008).

It is beyond the scope of this chapter to discuss genetics, epigenetics and the more recent advances in gene-editing technologies and their influence on optimizing speed in the population of young athletes. However, the reader should be aware of progress in these somewhat embryonic fields and the advantages they may soon bring.

Accelerated trainability phases

Children can be strategically speed trained during three distinct maturation periods. Being cognisant of these distinct periods, coaches can use them to integrate simple soccer-specific drills that will help develop key speed qualities, and reduce injury risk and dropout rates (Balyi and Way, 2005). Coaches can also be more specific to the demands of the game and the needs of their players depending on which maturational training window they are in. As set out by Balyi and Hamilton (2004) these three windows are:
• sampling years: 5–11 years of age
• specialization years: 10–16 years of age
• investment years: 15–18 years of age.
For the purpose of this of this chapter, we will only deal with the first two stages.

Sampling years: 5–11 years of age

Speed focus for the sampling years
Agility: a physical skill allowing athletes to slow down, change direction, or accelerate in response to a task-relevant cue.

Fun and learning to train phase

There are numerous terms that can be used to describe this period: prepubescent, middle childhood, preteen, etc. However these authors feel that using the taxonomy of 'sampling' best reflects the purpose of this fleeting period of a child's life (Balyi and Hamilton, 2004). *Sampling* lends itself naturally to the idea that children should experience as many different sports and learning environments during this period as possible to build sound basic physical movement patterns. Soccer, unlike gymnastics, is a late specialization sport and therefore Balyi's use of the term 'sampling' to describe this period seems very apt.

This phase should always centre on fun with the emphasis being on the development of the child's fundamental movement skills, such as stopping, starting, changing direction, jumping, landing and single leg balance (Balyi and Hamilton, 2004). From a psychosocial perspective, we should have a bias towards delivering sessions that promote intrinsic motivation, by centring around the young person's own meanings and goals.

Even at this early age children still have basic needs that need to be considered when developing athletic qualities:
• *Competency*, the need to believe that they are good at a task (positive reinforcement from coach when shuffling in and out of a ladder drill).
• *Autonomy*, that there is a degree of control (ability to make decisions in practice session such as during 1v1 or 2v2 scenarios).
• *Relatedness*, the need for meaning and purpose (the child understands why they are carrying out a particular drill or game and how it can help them improve at their sport).
It is theorized that all are correlated and all needs should be satisfied in order to optimize intrinsic motivation and optimal performance outcome (Reinboth et al., 2004; Ryan and Deci, 2000). Furthermore, from a neurological standpoint, the area in the brain known as the reticular activating system (RAS) is extremely sensitive to novelty and activities that arouse curiosity (Steriade, 1996). So, whenever a young athlete encounters an exercise that is novel, enjoyable and stress free, the RAS is alerted to pay more attention to the task, which helps when learning new skills.

During this window of accelerated trainability, research suggests that tasks should target the neural system to improve coordination, movement efficacy and speed of movement to develop high levels of agility (Fig. 33.1) (Van Praagh, 1998).

What is agility?

Technically agility is difficult to define. Some have traditionally defined it as the physical action of changing direction, stopping and starting – without any recognition for the integral role how the brain and the ever-changing dynamic nature of soccer can affect agility performance. While there are several definitions for agility, we like the way Verstegen and colleagues (2001) define agility as a physical skill in which players can slow down, change direction, or accelerate in response to a task-relevant cue such as an opponent or in anticipation of a pass from a teammate.

What is not agility

A simple search for examples of agility drills on the Internet will produce a whole host of entertaining clips of players performing different movements at pace and with exceptional coordination through ladders, cones, poles, obstacle courses, etc. While these drills are excellent for developing coordination and qualities such as improving stride frequency (fast

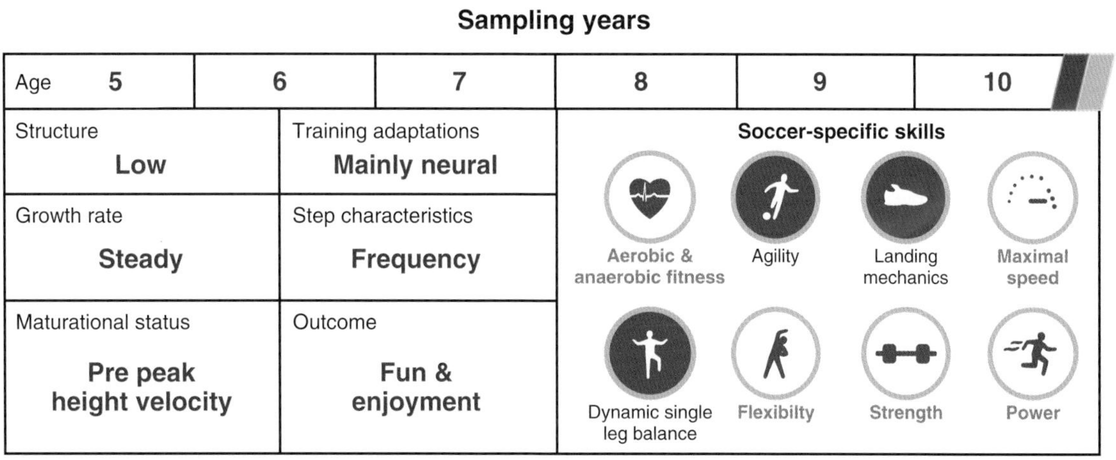

Sampling years

Age	5	6	7	8	9	10

Structure **Low**	Training adaptations **Mainly neural**	Soccer-specific skills

Growth rate **Steady**	Step characteristics **Frequency**	Aerobic & anaerobic fitness	Agility	Landing mechanics	Maximal speed

Maturational status **Pre peak height velocity**	Outcome **Fun & enjoyment**	Dynamic single leg balance	Flexibilty	Strength	Power

Fig. 33.1 Sampling years. (Adapted from Balyi, I., Hamilton, A., 2004. Long-Term Athlete Development: Trainability in Childhood and Adolescence: Windows of Opportunity, Optimal Trainability. National Coaching Institute British Columbia and Advanced Training and Performance Ltd, Victoria, Canada.)

feet), they do not necessarily help to improve a player's agility performance. This is not to say that these practice drills should be removed from practice sessions. Far from it, they should be embraced as they certainly help players develop fundamental movement qualities which will enable them to excel at sport. However, preplanned movements such as turning at a cone or shuffling laterally over a ladder very rarely occur during the game.

Why train agility?

In soccer, direction changes, stops and starts are usually in response to an external stimulus –they are unplanned, chaotic and can occur in an instant, e.g., trying to evade or beat an opponent in a 1v1, 2v1 or 1v2 situation. In these scenarios, players need to process a whole host of information and then decipher which option will lead to the desired outcome. But more than that, they need to make this decision faster than their opponent; they need to develop the ability to think fast to move fast.

Therefore, if we truly wish to improve a player's agility performance, we must include activities that obligate the player to recognize and react appropriately to unplanned scenarios, replicating the game as much as possible, such as reactive drills and small-sided games (Sheppard and Young, 2006).

Agility practice to help reduce injury incidence

Research indicates that if coaches include activities that the players are not able to plan for and instead have to react to, not only does this improve their agility but it also reduces

their likelihood of getting injured, as unplanned movements are a known injury risk factor in soccer (Besier et al., 2001). Therefore training agility performance in children is key for success in soccer.

How do we train agility

A simple way of incorporating agility activities into practice sessions is by dividing the activities into three stages. During the sampling years: plyometrics.

Stage 1: planned movements

- Changing direction/accelerating/decelerating
- Submaximal plyometrics:
  - Submaximal jumping and landing activities: These activities can be introduced safely by ensuring all jumping is submaximal in effort with the emphasis on landing 'quietly' (with good control). These *low-threshold* (submaximal) plyometrics can help improve a child's power profile (imperative for agility) as well as reduce their risk of noncontact injury, especially when landing from a height on to a single leg
- Focus on stride frequency, i.e., length of time foot is in contact with the ground (fast feet)
- Use of cones/poles/ladders/instruction/whistle, etc.
- 2–4 drills per session
- 1–2 repetitions per drill
- 2–10 seconds per drill
- 5–15 seconds rest between each drill
- Total time for stage 1 practical application: 2 to 3 minutes.

Stage 2: reactive movements

- Competitive drills: mirror/tag/shadow and dodging activities
- 1–3 drills per session
- 1–3 repetitions per drill
- 10–20 seconds per drill
- 10–30 seconds rest between each drill
- Total time for stage 2 practical application: 2 to 4 minutes.

Examples of agility training activities in the sampling years

Stage 1: planned physical movements

Changing direction

- Weave through 4 cones/poles/gates as fast as possible
- Repeat 3 times
- 5-second rest between each repetition

Stage 2: reactive physical movements

Partner reactionary agility activity

This exercise stresses both psychological capacity and physical structure by exposing the child to multiple high-speed cuts, checks, decelerations, accelerations, lateral movements, backpedalling, turns and short sprints. Multiple coloured cones are spread randomly around a 10 × 10 yd area or 7 × 7 yd area with a central cone in the middle of the area. One child walks around the working area and calls a colour. The child performing the activity reacts to the colour called and sprints to the cone, touches the cone with his/her hand and sprints back to the central cone and waits for another colour to be called.

Progressions/regressions: a world of endless opportunities

- Multiple cues:
  - Call three colours and see if the individual performing the activity can remember the colour sequence called as they are participating
  - Call red and player must go to blue, etc.

Stage 3: small-sided games (SSG)

SSG combine a multitude of agility-based tasks through fun games that are cognitively and physically challenging. Examples can include tag rugby, shadow games, and 1v1s, 2v2s with and without ball. These SSG can be performed as part of the warm-up, in the body of a practice session or during the cool down. The coach can adjust the complexity of the games depending on the children's ability to understand what is being requested of them, making it simpler if they do not understand or increase the cognitive challenge if they are finding it too easy. All exercises/games can be adapted to the coordination capacity of the children and should, where possible, be performed at full speed.

Stage 3: small-sided games

- 1v1/2v2/3v2/5v5, etc. (size of pitch to be appropriate to number of players)
- 5–10 drills per session
- 1–3 repetitions per drill
- 20 seconds to 4 minutes per small-sided game.

Exercise prescription

In general, very little periodization need to takes place during this phase of trainability. However, all programmes should still be structured and monitored. According to the US Department of Health (2018), children between the ages of 5 and 11 years should accumulate at least 60 minutes of moderate to vigorous physical activity daily, including vigorous activity at least 3 days per week, in order to achieve health benefits. With respect to agility-based tasks, these should ideally last between 5 and 10 seconds to ensure high-quality repetitions and that the focus is on building the mind–body connection rather than an aerobic or anaerobic base. In terms of ratio between practice and competition, eminent researchers in this field such as Faigenbaum (2002) and Balyi (2005) suggest a 70% practice and 30% competition split.

Measuring heart rate response during the sampling years

These authors believe that since highly structured practice may not be necessary during the sampling years, and due to the immaturity of the cardiovascular system, the use of heart rate to monitor exercise intensity is not required for children between 5–10 years of age.

Measuring active participation during the sampling years

During the sampling years, fun and enjoyment should be at the forefront of any session outcomes. While this is often best measured by way of dialogue and auditory feedback between players and coaches, there is potential to correlate these fun and enjoyable playing experiences with certain quantitative data measurements.

Active participation (AP) is a metric that provides a means of quantitatively analysing energy expenditure through measuring the metabolic equivalent of tasks (METs) via wearable technology. An MET is continuously recorded throughout the session. The MET is categorized into three AP zones: (1) low (1–3 METs), (2) moderate (3–6 METs) and (3) vigorous (6+ METs) (Haskell et al., 2007). This metric provides coaches with a percentage of how active the children were during a practice session and how intense the session was by highlighting how much time is spent operating in the low, moderate and vigorous physical activity zones. For example, if a child is on the move for 75% of the practice session then their AP percentage is 75%. This 75% will then be broken down to show what percentage was low, medium and vigorous activity. However, if the child only moved for half of the session, the AP would be 50% and again is broken down into low, moderate and vigorous activities.

Specialization years: 10–16 years of age

Speed focus for the specialization years

- Maximal velocity
- Acceleration
- Deceleration
- Repeated sprint performance

Training to train phase

This phase has been coined the 'specialization years' as it represents a period where children can focus on deliberate practice to improve soccer-specific skills, as most are developmentally ready to acquire such sport-specific skills (Balyi and Hamilton, 2004). This is a key period, as it also marks the onset of strength and power development in children. This occurs because of significant physiological changes in the musculoskeletal and neuromuscular systems mainly due to maturational influences (rise in growth hormone levels associated with puberty) (Beunen and Malina, 1988; Venturelli et al., 2008). During this phase children will experience rapid gains in bone mass, muscle mass and physical stature (height) (Bass et al., 1999). Therefore, research posits that the focus of speed training for this age group should be around a strength intervention to capitalize on this naturally occurring increase in growth hormones (Balyi and Hamilton, 2004). Note that children can also be introduced to aerobic training with the onset of peak height velocity (PHV; a major growing spurt) (Balyi and Way, 2005). However this is outside the remit of this chapter.

Developing speed qualities in boys and girls

During this phase, boys and girls will generally follow comparable rates of development in growth and maturation as well as similar rates for strength, power, speed, aerobic endurance and neuromuscular control (Beunen and Malina, 2005). As a result, from a training perspective, both boys and girls can follow similar training programmes during this window of trainability (Lloyd et al., 2011). Typically, the onset of the adolescent growth spurt occurs around 2 years earlier in girls than in boys (~10 years in girls vs. ~12 years in boys). Girls will also experience PHV at an earlier age than boys (12 years vs. 14 years) (Beunen and Malina 1988; 2005).

Stride characteristics for developing speed

While the sampling years focused on developing *stride frequency* through a neural intervention, activities to improve *stride length* (distance between toe off and touchdown) are also added in this phase of accelerated training by focusing on a strength and power stimulus (Fig. 33.2) (Cavanagh et al., 1989). These authors believe that it is critical to develop these characteristics in youth soccer players so that they can utilize stride frequency for agility-based activities such as evading an opponent and utilize stride length for longer, linear-based activities such as a counterattack over 40 m (Rompotti et al., 1975). Increases in stride length will occur naturally as the athlete's muscle mass increases during the pubertal phase. This correlates with an increase in force production and the resultant increase in the distance between toe off to touchdown (Hunter and Smith, 2007). However, through deliberate practice during the specialization years, youth athletes can further improve their stride length through the following interventions (Tucker et al., 2012):

Resistance training

Research suggests that as the strength profile of a child athlete develops rapidly through puberty, this will naturally have a positive influence on maximal speed. However, it also cautions that coaches should not rely on growth and maturation to solely improve speed-based qualities during this window of accelerated trainability (Faigenbaum et al., 2016; Lesinski et al., 2015; Rumpf et al., 2012). Instead, coaches should incorporate resistance training as part of their practice sessions to improve force production, which is associated with enhanced sprint performance in youth athletes (Christou et al., 2006). Regression modelling suggests that a modest improvement of 10% in strength in boys can result in up to a 4.2% increase in sprint performance (Faigenbaum et al., 2016). Meanwhile Meylan (2014) has illustrated that a 10% improvement in jump height may elicit a 2% improvement in sprint performance in youth athletes, thus highlighting the positive impact that a strength and power programme can have on sprint performance in youth. Plyometrics have been shown to improve strength

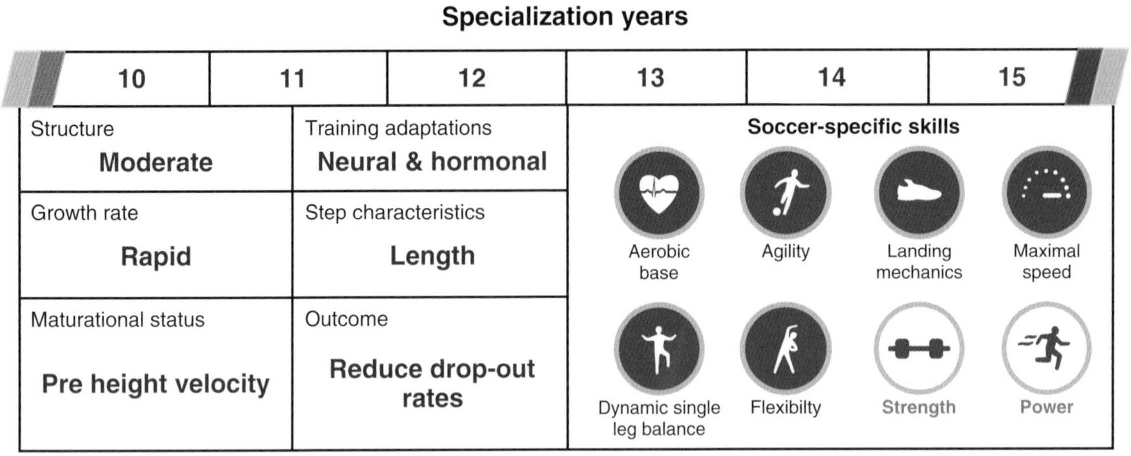

Specialization years

10	11	12	13	14	15

Structure **Moderate**	Training adaptations **Neural & hormonal**	Soccer-specific skills			
		Aerobic base	Agility	Landing mechanics	Maximal speed
Growth rate **Rapid**	Step characteristics **Length**				
Maturational status **Pre height velocity**	Outcome **Reduce drop-out rates**	Dynamic single leg balance	Flexibilty	Strength	Power

Fig. 33.2 Specialization years. (Adapted from Balyi, I., Hamilton, A., 2004. Long-Term Athlete Development: Trainability in Childhood and Adolescence: Windows of Opportunity, Optimal Trainability. National Coaching Institute British Columbia and Advanced Training and Performance Ltd, Victoria, Canada.)

and power profiles of youth athletes. They are relatively safe and convenient activities that can be carried out at the end of the warm-up during practice sessions. Plyometrics can help improve speed qualities such as agility, linear speed and maximum velocity in youth athletes in the following way:

Plyometrics. Multidirectional jumping exercises, otherwise known as plyometrics, are an excellent medium for developing agility and familiarization with unanticipated changes of direction, as well as improving maximal velocity in children (Besier et al., 2001). By incorporating simple plyometric exercises at the end of warm-up in practice sessions twice weekly over as short a period as 6 weeks, it has been shown that jump height, acceleration speed over 5 m, maximal speed over 20 m, agility performance with and without the ball and maximal ball striking ability can all be improved significantly (Villarreal et al., 2015). Weighted plyometrics (use of medicine ball) have also been shown to develop speed performance (Faigenbaum, 2002).

High-speed running

To improve sprint performance in young athletes it is imperative to expose them to high-speed running activities such as sprinting maximally or resisted runs to promote an anabolic response to help increase power output (Rumpf et al., 2012). By incorporating sprint-based activities in the warm-up and the body of the practice session, children build key physiological elements that are imperative to developing speed performance.

> **Examples of speed performance training activities for the specialization years**
>
> - Improve *acceleration* performance by practising running at maximal effort over 5 m and by carrying out maximal effort horizontal bodyweight plyometric jumps.
> - Improve *maximal velocity* by running as fast as possible over 20–30 m and through maximal vertical bodyweight and weighted (10–30% of 1 repetition max) plyometric jumps.
> - Improve *agility* performance by introducing activities that require players to think fast and move fast by obligating them to react to an unplanned external stimulus.
> - Improve *repeated sprint ability* (anaerobic power) by increasing duration of sprint-based activities (up to 20 s) to start building anaerobic capacity in youth soccer players of 15–16 years of age (average and early maturers).
>
>   For a more in-depth discussion on the mechanism and the practical application of sprint-based activities, please see Chapter 18.

Exercise prescription

The specialization years, especially 14–16 years of age, are characterized by a high amount of deliberate practice (Coté and Vierimaa, 2014). In this phase, load monitoring starts to become an important component in the athlete's periodization – monitoring intensity and volume of the exercise in order to prevent overtraining and injury.

When introducing youth athletes to activities with the goal of improving physical athletic qualities such as speed, it is always better to underestimate their physical capabilities and gradually increase the volume and intensity of the intervention rather than to overestimate their abilities and potentially increase their risk of injury. A sensible staring point would be 1–3 sets of 6–10 repetitions on one lower body exercise twice a week on nonconsecutive days, an example being 1 set of 6 reps of squat jumps at the end of the warm-up.

It is also worth noting that it may be necessary to decrease the volume and intensity of practice sessions during periods of rapid growth to reduce risk of growth-related injuries such as apophyseal injuries (e.g., Osgood–Schlatter disease, Sever's disease, Sinding-Larsen Johansson syndrome). Therefore, exposing children to appropriately designed exercise programmes of moderate- to high-load intensity, which flex to the maturational status of the child and with appropriate technical competency, can help greatly to improve their athletic physical profile (Kelly et al., 1990; Nelson et al., 1994).

For health benefits, children in this phase should accumulate at least 60 minutes of moderate to vigorous physical activity daily, which should also include vigorous intensity activities at least 3 times a week (Pescatello, 2014). Practice-to-competition ratio is recommended to be 60% practice versus 40% competition and competition-specific practice (Balyi and Hamilton, 2004).

Monitoring during the specialization years

Monitoring heart rate response

The circulatory system is vital to human function at rest as well as being integral to the ability to adjust to the demands of acute and chronic exercise. Together with the respiratory system, the cardiovascular system is responsible, via the bloodstream, for delivering oxygen and nutrients to the active tissues (Stanfield, 2012). During an acute exercise bout, the cardiovascular system will increase oxygen and substrate delivery to the working muscles in order to match the adenosine triphosphate (ATP) requirements of the exercise (Stanfield, 2012). There exists a linear relationship between exercise intensity and heart rate. As exercise workload increases, so does heart rate response (Pescatello, 2014). Cardiovascular endurance reflects one's ability to sustain vigorous activity. It is important for two reasons: (1) participation in many physical activities demands sustained vigorous exertion and (2) the health of the cardiac and respiratory systems is related to endurance levels, largely because training that improves the fitness makes these systems more efficient.

Using heart rate to help prescribe practice sessions

Intensity levels of physical activity in the research laboratory are often expressed relative to maximal oxygen consumption ($\dot{V}O_{2max}$). However, this measure is expensive and not always feasible or practical outside the laboratory (Warburton et al., 2006). Alternative methods of calculating optimal exercise intensity in children are available. Heart rate (HR) is a practical, objective and valid measure of exercise work rate. The adult formula '220 − age' is often used to prescribe exercise intensity for children. However, as stated by Rowland (1990), HR_{max} determined by maximal treadmill and maximal cycle ergometer test remains constant across the paediatric years. Therefore the use of an adult formula that is strongly dependent on age may not be appropriate. Although exercise is critical for children's health, measuring HR_{max} for children the same way we measure it for adults can put children at risk for overtraining and other negative effects such as dyspnoea and dizziness (Alleyne, 1998). Another equation used to predict HR_{max} in a population is $208 − (0.7 \times age)$ proposed by Tanaka et al. (2001). Given that this formula is slightly less age dependent, it has been shown to be more reliable when measuring maximal heart rate in children (Mahon et al., 2010; Verschuren et al., 2011).

When using heart rate to measure exercise intensity in activities that build physical capacities and mental capabilities during the late phase of the specialization group, there are a few points to consider. The intensity and duration of exercise activities need to be based on the maturity of the child, the medical background, and previous experiences with exercise. Also, regardless of age, the exercise intensity should always start low and progress gradually.

The guidelines for measuring exercise intensity in children during the late specialization phase are as follows:
- Moderate-intensity physical activity: 55–69% of HR_{max} and 40–59% of heart rate reserve.
- Vigorous-intensity physical activity: >70% of HR_{max} and >60% of heart rate reserve.

Challenges

One of the difficulties in this area is that there is still so much unknown about human growth, especially through these formative years. Children are not mini adults and principles that pertain to adults for developing speed qualities may not be appropriate for the child cohort. We must be cautious when applying any scientific principles that were founded on an adult population to children.

Developing speed qualities in children should be looked at from a long-term point of view, relating to a period of years, rather than weeks and months. Therefore, it is important that all speed interventions are tracked, recorded and monitored throughout to ensure continuity and progression. The challenge here is that children may fall out of love with sport for a time, or change school or club or sport, making it not always possible to keep continuous records. One solution may be to apply wearable technology that travels with the child, no matter what changes they face, so that all interventions can be recorded and downloaded to a central database. This could then be accessed by the child, the coach, the parents, etc., to ensure the child's exposure to a speed stimulus and any other physical activity is continuous and progressive.

Conclusion

Although the central theme of this chapter is the development of speed qualities in children, the authors acknowledge that the wellbeing of the child is the most important factor and strongly advocate for the healthy development of the child over performance outcomes.

This chapter aims to assure coaches and clinicians that it is possible to train speed qualities in children, and that it is possible from as early as 5 years of age. The key is to develop these qualities over the entire period of childhood and adolescence, with a sound understanding of the child's maturational status and match this with an appropriate training stimulus.

Perhaps then, when planning speed activities, we should consider various approaches to learning, and a more heuristic athlete-centred solution. Exercise selection should be based around the capability of the child, both physically and mentally, and also around the functional demands of the sport within a creative and enjoyable environment. To develop sport-specific speed qualities such as agility we should actively seek the most random and unpredictable scenarios and aim to sustain activation and complex skill acquisition within them. By adopting this methodology, the young athlete will be prepared to adapt to the unexpected stressors of sport.

References

Alleyne, J.M., 1998. Safe exercise prescription for children and adolescents. Paediatrics and Child Health 3 (5), 337–342.

Balyi, I., Hamilton, A., 2004. Long-Term Athlete Development: Trainability in Childhood and Adolescence—Windows of Opportunity—Optimal Trainability. National Coaching Institute British Columbia and Advanced Training and Performance Ltd, Victoria, Canada.

Balyi, I., Way, R., 2005. The role of monitoring growth in the long-term athlete development. Canadian Sport for Life.

Bass, S., Delmas, P.D., Pearce, G., Hendrich, E., Tabensky, A., Seeman, E., 1999. The differing tempo of growth in bone size, mass and density in girls is region-specific. Journal of Clinical Investigation 104, 795–804.

Besier, T.F., Lloyd, D.G., Ackland, T.R., Cochrane, J.L., 2001. Anticipatory effects on knee joint loading during running and cutting manoeuvres. Medicine & Science in Sports & Exercise 33, 1176–1181.

Beunen, G.P., Malina, R.M., 1988. Growth and physical performance relative to the timing of the adolescent spurt. Exercise and Sport Sciences Reviews 16, 503–540.

Beunen, G.P., Malina, R.M., 2005. Growth and biological maturation: relevance to athletic performance. In: Bar-Or, O. (Ed.), The Child and Adolescent Athlete. Blackwell Publishing, Oxford, pp. 3–17.

Cavanagh, P., Kram, R., 1989. Stride length in distance running: velocity, body dimensions, and added mass effects. Medicine & Science in Sports & Exercise 21, 467–479.

Christou, M., Smilios, I., Sotiropoulos, K., Volaklis, K., Pilianidis, T., Tokmakidis, S.P., 2006. Effects of resistance training on the physical capacities of adolescent soccer players. Journal of Strength and Conditioning Research 20, 783–791.

Côté, J., Vierimaa, M., 2014. The developmental model of sport participation: 15 years after its first conceptualization. Science & Sports Volume 29, Supplement, S63–S69.

Elert, G., 2017. Speed and velocity. The Physics Hypertextbook. Available at: https://physics.info/velocity/.

Ericsson, K.A., 2008. Deliberate practice and acquisition of expert performance: A general overview. Academic Emergency Medicine 15 (11), 988–994.

Ericsson, K.A., Krampe, R. Th., Tesch-Romer, C., 1993. The role of deliberate practice in the acquisition of expert performance. Psychological Review 100, 363–406.

Faigenbaum, A., Chu, D., 2017. Plyometric training for children and adolescents. In: American College of Sports Medicine, Indianapolis.

Faigenbaum, A., 2002. Resistance training for adolescent athletes. Athletic Therapy Today 7 (6), 30–35.

Faigenbaum, A.D., Lloyd, R.S., MacDonald, J., Myer, G.D., 2016. Citius, altius, fortius: beneficial effects of resistance training for young athletes. British Journal of Sports Medicine 50, 3–7.

Haskell, W.L., Lee, I.M., Pate, R.R., Powell, K.E., Blair, S.N., Franklin, B.A., et al., 2007. Physical activity and public health: updated recommendation for adults from the American College of Sports Medicine and the American Heart Association. Medicine and Science in Sports and Exercise 39 (8), 1423–1434.

Hunter, I., Smith, G.A., 2007. Preferred and optimal stride frequency, stiffness and economy: Changes with fatigue during a 1-h high-intensity run. European Journal of Applied Physiology 100, 653–661.

Kelly, P.J., Twomey, L., Sambrook, P.N., Eisman, J.A., 1990. Sex differences in peak adult bone mineral density. Journal of Bone and Mineral Research 5, 1169–1175.

Lesinski, M., Prieske, O., Granacher, U., 2015. Effects and dose–response relationships of resistance training on physical performance in youth athletes: a systematic review and meta-analysis. British Journal of Sports Medicine 1–17.

Lloyd, R.S., Oliver, J.L., Hughes, M.G., Williams, C.A., 2011. The influence of chronological age on periods of accelerated adaptation of stretch-shortening cycle performance in pre-and postpubescent boys. Journal of Strength and Conditioning Research 25, 1889–1897.

Mahon, A.D., Marjerrison, A.D., Lee, J.D., Woodruff, M.E., Hanna, L.E., 2010. Evaluating the prediction of maximal heart rate in children and adolescents. Research Quarterly for Exercise and Sport 365 (81), 466–471.

Meylan, C.M.P., Cronin, J., Oliver, J.L., Hopkins, W.G., Pinder, S., 2014. Contribution of vertical strength and power in sprint performance in young male athletes. International Journal of Sports Medicine 35, 749–754.

Mulvany, S., Wilson, J., 2018. Complex Adaptive Modelling in Sport Science and Sports Medicine. Available at: https://wilsonmulvany.wordpress.com/2018/10/18/model-number-1-neuromuscular-systems-conditioning-nsc-advantaged-stacked-over-preparedness-for-sport-specific-demand/.

Nelson, M.E., Fiatarone, M.A., Morganti, C.M., Trice, I., Greenberg, R.A., Evans, W.J., 1994. Effects of high-intensity strength training on multiple risk factors for osteoporotic fractures. Journal of American Medical Association 272, 1909–1914.

Pescatello, L.S., 2014. ACSM's Guidelines for Exercise Testing and Prescription, ninth ed. Wolters Kluwer/Lippincott Williams & Wilkins Health, Philadelphia.

Reinboth, M., Duda, J.L., Ntoumanis, N., 2004. Dimensions of coaching behavior, need satisfaction and the psychological and physical welfare of young athletes. Motivation and Emotion 28, 297.

Rompotti, K., 1975. A study of stride length in running. In: Canham, D., Diamond, P. (Eds.), International Track and Field Digest. Champions on Film, 1975, Ann Arbor, MI, pp. 249–256.

Rowland, T.W., 1990. Exercise and Children's Health. Human Kinetics, Champaign, IL, pp. 27–83.

Rumpf, M.C., Cronin, J.B., Pinder, S.D., Oliver, J., Hughes, M., 2012. Effect of different training methods on running sprint times in male youth. Pediatric Exercise Science 24, 170–186.

Ryan, R.M., Deci, E.L., 2000. Intrinsic and extrinsic motivations: classic definitions and new directions. Contemporary Educational Psychology 25, 54–67.

Sheppard, J.M., Young, W.B., 2006. Agility literature review: classifications, training and testing. Journal of Sports Sciences 24, 919–932.

Stanfield, C.L., 2012. Principles of Human Physiology, fifth ed. Benjamin Cummings, San Francisco, CA.

Steriade, M., 1996. Arousal: revisiting the reticular activating system. Science 272 (5259), 225.

Tanaka, H., Monahan, K.D., Seals, D.R., 2001. Age-predicted maximal heart rate revisited. Journal of the American College of Cardiology 37, 153–156.

Tucker, R., Collins, M., 2012. What makes champions? A review of the relative contribution of genes and training to sporting success. British Journal of Sports Medicine 46, 555–561.

US Department of Health and Human Services, 2018. Physical Activity Guidelines for Americans, 2nd edition. Washington, DC: US Department of Health and Human Services.

Vaeyens, R., Lenoir, M., Williams, A.M., et al., 2008. Talent identification and development programmes in sport: current models and future directions. Sports Medicine 38, 703–714.

van Praagh, E., 1998. Paediatric Anaerobic Performance. Human Kinetics Publisher, Inc, Champaign, IL.

Venturelli, M., Bishop, D., Pettene, L., 2008. Sprint training in preadolescent soccer players. International Journal of Sports Physiology and Performance 3, 558–562.

Verschuren, O., Maltais, D.B., Takken, T., 2011. The 220-age equation does not predict maximum heart rate in children and adolescents. Developmental Medicine & Child Neurology 53, 861–864.

Verstegen, M., Marcello, B., 2001. Agility and coordination. In: Foran, B. (Ed.), High Performance Sports Conditioning. Human Kinetics, Champaign, IL, pp. 139–165.

Villarreal, E., et al., 2015. Effects of plyometric and sprint training on physical and technical skill performance in adolescent soccer players. Journal of Strength and Conditioning Research 29 (7), 1894–1903.

Warburton, D.E., Nicol, C.W., Bredin, S.S., 2006. Prescribing exercise as preventive therapy. Canadian Medical Association Journal 174 (7), 961–974.

Chapter 34

Conditioning for the battle of momentum: a practical use of GPS technology for conditioning strategies

Adam Sheehan

Introduction

Momentum is a funny thing in a rugby game. They are moments even the most novice of fans can spot with the same accuracy as the wisest coach. The momentum moments in rugby are often big physical and psychological battles of will, those passages of play that make the back pages of the Sunday papers. They are the moments that can arise from a water-tight defence which cause a team to rise and repel a dominant opponent, or they can be attacking moments where giants bring a crushing blow to a minnow through a lethal counterattack.

This chapter will seek to explain how teams develop the physical qualities to not only survive these battles but win them. Specifically, we will explore the use and implementation of global position systems (GPS) technology to maximize players' physical development to the attributes of that specific team.

GPS introduction

The advancement of GPS technology coupled with the ease of data visualization through bespoke platforms has caused a proliferation of uses for GPS. GPS is currently in use by a large number of teams across professional and elite sport (Cummins et al., 2013). Teams are typically using GPS to aid in the monitoring and understanding of the demands of their sport. The ease of use and large amount of data points collected has been instrumental in providing a deeper understanding to all sports. Much like any journey

of discovery, in the beginning you are just scrutinizing the map before you start to make decisions on where to go, before finally working out how long it will take to get to certain points on that map. An overview of the big milestones along the GPS journey are given here.

1. **Data collection stage.** The initial introduction of any new technology will naturally allow for an acclimatization period where the primary goal of the new technology is data collection. GPS technology is no different. Users can assess published research within a given sport, but the benefit of GPS collection within a team is its delivery of a perspective that is unique to that specific team. This initial phase correlates to identifying the edges of the map, so to speak. It provides general insight into the demands of training phases, week-to-week demands, session types and demands of specific drills.

2. **Comparison stage.** This stage utilizes the data that has been collected to run comparisons between session types, on sessions versus games, and positional group differences or player/athlete-type differences or traits.

3. **Implementation stage.** The information gathered is extrapolated to draw meaningful conclusions about training or games. This could be as simple as comparing the effectiveness of similar sessions or using the game as a benchmark and then basing training on game demands. It can also be used to look at total weekly loading across weeks with respect to the turnaround (days between games – and the effect of recovery days available) for that training.

4. **Forecasting stage.** Whether this phase is ever truly attained is a point of contention due to the unpredictable chaotic environment of sport; it is certainly the most difficult of the stages. Forecasting training demands

is both obvious in its usefulness but difficult in its implementation. Basing the weekly training on a contextual history of previous weeks – using this data to highlight the need for high-load or low-load sessions – can help in the construction of an effective training week. This data can be further refined by identifying which individuals are being over- or underworked, which is important in the management of a playing squad and not just a playing team. Finally, GPS information can be used to accurately focus physical development, e.g., where a player is deficient or in helping to assess an individual's workload based on their capacity for that work at that specific time point; this utilizes some of Gabbett's work on acute:chronic ratios (Gabbett, 2012). It mitigates injury risk, helps provide a healthy level of player availability to aid in squad competition, and aids coaches' selection choices to optimize overall team performance.

Much of this work can be performed with some of the basic plug-and-play metrics that are common on all GPS platforms. The usage of GPS platforms often develops with the team's and practitioners' familiarity with it and usage of the information. Therefore the need to answer ever-more specific or detailed questions tends to arise. Top-tier elite GPS systems allow for a far greater amount of customization. This gives more control and autonomy to the end-user to interpret and infer meaning from a greater scope of metrics. The setup is highly dependent on the system chosen, but all systems will operate with some general categories. Depending on your sport, the priority of these parameters will change, but all sports will have a combination of categories and subbandings of those categories which, when configured, can give some meaningful insight into the sport in question and develop a better contextual picture for that sport.

All systems have the three basic categories of information:

- *velocity* – running-based demands
- *acceleration* – change of velocity demands
- *impact* – G-force measurement of impacts.

When using these parameters most systems will allow for the setup of multiple bands within these categories. This allows for more in-depth assessment and for framing some of the contextual nature of the information. There is already a body of research identifying bands for each of the parameter categories listed above. Fig. 34.1 shows some typical bandings seen in the different categories within the author's setting, the reasons for defining the bands in this way and also the potential application of these bands.

Velocity

The velocity category will encompass all running-based movements through GPS. Some of the simple metrics that are most often used are 'distance', 'metres per minute' or 'high-speed running'. The ability to customize the bands by different velocities allows for a greater understanding as to the running demands and efforts for any given session. Velocity bands were previously used as either an absolute or relative banding method. This meant that teams could decide to look at all individuals by absolute bands assessing everyone by the same absolute maximal velocity or they could chose to look at everybody relative to an individual percentage of maximal velocity. Most elite systems now have the ability to perform both of these assessments and it is an excellent method for not only assessing performance of an individual through absolute speed but also assessing an individual against their own individual maximal velocity.

Acceleration

The acceleration category will encompass all change of velocity movements recorded through the accelerometer; this will include both acceleration and deceleration events. By using this category coaches can identify change of direction demands. This will include not only the total number of acceleration and declarations but also the distance for each of these events and through use of the intensity bands will drill down into the severity of change of direction events. This information can be used to determine typical demands as well as highlight significant differences between positional groups and even within-group differences for frequency of efforts or differences in distances covered in acceleration or declaration zones.

Impact

Impacts are recorded through the integrated accelerometer and measured in G-force. This function is available within most elite-level devices. This information is of particular importance in rugby union or other contact-based sports as often the single biggest determining factor in game intensity is the severity and frequency of impact events. Most elite systems also run algorithms with the impact data to further identify collision events. These collision events are often detected through a combination of the accelerometer data, orientation of the gyroscope and the impact recorded in G-force data. This combination gives more stringent criteria for collision detection.

Velocity

Band	Band 1	Band 2	Band 3	Band 4	Band 5	Band 6	Band 7
Absolute	0–2.2m/s	2.2–4.4m/s	4.4–5.5m/s	5.5–7.0m/s	7.0–8.0m/s	8.0–9.0m/s	9.0–11m/s
Rational	Walking	Jogging	Running	High-speed running	Very HSR	Sprint dist	Max velocity
Relative	0–20%	20–40%	40–55%	55–70%	70–85%	85–90%	90–110%
Rational	Low-grade running zone		Conditioning running zone	High-intensity running zones		Sprint zone	Max sprints

HSR, High-speed running

Acceleration

	Deceleration			Midpoint	Acceleration		
Band	Band 1	Band 2	Band 3	Band 4	Band 5	Band 6	Band 7
Absolute	–10m/s to –6m/s	–6m/s to –4m/s	–4m/s to –2m/s	–2m/s to 2m/s	2m/s to 4m/s	4m/s to 6m/s	6m/s to 10m/s
Rational	Severe deceleration	High deceleration	Moderate deceleration	Low acceleration and deceleration	Moderate acceleration	High acceleration	Severe acceleration

Impacts

Band	Band 1	Band 2	Band 3	Band 4	Band 5	Band 6	Band 7	Band 8
G-force	1–2g	2–4g	4–5g	5–6g	6–7g	7–8g	8–9g	9–15g
Rational	Micro impacts	Low-grade impact	Moderate impacts		Heavy impacts		Severe impacts	

Fig. 34.1 Some typical velocity, acceleration and impact bandings seen in GPS systems.

Demands

General demands

Irrespective of the level of play, rugby is a simple game. The general physical demands for all players are to run, jump, evade and either avoid or make a tackle. As a field-based 80-minute raid game, the general demands are also simple. For the duration of the game a player seeks to expose space in attack and reduce space in defence. These demands are like those in many other field sports. Where rugby differs to other sports is the physical and confrontational nature of the collisions and set-piece battles (Table 34.1). When developing the physical demands needed to play the game we can categorize these to three generic groups.

Running. The need to have highly developed ability to hit top speed and to repeat this often; the need to run typically 6 km over the course of a game and to have a proportion of this distance at high speed.

Change of direction. The ability to accelerate and decelerate frequently and at high speeds. Typically, these acceleration and declaration events are highly position specific regarding intensity and frequency of efforts.

Collisions. Collisions are an integral part of rugby union. The contact nature of the game is a key attribute in its

Table 34.1 Comparison of distance, velocity, load and efforts metrics for different rugby positions

Figures given are per session (i.e., game) averages

Position	Avg dist (m)	Meterage per minute (m/min)	Avg PL	Avg PL (slow session)	Avg cond dist (m)	Avg HSR (m/s)	Avg tot COD	Avg collisions	Avg tot eff	RHIE
Prop	4282	63	463	250	181	38	45	31	93	2
Lock	4905	65	546	265	361	67	64	45	140	4
Hooker	5074	68	529	247	431	112	56	38	131	6
Back row	5842	68	644	307	576	163	79	55	185	9
Fly half	5125	75	481	199	605	199	47	24	118	9
Centre	5784	73	571	235	855	346	55	33	158	16
Scrum-half	6269	74	625	248	1158	422	68	35	183	16
Back 3	6006	71	543	230	918	471	49	28	153	17

Avg dist, Distance covered for the session in metres; meterage per minute, total distance divided by time; avg PL, average PlayerLoad of the session (PlayerLoad is a Catapult custom metric to assess overload demand); avg cond dist, a custom metric of total distance covered at ≥4.4 m/s; avg HSR, total distance covered at ≥5.5 m/s and above (i.e., high-speed running); avg tot COD, total number of change of direction efforts/ acceleration and deceleration events; avg collisions, total number of collision events greater than 4 G; avg tot eff, a combination of all high-intensity running, change of direction and collision efforts; RHIE, total number of repeated high-intensity efforts for the session.

spectacle. A rugby player has the need to not only produce collision efforts to stop an opponent in defence but also be robust enough to enter collision efforts in attack. There are noticeable profiles to the collision demands of the different positions of a rugby team and there is little doubt that this has kept the diversity of athletic shape playing on a rugby pitch. Forward positions typically have a greater number of collisions when compared to the back positions. Interestingly and as a byproduct of how collisions are assessed, it is often the backs who have a greater proportion of their collisions within the higher acceleration zones. This is due primarily to the entry velocity into collision events.

Specific demands

Training specificity is a key training variable and a central tenet of performance improvement (Gabbett et al., 2012). The need for training to have high degrees of specificity escalates as the playing level rises. At the top-level, specificity and the transferability of physical conditioning is of paramount importance to success in a given sport. The emphasis on this is further exaggerated by the continual figurative 'arms race' in terms of performance improvement. GPS technology can help by highlighting the specific physical demands of a team's games and it provides a means by which to assess the training for those games. The general level of fitness is developed as a player rises through the ranks into professional

sport; the key distinguishing factor at all levels is the player's technical ability. Yet because there are now many structures in place for physical development across ages, at the top level the fitness is specific and unique to the team in question.

General aerobic fitness is developed from a young age, with additional strength development and power development occurring as the player becomes older. At academy level within rugby, between the ages of 18 and 22 years, maximal strength development and power development are combined with anaerobic capacity as the key physical qualities to come to the fore. Before anaerobic power is developed, maximal power and maximal speed development are essential to develop at senior level. At international level all these qualities are usually already at their peak and so the focus is on the optimization of ways to reduce fatigue that allow for peak performance. This reflects the fact that most international players are physically well developed and have high level technical and tactical skill. The mitigation of fatigue for the benefit of freshness is more important than further physical development as it is already high and the competition windows are often too short for true physical development to be the primary focus.

Positional needs differ the more specialized the playing level becomes. Within an elite team environment you can often have some distinctive differences between players, even between those playing the same position. This can produce a level of complexity and time-sensitive decision making with respect to which traits to prioritize and what fitness qualities to focus on. It is important to have a deep understanding of the demands of training and games day and facilitate the development of supplementary fitness qualities in or around training demands. This deep-rooted understanding of the training demands will provide greater accuracy and specificity to the delivery of key physical improvements and when to approach these.

Currently GPS technology is the only practical means to ascertain this granular level of individual fitness. Underscoring the need for a high degree of specificity is the fact that time is a limited resource at elite level due to fixture congestion and the high priority placed on recovery. Having specific focuses at different time points throughout the year is essential due to the week-to-week nature of an almost year-long season in conjunction with the physical toll on players due to the demanding and confrontational nature of the game. In this context, GPS can be used as a tool to assess the continual demands on the team inseason, with the ability to focus in on the demands of the training schedule overall, as well as the training demands in any given week. By utilizing this data, appropriate increases in training volume, intensity or density of work can be planned and implemented into the competitive season week and increased further in weeks where no game occurs. Emphasis must be given to the time needed for a team's training to provide the physical stimulus for long-term sustainability inseason.

By having an understanding as to the typical patterning of physical demands in games, a team's training can be designed to simulate these events, allowing for a detailed fitness quality to be derived from the technical and tactical planning of the week. Leveraging a physical fitness quality to a specific technical drill will result in its development from merely technical execution to the ability to perform these technical skills under fatigue.

GPS: role in planning

Planning the training week is one of the key areas where GPS can be used in conjunction with players' rate of perceived exertion (RPE) data and information gather through wellness and monitoring questionnaires. This provides the trinity of information as to the current state of fatigue and preparedness. While dealing with the chaos and congestion of weekly match day fixtures, quick and usable insights into the readiness of the team is made available.

There are three simple ways to approach navigating a season with up to 32 competitive games excluding the international windows for test matches.
1. *Planning the weekly load based on average weekly demands and the turnaround available before the next competitive fixture.* This can be done through the use of volume,

intensity and density measures taken directly from the GPS. Examples of this might be: total average player load/dynamic stress load (both off-the-shelf metrics with Catapult and Statsports, respectively) for each session within the week including the game. This method allows for the balancing of training days available against the fatigue of training, thus optimizing training within a given week. A simple division of workload completed for the typical match day turnaround period (i.e., 7 days apart during the inseason week) can allow for the making of appropriate modifications, e.g., reducing workload in weeks with shorter turnaround or increasing training demands in weeks with a longer turnaround. The decision might also be made to increase recovery time through additional rest days when applicable.
2. *Using acute:chronic (A:C) ratios to understand the fluctuations in training demands at a given time point within a team.* A:C ratios, as popularized by Hulin et al., 2016, can be used in conjunction with a team's monitoring information to assess the risk of injury to a given player within the squad. Whilst the relative risk as proposed by Gabbett is not proven, the main principles of this work are the cornerstone of any type of physical training; that is, too little or too much training is detrimental and any quick change results in physical soreness and decreased performance. One caveat is that one must continually benchmark the A:C ratio against the absolute amount of work completed.
3. *Averages and percentage change.* On either a team or individual level these metrics can be used as a traffic light system to provide some quick and actionable information on the training demands on the team at any level of analysis. This may be at a weekly level, session or training day level, or with enough information and consistent training time, specific training drills. Average sets can be used across some key metrics to ascertain the training demand and natural fluctuation in training, but when combined with a simple traffic light system, can also give the coach guidance on curtailing or increasing the volume or intensity of a given week, session or drill.

GPS: role in conditioning

The rise and ease of use of monitoring technology has allowed for an unprecedented level of analysis and interpretation of game and training demands. This information is increasingly being used to develop not only global conditioning strategies for the team, but also for positional groups, game differences, training versus game demands and key critical moments within games. This ease of use and the proliferation of GPS has allowed an ever-more

Table 34.2 Levels of granularity at which game play in rugby can be assessed with GPS

Game	Training
Half by half	Drill by drill
Segmental time analysis: 10-, 5- or 3-min blocks	Drill variants
Multiphase passages	Concurrent passages
PoS/WCS	Ball
Minute-by-minute analysis	

PoS, Passages of significance; *WCS*, worst-case scenarios.

detailed and specific conditioning dose to be given to the team and modelled against scheduling demands and training requirements, as mentioned previously.

This ability to increase the specificity of training volume, intensity and density and marry this with game demands and the context in which these demands occur has provided direction to enable the development of some key physical qualities that improve team performance. GPS technology can provide some of the most detailed information we have on the physical qualities needed at the elite level. GPS technology can often be misinterpreted as only being a monitoring tool, and we have to remember that it is also a performance enhancement tool. The GPS toolkit has allowed the integration of multiple information points to help create a complete contextual picture. As well as combining information on the specific and general demands to create the scenarios where physical improvement and skill improvement intersect, it can also feedback information to the athlete and coach regarding performance.

Using GPS to assess performance can be done in a number of ways. Typically, coaches like to understand the demands of the game at every level, from a 'wide-angled view' of the game and drilling down to the minutest detail of every passage or game. This telescopic approach works best when assessing demands (Table 34.2). Each level invites further analysis and interpretation regarding the specific context, etc.

Worst-case scenarios

Worst-case scenarios (WCS) were brought to prominence by Tim Gabbett (Austin et al., 2011a; Delaney et al., 2017). WCS are specific passages of play that identify the ceiling for a conditioning coach's physical preparation model. WCS are, by definition, game events where peak/maximal demands are placed upon the team or group. WCS are excellent at defining the upper limits to one's conditioning

framework and can be easily categorized based on physical quality (running, acceleration or collisions), duration or effort type. This allows the coach to tailor the conditioning to realistic opposition scenarios.

Like any maximal training event they are best used sparingly. WCS are extremely fatiguing bouts of work to demand from a team training session on a regular basis. The use of WCS bouts is not suitable as a means of developing fitness in the same way that absolute maximal strength training is not a reasonable means of gradual improvement; extreme fatigue is inherent in these methods. Yet with the necessary foundation of fitness, WCS are a means to supramaximally overload players and can form a key ingredient to the planning of preseason.

Passages of significance

Passages of significance (PoS) are passages of play that are greater in duration or intensity than those that typically occur within a game. They can be used in tandem with the biggest outlier of this data set – the WCS. An example might be the use of an artificially extended passage of training mimicking game demands to the point where fitness levels can tolerate the single largest passage, the WCS (Austin et al., 2011b). PoS can be further subdivided to highlight the trends within specific patterns of play or for simple attack-versus-defence assessment of high intensity. Because PoS cumulate continually it is also possible to highlight the difference between a team and opposition level or your own training versus game demands. This provides insight into the specific passages of play that make up a game. Thus, PoS effectively highlight the need to have passages in training that mimic not only the typical time and intensity but also the frequency of these longer passages within games against top-rated opposition.

The premise for using PoS to aid conditioning relates to the idea that as a team's ability level rises, team members become more comfortable within the systems and tactics they mobilize against an opposition team in attack or defence. This is also linked to a higher standard of player and a great contingent of those players on the same team. Furthermore as a team's ability to attack and defend for longer and with more accuracy rises, so does:

• the need for capacity to tolerate the increased physical demand of each passage, and
• the need to back up and replicate these types of passages with reduced rest time.

These passages can be aggregated to highlight the differences in trends across different teams, competition and play styles. It is hard for teams not to have a fingerprint style of play which effects these passages. The way they play is also the way they train, reflecting the training adage that a team gets better at what it does often. If a team is uncomfortable with the duration, frequency or intensity of these

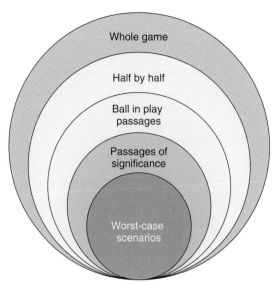

Fig. 34.2 A visual means of understanding the telescopic approach to granular game demands.

passages, most often it will try and return to its own specific norm when in possession. This is often what people perceive to be different play styles, such as:

• tactical position and structured attack
• counterattack
• continuity and unstructured attack.

Creating these passages

By using current GPS platforms, conditioning coaches now have some effective means of assessing PoS across games and training. A game or training session can be viewed overall or broken down into ever-smaller segments to analyse more detail (Fig. 34.2). This granular approach allows for better understanding as to the constituent makeup of any game.

A game can be split into halves or quarters; theses halves or quarters are made up of moments of play. Ball-in-play time is merely the removal of transitional or dead time within a half. By looking at all these passages of ball-in-play time, an outline of passage demand can be made for a whole game. Passages of significance are the passages that are longer in duration than the average passage length. Often it is these passages of greater duration that physically stress a player. A worst-case scenario is merely the single largest passage of play within a game or, as previously described, from a season's worth of games.

Creating comparative databases of this information for analysis can guide the conditioning coach with regard to the effectiveness or level of intensity of a training drill in its replication of game intensity. Further expansion of this may look at replicating passages which occur in game within

training. Having this type of game simulation within training whilst also connecting the technical element of game play is the eternal goal in creating information which is not only physically relevant but contextually relevant to the game from a technical and tactical viewpoint. .

Data can be broken down further to assess positional groups and even individual player traits. This information can be used in combination with performance analysis measures (pass accuracy, tackle completion, number of carries, etc.) to provide a holistic view of the demands, actions and effort of individuals within specific passages of play.

Repeated high-intensity efforts

Repeated high-intensity efforts (RHIE) are another excellent means of assessing where peak physical demands occur.

Repeated high-intensity efforts

Definition

A bout that involves three or more contact, acceleration, or high-speed running efforts with less than 21 seconds between each effort.

Austin, D., Gabbett, T., Jenkins, D., 2011c. The physical demands of Super 14 rugby union. Journal of Science and Medicine in Sport, 14 (3), 259–263.

RHIE can be a mix of these three components or solely comprise running, acceleration or impact; however, a mix is more common due to the nature of game play (Austin et al., 2011c). The level of the effort is typically set so that only high efforts are recorded. Across a game, trends and differences can be seen in relation to opposition, result, half by half, position or even individuals within similar positional groups.

RHIE have been described in the research literature as being critical to performance and team success (Austin et al., 2011a). RHIE take into account the three primary effort actions of rugby union, the high-intensity efforts of running, change of direction and/or collisions. These efforts comprise the general physiological basis of all actions occurring within a game of rugby excluding static-based events such as mauling or scrummaging. The typical demands of match play can be assessed by understanding the typical effort type and frequency of those high-intensity efforts at multiple levels, including:

• the team demands as a whole, by training session or game
• positional group differences, generally found between forwards and backs, and at a per position level
• for individual athletes within similar positions and/or by individual.

An example of this might be a detailed look into the RHIE makeup of the centre partnerships in rugby union. Often the 12 (inside centre) is more collision-focused, both in

Table 34.3 Comparison of RHIE and effort metrics for different rugby positions

Figures given are per session (i.e., game)

Position	Max RHIE bouts	Max no. efforts	Avg no. efforts	Max effort duration	Avg effort duration
Prop	7	8	6	00:00:17	00:00:03
Hooker	11	9	7	00:00:11	00:00:03
Lock	12	9	7	00:00:09	00:00:03
Back row	20	11	7	00:00:12	00:00:04
Scrum-half	23	14	9	00:00:16	00:00:05
Out half	18	15	6	00:00:11	00:00:02
Centre	26	14	8	00:00:21	00:00:02
Back 3	24	14	6	00:00:13	00:00:02

RHIE, Repeated high-intensity efforts; *max no. efforts*, maximum number of efforts per RHIE bout; *avg no. efforts*, average number of efforts per RHIE bout.

attack and defence, and so may have a very different collision profile to the 13 (outside centre), who is often more a strike runner and defensive reader of play, and therefore might have more acceleration efforts and running efforts compared to the 12.

A breakdown of this information may highlight differences between individual players within a similar position. Within rugby, a coach might intentionally have a variety of traits apparent in their selection choices. This is often readily seen in the composition of the back row. The RHIE profile of each of the three players might be markedly different based on the skill traits and physical makeup of the individual players, e.g., a ball-carrying number 8, a poach threat 7 and a lineout-focused 6. The RHIE composition will be heavily influenced by the mission each of these players is tasked with completing. An understanding as to the physical demand and effort profile combined with the contextual game plan can aid in the delivery of conditioning strategies for each of these subpositions.

There is no upper limit to the number of efforts involved or timeframe for which a single bout can exist, as long as each effort is connected to the previous effort within a 21-second window. Because of this, RHIE can be extremely relevant to play, as this basic effort demand is often woven directly into all game play actions, and the duration of a passage of play can open the opportunity for an athlete to produce high-effort bouts as well as bouts of longer duration. The converse may also be true when an athlete's lack of ability to produce continual high-intensity efforts results in technical errors causing play to stop.

Typically the average number of RHIE bouts within a game is 17 ± 7. Differences can be seen within the data

due to the varying tactical roles within positions and the varying physical traits attributed to these positions. These variations can be seen in total number of bouts, average number of efforts per bout and maximum effort duration.

The backs positional group often have more RHIE bouts when compared to forwards (Table 34.3), although the average number of efforts does not differ significantly. Often the differences are that the backs pick up smaller effort bouts in brief contesting of play, but in long-duration passages all positions are demanded to repeat efforts in either attack or defence. This, in part, explains how the forwards can gather a similar number of efforts when called upon. The typical bout of a forward also tends to be shorter in duration and often the time between efforts is longer than that seen by backs regarding acceleration and velocity efforts. However, impacts often make up a greater contribution of the forwards' bouts when compared to backs', who can have a high number of bouts but with no impact efforts recorded. These are typically seen in supporting attack play.

Considerations

GPS technology is not without its flaws. There are varying degrees of error depending on what parameters you chose to use as your key determinants of assessment. Like all GPS systems, the accuracy of the data is based on the quality of signal being received. Simple parameters like distance covered and time breakdown of distance parameters are quite accurate. However, the greater the speed at which the parameter is measured, the more opportunity for data collection error. Thus metrics such as total distance and distance covered in zones of lower speed are quite accurate, but high-zone accelerations are more prone to error.

Elite-level systems have the hardware and software processing capability to more accurately detect micromovements like change of direction and high changes in velocity. They also have the price tag to accompany this. Impacts and collision data require additional post-download analysis and are only available on elite-level systems that have both the high-sampling accelerometer and gyroscope hardware on board and the algorithms to assess the accuracy and validity of the data collected.

Your given sport will be a key consideration when choosing a GPS platform provider, as top platforms now come with sport-specific algorithms, for example:
- Catapult has goalkeeper number of dives, scrum analysis for rugby, RHIE specific to hockey or jumping events.
- Statsport has kick count as well as scrum and collision analysis for rugby union.

Machine learning is the next frontier for the generation of more sport-specific algorithms and analysis. Examples here include automatic drill detection or gait analysis of individual players, where the algorithm can make inferences based on historical data unique to that player in question.

One of the leading-edge benefits that GPS technology is starting to provide is the ability to combine sport-specific performance markers with a capacity to contextualize performance through the integration of multiple information sources. This ability to link multiple layers of information – ranging from subjective wellness information provided by athletes, to the internal and external objective response to training garnered by GPS and heart rate, to the assessment of performance harvested through performance analysis and coaching insights – is key. It is this synergy of information that will provide some of the main avenues for progression in the near future.

Conclusion

The aim of this chapter has been to provide insight into the practical application of GPS, not only as a monitoring tool but also as a performance-enhancement platform. GPS has risen to prominence because of its ability to gather physical insights into the captivating world of sport. The information presented here is hopefully a means by which a conditioning coach can use GPS to both monitor how a team is training and performing compared to results and to assess individual's contribution to those performances. This can be undertaken through an analysis of the effort demands on and output of individuals as assessed by high-intensity efforts or RHIE bouts.

GPS can also be used as a shared platform to assess training design and output within a multidisciplinary team through the use of replicating game intensity passages of play to make training as specific as possible to the context of the game. This ensures the delivery of training in which physical, technical and tactical development occurs at a relevant intensity. The techniques outlined here, it is hoped, will help to maximize performance in those occasional but rewarding moments within games where the momentum play wins you the day.

References

Austin, D.J., Gabbett, T.J., Jenkins, D.J., 2011a. Repeated high-intensity exercise in a professional rugby league. The Journal of Strength and Conditioning Research 25 (7), 1898–1904.

Austin, D.J., Gabbett, T.J., Jenkins, D.J., 2011b. Repeated high-intensity exercise in professional rugby union. Journal of Sports Sciences 29 (10), 1105–1112.

Austin, D., Gabbett, T., Jenkins, D., 2011c. The physical demands of Super 14 rugby union. Journal of Science and Medicine in Sport, 14 (3), 259–263.

Cummins, C., Orr, R., O'Connor, H., West, C., 2013. Global positioning systems (GPS) and microtechnology sensors in team sports: a systematic review. Sports Medicine 43 (10), 1025–1042.

Delaney, J.A., Thornton, H.R., Pryor, J.F., Stewart, A.M., Dascombe, B.J., Duthie, G.M., 2017. Peak running intensity of international rugby: implications for training prescription. International Journal of Sports Physiology and Performance 12 (8), 1039–1045.

Gabbett, T.J., 2012. Sprinting patterns of national rugby league competition. The Journal of Strength and Conditioning Research 26 (1), 121–130.

Gabbett, T.J., Jenkins, D.G., Abernethy, B., 2012. Physical demands of professional rugby league training and competition using microtechnology. Journal of Science and Medicine in Sport 15 (1), 80–86.

Hulin, B.T., Gabbett, T.J., Lawson, D.W., Caputi, P., Sampson, J.A., 2016. The acute:chronic workload ratio predicts injury: high chronic workload may decrease injury risk in elite rugby league players. British Journal of Sports Medicine 50 (4), 231–236.

Chapter | 35 |

Managing the overhead athlete

Steve McCaig

Introduction: what is 'the overhead athlete'?

Sports such as baseball, tennis, softball, cricket, volleyball, handball and water polo can be considered overhead sports. These sports all involve activities where one hand either throws a ball or hits a ball overhead, with or without an implement, such as a racquet, in hand. Although there are many differences between these sports, the motion that occurs at the upper limb during these tasks is broadly similar (Fleisig et al., 1996; Wagner et al., 2014), as are the upper limb injuries sustained (McCaig and Young, 2016). Therefore similar principles can be applied when managing these athletes.

Throwing arm pain

Throwing arm pain (TAP) has been used to describe the collection of shoulder and elbow conditions reported in overhead sports (McCaig and Young, 2016). These sports cause similar upper limb conditions as they have similar intrinsic and extrinsic factors, such as technique, workload, physical and psychosocial factors, that contribute to injury. To manage the overhead athlete, it is vital to understand the biomechanics of overhead activity, including pathomechanics and the associated physical adaptations

Biomechanics of the overhead activity

The biomechanics of a baseball pitch and a tennis serve have been well described, as have other overhead activities (Cook and Strike, 2000; Fleisig et al., 1996; Kovacs and Ellenbecker, 2011; Wagner et al., 2014). They all have a preparation phase, an acceleration phase and a deceleration phase (Table 35.1). While there are many differences between these sports, the motions of the upper limb vary little (Fleisig et al., 1996; Wagner et al., 2014). The physical qualities required for each phase of overhead activity are described in Table 35.2 and the key factors in throwing performance and injury risk are described in Table 35.3.

Preparation phase

The preparation phase includes all actions taken to place the body into position to achieve maximum external rotation (MER) of the shoulder during the arm cocking stage (Fleisig, 2010). The stages involved during the preparation phase vary between sports, but all end in an arm cocking stage. In some scenarios the athlete will start with the ball in hand, such as for a baseball pitch or tennis serve, while in others the player is required to move into position to gather or hit the ball, such as a baseball outfielder or outside hitter in volleyball. It is important to recognize that other factors, such as the base of support, e.g., water polo versus baseball pitching, time and decision-making constraints, e.g., tennis serve versus quarterback about to be tackled, will also influence the preparation phase.

Arm cocking stage

During the cocking phase the dominant shoulder moves into MER, which is critical for performance (Fortenbaugh et al., 2009; Whiteley, 2007). The pelvis, followed quickly by the trunk, rotates towards the target, which forces the upper limb into MER, which can reach up to 200 degrees (Werner et al., 1993). MER is a combination of glenohumeral joint (GHJ) external rotation (ER), scapula posterior tilt and external rotation, trunk extension and elbow valgus (Miyashita et al., 2010).

Table 35.1 Comparison between the biomechanical phases of baseball pitching and tennis serving

Phases of overhead activities in sport		Stages of baseball pitching		Stages of tennis serve	
1. Preparation phase	Starts with the first movement and ends in maximum external rotation (MER) of the shoulder	1. Wind-up	Begins when the pitcher lifts the front leg off the ground and ends at maximum hip flexion of the front leg	1. Start	Both the ball and racquet are at rest
		2. Stride	Begins when the front leg starts to move forward and ends when it contacts the ground (foot contact; FC)	2. Release	Starts from the initial movement of ball and racquet until the ball is released from the nonserving hand
		3. Arm cocking	Begins at FC and ends at MER	3. Loading	From release until the lower body is fully loaded in maximum knee flexion
				4. Arm cocking	Begins at end of loading stage and finishes in MER, which results in the racquet head point towards the ground
2. Acceleration phase	Begins at MER and ends at either ball impact or release	4. Acceleration	From MER until the ball is released	5. Acceleration	From MER until ball contact
				6. Contact	The brief period where the racquet is in contact with the ball
3. Deceleration phase	Begins immediately after ball release or impacts and finishes when the next motor skill begins	5. Deceleration	Following contact until maximum internal rotation (MIR) of the shoulder	7. Deceleration	Following contact until MIR
		6. Follow through	Any continued movement after MIR until the next motor skill begins	8. Follow through	Any continued movement after MIR until the next motor skill begins

Adapted from Kovacs, M., Ellenbecker, T., 2011. An 8-stage model for evaluating the tennis serve: implications for performance enhancement and injury prevention. Sports Health 3, 504–513.

Table 35.2 Key physical qualities required for overhead throws

Phase of overhead action	Region	Range of motion	Soft tissue length	Muscle activity
Preparation	Lower limb	DOM leg hip ext. and abd.	DOM leg hip flexor length	DOM leg con. triple ext.
		DOM and NDOM leg hip ER	DOM leg hip adductor length	DOM leg conc. hip abd.
				NDOM leg triple ext. stiffness
	Trunk	DOM side thoracic rot.		Ecc. then con. oblique abdominal activity
		Thoracic ext.		Ecc. then con. trunk flexors
	Upper limb	DOM shoulder ER	Pectoralis minor length	Ecc. DOM shoulder IR and hor. flex.
		DOM scapula ret.		Ecc. CFO muscles
Acceleration	Lower limb	DOM hip ER and IR		NDOM leg triple ext. stiffness
				NDOM concentric knee ext.
	Trunk			Con. oblique abdominal activity
				Con. trunk flexors
	Upper limb			Rapid con. DOM shoulder IR and hor. flex.
				Concentric DOM scapula protractors
Deceleration	Lower limb	NDOM hip flex. and IR	NDOM hamstring length	Ecc. NDOM hip extensors and ER
		DOM hip IR and abd.		NDOM knee stiffness
	Trunk	NDOM thoracic rot.		Ecc. thoracolumbar extensors
		Trunk flex.		
	Upper limb	DOM shoulder IR and hor. flex.		Eccentric DOM shoulder ER and hor. ext.
		DOM scapula prot.		Ecc. DOM scapula retractors
		DOM Elbow ext. and pron.		Ecc. DOM elbow flexors and supinators
				Ecc. DOM LH biceps

abd., Abduction; *CFO*, common flexor origin; *con.*, concentric muscle activity; *DOM*, dominant side; *ecc.*, eccentric muscle activity; *ER*, external rotation; *ext.*, extension; *flex.*, flexion; *hor.*, horizontal; *IR*, internal rotation; *NDOM*, nondominant side; *pron.*, pronation; *prot.*, protraction; *ret.*, retraction; *rot.*, rotation

Acceleration phase

This phase begins after MER and ends at ball release or ball contact and is the fastest joint motion in all sports, with the shoulder rotating at up to 7000 degrees/s, which is the equivalent of the shoulder completing around 18 full rotations in a second, and the elbow extends at 2500 degrees (Fleisig et al., 1995).

Deceleration phase

This begins after ball release or contact and finishes when the next motor skill begins. The deceleration phase is crucial to dissipate the forces generated during acceleration. However each sport will have varying constraints that effect this phase, e.g., volleyball net during a spike.

Table 35.3 Key factors for throwing performance and injury risk

Key factors for performance (velocity and accuracy)	Key factors for injury risk (reducing joint loads)
Increased stride length	Stride length
Foot to target at foot contact	Foot to target at foot contact
Timing between pelvis and trunk rotation during cocking phase	Timing between pelvis and trunk rotation during cocking phase
Range of maximum external rotation at end of cocking phase	Shoulder abduction during cocking and acceleration
Trunk flexion during acceleration	Elbow flexion during cocking phase
Slight knee extension during acceleration	Horizontal extension during cocking phase
Follow through towards target	Shoulder external rotation at foot contact
	Trunk lateral flexion
	Follow through towards target

From Fleisig, G.S., 2010. Biomechanics of overhand throwing: implications for injury and performance. In: Portus, M. (Ed.) Conference of Science, Medicine and Coaching in Cricket. Conference Proceedings. Brisbane: Cricket Australia; Fortenbaugh, D., Fleisig, G.S., Andrews, J.R., 2009. Baseball pitching biomechanics in relation to risk and performance. Sport Health 1, 314–320; Whiteley, R., 2007. Baseball throwing mechanics as they relate to pathology and performance: a review. Journal of Sport Science and Medicine 6, 1–20.

Pathomechanics of overhead activity

The development of TAP is thought to be related to the stresses experienced at the upper limb during key phases and stages of overhead activity (Fleisig et al., 1995; Fortenbaugh et al., 2009; Wassinger and Myers, 2011).

Cocking/acceleration phase

Extreme ranges of MER can contribute to the development of TAP through both internal impingement and the 'peel back' phenomenon (Wassinger and Myers, 2011). Internal impingement is where the articular surface of the postero-superior rotator cuff and glenoid labrum gets compressed between the greater tuberosity of the humerus and the glenoid fossa (Burkhart et al., 2003a; Edelson and Teitz, 2000; Walch et al., 1992) (Fig. 35.1B). Although this is a normal phenomenon that occurs during end-range external rotation in abduction (Edelson and Teitz, 2000), the repetitive stress from high forces that occur during overhead sports can result in pathological changes in the rotator cuff and glenoid labrum. The peel back phenomenon is where the long head of biceps tendon twists during MER; when combined with muscle activity, this results in the labrum being 'peeled back' from the glenoid (Burkhart et al., 2003b). This is thought to contribute to the development of biceps tendinopathies and superior labral lesions (e.g., SLAP, superior labral tear from anterior to posterior) (Burkhart et al., 2003b) (Fig. 35.1C).

During MER valgus forces can exceed the tensile strength of the ulna collateral ligament (UCL) (Fleisig et al., 1995), which can lead to attenuation of or acute injuries to the UCL. The resulting laxity in the UCL can lead to the radial head being compressed against the capitellum and the olecranon which impact upon the olecranon fossa medially during valgus stress. This process, and the pathologies associated with it, is known as valgus extension overload (VEO) (Cain et al., 2003) (Fig. 35.2). The muscles of the common flexor origin (CFO) act as secondary stabilizers to valgus stress (An et al., 1981; Davidson et al., 1995) and increased load on the CFO due to UCL laxity can lead to CFO tendinopathy. Valgus laxity can also compress the ulnar nerve in its groove posterior to medial condyle resulting in ulnar nerve irritation and neuropathy (Cain et al., 2003).

Deceleration phase

During deceleration, high levels of eccentric muscle activity occur in the posterior cuff and biceps to control shoulder and elbow motion, although the whole kinetic chain should function to absorb these forces (Chu et al., 2016). Inadequate trunk flexion and contralateral rotation, and hip flexion and internal rotation (IR) during deceleration increase the stress on the shoulder and elbow, which can lead to the development of TAP (Chu et al., 2016).

Adaptations to overhead sport

The musculoskeletal adaptations to overhead sport are well documented and are likely to be necessary for high performance. However they may also lead to increased injury risk (Borsa et al., 2008; Whiteley et al., 2012). These adaptations include specific postural, mobility and strength changes in the dominant upper limb (Borsa et al., 2008; Forthomme et al., 2008; Whiteley et al., 2012). When assessing the overhead athlete, it is important to be aware that these findings are common in asymptomatic athletes.

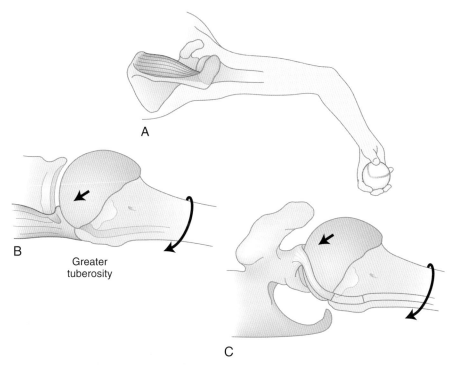

Fig. 35.1 Internal impingement and the 'peel back' phenomenon. (A) Shoulder in maximum external rotation during cocking phase; (B) internal impingement; (C) 'peel back' phenomenon. (Adapted from Fig. 10 in Chang, I.Y., Polster, J.M., 2016. Pathomechanics and magnetic resonance imaging of the thrower's shoulder. Radiologic Clinics of North America 54 (5), 801–815.)

Scapula

The dominant scapula commonly sits in depression, downward rotation and internal rotation (protraction) relative to the nondominant side in overhead athletes (Forthomme et al., 2008; Oyama et al., 2008). This is due to increased muscle bulk and tightness in the pectoralis minor and major and latissimus dorsi. Scapula dyskinesis is commonly found in overhead athletes (Burn et al., 2016) and has been proposed to be a risk factor for TAP. However there is conflicting evidence to support this (Hickey et al., 2017; Myers et al., 2013; Struyf et al., 2013).

GHJ rotation range of motion

In the asymptomatic overhead athlete, the dominant shoulder usually displays a gain in external rotation (ERG) and a decrease in internal rotation (glenohumeral internal rotation deficit, GIRD) range of motion (ROM) when measured in 90 degrees abduction. Total rotation ROM (TRROM) (TRROM = ER + IR) being similar on the dominant (DOM) and nondominant (NDOM) sides (Borsa et al., 2008; Whiteley and Oceguera, 2016). The increase in ER ROM is thought to be crucial for throwing speed

performance as it may allow for greater MER (Fortenbaugh et al., 2009; Whiteley, 2007).

These changes in ROM are thought to occur due to either soft tissue or bony changes (Borsa et al., 2008). Soft tissue changes include acquired laxity in the anterior capsule and tightness in the posterior capsule of the shoulder and are thought to contribute to the development of ERG and GIRD, respectively (Borsa et al., 2008). Alterations in the degree of humeral torsion, which is the degree of twist in the long axis of the humerus, have been consistently observed in overhead athletes (Whiteley et al., 2009; Yamamoto et al., 2006). The DOM humerus in the overhead athlete displays increased human retroversion compared to the NDOM side and these changes would account for any observed ERG and GIRD in overhead athletes (Chant et al., 2007; Crockett et al., 2002; Whiteley and Oceguera, 2016). Increased humeral retroversion is thought to both improve performance and reduce the risk of shoulder pain, as less stress will be placed on the soft tissues as more ER range is allowed due to the bony geometry (Whiteley et al., 2009).

Several studies have found that increased GIRD, lack of ERG, reduced TRROM and shoulder flexion have been found to associated with TAP (Camp et al., 2017; Clarsen et al., 2014; Shanley et al., 2011; Wilk at al., 2014; Wilk et al., 2015a,b), although others found no association (Oyama et al., 2017). Accurate measurement of shoulder range of motion is crucial when assessing overhead athletes, and many methods exist. However the shoulder range measured will vary significantly depending upon the method used, be it active or passive, and with or without scapula stabilization (Wilk et al., 2009). For a single practitioner we find that measuring GHJ rotation ROM passively with scapula stabilization with an inclinometer to be a reliable method (Figs 35.3 and 35.4).

GHJ strength

Overhead athletes consistently demonstrate increased IR strength on the DOM shoulder and increased IR:ER strength ratio, while the external rotators demonstrate no change in strength or may have a reduction in strength compared to the NDOM shoulder (Whiteley et al., 2012). The internal rotators make a significant contribution to throwing velocity (Roach and Lieberman, 2014); however, weakness in the ER and marked increases in IR:ER ratio (>1.5) have been associated with increased risk of developing TAP (Byram et al., 2010; Clarsen et al., 2014). Increased IR:ER ratio can result in the external rotators being unable to control the acceleration forces generated by the internal rotators during the deceleration phase, which increases the risk of TAP (Whiteley et al., 2012).

Whilst isokinetic testing is considered the gold standard for assessing rotator cuff strength (Whiteley et al., 2012), we find handheld dynamometry to be useful for the clinician given its ease of use, portable nature and relative inexpensiveness. Testing of GHJ rotation strength can be completed as either a 'make' or a 'break' test. In a 'make' test the subject is asked to push as hard as possible into the therapist who matches their force and the dynamometer measures their maximal isometric contraction. In a 'break' test the therapist asks the subject to stay still and then gradually increases their force until the subject is no longer able to hold this position. This measures their maximal eccentric contraction and can be provocative in irritable shoulders. Testing shoulder strength in 90 degrees of abduction is a

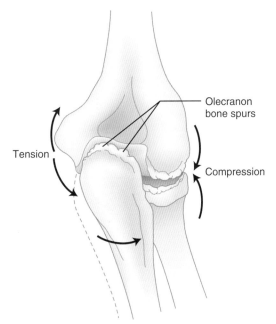

Fig. 35.2 Valgus extension overload. (Adapted from Fig. 35.1 in Abrams, G., Safran, M., 2011. Valgus extension overload. In: Miller, M.D., Sanders, T.G. (Eds.), Presentation, Imaging and Treatment of Common Musculoskeletal Conditions: MRI – Arthroscopy Correlation. Elsevier Saunders, Philadelphia, PA.)

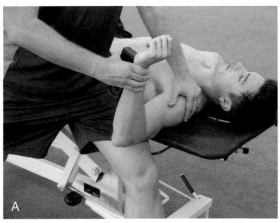
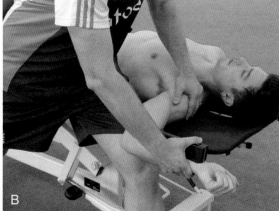

Fig. 35.3 Measuring glenohumeral joint external rotation ROM passively. (A) Start position. (B) End position.

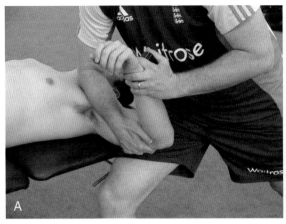
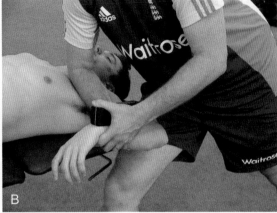

Fig. 35.4 Measuring glenohumeral joint internal rotation ROM passively. (A) Start position. (B) End position.

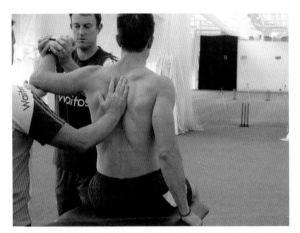

Fig. 35.5 Measuring external rotation strength with handheld dynamometer.

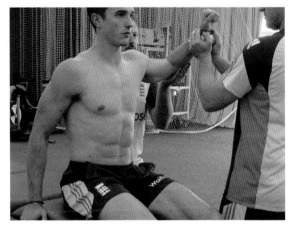

Fig. 35.6 Measuring internal rotation strength with handheld dynamometer.

more functional position for the overhead athlete (Figs 35.5 and 35.6); it can be provocative to some athletes who may need to be assessed in 0 degrees of abduction.

Elbow range of motion

It is not uncommon for overhead athletes to have reduced elbow extension and increased carrying angle (Chang et al., 2010; Wright et al., 2006). However few studies have investigated any injury risk associated with this.

The kinetic chain (trunk and lower limb)

The entire kinetic chain is utilized during overhead activities and its effective function is crucial for performance and

reducing injury risk (Chu et al., 2016; Fortenbaugh et al., 2009). The role of the kinetic chain is to channel forces generated from the lower limb and trunk to the upper limb to increase the velocity of shoulder internal rotation, as well as to absorb these forces. Several lower limb and trunk muscle performance tests have been found to correlate with throwing velocity, such as a lateral leap and medicine ball side toss (Freeston et al., 2016; Lehman et al., 2013).

Total athlete management of the overhead athlete

Total athlete management is the ongoing process of 'plan, do, review' applied to all aspects of the athlete to optimize performance and minimize risk of injury. It encourages clinicians to be proactive rather than reactive to injury (Newton et al., 2011). It is important the practitioner considers all factors that may impact on the athlete's ability to train and compete. The total athlete management plan should be adjusted according to the demands of the specific training or competitive phase.

Offseason management

All athletes need a recovery phase at the end of their competitive season; however, the length of this period depends upon the intensity and duration of both the previous season and the preparation time required for the upcoming season. While a period off from overhead activity is crucial to physically and psychologically recover, it is important the athlete maintains the physical qualities required for overhead activity during this phase. If they become deconditioned they will be vulnerable to injury, as there may then be insufficient time available to prepare them for the demands of the upcoming competitive season.

Past history of injury is a significant risk factor for injury. This may be because the injury was never fully resolved or the contributing factors to that injury were not addressed (Finch and Cook, 2014). Lower limb and spinal disorders can affect the function of the kinetic chain, which can increase the load on the upper limb during throwing, increasing the risk of TAP (Chu et al., 2016). The preseason periodic health check should involve a thorough review of any previous musculoskeletal disorders and any conditions identified should be managed appropriately during the offseason.

The value of preseason screening has been questioned (Bahr, 2016; Whiteley, 2016), particularly with regard to injury prediction. We prefer the term 'profiling', which describes the process of gathering information to better understand the athlete to inform their management. This information is used to help inform each player's preparation programme, establish squad benchmarks and determine clinical and functional baselines, which can be used to help determine readiness to return to play postinjury. Profiling of the overhead athlete should include an assessment of all the key physical requirements for throwing as well as the specific work capacity requirements of the sport, using tests with established reliability and validity. Upon the completion of profiling, support staff should develop an individualized preparation programme based on these results, in consultation with both athlete and coaching staff, as this will improve compliance.

Any technical deficiencies identified should be addressed during the offseason with a focus on drills that address the technical factors relating to performance and injury risk (see Table 35.3). Although 3D motion analysis is the gold standard for assessing throwing biomechanics

it is not practical for most sports as it requires expensive equipment and is time consuming (McCaig and Young, 2016). High-speed footage can be used by coaches and support staff to identify areas for development based on a sound understanding of an optimal technical model. Any technical work should be completed as part of a graded return to overhead activity based on preparing the athlete for the demands of the competitive season. It is crucial that the athlete develops the physical capacity to tolerate the workload of their sport; fatigue can result in technical alterations that can increase stress on the upper limb, increasing susceptibility to injury (Erickson et al., 2016; Gabbett, 2016).

Inseason management

During the competitive season it is important that practitioners monitor the throwing athlete's workload (external load) and their response to this workload (internal load). The relationship between throwing workload and increased injury risk in overhead sports is well established (Black et al., 2016). Higher volumes of throwing on a daily and weekly basis, reduced rest days and increases in acute:chronic workload ratio (ACWR) have all been shown to increase the risk of developing TAP (Black et al., 2016). The number of throws the athlete performs should be recorded where possible, as well as any other sports and training loads. Unfortunately, monitoring throwing workload can be challenging; players cannot accurately remember how many throws they did each session, nor can the intensity of each throw be quantified. Advances in technology such as global positioning systems (GPS) and inertial measurement units (IMU) are making it easier to monitor throwing loads (Murray et al., 2017). However the costs are high, technological problems can occur, it requires significant human resources and some athletes may not wish to wear the units (Warren et al., 2018). We have found calculating arbitrary units (AU) by multiplying session ratings of perceived exertion (RPEs) and the duration of the session to be a practical way of monitoring workload. Furthermore, we have found an increased risk of injury and illness in throwing athletes with higher daily and weekly loads and increased ACWR.

Daily wellness questionnaires can be used to monitor the athlete's response to workload and should collect information such as sleep duration and quality, muscle soreness, cold symptoms, mood and stress levels, with the scores anchored around what is normal for that individual (Saw et al., 2017). This information can be collected either manually from the athlete or via text messages or apps. Soreness and fatigue can often precede TAP; therefore any deviation from the athlete's normal responses should be discussed with that athlete and management implemented as indicated.

Acute and chronic bouts of throwing result in changes to a throwers musculoskeletal profile. These changes include reductions in shoulder internal rotation and elbow range of motion (Dwelly et al., 2009; Kibler et al., 2012; Laudner et al., 2013; Reinold et al., 2008), and reductions in shoulder external rotation strength (Whiteley, 2010). Athletes at risk of developing TAP should be monitored for changes in upper limb function regularly over the course of a season (Whiteley, 2010). As lower limb power is crucial to throwing, this should be monitored as well and this can be done via a countermovement jump on a jump mat or force platform (Cormack et al., 2006; Laffaye et al., 2014). If resources are limited athletes can be taught a self-check routine which may include specific mobility exercises such as the horizontal flexion stretch, thoracic rotation, overhead squat, split squat and lateral split squat. These can be performed daily as part of a warm-up to other activities.

Any physical monitoring should be done on a consistent basis at the same stage in competition, either after a rest day before beginning training that day or the day after a match, depending on that sport's competitive phase (Whiteley, 2010). Regular monitoring allows the practitioner to understand what is the normal for that athlete, which can then be used to identify when these changes exceed normal variation. Athletes must be given regular feedback on any information they share, which is crucial to gain their 'buy in'. If any significant changes are noted, the practitioner should look to modify either the athlete's training or competitive workload, add specific recovery methods, such as soft tissue therapy or extra mobility sessions, or add strength sessions where appropriate (Gabbett et al., 2017). However, any changes to the athlete's programme, especially during their competitive schedule, needs to be done in careful consultation with the athlete and coach and should be informed by the best available evidence from athlete monitoring (Gabbett et al., 2017).

During the competitive season it is important that the athlete continues to train to maintain the physical qualities necessary for optimal performance and to maintain robustness. This training should be similar to their offseason programme, but the volume of sets and loads is reduced according to the other demands of their sport. These sessions should be programmed as part of the athlete's weekly schedule with consideration given to their match and training schedule. An easy way to implement these is to include some of these exercises as part of warm-up and recovery sessions.

Assessing the injured overhead athlete

Any overhead athlete with TAP should be carefully assessed and the practitioner should have a thorough understanding of that athlete's pain presentation prior to initiating a management plan. The following questions are crucial to this:

1. Are any red flags present?
2. Is the presentation consistent with a specific or nonspecific disorder?
3. What is the stage of the disorder? Acute, persistent, acute on persistent?
4. Is the pain presentation mechanical, nonmechanical or mixed?
5. Does the pain presentation respond to improvement testing?
6. What are the contributing factors (intrinsic and extrinsic) and are they modifiable?

Red flags

The presence of red flags, although uncommon, should be screened in all patients, including overhead athletes, and the practitioner must continue to be vigilant during the management process. The presence of red flags should result in immediate medical referral for further investigations (Lewis et al., 2015). When assessing the overhead athlete, it is important to look for a history of trauma to the shoulder, particularly from diving or contact with an opponent, prior to developing TAP.

Specific versus nonspecific pain

The finding of abnormalities during investigations of asymptomatic overhead athletes in very common (Connor et al., 2003; Jost et al., 2005; Miniaci et al., 2002) and this can make interpreting the results of any investigation in the athlete with TAP challenging. This phenomenon is also common in other areas of the body and has led to the concept of specific and nonspecific conditions (O'Sullivan et al., 2015). Specific conditions are where the pain presentation is consistent with the pathology found upon investigation. Specific shoulder and elbow conditions include GHJ dislocations and subluxations, acute tears in the UCL, fractures of the upper limb, massive rotator cuff tears, acute capsule–labral injuries to the shoulder and ligamentous injuries to the elbow; these conditions may require specific medical management. In the younger overhead athlete these specific conditions are usually the result of trauma. However, partial rotator cuff tears and tendinopathies, shoulder bursitis, long head of biceps tenosynovitis and SLAP lesions are commonly found in asymptomatic overhead athletes (Connor et al., 2003; Jost et al., 2005; Miniaci et al., 2002) and these may be considered nonspecific. In these conditions, management should be based on addressing the presentation dysfunctions and contributing factors, not the diagnosis.

Table 35.4 Potential contributing factors to throwing arm pain

Intrinsic factors	
Nonmodifiable	
General	Gender, age, maturation status, genetics, injury history, anatomical structure
Potentially modifiable	
Motor control	Sport-specific activities and technique, throwing, serving, hitting; habitual postures and movement patterns
Mobility and flexibility	Specific upper limb, trunk and lower limb joint ROM and muscle length required for the task
Conditioning	Strength qualities required: max force, RFD, work capacity; general aerobic and local muscle endurance, sport-specific conditioning
Physiological	General health, other medical conditions, fatigue, sleep
Psychological	Injury and illness beliefs, fear and anxiety, coping strategies, self-efficacy, depression and stress
Extrinsic factors	
Training-related	Volume, intensity, frequency and training type; competition and training schedule; rest and recovery
Environmental	Coaches, team mates, support staff, medical specialists, family, team selection and contract issues, work, other activities, travel, sponsors
Social factors	Teammates, coaches, families, agents, work
Other	Previous treatments, diet, supplements, medications

RFD, Rate of force development; *ROM,* range of motion.
Adapted from Mitchell, T., Burnett, A., O'Sullivan, P., 2015. The athletic spine. In: Joyce, D., Lewindon, D. (Eds.), Sports Injury Prevention and Rehabilitation: Integrating Medicine and Science for Performance Solutions. Routledge, Oxon, UK.

Pain presentation and stage of the disorder

Most presentations of TAP are mechanical. However changes in central sensitivity may occur in athletes with a prolonged history of TAP or other musculoskeletal conditions and has been observed in tendinopathies (Lewis et al., 2015). The presence of widespread symptoms, mechanical hyperalgesia and allodynia should alert the clinician to the possibility of central changes. Psychosocial factors such as hypervigilance, fear and anxiety and issues around selection can influence an athlete's pain presentation and should be considered as a potential factor in every athlete's pain presentation (Mitchell et al., 2015; Puentedura and Louw, 2012).

Improvement testing

Improvement testing involves applied external forces or self-applied forces to either the thorax, scapula, humeral head, elbow or cervicothoracic spine during an aggravating

activity and observing the effects of this force (Lewis, 2009; Lewis et al., 2015). It can often result in immediate improvement in symptoms and if this occurs the intervention may then be included in a management plan. Due to speeds of motion during overhead sports it is often difficult to conduct improvement testing during actual sporting tasks. However it can be applied to components of the task or other aggravating activities, e.g., manually altering scapula or humeral head position during resisted ER at 90 degrees of abduction.

Contributing factors

All pain presentations are associated with a variety of contributing factors unique to that individual and condition (Lewis et al., 2015; Mitchell et al., 2015; O'Sullivan et al., 2015). Some of these factors are described in Table 35.4. During the examination the clinician must consider the relevance and significance of these factors in relation to that individual's condition and determine which ones are potentially modifiable, as this will guide management.

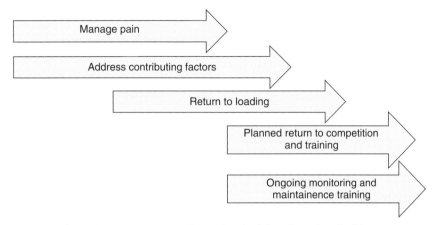

Fig. 35.7 Management pathway for the injured overhead athlete.

Managing the injured overhead athlete

If any red flags are identified or if the athlete has a specific pain presentation they should be referred to a medical practitioner, ideally one that is familiar with overhead athletes, for further investigation. In the absence of red flags or specific disorders, a management pathway for the overhead athlete is described in Fig. 35.7. The pathway is similar for specific disorders but will vary depending upon the specific medical management required. The components of this management plan should not be considered as separate entities, as there is considerable overlap between each component. It is crucial that the athlete is at the centre of this plan and understands it and that all other stakeholders (coaches, other support staff, agents) are supportive of the plan. This is essential for any management plan to be effective. It is important that the language used to explain the athlete's condition does not contribute to any unhelpful injury beliefs, as this can be detrimental to outcome (Saw et al., 2017).

Manage pain

Most TAP is only painful during overhead activity and often settles quickly with load modification. Some athletes may continue to play despite TAP and may require medical interventions such as medications or injections to manage symptoms to allow this. If improvement testing is effective, these techniques can be integrated into management to help control symptoms; in addition, taping that replicates these techniques can also prove effective (Lewis, 2009; Lewis et al., 2015).

Address contributing factors and return to loading

Targeted interventions aimed at addressing the contributing factors relevant to that athlete's specific presentation should be introduced immediately (Lewis, 2009). Specific mobility exercises and manual and soft tissue therapy should target any identified movement restrictions. Motor retraining should be introduced to address any specific control impairments and specific strengthening exercises should address any rotator cuff or scapula muscle strength deficits (Lewis, 2009; Lewis et al., 2015; Mitchell et al., 2015; O'Sullivan et al., 2015). Any relevant exercises to improve movement and control impairments and strength deficits in the trunk and lower limb should be introduced immediately regardless of the severity of TAP, as can general and specific conditioning exercises. It is vital that the athlete has the physical qualities required for throwing prior to resuming a return-to-throwing programme. Education and sometimes psychological support may be necessary to address any unhelpful thoughts, beliefs and feelings that may be influencing their pain presentation (Mitchell et al., 2015; O'Sullivan et al., 2015; Saw et al., 2017).

Planned return to competition and training

When, according to clinical examination, the athlete's symptoms have settled and they have regained the physical qualities required for throwing, a graded return-to-throwing programme should be initiated. This programme should follow a similar structure to the preseason throwing programme. However the athlete may need to progress more slowly. If technique was considered a significant contributing factor, specific interventions to address this should be included as part of this programme, but only in consultation with coaching staff. It is important that distance thrown is gradually increased and then intensity added over shorter distances when the athlete can throw near their maximal distance (Axe et al., 2009; Reinold et al., 2002). The volume of throws should reflect the demands of normal competition and training, but the athlete should be monitored for signs of fatigue, such as alterations in technique, during each session (Axe et al., 2009; Reinold et al., 2002). Clinical signs should continue to be normal as the programme progresses. The presence of any soreness or pain is an indication that the programme is being progressed too quickly and should be adjusted accordingly (Axe et al., 2009; Reinold et al., 2002).

Ongoing monitoring and maintenance rehabilitation

Once the athlete has returned to full training and competition they should continue to be observed closely as recurrent episodes of TAP are common. Throwing and overall workload should be monitored, as should the athlete's response to this load (Gabbett et al., 2017; Whiteley, 2010). The presence of fatigue, soreness, reductions in GHJ ROM and strength can indicate that the athlete is not coping with this workload and may be at risk of TAP recurrence (Whiteley, 2010). The athlete should continue with key aspects of their rehabilitation programme to maintain the physical qualities required for throwing and some athletes may benefit from ongoing manual or soft tissue therapy to address any movement restrictions or muscle soreness.

Conclusion

To manage any overhead athlete, regardless of their sport, it is critical the practitioner has a thorough understanding of the specific biomechanics of that sport and associated pathomechanics, as well as the physical qualities and associated adaptations that occur in the overhead athlete. The clinician needs to ensure that the athlete is prepared for the specific competitive and training demands of their sport, including both overhead and general activity. Abnormalities are commonly found in the upper limb in asymptomatic overhead athletes during investigations, which can make interpreting these scans in an athlete with TAP challenging. The management of an overhead athlete with TAP should address the contributing factors specific to that athlete's pain presentation. When these factors have been addressed and their pain is under control they should be reintroduced to overhead activity in a planned and graded way, with continued monitoring throughout this process.

References

An, K.N., Fui, H.C., Morrey, B.F., 1981. Muscles that cross the elbow joint: a biomechanical analysis. Journal of Biomechanics 14, 659–669.

Axe, M., Hurd, W., Synder-Mackler, L., 2009. Data based interval throwing programs for baseball players. Sport Health 1, 145–153.

Bahr, R., 2016. Why screening tests to predict injury do not work – and probably never will …: A critical review. British Journal of Sports Medicine 50, 776–780.

Black, G.M., Gabbett, T.J., Cole, M.H., Naughton, G., 2016. Monitoring workload in throwing dominant sports: a systematic review. Sports Medicine 46, 1503–1516.

Borsa, P.A., Laudner, K.G., Sauers, E.L., 2008. Mobility and stability adaptations in the shoulder of the overhead athletes. a theoretical and evidence-based perspective. Sports Medicine 38, 17–36.

Burkhart, S.S., Morgan, C.D., Kibler, W.B., 2003a. The disabled shoulder: spectrum of pathology. part I: patho-anatomy and biomechanics. Arthroscopy 19, 404–420.

Burkhart, S.S., Morgan, C.D., Kibler, W.B., 2003b. The disabled shoulder: spectrum of pathology. part II: evaluation and treatment of SLAP lesions in throwers. Arthroscopy 19, 531–539.

Burn, M., McCulloch, P.C., Lintner, D.M., Liberman, S.R., Harris, J.D., 2016. Prevalence of scapula dyskinesis in overhead and nonoverhead athletes. a systematic review. The Orthopaedic Journal of Sports Medicine 4 (2), 2325967115627608.

Byram, I.R., Bushnell, B.D., Dugger, K., Charron, K., Harrell Jr., F.E., Noonan, T.J., 2010. Preseasons shoulder strength measurements in professional baseball pitchers: identifying players at risk for injury. American Journal of Sports Medicine 38, 1375–1382.

Cain, E.L., Dugas, J.R., Wolf, R.S., Andrews, J.R., 2003. Elbow injuries in throwing athletes: a current concepts review. American Journal of Sports Medicine 31, 621–635.

Camp, C.L., Zajac, J.M., Pearson, D.B., Sinator, A.M., Spiker, A.M., Werner, B.C., et al., 2017. Decreased shoulder external rotation and flexion are greater predictors of injury than internal rotation deficits: analysis of 132 pitcher-seasons in professional baseball. Arthroscopy 33, 1629–1636.

Chang, H.Y., Chang, B.F., Jong, Y.J., 2010. Characteristics of elbow range of motions and dependent position comparison in high school baseball players. Formosan Journal of Physical Therapy 35, 284–291.

Chant, C.B., Litchfield, R., Griffin, S., et al., 2007. Humeral head retroversion in competitive baseball players and its relationship to glenohumeral rotation range of motion. Journal of Orthopaedic and Sports Physical Therapy 37, 514–520.

Chu, S.K., Jayabalan, P., Kibler, W.B., Press, J., 2016. The kinetic chain revisited: new concepts on throwing mechanics and injury. Physical Medicine and Rehabilitation 8, S69–S77.

Clarsen, B., Bahr, R., Haugsboe Ndersson, S., Munk, R., Myklebust, G., 2014. Reduced glenohumersal rotation, external rotation weakness and scapula dyskinesis are risk factors for shoulder injuries among elite male handball players: a prospective cohort study. British Journal of Sports Medicine 48, 1327–1333.

Connor, P.M., Banks, D.M., Tyson, A.B., Coumas, J.S., D'Alessandro, D.F., 2003. Magnetic resonance imaging of the asymptomatic shoulder in overhead athletes. American Journal of Sports Medicine 31, 724–727.

Cook, D.P., Strike, S.C., 2000. Throwing in cricket. Journal of Sport Sciences 18, 965–973.

Cormack, S.J., Newton, R.U., McGuigan, 2006. Neuromuscular and endocrine responses of elite players to an Australian rules football match. International Journal of Sports Physiology and Performance 3, 359–374.

Crockett, H.C., Gross, L.B., Wilk, K.E., et al., 2002. Osseous adaptation and range of motion at the glenohumeral joint in professional baseball pitchers. American Journal of Sports Medicine 30, 20–26.

Davidson, P.A., Pink, M., Perry, J., et al., 1995. Functional anatomy of the flexor pronator muscle group in relation to the medial collateral ligament of the elbow. American Journal of Sports Medicine 23, 245–250.

Dwelly, P.M., Tripp, B.S., Tripp, P.A., Eberman, L.E., Gorin, S., 2009. Glenohumeral rotational range of motion in collegiate overhead-throwing athletes during an athletic season. Journal of Athletic Training 44, 611–616.

Edelson, G., Teitz, C., 2000. Internal impingement in the shoulder. Journal of Shoulder and Elbow Surgery 9, 308–315.

Erickson, E.J., Sgori, T., Chalmers, P.N., Vignona, P., Lesniak, M., Bush-Joseph, C.A., et al., 2016. The impact of fatigue on baseball pitching mechanics in adolescent male baseballers. Arthroscopy 32, 762–771.

Finch, C.F., Cook, J., 2014. Categorising sports injuries in epidemiological studies: the subsequent injury categorisation (SIC) model to address multiple, recurrent and exacerbation of injuries. British Journal of Sports Medicine 48, 1276–1280.

Fleisig, G.S., 2010. Biomechanics of overhead throwing: Implications for injury and performance. In: Portus, M. (Ed.), Conference of Science, Medicine and Coaching in Cricket. Conference Proceedings. Brisbane, Cricket Australia.

Fleisig, G.S., Andrews, J.R., Dillman, C.J., Escamilla, R.F., 1995. Kinetics of baseball pitching with implications for injury mechanisms. American Journal of Sports Medicine 23, 233–239.

Fleisig, G.S., Escamilla, R.F., Andrews, J.R., Tomoyuki, M., Satterwhite, Y., Barrentine, S.W., 1996. Kinematic and kinetic comparison of baseball pitching and football passing. Journal of Applied Biomechanics 12, 207–224.

Fortenbaugh, D., Fleisig, G.S., Andrews, J.R., 2009. Baseball pitching biomechanics in relation to risk and performance. Sport Health 1, 314–320.

Forthomme, B., Crielaard, J.M., Crosier, J.L., 2008. Scapula positioning in athlete's shoulder: particularities, clinical measurements and implications. Sports Medicine 38, 369–386.

Freeston, J.L., Carter, T., Whitaker, G., Nicholls, O., Rooney, K.B., 2016. Strength and power correlates of throwing velocity in sub-elite male cricket players. Journal of Strength and Conditioning Research 30, 1646–1651.

Gabbett, T.J., 2016. The training–injury prevention paradox: shoulder athletes be training smarter and harder? British Journal of Sports Medicine 50, 273–280.

Gabbett, T.J., Nassis, G.P., Oetter, E., Pretorius, J., Johnston, N., Medina, D., et al., 2017. The athlete monitoring cycle: a practical guide to interpreting and applying training monitoring data. British Journal of Sports Medicine 51, 1451–1452.

Hickey, D., Solvig, V., Cavalheri, V., Harrold, M., McKenna, L., 2017. Scapula dyskinesis increases the risk of future shoulder pain by 43% in asymptomatic athletes: a systematic review and meta-analysis. British Journal of Sports Medicine 52, 102–110.

Jost, B., Zumstein, M., Pfirrmann, C.W., Zanetti, M., Gerber, C., 2005. MRI findings in throwing shoulders: abnormalities in professional handball players. Current Orthopaedic Practice 434, 130–137.

Kibler, W.B., Sciascia, A., Moore, S., 2012. An acute throwing episode decreases shoulder internal rotation. Clinical Orthopaedics and Related Research 470, 1545–1551.

Kovacs, M., Ellenbecker, T., 2011. An 8-stage model for evaluating the tennis serve: implications for performance enhancement and injury prevention. Sports Health 3, 504–513.

Laffaye, G., Wagner, P., Tombleson, Y., 2014. Countermovement jump height: gender and sport-specific differences in the force–time variables. Journal of Strength and Conditioning Research 28, 1096–1105.

Laudner, K., Lynall, R., Meister, K., 2013. Shoulder adaptations among pitchers and position players over the course of a competitive baseball season. Clinical Journal of Sports Medicine 23, 184–189.

Lehman, G., Drinkwater, E.J., Behm, D.G., 2013. Correlation of throwing velocity to lower body field tests in male college baseball players. Journal of Strength and Conditioning Research 27, 902–908.

Lewis, J., McCreesh, K., Jean-Sebastien, R., Ginn, K., 2015. Rotator cuff tendinopathy: navigating the diagnosis management conundrum. Journal of Orthopaedic and Sports Physical Therapy 45, 923–937.

Lewis, J.S., 2009. Rotator cuff tendinopathy/subacromial impingement syndrome: is it time for a new method of assessment? British Journal of Sports Medicine 43, 259–264.

McCaig, S., Young, M., 2016. Throwing mechanics in injury prevention and performance rehabilitation. In: Joyce, D., Lewindon, D. (Eds.), Sports Injury Prevention and Rehabilitation: Integrating Medicine and Science for Performance Solutions. Routledge, Oxon, UK.

Miniaci, A., Mascia, A.T., Salonen, D.C., Becker, E.J., 2002. Magnetic resonance imaging of the shoulder in asymptomatic professional baseball players. Journal of Sports Medicine 30, 66–73.

Mitchell, T., Burnett, A., O'Sullivan, P., 2015. The athletic spine. In: Joyce, D., Lewindon, D. (Eds.), Sports Injury Prevention and Rehabilitation: Integrating Medicine and Science for Performance Solutions. Routledge, Oxon, UK.

Miyashita, K., Kobayasi, H., Koshida, S., Urabe, Y., 2010. Glenohumeral, scapular, and thoracic angles at maximum shoulder external rotation in throwing. American Journal of Sports Medicine 38, 363–368.

Murray, N.B., Black, G.M., Whiteley, R.J., Gahan, P., Cole, M.H., Utting, A., et al., 2017. Automatic detection of pitching and throwing events in baseball with inertial measurements sensors. International Journal of Sports Physiology and Performance 12, 533–537.

Myers, J.B., Oyama, S., Hibberd, E.E., 2013. Scapular dysfunction in high school baseball players sustaining throwing-related upper extremity injury: a prospective study. Journal of Shoulder and Elbow Surgery 22, 1154–1159.

Newton, R.U., Cardinale, M., Nosaka, K., 2011. Total athlete management (TAM) and performance diagnosis. In:

Strength and Conditioning – Biological Principles and Applications. Wiley-Blackwell, Oxford, UK.

O'Sullivan, P., Dankaets, W., O'Sullivan, K., Fersum, K., 2015. Multidimensional approach for the targeted management of low back pain. In: Jull, G., Moore, A., Falla, D., Lewis, J., McCarthy, C., Sterling, M. (Eds.), Grieve's Modern Musculoskeletal Physiotherapy, fourth ed. Elsevier Ltd, Oxford.

Oyama, S., Hibberd, E.E., Myers, J.B., 2017. Preseasons screening of shoulder range of motion and humeral retrotorsion does not predict injury in high school baseball players. Journal of Shoulder and Elbow Surgery 26, 1182–1189.

Oyama, S., Myers, J.B., Wassinger, C.A., Ricci, D., Lephart, S.M., 2008. Asymmetric resting scapula posture in healthy overhead athletes. Journal of Athletic training 43, 565–570.

Puentedura, E.J., Louw, A., 2012. A neuroscience approach to managing athletes with low back pain. Physical Therapy in Sport 13, 123–133.

Reinold, M.M., Wilk, K.E., Macrina, L.C., Shehane, C., Dun, S., Fleisig, G.S., et al., 2008. Changes in shoulder and elbow passive range of motion after pitching in professional baseball players. American Journal of Sports Medicine 36, 523–527.

Reinold, M.M., Wilk, K.E., Reed, J., Crenshaw, K., Andrews, J.R., 2002. Interval sport programs: guidelines for baseball, tennis, and golf. Journal of Orthopaedic and Sports Physical Therapy 32, 293–298.

Roach, N.T., Lieberman, D.E., 2014. Upper body contributions to power generation during rapid, overhead throwing in humans. Journal of Experimental Biology 217, 2139–2149.

Saw, A., Kellmann, M., Main, L.C., Gastin, P.B., 2017. Athlete self-report measures in research and practice: considerations for the discerning reader and fastidious practitioner. International Journal of Sports Physiology and Performance 12, S127–135.

Shanley, E., Rauh, M.J., Michener, L.A., Ellenbecker, T.S., 2011. Shoulder range of motion measures as risk factors for shoulder and elbow injuries in high school softball and baseball players. American Journal of Sports Medicine 39, 1997–2006.

Struyf, F., Nijs, J., Roussel, N.A., Mottram, S., Truijen, S., Meeusen, R., 2013. Does scapular positioning predict shoulder pain in recreational overhead athletes? International Journal of Sports Medicine 35, 75–82.

Wagner, H., Pfusterschmied, J., Tilp, M., Landlinger, J., von Duvillard, S.P., Muller, E., 2014. Upper-body kinematics in team-handball throw, tennis serve, and volleyball spike. Scandinavian Journal of Medicine and Science in Sports and Exercise 24, 345–354.

Walch, G., Boileau, P., Noel, E., Donnell, S., 1992. Impingement of the deep surface of the supraspinatus tendon on the posterior superior glenoid rim: an arthroscopic study. Journal of Shoulder and Elbow Surgery1 238–245.

Warren, A., Williams, S., McCaig, S., Trewartha, G., 2018. High acute:chronic workloads are associated with injury in England & Wales cricket board development programme fast bowlers. Journal of Science and Medicine in Sport 21, 40–45.

Wassinger, C.A., Myers, J.B., 2011. Reported mechanism of shoulder injury during the baseball throw. Physical Therapy Reviews 16, 305–309.

Werner, S.L., Fleisig, G.S., Dillman, C.J., Escamilla, R.F., 1993. Biomechanics of the elbow during pitching. Journal of Orthopaedic and Sports Physical Therapy 17, 274–278.

Whiteley, R., 2010. Throwing mechanics, load monitoring and injury: perspective from physiotherapy and baseball as they relate to cricket. In: Portus, M. (Ed.), Conference of Science, Medicine and Coaching in Cricket. Conference Proceedings. Brisbane, Cricket Australia, pp. 21–24.

Whiteley, R., 2007. Baseball throwing mechanics as they relate to pathology and performance – a review. Journal of Sport Science and Medicine 6, 1–20.

Whiteley, R., 2016. 'Moneyball' and time to be honest about preseason screening: it is a sham making no inroads on the 1 billion dollar injury costs in baseball. British Journal of Sports Medicine 50 (14), 835–836.

Whiteley, R., Oceguera, M., 2016. GIRD, TRROM and humeral torsion-based classification of shoulder risk in throwing athletes are not in agreement and shoulder be used interchangeably. Journal of Science and Medicine in Sport 19, 816–819.

Whiteley, R., Oceguera, M.V., Valencia, E.B., Mitchell, T., 2012. Adaptations at the shoulder of the throwing athlete and implications for the clinicians. Techniques in Shoulder and Elbow Surgery 13, 36–44.

Whiteley, R.J., Ginn, K.A., Nicholson, L.L., et al., 2009. Sports participation and humeral torsion. Journal of Orthopaedic and Sports Physical Therapy 39, 256–263.

Wilk, K.E., Macrina, L.C., Fleisig, G.S., Aune, K.T., Porterfield, R.A., Harker, P., et al., 2014. Deficits in glenohumeral passive range of motion increase risk of elbow injury in professional baseball pitchers. American Journal of Sports Medicine 42, 2075–2081.

Wilk, K.E., Macrina, L.C., Fleisig, G.S., Aune, K.T., Porterfield, R.A., Harker, P., et al., 2015a. Deficits in glenohumeral passive range of motion increase risk of shoulder injury in professional baseball pitchers. American Journal of Sports Medicine 43, 2379–2385.

Wilk, K.E., Macrina, L.C., Fleisig, G.S., Porterfield, R.A., Simpson II, C.D., Harker, P., et al., 2015b. Correlation of glenohumeral internal rotation deficit and total rotational range of motion to shoulder injuries in professional baseball pitchers. American Journal of Sports Medicine 39, 329–335.

Wilk, K.E., Reinold, M.M., Macrina, L.C., et al., 2009. Glenohumeral internal rotation measurements differ depending on stabilization techniques. Sports Health 1, 131–136.

Wright, R.W., Steger-May, K., Wasserlauf, B.L., O'Neal, M.E., Weinberg, B.W., Paletta, G.A., 2006. Elbow range of motion in professional baseball pitchers. American Journal of Sports Medicine 34, 190–193.

Yamamoto, N., Itoi, E., Minagawa, H., et al., 2006. Why is the humeral retroversion of throwing athletes greater in dominant shoulder than in nondominant shoulders? Journal of Shoulder and Elbow Surgery 15, 571–575.

Chapter 36

Treatment and management of soft tissue injuries

Graham Smith

Introduction

Everyone who participates in sport runs the risk of suffering a soft tissue injury. How that injury is treated will determine its eventual outcome. The aims of this chapter are to give an overview of the principles that the author believes should be followed for managing soft tissue injuries and, hopefully, to dispel many of the myths and misconceptions that have built up over recent years with regard to this extremely important area of musculoskeletal medicine.

Classification of injuries

Over recent years there have been many articles published that have focused on finding 'the holy grail' for the treatment and management of soft tissue injuries. Consequently, there has been a proliferation in the treatment options available, all aiming to accelerate the healing process and subsequent return to activities. Without wishing to criticize this research, there is nothing that can realistically change the basic pathophysiological responses that will occur after a soft tissue injury. That is why an understanding of these responses is integral to the successful treatment and management of these injuries. This information is taught to all healthcare and medical practitioners during their training but usually at a time when its clinical and functional implications is not fully understood. It is also assumed that, once taught, there are no reasons as to why it should be revisited. However, an understanding of these pathophysiological responses and their clinical presentation is imperative for anyone responsible for the treatment

and management of soft tissue injuries, no matter the level at which they work in the sports medicine field.

These pathophysiological responses to injury are inherent and the patient will present in one of three clearly defined stages:

1. acute (inflammatory) phase
2. subacute (remodelling) phase
3. chronic (unresolved and/or repetitive trauma) phase.

When this material is taught, specific timescales as to when the patient will present in each phase is often given. This can lead to a misunderstanding as to which specific phase the patient is in; consequently, inappropriate measures are taken to manage it. It is the clinical and functional response in each pathophysiological phase and the way that this presents that should be determined and managed, rather than the time since injury.

Acute phase

An acute inflammation is a one-off stimulus that has a clearly defined pathophysiological response: heat, swelling, pain, discolouration (often described as redness) and a reduction in range of movement/function. The response will also be time limited, which is often given as 36–48 hours. This timescale should be disregarded as it will be totally dependent on the size and area that has been affected. For example, if an interphalangeal joint of a finger is injured, then the acute inflammatory response will likely be 2–3 hours. However, studies have shown that where there is trauma to a much bigger joint such as the knee or a direct blow to the anterior aspect of the thigh, the acute phase can last 72–90 hours. This is also on the proviso that there is no further trauma to the area. This is important in the understanding of acute inflammation – of not only how it presents but how it should be treated.

For clarification, an acute inflammation is a pathophysiological response to a *one-off* stimulus or injury and any other trauma that may occur during this phase will alter the pathophysiological response. This is discussed later as is the management of acute injuries.

Subacute phase

Assuming that there is no further trauma, the next stage that the injury will progress to is a subacute or remodelling phase. This is when healing tissue of a similar structure to that which was traumatized will be laid down but within a collagenous framework. Whilst this tissue may be of a similar nature, it will not have the strength of the original structures. It has also been hypothesized that the maximum strength will be 80% of what it was before (Lin et al., 2004; Mercandetti and Cohen, 2017; Watson, 2016). Consequently, this should always be considered both in rehabilitation and in returning to functional activities. It is also one of the main reasons for 'maintenance' programmes, even when the patient returns to sporting activities. It may also explain why many athletes suffer reinjury, not necessarily when they return to sport but in the following season when they stop their rehabilitation programme that enabled them to do so.

The other misconception about this phase is that it is limited to a 7–10 day period. This should be disregarded immediately as the healing process can continue for up to 120 days or more (Gillquist, 1993; Hardy,1989; Watson, 2016).

The clinical presentation of the patient, rather than the time since injury, confirms whether they are still in the subacute phase. Patients in this phase have a clearly defined presentation. They have an ease of movement within the range that is available with discomfort and restriction at its limits. This ease of movement is always on the proviso that:

• movements are performed in anatomical directions
• there is no further trauma.

Consequently, subacute patients should be advised to move their joint/limb in an anatomical direction on a repetitive basis but without pushing it through its limits (Brukner and Khan, 2017; Smith,1998). They should also be advised that this is their clinical indicator to determine how they are progressing. Range of movement, strength and function should improve as the healing tissue is laid down in an anatomical alignment provoked by correct patterns of movement. These principles should be applied until full, normal, comparative anatomical movement is obtained with no pain, discomfort or restriction, and regardless of the time from the original one-off trauma.

Chronic phase

Chronic inflammation has frequently been defined as either a nonresolved subacute inflammation or one that has been subjected to repetitive minor trauma (Hurley,

1985; Smith, 1999; Watson, 2016). This phase is characterized by an excessive collagenous response where collagen is laid down in a haphazard formation. This is primarily to protect and strengthen the structures that are either being repetitively traumatized or not being subjected to movements within anatomical directions to promote healing.

In this phase, patients will complain of stiffness and discomfort after periods of inactivity which then eases with movement. For example, patients with chronic ankle problems will report stiffness in the morning but by the time they have walked a little it eases. Consequently, the activity that gives the reduction of stiffness is also the underlying aggravating activity that provokes the minor repetitive trauma. Hence the reason for determining the aggravating activity as quickly as possible so that it can be modified accordingly.

There are three clearly defined pathophysiological phases of inflammation each with their own specific clinical presentation. Each phase has its own specific management regime, which if applied incorrectly or to the wrong phase has implications that can delay a return to normal function or sports. These problems often arise when treatment and rehabilitation measures are applied with respect to timeframes only, rather than the specific inflammatory phase. The take-home message is to concentrate on the clinical presentation and given less importance to timeframe.

To illustrate this, a case study is presented below. Whilst the case is a simplistic, hypothetical example, it shows many of the problems that can occur if the normal pathophysiological responses are not understood and inappropriate management regimes are applied. However, it is acknowledged that in competitive sport it is not feasible for every player to leave the field of play if they sustain a minor injury.

Case study

Two hockey players sustain identical inversion injuries to their ankle 10 minutes into a match. Neither have had injuries before and, as such, these can be determined as one-off first-time problems. One of the players leaves the field of play immediately while the second player remains on the field of play for the remainder of the match.

Both players are in the treatment room on adjacent plinths 10 minutes after the game. What pathophysiological stage is the player who left the field of play at now? Similarly, what phase is the player who remained on the field at?

The answers to both are simple and logical: The player that left the field of play immediately will be in the acute phase of inflammation as they sustained a *one-off* injury, whereas the one who remained will already be in the chronic phase. The reason that the latter is in the chronic phase is because they will have continued to invoke minor repetitive traumas to the initial injury, therefore provoking a collagenous response, regardless of the fact that it is only 90 minutes since the initial trauma.

Both players are treated, given advice as to what they should do overnight and are instructed to report back the following day.

The following morning both players are reassessed. The strapping and support is removed from the ankle of the player who was taken from the field of play immediately and he is asked to move his ankle up and down. Whilst initially reluctant he is able to move the joint comfortably without any pain or discomfort but with a restriction in range. There is also a noticeable lack of swelling. Consequently, the injury is moving into the subacute phase and will have minimal acute symptoms.

The ankle of the player who remained has minor pitting oedema around the joint margins and when requested to move, it has stiffness and discomfort, which ease with repetition. Already the player is in the chronic phase of inflammation, even though it is less than 24 hours since the incident. So, if this injury was treated as being in the acute inflammatory phase, the patient would be advised to rest and not move it for 36–48 hours. This may lead to a highly organized oedema (swelling) with an extremely stiff joint, both of which would require time to treat and resolve before the player could even consider returning to hockey. Conversely, the player who left the field and is now subacute will have a completely different management regime which will give him a much better chance of an earlier return to sport.

Management of subacute and chronic inflammatory injuries are significantly different to acutely injured soft tissue structures. Therefore, in spite of being less than 24 hours following injury, both players will require a different regime.

Determining the phase

The following questions should be asked as a matter of course on initial presentation:

1. **What happened?** Can the patient explain the mechanism of injury, which will help to determine structures that may have been damaged.

2. **What did you do immediately following the injury?** Was the patient able to continue activities or forced to stop? This will then determine whether it was a one-off trauma that was immediately protected from further injury or something that was subjected to continued repetitive trauma. This will help determine the pathophysiological phase of the injury.

3. **Was there swelling and when was it first noticed?** If the patient felt throbbing and noticed swelling immediately and that the injured area was hot and tense to touch, the practitioner should suspect bleeding into the area. If it is a joint injury then it is likely to have been a haemarthrosis (bleeding into the joint space) and must be regarded as a clinical emergency. It will have a high cellular

component with an increased metabolic activity within the joint that will generate heat. A high cellular component in any confined space will also cause pain. However, if the patient did not notice any significant swelling until several hours after the injury and there is no reported heat or pain it is likely that they have a synovial effusion if it is a joint problem or tissue fluid if in soft tissue.

4. **What happened immediately following the injury?** What did the patient do immediately following the injury? Did they receive any treatment? Have they taken any medication? All of these factors determine where the patient sits within the inflammatory spectrum so that appropriate treatment measures can be planned.

5. **How are they now and what are their problems?** At this point it is necessary to determine the degree of disability that the patient has on presentation, regardless of how long it is since the injury occurred. It is this determination that will help to classify the phase of inflammation and, subsequently, the stage of rehabilitation. This will ensure that appropriate treatment measures for inflammation are applied and the correct exercises are commenced.

Knowledge of the pathophysiological responses to injury allows the practitioner to follow the following specific aims for each inflammatory stage:

Acute inflammation. Management strategies will be covered in greater detail after the following two sections.

Subacute inflammation. The main aims in this phase of inflammation are to:

1. Increase range of movement within the limits of pain and discomfort and through normal anatomical directions.

2. Increase strength of muscles acting about the injured area within the limits of pain and discomfort and without applying excessive forces to them. Movements should be anatomically directed.

3. Restore and improve proprioception within the limits of pain and discomfort. Proprioception is joint awareness and reeducating this as early as possible, even in a non-weight-bearing position, is imperative.

Chronic inflammation. The aims in this phase of inflammation are to:

1. Identify and stop/minimize the aggravating activities. If the patient is unable to stop the aggravating activity, it is best to advise the patient on how to manage the responses to the aggravation. Advice on how to prepare for the activities and minimize chronicity is also required.

2. Maintain range of movement that is available without aggravating or provoking further minor trauma.

3. Reduce any chronic swelling in the surrounding areas by utilizing physical therapy measures that may include massage and soft tissue mobilizations. Increase range of movement, strength and proprioception without provoking further trauma and always within anatomical movement patterns.

Finally, what might present as being in one inflammatory phase at one point may soon move to another. Not only should practitioners be cognisant of this but patients too. When patients are given exercise programmes, they must also be instructed how to assess if there have been any changes to their inflammatory status. For example, if on one day the patient is given exercises that are appropriate to the subacute stage but the following morning wakes up with stiffness and discomfort then they have now moved into the chronic stage. Consequently, it is important that the patient knows what they should do if this occurs so that they can manage it correctly without provoking further trauma until such time as they can be reassessed and advised accordingly. They must also be counselled as to how frequently this occurs and that it is not unusual. Thus, it is easy to see how problems occur when the pathophysiology is not fully understood and treatment measures are inappropriately applied.

Treatment and management of acute injuries

This is one of the most misunderstood areas of injury management. Despite significant research in this field, principles that have been proven as being ineffective are still being taught and applied. More worryingly, basic pathophysiological principles, including tissue responses to trauma, are often ignored with many of the treatment strategies taught being anecdotal and outdated.

As stated previously, acute inflammation is a pathophysiological response to a one-off stimulus or trauma that results in the area becoming hot, painful, discoloured (red), swollen and, as such, there is a loss of function. This response starts immediately.

Swelling. Damage to the semipermeable membranes of tissues within the area will allow fluid exudate and in some cases blood to enter the tissue spaces immediately. This fluid will have a high cellular component that includes blood cells and platelets.

Heat. Release of cells into the tissue space promotes cellular activity and metabolism including clotting and laying down of collagen within the area. This metabolism also generates heat.

Pain. As the swelling progresses and the cellular content increases the pressure exerted rises and pain and discomfort are provoked.

Discolouration (redness). Increased metabolism and heat also increases circulation to the peripheral vessels thereby giving an erythema reaction on the surface of the skin, which may either be seen as redness or discolouration, depending on the skin tone.

Loss of function. As pain and swelling increase, movement within the area becomes impaired and, as such, function is compromised.

Whilst the above is taught on most courses, it is frequently ignored when applying treatment strategies during this stage of inflammation. Consequently, if exudate in the tissue spaces is primarily responsible for all of the above then this must be stopped or minimized. Importantly, if swelling is allowed to become established it is not only going to cause pain but also prevent progression of rehabilitation. As Brukner and Khan (2017) assert, 'the process of rehabilitation starts immediately to control, minimize and alleviate swelling'. The priority of treatment must be:

1. compression
2. elevation
3. cooling
4. reduce activity.

Compression

Prioritize the application of compression as early as possible to minimize the space available for the fluid to enter and so that it can absorb the outward pressure that is going to be exerted by the fluid trying to enter the tissue spaces. Compression applied should be sustained for as long as there is a potential for swelling to occur. In a large area, such as the quadriceps or knee joint, compression should be retained, wherever possible, for up to 90 hours following injury. This principle is controversial but has evidence to support its application (Schröder and Pässler, 1994; Shelbourne et al., 1994) and builds on the evidence relating to postoperative care for ACL reconstruction. Additionally, pathophysiological responses do not stop at night; they continue throughout the 24-hour cycle. The following key points should be considered:

- Compression should be applied to cover the whole area that has been injured with an overlap too. For example, with the knee joint the compression should extend from 2.5 cm above the suprapatella bursa to below the tibial tuberosity. As a guideline it should extend for at least 2.5 cm above and below the affected part.
- Compression should be applied with something that will absorb the outward pressure from within the injured area. Two examples of equipment that apply these principles include the Cryocuff and Game Ready. However, if this equipment is not available then wrapping the injured part in a towel and then securing this in place with a crepe bandage will suffice. This is a compression bandage that follows the principles of the Robert Jones compression bandages that were used many years ago. A direct application of adhesive elastic tape is *not* appropriate as it is likely to wrinkle and allow for areas where the swelling can push through. This then becomes extremely painful for the patient and does not

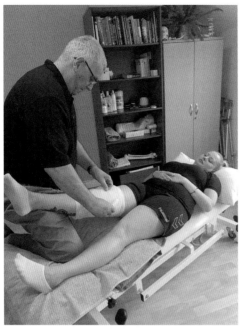

Fig. 36.1 The application of compression (the priority) with cotton wool or towel and bandage.

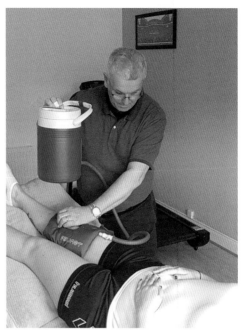

Fig. 36.2 Compression (priority), elevation (secondary) and cooling via a Cryocuff or similar product.

achieve the required effect. Similarly, utilizing stocki-nette-style bandages is not appropriate either, as these still allow swelling to occur and, if folded over, the fold has the potential to act as a tourniquet. Examples of a compression bandage being applied using a towel (Fig. 36.1) and a Cryocuff (Fig. 36.2) are shown.

The application of compression to minimize swelling is a priority. Swelling must not be allowed to become established as it causes pain, which adds the following associated problems:
- local neuromuscular inhibition
- reduced movement
- reduced strength
- compensatory movement patterns
- the area does not feel 'normal' to the patient.

The sooner compression is applied the better. However, if it is days, weeks or even months after the initial injury when the patient is first assessed and they still have swelling, it is likely to be very chronic, and the reduction of it, as a priority, remains. In the management of all soft tissue and joint-related problems remember: swelling is the practitioner's enemy!

Elevation

Once compression has been applied, the injured part should be elevated. Ideally this elevation should be above the heart or as high as possible. Elevation reduces the hydrostatic pressure of blood flow into the area. The normal production and reabsorption of tissue fluid is dependent upon the ratio between hydrostatic and osmotic pressures and this is compromised when the semipermeable membranes are disrupted with trauma. Any measure that reduces hydrostatic pressure, such as elevation, will assist in minimizing inflammatory exudate entering the tissue spaces. If elevation is high enough it is also one of the main factors that allows compression to be sustained.

Cooling

The application of ice to the skin does not stop swelling! The effects of ice are extremely superficial and have no immediate effect on semipermeable membranes that have been damaged. The direct application of ice to stop swelling is both ineffective and inappropriate.

However, cooling the area over a sustained period does have a beneficial effect and wherever possible should be applied. Importantly, the compression should not be removed to allow the cooling to be applied. Equipment such as the Cryocuff and Game Ready machines allow cold water to be contained in or passed through the compression garment, cooling the underlying structures gradually. This means that there is no vascular response in the peripheral blood vessels, often described as a vasoconstriction and

449

vasodilatation effect. If the injured part has a compression bandage on it then this can be soaked with cold water to apply the same principles. Putting an icepack underneath the compression garment is not advised as this allows potential areas for swelling to occur.

Sustained cooling will, over a period of time, reduce the metabolic activity within the tissues, reducing blood flow to the area and thus minimizing swelling. There is also the supplementary benefit of reducing the risks of secondary hypoxia. Therefore, the application of cold has a beneficial effect but it results from gradual cooling rather than the intensity associated with direct application of icepacks. However, cooling is not a major priority and should not be applied before compression and elevation.

Reduce activity

The guidelines often describe this as 'rest'. Whilst it is important to stop moving the area and aggravating it, it is also advisable for patients to try to gently move the injured part through pain-free range that is available at least once an hour. This requires the compression to be taken off for a short period of time so that so that the patient can do 2–3 gentle active pain-free movements. Compression should then be reapplied immediately, along with elevation. If the injured part is anatomically very small then the length of time the compression should be applied will be significantly shorter than if it is a larger area. Consequently, modified rest is the principle to follow rather than complete inactivity.

The other key principles to consider with regards to the treatment of acute injuries are protect and prevent. Therefore, the injured part should be protected by preventing the patient from undertaking activities that could cause further trauma.

Understanding the pathophysiological responses of inflammation will significantly help the practitioner to apply appropriate management strategies for soft tissue injuries. It is important that patients are classified to the appropriate stage of inflammation, not only on the first occasion that they are seen, but at each subsequent consultation. Similarly, it is also necessary to classify what stage of rehabilitation the patient should be working at, to ensure a successful outcome.

Whilst this chapter will not focus extensively on rehabilitation, a brief overview of the stages of rehabilitation and criteria that determine what level and activities the patient should be performing are given below. It also helps to understand when patients should progress through to the next stage.

Stages of rehabilitation

There are four main stages of rehabilitation after soft tissue injury, each with its own specific criteria and activities. These are:

Early-stage rehabilitation

Frequently described as the non-weight-bearing stage, the main aims are to:

- increase pain-free range of movement
- increase strength and proprioception within limits of pain and discomfort.

These principles should be applied to the injured limb within the acute and subacute phases of inflammation.

Patients should not progress to full weight-bearing until they have achieved the criteria necessary to progress to the intermediate stage of rehabilitation. These are the establishment of:

- at least two-thirds of the normal anatomical active range of movement (i.e., as compared to the other limb)
- eccentric and concentric control throughout available range
- full pain-free movement
- no or minimal swelling.

If the patient meets all these criteria they can progress to the next stage.

Intermediate-stage rehabilitation

Frequently described as the progressive stage of rehabilitation, this stage starts with a deficient limb but progresses to the point where the patient's limbs are considered as bilateral entities. It is the stage where, if the injury is on the lower limb, walking reeducation becomes an integral part of the activities undertaken. Similarly, as with the early stage, no rotational forces should be applied to the injured limb. No running should be undertaken during this stage. Running can be introduced only when the patient has progressed to the 'late stage' and this can only occur when the following have been achieved:

- full active pain-free range compared to the opposite side
- ability to control movement both eccentrically and concentrically
- no or minimal swelling
- normal gait (lower limb injury only); if the patient is allowed to progress with an abnormal walking pattern this will be exaggerated when running commences.

During this stage, patients may be either in the subacute or chronic phases of inflammation but not the acute. The patient can then progress to the late stage of rehabilitation once the above criteria have been achieved.

Late-stage rehabilitation

Frequently described as the dynamic stage of rehabilitation, it is the stage at which the patient should be undertaking dynamic bilateral activities. Running, jumping, twisting, turning and rotational forces can commence during this stage. It is also the stage where all of the exercises and activities performed should be functional and appropriate to whatever activity the patient is hoping to return to.

Patients will be relearning movement patterns during this stage. Wherever possible, these movement patterns should be within the environment that the patient is returning to or as close to it as possible. It is also the stage where patients should not be having any inflammatory responses and definitely not presenting with those of a chronic nature. If a patient complains of stiffness and discomfort the morning after undertaking late rehabilitation exercises then they have been working at an inappropriate level and subjecting the injury to minor repetitive trauma. This is why patients must be reassessed and classified *on a daily basis*.

Predischarge stage of rehabilitation

The final stage is the predischarge stage. The aim is to specifically identify any deficiencies at the end of the rehabilitation process. Whilst the early, intermediate and late stages of rehabilitation are progressive and 'caring' in nature, the predischarge stage needs to be much more aggressive. Consequently, it is a stage that is only applicable to certain patients – those that have been injured for a reasonable length of time and are expected to return to dynamic activities or high levels of occupational fitness.

Importance of classification

The phases of inflammation and their pathophysiological responses, together with the use of the relevant stages of rehabilitation, are integral to the effective management of any soft tissue or joint-related problem. The classification of a patient's pathophysiological phase should therefore be done every time the patient is seen by a practitioner or on a daily basis by the individual themselves. This analysis will help to avoid problems with treatment, clarify why things may be going wrong or why they are not responding as anticipated. For example, if the patient has not achieved

the criteria required to be in the late stage of rehabilitation but they are continuing to run and report ankle stiffness every morning, then they are carrying out activities that are inappropriate to their pathophysiological phase. They are provoking a chronic inflammatory state through repetitive trauma.

Take-home points

Understanding the pathophysiological processes related to the three key phases of inflammation is imperative to allowing the practitioner to assess soft tissue injuries appropriately and apply effective management strategies.

Having an understanding of the stages of rehabilitation and the criteria required for progressing through each stage will help to clarify why some management regimes fail.

Classification of a patient's inflammatory phase and rehabilitation stage – regardless of length of time since the injury or previous interventions – should be carried out by the patient daily and on each occasion they are seen by the practitioner to ensure a successful outcome.

In summary, the overall management of soft tissue injuries should be based on the following six principles:

1. Minimize the extent of the initial damage and swelling wherever possible.
2. Reduce and control any associated inflammation and pain.
3. Promote healing of damaged tissue.
4. Maintain, or restore, range of movement, strength, proprioception and general fitness, especially during the healing (subacute) phase.
5. Functionally rehabilitate the injured patient to enable them to have a safe return to sport.
6. Assess and correct any predisposing factors to reduce risk of recurrence.

References

Brukner, P., Khan, K., 2017. Brukner & Khan's Clinical Sports Medicine, fifth ed. McGraw-Hill, New York.

Gillquist, J., 1993. iii. Principles of repair. Current Orthopaedics 7 (3), 90–93.

Hardy, M.A., 1989. The biology of scar formation. Physical Therapy 69 (12), 1014–1024.

Hurley, J., 1985. Inflammation. In: Anderson, J.R. (Ed.), Muir's Textbook of Pathology, twelfth ed. Edward Arnold, London.

Lin, T.W.T., Cardenas, L., Soslowsky, L.J.L., 2004. Biomechanics of tendon injury and repair. Journal of Biomechanics 37 (6), 865–877.

Mercandetti, M., Cohen, A.J., 2017. Wound healing and repair (update). Medscape.

Schröder, D., Pässler, H.H., 1994. Combination of cold and compression after knee surgery. A prospective randomized study. Knee Surgery, Sports Traumatology, Arthroscopy 2 (3), 158–165.

Shelbourne, K.D., Rubenstein, R.A., McCarroll, J.R., Weaver, J., 1994. Postoperative cryotherapy for the knee in ACL reconstructive surgery. Orthopaedics International 2 (2), 165–170.

Smith, G.N., 1999. Sports Medicine – Clinical Update Royal College of General Practitioners Members Reference Book (1999–2000). Camden Publishing, London.

Smith, G.N., 1998. Return to fitness. In: Tidswell, M. (Ed.), Orthopaedic Physiotherapy. Churchill Livingstone, Edinburgh.

Watson, T., 2016. Soft Tissue Repair and Healing Review. Available at: http://www.electrotherapy.org/modality/soft-tissue-repair-and-healing-review.

451

Chapter | 37 |

The inseason strength programme: a professional rugby perspective – programming through the season

Aidan O'Connell

Introduction

Professional rugby is a pressurized, high-stakes environment where optimization of strength, power and speed provides a definitive performance edge. Developing and sustaining these qualities across the preseason can be straightforward. However, the unpredictability and volatility inherent in a 40-game inseason combined with transient nonlinear individual responses to this environment creates one of coaching's greatest challenges. This chapter examines how we tackle this problem at a professional rugby team and programme strength throughout the season.

> *The human organism was not designed to play rugby.*
>
> Craig White

Rugby is a physical game. Tactically, rugby can also be as subtle as a game of chess until it explodes into life with big momentum-shifting plays. These game-breaking moments, from an explosive sidestep to a ferocious tackle, require the players to be technically, tactically, mentally and physically adept. It is the job of strength and conditioning coaches to work with the rugby coaches and medical team to prepare the players so that they can operate successfully in this environment. More specifically, strength and conditioning coaches develop the player's game-breaking strength, speed and power and their ability to do this repeatedly during the game. Optimizing these physical characteristics allows the player to not just survive in the combat zone but to dominate.

Bigger, stronger and more powerful players recover faster between games and acutely between collisions, thereby enhancing their fitness profile. From a psychological perspective, increased strength levels bolster confidence in their physicality. Furthermore, and crucially in professional sport, stronger players are injured less frequently – and this, in turn, has a positive effect on player availability. The correlation between player availability and the win/loss ratio in sport is well established. Creating an environment whereby the players train and play more is one of the primary performance drivers in professional sport.

Strength training, injury risk profiling, a recovery/lifestyle programme and a sensitive training monitoring system are potent weapons in the availability war. Strength training primarily serves to better protect the players against the violent nature of the game. It also builds robustness by increasing the stress tolerance of the musculoskeletal system to load. Additionally, strength gains improve movement efficiency by correcting energy leaks caused by lagging stabilizers and joint instability. This mechanism not only protects the body against injury risk but also minimizes poor patterns of movement that rob players of strength, power, speed and endurance.

The biggest window of opportunity for professional rugby players to get strong is through the malleable teenage years via the school system and the subsequent academy system. The steep strength gains of the teenage years lessen as players transition through their professional career, where windows of opportunity for strength development are few and far between. However, on an annual basis, the 6- to 8-week preseason offers a golden opportunity to get stronger. Preseason and strength gains

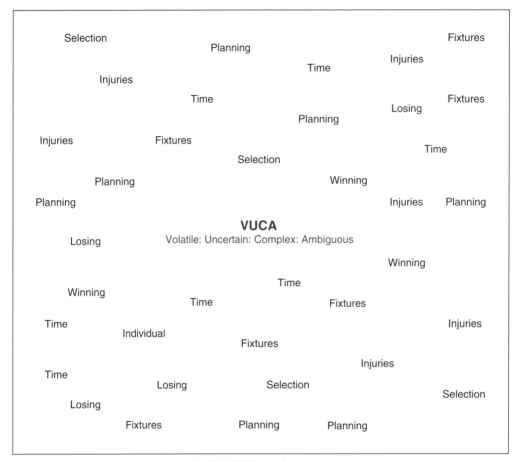

Fig. 37.1 VUCA environment.

go hand in hand as this stable environment is designed for it. Session intensity, session volume and session dosage can all be manipulated in concert with the wider training process to build size, strength, power and speed. Strength development inseason is, however, a different proposition.

From the initial kick-off of the opening game of the season, a battle ensues every week for 40 weeks. Coaches are flung from a stable preseason environment into the VUCA (volatile, uncertain, complex, ambiguous) (Fig. 37.1) environment of the inseason. The precision and accuracy of the strength training prescription becomes very difficult under these conditions. For example, in any one week one could be preparing the squad players for up to three competitions: European or League competition, B team competition and domestic second-tier competition. Logistically, these games may be home or away, which may involve extensive travel. The turnaround between games can vary and may range

from 5 to 8 days. From a raw performance perspective, the team is required to peak or operate close to peak every week. These plans need to be further individualized based on selection, age, injury status, monitoring status and individual needs analysis. Add the emotional factors caused by selection, winning or losing, injury, physical and mental fatigue, and other external stressors into the equation and you have a potent mix that if not managed has the potential to derail a season.

Nevertheless, in every difficulty there is an opportunity. Peak performance in a high-stakes environment is about being on this edge, acknowledging uncertainty, anticipating roadblocks, taking calculated risks, thinking about possibilities and finding effective solutions through the foggy haze. Manage the VUCA environment successfully and your team can gain a significant competitive advantage over the opposition. The following section will examine solutions that can optimize the inseason strength training process.

Adaptive periodization model

An effective inseason strength training process needs to be based on a stable philosophical and strategic platform, whilst having the flexibility and adaptability to deliver the programme with accuracy. Philosophical alignment with the rugby coach, operation alignment with all departments to form integrated performance teams, and sensitivity to the environment are central to its effectiveness. An adaptive training blueprint provides systematic inbuilt agility into the training programme so that it can adapt swiftly and respond appropriately to the ever-changing scenarios that are presented. This adaptive process allows one to manoeuvre in an unpredictable complex environment.

Adaptive periodization is based on the premise that every player will have a unique biological response to the training process, and that the strength programme must respond to these changes and the current environmental conditions. Every individual, every team and every environment is unique and their interactions are unique. Adaptive periodization is characterized by:

1. scenario planning
2. short planning cycles
3. 'what if' analysis
4. inbuilt flexibility
5. embedded testing
6. multiple feedback loops
7. informed decision making
8. habitual reviewing
9. 'multidepartmental performance solutions'.

There are five stages to the adaptive periodization model (Fig. 37.2). Each stage complements and builds on the previous stage. Optimizing each stage upregulates the entire process.

Stage 1: general strategy – the alignment process

Adaptability and the ability to respond to change are of paramount importance when programming in a VUCA environment. However, the effectiveness of this process will depend on the strength of the framework on which it is built. General strategies that stabilize this environment include not only a strong and resolute inseason strength training philosophy and model, but they also align and integrate with the head coach's rugby training philosophy and the broader training process. The strength training programme should complement the (rugby) programme rather than try to *be the programme*.

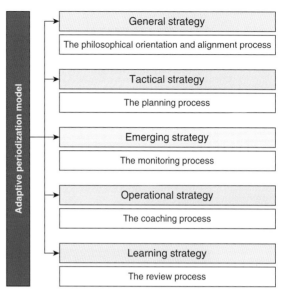

Fig. 37.2 Adaptive periodization model.

Strength training philosophy

A first step in building an effective strength programme and reinforcing the stability of the environment is to have an unwavering inseason strength training philosophy. The author's inseason strength training philosophy is simply to optimize player availability and build confidence by making them strong and robust enough to meet the intense physical demands of the game. Confidence is the currency of high-performance sport, and strength sessions are designed to inflate this valuable commodity.

Central to this philosophy is the mantra that we are getting bigger, stronger, faster and more powerful inseason. We are not merely maintaining performance levels. A maintenance mindset over a 40-week inseason will not only lead to mental stagnation and demotivation, but also to physical detraining and degradation over time. Importantly, the programme recognizes that this development must add value to the larger rugby training process. Striking a balance between sustained development in the gym, while leaving enough 'juice in the tank' to train and play, is a tricky balance. All players have limited time to train and recover. Therefore, we must spend our precious strength training time wisely on what the players need and what gives the best return.

Strength training model

The inseason strength training model is a contact–running-based strength model (Fig. 37.3). It is built on the premise that improving these strength characteristics will improve performance directly and also indirectly

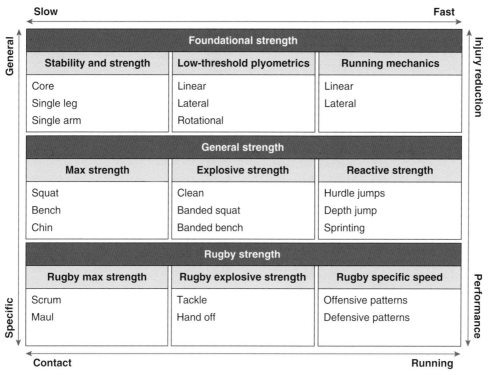

Fig. 37.3 Strength model.

through injury reduction. The degree to which a player is exposed to either contact-based strength or running-based strength requirements, and whether this exposure targets performance or injury reduction, will depend on their strength profile, injury history, playing position, etc. The model has three distinct streams; they complement each other and prepare the player for the next level by moving from general to specific and from simple to complex. Furthermore, within each stream the player is progressed in terms of speed from slow to fast and from low force to high force.

Foundational strength stream

The foundational or movement strength stream serves to lay solid foundational strength to reset, activate and stimulate the body prior to more strenuous exercise. It prepares the body to produce and reduce high forces more effectively. This movement stream is subdivided into three sections:

- The core and single limb strength exercise role is to fix energy leaks and inefficient movement patterns by correcting muscle imbalances and activating lagging stabilizers, primarily in the lateral hip and rotator cuff. Soft

tissue quality is also reinforced, thus maximizing the stress tolerance of the kinetic chain.
- Low-threshold plyometrics or single limb landing mechanics also improve inefficient movement patterns through the mechanism of improving control and force absorption.
- Running mechanics improve running-specific strength directly by targeting the strength and stiffness at the ankle, lateral hip and core. As a byproduct, these drills may also reduce injury potential and enhance running performance by teaching correct posture, hip height, foot placement, coordination and running rhythm.

Movement strength exercises together with mobility exercises form the movement system at Munster Rugby. Together these exercises are systematically programmed in movement preparation sessions at the beginning of each training day or in movement warm-ups prior to strength and field sessions. The core and single limb exercise may also live in the main strength training programme. This distribution of work across multiple training platforms allows all aspects of strength to be comprehensively covered during the busy and time-poor inseason period.

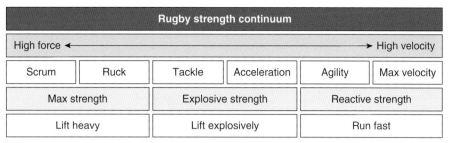

Fig. 37.4 Rugby strength continuum.

General strength stream

This stream aims to build strength through maximum strength, explosive strength and reactive strength methods:

- Maximum strength is built through the three 'big rock' exercises of: squat, bench, chin and their derivatives. These exercises are chosen because of their 'bang for buck' ability to develop not only strength but, with manipulation, power and lean mass. The operational bandwidth inseason is set between 75–90% of maximum intensity.
- Explosive strength is primarily developed through the clean and its variants, or alternatively through the dynamic squat. These explosive strength exercises are programmed based on intent and quality of speed of movement, with intensity ranging from 60% to 80% of maximum.
- Reactive strength is trained primarily through rugby training and specially designed drills that expose the players to maximum-velocity running. Extra high-velocity running work is given to players who lack exposure as highlighted through either global positioning system (GPS) or subjective feedback from a coach or the player themselves. Backs are also programmed with reactive plyometrics periodically inseason, both to feed their psychological need for speed and to top up on their ankle stiffness as pitches soften during the winter months.

Rugby strength stream

The rugby strength stream (Fig. 37.4) recognizes that training or playing rugby provides an inherent strength stimulus during the inseason. Significant specific force-generating and force-reducing capacities are trained week-in and week-out. Whilst it is difficult to quantify the extent and magnitude of this exposure, careful monitoring of training load, GPS data and rugby performance analysis can help shed some light. This information is then used to further influence strength programme design, as it highlights strength qualities that are either over- or underexposed through rugby training and matches.

Philosophical and training alignment

A central strategy in shaping and bringing the strength model to life is to align it with the head coach's rugby training philosophy. For example, tactical information regarding rugby style, or whether the coach has a running- or contact-based philosophy, adds depth to the strength programme as it shines a light on the strength characteristics that will complement and add value to the game plan. The length of time that the coaching team gets to foster this alignment in the volatile world of professional sport is also extremely important. A stable coaching setup not only provides a strong backbone to buffer against this turbulence, but also allows relationships, systems and processes to grow, develop and evolve together with time.

The next step in the alignment process is to manage and stabilize the wider rugby training process and find within it a consistently secure home to launch the programme every week. In this regard, we use *tactical periodization*, a periodization model developed for football by Vítor Frade, a lecturer at the University of Porto. Tactical periodization recognizes that performance is a function of tactical, technical, psychological and physical preparation, and that to optimize these components in the time-strapped inseason it is best to integrate and train all components together. This process of workload synchronization reduces the complexity but not the intensity of training.

Tactical periodization utilizes the head coach's tactical philosophy as the design platform for the training week. For example, the central tactical elements of attack, defence and transitions can be overloaded and stress-tested on specific days every week. These sessions are characterized by an intensity that stretches the players' decision-making ability, concentration levels, tactical skills, and fitness. Whilst stretch practice promotes the quality of the session, the training stress dial can be turned up or down per session, or per week, through volume manipulation. This manipulation and the stability that a fixed training week provides, create a rugby training model that facilitates consistency of performance over a 40-week season. It also provides a solid framework in which the strength programme can be

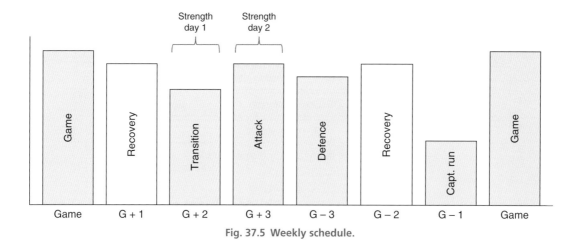

Fig. 37.5 Weekly schedule.

consistently housed every week. Additionally, strength sessions can be designed to complement the rugby sessions being trained on any day.

In a typical week (Fig. 37.5) with a game from Saturday to Saturday, strength training is programmed at best twice a week. Sessions are embedded into the weekly structure on game day + 2 and game day + 3. The strength sessions have a vertically integrated design targeting multiple strength qualities in a single session. At the time of writing our training week is as follows:

Strength session 1: total-body strength day

It targets double and single leg strength, upper body pull strength, and upper body pull size. From a rugby training perspective, game day + 2 is a heavy day in terms of learning but a light day in terms of rugby-specific contact and running load. Physical restoration is the order of the day. In most programmes, placing leg work appropriately into the programme is one of the biggest conundrums. We place it on this day because it is the lightest day in terms of rugby load. Furthermore, anecdotal evidence suggests that this leg-dominant day accelerates the recovery process by helping the body to reset and recalibrate postgame. This day is also a pull-dominant day primarily to balance the flexion pattern dominance of match play and training, and also because the anterior shoulder structures can be still 'banged up' postgame.

Strength session 2: total-body power and upper body strength day

The focus is more specifically on explosive strength, upper body push strength, and upper push/pull size. Game day + 3 is the main rugby training day. It is mentally and physically

taxing on all fronts, particularly with regard to contact and extensive running parameters. Consequently, the legs are spared and upper body push strength is prioritized. Game day + 3 can also provide a window of opportunity to train explosive strength, as the players are at their optimal readiness for this stimulus. Furthermore, this stimulus activates them for the big day ahead, without debilitating fatigue bleeding out onto the pitch.

As mentioned earlier, we can adjust the dial on these sessions depending on how the players or the environment are presenting. Sessions can easily switch between a resetting, building or stimulating focus depending on the emerging landscape. Importantly, game day + 2 and game day + 3 strength sessions can be switched, or sections of a session can be switched and 'mixed and matched' to suit an individual's needs. This agility or flexibility is a vital component of programming inseason and we will explore this in greater detail in the next section.

Stage 2: tactical strategy – optimizing the planning process

The inseason period is the dominant training period for professional rugby. Our focus is to develop and preserve strength, power and size across the entire season, and from season to season. Developing and protecting the strength stimulus inseason is indeed a challenging process given the fact that the players have a finite amount of time and energy to strength train. We therefore need to maximize the 'juice from the squeeze'.

Our primary tactic inseason is that we 'plan short and plan often' in mini blocks of three to four games. We plan as needed in short cycles, given the inaccuracies of forecasting

		Inseason strength programme						
Phase		Block A			Block B			
Focus 1		Max strength			Explosive strength			
		Light	Medium	Heavy	Light	Medium	Heavy	
Squat		Regular			Regular +25% band weight			
	% 1RM / V(m/s)	75–80% .55–.6m/s	80–85% .5–.55m/s	85–90% .45–.5m/s	60–65% .7–.75m/s	65–70% .65–.7m/s	70–75% .6–.65m/s	
	Reps	3–4	2–3	1–2	3–4	2–3	1–2	
	Sets	2–4	3–5	4–6	2–4	3–5	4–6	
Bench		Regular			Regular +10% band weight			
	% 1RM / V(m/s)	75–80% .55–.65m/s	80–85% .45–.55m/s	85–90% .35–.45m/s	65–70% .65–.7m/s	70–75% .6–.65m/s	75–80% .55–.6m/s	
	Reps	5–6	4–5	2–3	4–5	3–4	1–2	
	Sets	2–3	3–4	4–5	2–3	3–4	4–5	
Chin		Regular			Regular +5% band weight			
	% 1RM	75–80%	80–85%	85–90%	65–70%	70–75%	75–80%	
	Reps	5–6	4–5	2–3	4–5	3–4	1–2	
	Sets	2–3	3–4	4–5	2–3	3–4	4–5	
Clean		Clean			Jump shrug			
	% 1RM	70–75%	75–80%	80–85%	55–60%	60–65%	65–70%	
	Reps	3–4	2–3	1–2	3–4	2–3	1–2	
	Sets	2–3	3–4	4–5	2–3	3–4	4–5	

Fig. 37.6 Inseason strength programme. *1RM*, 1-repetition maximum; *V*, velocity.

beyond this timeframe in an unpredictable environment. Secondly, the fundamental qualities of strength, power and size are trained constantly across all these blocks. The exercises used to drive these qualities are also kept consistent inseason with very little variability. This consistency facilitates improvement by narrowing the focus and avoids the stress caused by continual change and perturbation.

Consistency in the programme is not only expressed through exercise selection, but also through intensity. Intensity is kept consistently high inseason. This is made possible by working within strict operational bandwidths. For example, our intensity ranges for training maximum strength is kept between a narrow bandwidth of 75–90% of maximum. This strength 'sweet spot' gives us the manoeuvrability to develop strength week-in and week-out. Importantly, it adds further efficiency to the programme because it avoids the dead zones of training either too lightly or too heavily. The latter decreases technical performance and can lead to potential neural haemorrhaging, thereby outweighing any potential benefits. We therefore plan our programmes within a very stable operational bandwidth in terms of exercise selection and intensity. However, this space has enough variability to simulate adaptation over the course of the season.

Our ideal inseason strength programme as shown in Fig. 37.6 has two complementary strength blocks or cycles

of 3–4 games which run back to back throughout the season. Intensity is also cycled in a wave-like fashion within a block, and from block to block. The first strength block (block A) overloads the strength stimulus via high-force barbell resistance exercises, whilst the second strength block (block B) targets the strength stimulus through explosive strength using accommodating resistance. The primary difference between blocks is that block B is biased towards power. For example, in the strength block a barbell squat might be used to promote maximum leg strength, while in the explosive strength phase a banded variation could be used. The accommodating resistance provided by the band will not only overload the strength stimulus at the top end but will provide greater power output during the concentric initial portion of the lift.

The next layer in the planning process is to decide whether the block, be it a strength block or explosive strength–dominant block, is an opportunity to develop strength or a time to be more conservative and settle to preserve. Examining factors such as the fixture list, opponents, competition phase, game location, etc., informs this important decision. Current strength levels and trends are also factored into the equation. We can turn the dial up or down for a training block through exercise selection, volume manipulation and by using relative intensities. Exercise selection, a subtle but effective method, works by

Explosive strength programme									
		Tempo	Clock	Reps	Set 1	Set 2	Set 3	Set 4	Set 5
1a	Jump shrug / squat jump	2–0–X	3mins	3 Reps	2 @55%	2 @60%	2 @65%	2 @65%	
1b	Depth jump / hurdle jumps	X			3	2	2	2	
2a	Banded squat / banded hex	2–0–1	3mins	2 Reps	3 @55%	2 @60%	2 @65%	2 @70%	2 @>70%
2b	CMJ / box jump	X							
3a	Banded bench / football bar bench	2–0–1	3mins	2 Reps	5 @65%	4 @70%	3 @75%	3+ @75%	
3b	DB row / bench pull	2–0–1			5–8	5–8	5–8		
4a	DB incline / jammer press	3–0–1	3mins	2 Reps	8–12	8–12	8–12		
4b	Cable pull / band face pull	3–0–1			8–12	8–12	8–12		

Fig. 37.7 Agile inseason strength programme. Red sets are optional sets to be completed based on readiness. CMJ, Countermovement jump; DB, dumbbell.

choosing a less taxing concentric-orientated exercise over an eccentric-dominant one. Volume can be manipulated across reps, sets, sessions and blocks. Finally, the application of relative intensities also gives us great operational flexibility. For example, in the strength phase we can keep intensity high at 85% and protect the stimulus by either attacking and developing it with 4–5 reps or preserving it with 2–3 reps.

> *If you have to plan for a future beyond the forecast horizon, plan for surprise.*
>
> Philip Tetlock

Whilst it is important to shape the programme based on short-term forecasting, the accuracy of prescription for an individual on a given day can be further increased by embedding flexibility into the programme through contingency planning – in other words, 'planned unpredictability'. Contingency planning promotes autoregulation by providing the players with options such as open sets, plus sets, optional extra sets, exercise choice, rep ranges and intensity ranges to choose from depending on their readiness (Fig. 37.7). This flexibility is at the heart of the concept of adaptive periodization.

Stage 3: emerging strategy – optimizing the monitoring process

What is certain during the trials and tribulations of the inseason is that conditions will evolve beyond the assumptions made in the planning process. Planning based on predictability in a VUCA environment habitually goes awry due to the dynamic nature of the environment and variability in the individual response to training. For example, acute events that could redirect your programme may include red flags from objective and subjective 'readiness to train' markers, as well as load-monitoring data. Programme modification may also be warranted based on information from the medical department. From a more general perspective, a change of plan to the rugby training programming in the form of, for example, an impromptu scrumming session will also have a knock-on effect on the strength programme.

The ability of the strength programme to change and fit new circumstances lies in the sensitivity to these unfolding events. A comprehensive multidepartment monitoring system, driven by effective feedback loops and fluid communication channels, heightens this sensitivity. Quick, adaptive workflow systems that feed the pertinent data and information to the strength programme can be as simple as having daily multidepartment short meetings that identify broader programme deviations or individual changes as they occur in real time. These debriefs occur at the beginning and end of each day, as well as precede all strength and pitch training sessions. This process increases the accuracy of the training prescription by ensuring that information and data across all departments is current, circulated fluidly and moved to action.

Formal monitoring and communication loops (Fig. 37.8) are vital when managing the emerging environment. However, the picture is incomplete without player feedback and input. The players themselves are a powerful source of knowledge. A culture of respect and trust between the players and the coach will insure that players will volunteer information on their training needs and readiness. Adapting the programme based on their input will further strengthen this bond.

As coaches, we must talk to them, listen to them and observe them. We can glean important information from the players by watching and observing how they interact with each other and with the coaches. Are they quieter or more bubbly than usual? Watching how well they are moving in the warm-up/movement session prior to the gym session will also shine a light on whether any last-minute changes are warranted.

Adapting the strength programme to new and emerging circumstances during the inseason requires informed decision making based on both 'concrete' facts and 'gut feeling' intuition.

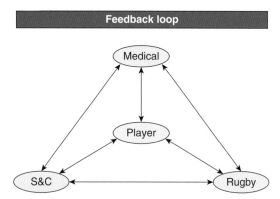

Fig. 37.8 Feedback loop. Reciprocal communication between S&C (strength and conditioning coaches), player, rugby coaches and medical team.

Stage 4: operational strategy – optimizing the coaching process

The effectiveness of the strength process in the inseason hinges on optimizing the coaching process. The planning and emerging strategies have to be complemented with strength training sessions that translate or realize programming into effective action. Central to augmenting this process is a strong performance culture that powers the implementation of the action plan. A performance culture can be defined as a set of expected behaviours that emulates from the group during every session. We promote a strong positive performance culture by setting high behavioural and performance standards, creating a competitive environment, and empowering the players through directed autonomy (Fig. 37.9).

High behavioural standards are set through an unwritten code of conduct. Train hard but smart, focus on the process, and perform the session with intent and technical excellence. Clear and transparent targets (Fig. 37.10) drive performance standards in the core strength qualities of power, strength and speed. These targets are based on international best practice per position and the minimal standards are set to stretch the player. This process provides the players and coaches with both a performance compass and fuel to ignite their competitive spirit. Leader boards, performance awards and specific goal setting all add spice. The players are, by nature, competitive animals and this instinct can be further fuelled by grouping players based on position or by proficiency in a particular exercise. Additionally, live in-session leader boards which feedback on velocity-based training scores or maximum efforts can

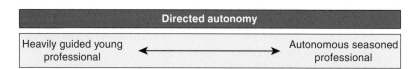

Directed autonomy		
Heavily guided young professional	⟷	Autonomous seasoned professional

Fig. 37.9 Directed autonomy.

Strength targets - Backs		
Squat		
Compete	Dominate	Annihilate
1.7–1.8 × BW	1.8–1.9 × BW	>1.9 × BW
Bench		
Compete	Dominate	Annihilate
1.2–1.3 × BW	1.3–1.4 × BW	>1.4 × BW

Fig. 37.10 Strength targets. *BW*, bodyweight.

all help electrify the atmosphere. Competition is healthy. However, there are sessions and blocks where the intensity that competition organically generates needs to be tempered. This valuable commodity may be of greater value elsewhere in the training process.

Central to an adaptive strength training programme is choice. Choices are offered to players around session type, exercises, intensity ranges and volume. Good choices are made by well-educated informed players who understand the *why* or rationale behind the programme. Choosing the right path for the right day is a collaborative process of mutual trust between the coaches and the players. This process of directed autonomy empowers and motivates the players by allowing them to shape their own programme. This fluid, two-way communication channel also facilitates feedback and 'on the fly' decision making during the session. For example, a session could be terminated early if a player communicates a problem; conversely, sessions can be extended if a player reports that they are 'feeling great' and wants to give it another go. However, it should be noted that directed autonomy should be a continuum whereby younger, newly recruited or less in-tune players are more heavily guided compared to the more autonomous approach given to seasoned professionals.

The performance culture provides the framework in which to coach. The essence of our job as coaches on the ground is to help guide and facilitate the players through the implementation of the programme. We do this by:

- talking to the players before the session to explain "the why" behind the programme; once they understand this, their intent goes up
- explaining and demonstrating 'the what' so that players understand the task at hand
- highlighting the core mantras of 'intent' and 'quality technical execution'
- delivering the coaching session with passion and energy
- coaching the session with focus and by providing quality instruction and feedback based on what you can see, feel and hear from the players.

To get the best out of every session our state of coaching preparedness, readiness and subsequent delivery must be of unwavering high quality. This consistency sets the tone for the players as they feed off our professionalism and energy. Once the session begins, mentally being in a state of concentrated attentive 'high alert' increases our sensitivity to how the players are performing. The ability to switch attention constantly from a narrow individual focus to 'hovering overhead' and soaking in the wider view allows us to coach more effectively. Combining the sensory feedback from what we can see, hear and feel with our intuition and gut informs our decision making and allows us to individually programme and reprogramme as we go.

Stage 5: learning strategy – optimizing the reviewing process

The only way to win is to learn faster than anyone else.

Eric Ries

The planning–doing–reviewing cycle gives us a performance and decision-making framework that helps us operate in the uncertainty of the inseason. As coaches, we love to plan and we love the intoxicating atmosphere of coaching the session. Closing the loop and reviewing is often less appealing. We either run out of time or run away from ego-depleting critical feedback. Reflecting on performance and checking our beliefs and assumptions on a routine and regular basis is a labour of love that has to be worked on.

The 'review habit' will give us the competitive advantage we desire, but as coaches we can be slow to nurture its undoubted powers. Upregulating this part of the coaching process and desensitizing fear through frequent exposures requires formalized and systemized operational reviews implanted throughout. Our review process is characterized by simple, short, checklist-style debrief postsession and more comprehensive reviews that take place at the end of a 3–4 game cycle.

The strength training sessions can be viewed as a giant monitoring laboratory where training is testing and testing is training. Simple trend analysis from session to session and block to block will allow us to analyse if strength indices are on track for the group and the individual. Goals can then be reassessed and the programme redirected where necessary. However, not only is it important to review the numbers; immediately postsession, simple 5-minute coach and player 'check-out' feedback forms are completed (Figs 37.11 and 37.12). From a coaching perspective, a simple sliding scale is used to reflect on session organization, design, flow and delivery. This 'check-out' document also contains a player list that allows us to quickly review each player's performance after the session. Brief notes are taken and all 'red flags' or information pertaining to player participation in subsequent sessions are immediately disseminated to the wider performance team.

A formal strength viva or review/preview takes place every month. The primary purpose of this review is to provide a forum to explain and examine the strength data from month to month. It also provides a platform to throw 'all the cards on the table' to defend the previous programme and outline and defend the next programme for coaching peers and the medical team. This process allows the programme to be stress tested before launch by auditing mistakes and highlighting strengths. Gathering and synthesizing other

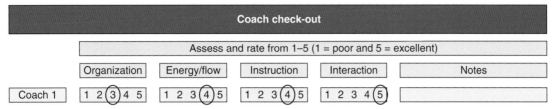

Fig. 37.11 Coaches' check-out.

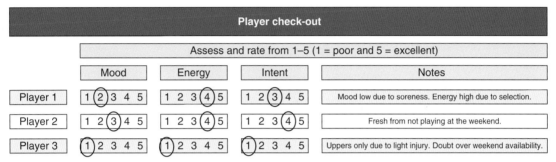

Fig. 37.12 Players' check-out.

perspectives adds value to the programme, not only by incorporating their technical expertize but also by buffering the programme against cognitive bias such as 'confirmation bias' and 'groupthink'. This open-minded, bias-sensitive review process facilitates perpetual programme growth and development in the VUCA world by helping us to recognize where we went wrong, get over ourselves quickly, learn and redirect.

Conclusion

The adaptive periodization model provides a stable philosophical and strategic platform to launch the strength programme while providing the agility to operate successfully in the VUCA environment. The driving force behind the model is strong technical, interpersonal and mental expertize. Technical proficiency ensures that the planning,

programming, coaching and reviewing processes have the requisite methodological knowledge to succeed. Interpersonal skills ensure that communication and feedback networks are aligned and free flowing. Strong mental skills not only give you the resilience to coach throughout the entire season, they also equip you with the correct dose of cognitive readiness as the war rages around you. Cognitive readiness provides the preparedness and agility needed to sustain coaching performance in a complex and unpredictable environment.

Successful inseason programming requires smart, agile, contingency-rich programmes guided by reflection and driven by deliberate 'stretch' practice. Victory through the fog of war is an artful science requiring deep questioning of both the process and direction taken at each and every juncture. The ability of the strength training programme to expect, adapt and thrive on unpredictability can be a real competitive advantage. In professional sport this can be the difference between wining and losing.

Chapter | **38** |

Movement analysis: science meets practice

David M. Clancy

> *Nothing is more revealing than movement.*
>
> Martha Graham (1894–1991),
> American modern dancer and choreographer

Introduction

This chapter will highlight the importance of movement analysis to achieve better results in the initial stages of rehabilitation, improvements in performance and reinjury prevention strategies.

Why is movement analysis important?

According to the literature, '… 35% of patients do not return to preinjury levels and 45% do not return to competitive sport' (Ardern et al., 2014). These startling figures are in relation to anterior cruciate ligament (ACL) returns; examples such as this have made the understanding of movement principles, neurophysiology and biomechanics of the utmost importance. It shows that we as clinicians and practitioners can all up our games and improve our clinical outcomes and results.

We think we are doing a good job. However, published work by Ardern and others highlight that we need to target deficiencies to a greater degree to effect significant change and get athletes back to their 'expected' preinjury level of play and/or performance.

Movement is fundamental to all biology, from the movement of blood cells in the circulatory system to movement of ions across a plasma membrane to immunity as a phagocyte moves towards an invading pathogen. At a macro level, when movement becomes impaired after an injury many fundamental aspects of living can be affected.

It is vital to include movement analysis in rehabilitation, as movement dysfunction is often a key factor in injuries: it may have been a contributor to the original injury or may have developed because of injury. As an example, movement dysfunction such as dynamic knee valgus is the main mechanism of injury to the ACL (Hewett et al., 2005) – a catastrophic sporting injury that can ruin sporting careers. One needs to understand the key factors that feed a valgus knee moment so that they can be addressed specifically.

Movement analysis can be a link between the early phases of rehabilitation and the final stages of on-field preparation for a safe return to play (RTP). The goal of movement analysis is to identify and correct movement dysfunction, restore neuromuscular function (brain-to-muscle connection) and enhance movement coordination. It appears to be integral to developing safe movement patterns prior to targeting sport-specific skills in preparation to full RTP and also to strategically reduce reinjury risk factors.

What is movement analysis?

Movement is both the goal and conclusion of the nervous system, which acts through bones, joints and muscles ending in a predetermined position in space. Analysing movement, therefore, is the process of assessing and evaluating the quality of a movement as it relates to a task, with the intent of optimizing the movement's ease and efficiency. There are multiple ways to assess movement from the use of the trained eye, to a camera phone, to force plates, right through to the very complex implementation of three-dimensional motion capture. All methods have the same goal: identify the dysfunction and then address this through targeted movement retraining.

Terms employed during movement analysis

A detailed analysis of movement is a complex activity and should involve the following:
1. A description of the movements that occur at the joints involved.
2. The plane(s) and axis/axes in which the movement occurs.
3. The muscles producing the movement.

A description of the movements involved

> **Example: analysis of a double leg squat**
> This involves the understanding that the squat is a compound, multijoint exercise designed to target many muscles of the lower limb and lumbopelvic–hip complex (pelvis, low back and abdominals). It occurs in the sagittal and frontal planes (Fig. 38.1).

The planes and axes in which the movement occurs

All body movements occur in different planes and around different axes (Fig. 38.2). A plane is an imaginary two-dimensional flat surface running through the body. An axis is an imaginary line at right angles to the plane, about which the body rotates (Hamill et al., 2015).

There are three planes of movement:
1. *Sagittal plane* – a vertical plane that passes through the centre of the body and divides the body into left and right sides. Flexion- and extension-types of movement occur in this plane (e.g., kicking a football, chest pass in basketball, walking, jumping, squatting).
2. *Frontal plane* – passes from side to side and divides the body into the front and back. Abduction and adduction movements occur in this plane (e.g., jumping jack exercises, raising and lowering arms and legs sideways, cartwheels).
3. *Horizontal or transverse plane* – passes through the centre of the body and divides the body horizontally in an upper and lower half. Rotation types of movement occur in this plane (e.g., hip rotation in a golf swing, twisting in a discus throw, pivoting in basketball).

There are three axes of movement around which the body or body parts rotate:
1. *Sagittal horizontal or transverse axis* – this line runs from left to right through the centre of the body (e.g., when

a person performs a somersault they rotate around this axis).
2. *Frontal or anterior–posterior axis* – this line runs from front to back through the centre of the body (e.g., when a person performs a cartwheel they are rotating about the frontal axis).
3. *Vertical or longitudinal axis* – this line runs from top to bottom through the centre of the body (e.g., when a skater performs a spin they are rotating around the longitudinal axis).

The muscles producing the movement

When analysing movement we need to consider the type of contraction (concentric, eccentric or isometric) and the function of the muscles involved – what are the agonists and antagonists, synergists and stabilizers? Box 38.1 provides definitions of the key terms.

Models of analysis

The three main methods of analysing the biomechanics of sport movements are:
- movement phases
- free body diagrams
- deterministic models.

Movement phases and free body diagrams are commonly used by coaches and sports scientists, whereas deterministic models are used in more complex movement analysis and therefore more often used in sports research.

Movement phases

A sport movement, especially for ballistic actions such as hitting, throwing and kicking, generally contains three main phases:
1. *Preparation* contains all the movements that prepare an athlete for the performance of the skill, such as the backswing during a golf swing and the run-up in long jumping.
2. *Execution* is the performance of the actual movement that often includes a point of contact with an object (e.g., contact between golf club and ball), the release of an object (e.g., discus) or a flight phase (e.g., long jump).
3. *Follow-through* refers to all the movements that occur after the execution phase (e.g., leg lift after striking a football) that slow the body's momentum to prevent injury, to get ready for another movement or both.

These three distinct movement phases are important to understand. If the athlete can improve their efficiency during each of these phases it may lead to a cumulative improvement of the gesture overall.

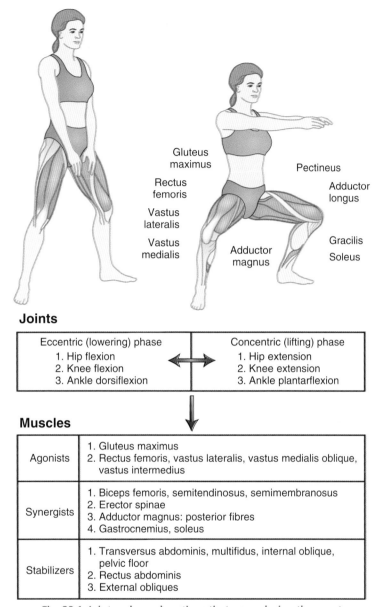

Joints

Eccentric (lowering) phase	Concentric (lifting) phase
1. Hip flexion	1. Hip extension
2. Knee flexion	2. Knee extension
3. Ankle dorsiflexion	3. Ankle plantarflexion

Muscles

Agonists	1. Gluteus maximus 2. Rectus femoris, vastus lateralis, vastus medialis oblique, vastus intermedius
Synergists	1. Biceps femoris, semitendinosus, semimembranosus 2. Erector spinae 3. Adductor magnus: posterior fibres 4. Gastrocnemius, soleus
Stabilizers	1. Transversus abdominis, multifidus, internal oblique, pelvic floor 2. Rectus abdominis 3. External obliques

Fig. 38.1 Joint and muscle actions that occur during the squat.

Free body diagrams

A free body diagram is a visual diagram of the expected or predicted movement pattern. This is usually drawn as a simple stick figure. Coaches and researchers often use the technique to describe a subphase or point of interest in a movement pattern. Coaches often use these for cueing aids for their athletes. Fig. 38.3 is a simple example of a squat free body diagram.

Deterministic models

A deterministic model is a modelling paradigm that describes the biomechanical factors determining a movement. This model starts with the primary performance factor(s) (e.g., jump displacement for long jump, race time in sprinting), followed by a breakdown into secondary factors (elements that contribute to the performance factor).

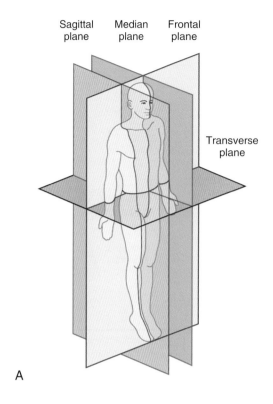

Sagittal plane Median plane Frontal plane

Transverse plane

A

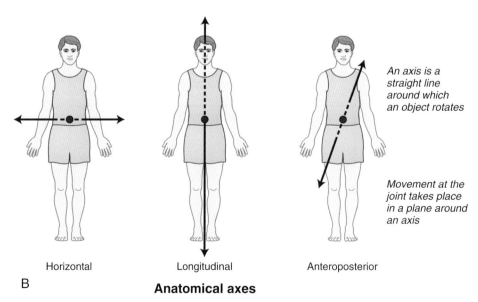

Horizontal

Longitudinal

Anteroposterior

An axis is a straight line around which an object rotates

Movement at the joint takes place in a plane around an axis

B

Anatomical axes

Fig. 38.2 (A) Planes and (B) axes of movement.

Box 38.1 **Glossary of muscle work terms**

Active insufficiency

The inability of a muscle that spans two joints to contract maximally across both joints at the same time, e.g., a powerful fist occurs with the wrist extended otherwise the finger flexors cannot contract across all the finger interphalangeal joints and wrist joint at the same time.

Antagonists

Antagonist muscles are the muscles that produce an opposing joint torque to the agonist muscles. Antagonism is merely the role that a muscle plays depending on which muscle is currently the agonist. For example, biceps sometimes acts as an agonist and at other times as an antagonist.

Agonists

Agonist muscles cause a movement to occur through their own activation; also interchangeably referred to as 'prime movers', since they are the muscles considered primarily responsible for generating or controlling a specific movement.

Coactivation/cocontraction

Sometimes during a joint action controlled by an agonist muscle the antagonist will be simultaneously activated, naturally.

Concentric contraction

Muscle is actively shortening.

Eccentric contraction

Muscle is actively lengthening.

Isometric contraction

The muscle generates tension but does not change in length, e.g., holding a weight out at arm's length.

Length–tension relationship

The observation that the isometric force exerted by a muscle is dependent upon its length when tested.

Muscle imbalance

The respective equality between the antagonist and agonist, required for normal muscle movement and roles.

Passive insufficiency

The inability of a muscle that spans two joints to stretch maximally across both joints at the same time, e.g., maximum dorsiflexion cannot be attained with an extended knee when gastrocnemius is stretched.

Reciprocal inhibition

The process of muscles on one side of a joint relaxing to accommodate contraction on the other side of that joint.

Synergistic action

Synergists are sometimes referred to as 'neutralizers' because they help cancel out, or neutralize, extra motion from the agonists to make sure that the force generated works within the desired plane of motion, e.g., when making a fist the wrist extensors contract to allow stronger finger flexion at the interphalangeal joints.

Synergistic dominance

The process by which the main agonist muscle of a movement is inhibited or weak, and the synergist (a helper muscle) becomes the main contributor to the movement.

The relationships between a movement outcome measure and all of these factors are considered. This allows one to examine the relative importance of various factors that influence the outcome of a movement (Peh et al., 2011). Fig. 38.4 examines flight distance as the primary performance factor, with the secondary factors being take-off height, take-off horizontal velocity and take-off vertical velocity (Bartlett, 2007).

Regardless of the technique employed, movement analysis requires careful planning. These techniques may also suit qualitative or quantitative analyses of movement. Qualitative analysis assesses the technical quality of the movement (e.g., rhythm, posture), whereas quantitative techniques assess the movement using numbers (e.g., angles, distance, speed, force).

> **Movement analysis models**
> Having a usable model to assess and coach movement is important for evaluating and improving movement quality.

Movement dysfunction

It is imperative to identify dysfunctional movement patterns via movement analysis and having done so, correct it with specific training elements. This is important for long-term health after an injury. An altered neuromuscular movement control pattern predisposes to a second injury to the ACL after an ACL reconstruction so it is vital to address dysfunction and maintain those principles (Paterno et al., 2010).

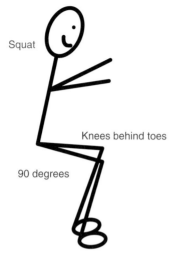

Squat

Knees behind toes

90 degrees

Fig. 38.3 Squat free body diagram.

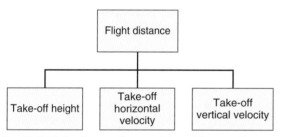

Flight distance

Take-off height

Take-off horizontal velocity

Take-off vertical velocity

Fig. 38.4 Flight distance factors. Adapted from Bartlett, R., 2007. Introduction to Sports Biomechanics. Routledge, London.

Often after an injury an individual learns a new way to move. The body will always seek the path of least resistance when it comes to movement, as this is metabolically most efficient. A body can organize itself functionally in an extraordinary way but what is most metabolically efficient may not necessarily be the most mechanically efficient in the long term (Buckthorpe and Roi, 2018).

Understanding these nuances and how they can contribute to the delaying of 'normal movement' is important so that they can be critically addressed and corrected. Movement dysfunction can lead to a cascade of issues. The most efficacious intervention strategies should aim to target these modifiable impairments to optimize movement control competency.

Fig. 38.5 shows the ideal technique for a single leg squat in the frontal view, as an example. The knee alignment does not show any medial displacement (absence of valgus), there is no pelvic tilt and the trunk remains vertical. For ideal frontal plane control to be exhibited, there needs to be a solid foundation of strength (peak torque) in hip abduction, knee flexion and knee extension as this is correlated with less motion into valgus (Claiborne et al., 2006).

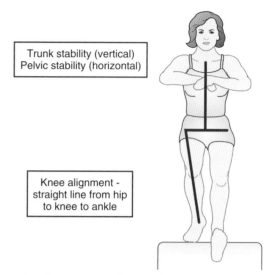

Trunk stability (vertical)
Pelvic stability (horizontal)

Knee alignment - straight line from hip to knee to ankle

Fig. 38.5 Ideal alignment for a single leg squat, frontal view.

Here are some of the most prevalent movement dysfunctions for the lower limb and knee in particular:

Deficit in limb stability

A lack of limb stability refers to an inconsistency of the knee position in the frontal plane, with medial knee displacement or any appearance in dynamic valgus, also known as ligament dominance (Di Stasi et al., 2013). This altered chain of kinematics of the knee joint is usually associated with a contralateral pelvic drop and mild foot intrarotation in cutting manoeuvres (Imwalle et al., 2009). This is a risk factor for a variety of different knee pathologies such as ACL disruption, medial collateral ligament sprain, medial compartmental loading, medial meniscus tears, fat pad impingement and so forth.

Fig. 38.6 shows where the right knee is in a valgus position, with hip internal rotation with foot eversion. The patient is also adopting a forward lean position thereby overloading the anterior compartment of the knee joint. This is a fine example of impaired lumbopelvic control.

As an aside, foot position is important in movement analysis. Whilst not displayed in Fig. 38.6, a 'toe in' posture usually results in increased hip adduction, increased knee abduction and increased knee internal rotation (angle and moment), all significant risk factors for a major knee injury such as an ACL tear (Tran et al., 2016).

Deficit in pelvic stability

This refers to misalignment in the frontal plane of the pelvic area, usually seen as a pelvic hike or hip drop

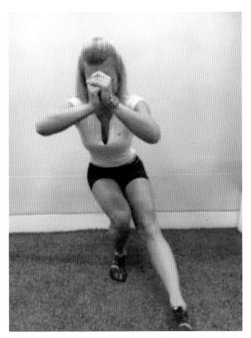

Fig. 38.6 Example of dynamic knee valgus on the right side.

(Jamison et al., 2012). This is frequently observed in combination with an associated knee valgus (Sigward and Powers, 2007).

Fig. 38.7 shows an anterior and posterior perspective revealing hip hiking on the right side. There is also minor knee medial displacement. Weakness of the right gluteus medius will cause the left hip to drop when standing on the right limb. Fig. 38.8 shows the Trendelenburg sign. This reveals weakness of the left hip abductors with subsequent drop on the right pelvis.

Deficit in trunk stability

This refers to the excessive deviation of the trunk from the median line with destabilization proximally (Zazulak et al., 2007). Ipsilateral trunk lean in cutting is commonly seen on analysis. Trunk lean on the right side with a present knee valgus at the knee joint during a single leg squat is shown in Fig. 38.9. The ideal technique for a single leg squat in the lateral view is given in Fig. 38.10. The knee alignment does not show any medial displacement (absence of valgus), there is no pelvic tilt and the trunk remains vertical.

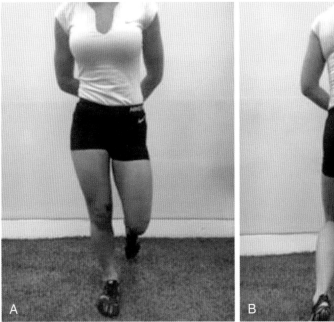

Fig. 38.7 (A) Anterior and (B) posterior views of hip hiking on the right side (observe the ripples on the T-shirt).

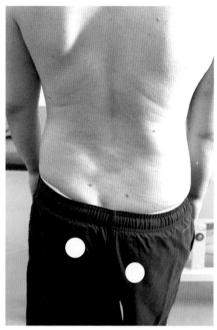

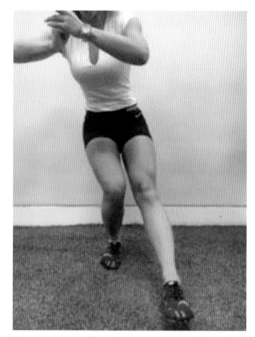

Fig. 38.8 **Trendelenburg sign.** The white circles mark the anatomical landmarks of the posterior superior iliac spines, which are the main bony sites to observe for this sign.

Fig. 38.9 **Example of trunk lean on same side as knee valgus stance.**

Deficit in shock absorption

This refers to an inability of the athlete to dissipate loads such as high ground reaction forces, usually seen with high knee angle in drop jumps and hopping manoeuvres (Leppänen et al., 2017). This can be measured using a force plate, which is a helpful adjunct. Upright postures tend to be commonly seen here and this can be known as adopting a 'knee strategy' whereby a stiffer landing involves increased knee extension, decreased hip extension and thus less gluteus maximus, as seen in Fig. 38.11 (Pollard et al., 2010).

Deficit in movement strategy

Deficit in movement strategy occurs in relation to altered global kinematics in the sagittal plane. Uneven load distribution and dissipation is usually seen with these deficits. Incorrectly loading forward onto the knees is a common fault seen with this, with weakness of the posterior muscle groups common.

Fig. 38.12 reveals excessive loading through the knee joints with poor knee position in relation to the toes. This is despite a relatively well-controlled core and upright stance posture.

Muscle imbalances

Movement dysfunction can be driven by muscle imbalances because of either muscle inhibition or resultant synergistic dominance (explained below) of a muscle group or due to relative strength deficits (weakness, but normal function) .

An example could be a weak and inhibited gluteus maximus being 'assisted' by the biceps femoris muscle, which can become overactive and dominant, during hip extension. This can be identified through muscle palpation techniques with an assessment in prone lying of the muscle bellies of the hamstrings and the glutes. The distinction between the two is important and will directly contribute to the success of a movement training programme.

If inhibition is present then it needs to be treated to effectively train a movement. If a muscle cannot be activated due to inhibition, then it cannot be trained in function and resultant compensation will occur in movement. If corrective training does not occur, then these compensations will be reinforced, and the faulty movement patterns will remain (Buckthorpe and Roi, 2018).

It is essential to ensure that harmonized movement training is built upon a solid foundation, and the correct movement pattern is utilized, trained and developed into unconscious sport-specific movement patterns.

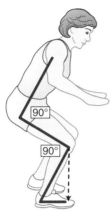

Trunk and knee position - equal knee bend and hip bend is favorable for 'hip strategy' approach, known as 'double flexion'

90°

90°

Knee position in relation to toes is important

Fig. 38.10 Ideal alignment for a single leg squat, lateral view.

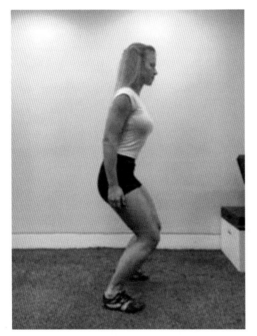

Fig. 38.11 Example of knee-dominant quad loading pattern, rather than loading through the hip joint and recruiting glutes better.

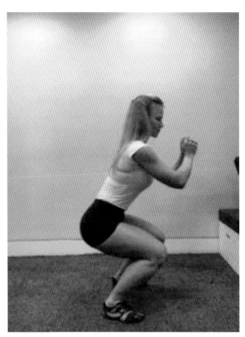

Fig. 38.12 Variable factors that can arise from dysfunctional movement patterns, such as excessive loading and shear through the knees, beyond the toes

An important concept here is to train effective conscious safe movement patterns. This may require some form of corrective retraining if this has not yet successfully been undertaken in the initial stage of the rehabilitation process. Therefore, initially identifying any underlying dysfunction through movement analysis is essential. An individual movement reeducation programme will need to be

developed to consider imbalances and an effective corrective programme implemented to address this, such as that outlined in the ensuing example.

Reciprocal inhibition describes the process of muscles on one side of a joint relaxing to accommodate contraction on the other side of that joint, such as the agonist producing an action whilst the antagonistic muscle relaxes (Hamill et al., 2015).

As an example, tightness of the psoas muscle may inhibit glute maximal activation; altered reciprocal inhibition can contribute to muscle imbalances and movement dysfunction, such as dynamic knee valgus during a single leg squat (see corrective programme below for more detail). This needs to be addressed to allow for movement complexity for functional strengthening and sporting movements.

Here is an example of a corrective programme for addressing knee instability referred to as dynamic knee valgus (a significant risk factor for injury to the ACL) (Hewett et al., 2005) during a squatting pattern, which targets maximal movement through the hip and knee joints.

Bear in mind that knee joint stability is attributed to passive and active constraints. The passive constraints are the ligaments and the joint capsule. The active constraints are the muscles, which provide stability to the joint in motion. Healthy and well-recruited muscles are very important to help reduce the risk of injury to the passive constraints of a joint such as that of the knee.

A corrective programme will address the vulnerability in a slower, controlled movement initially before introducing dynamic practice. The following outlines the process:

Identify contracted muscles. Psoas, tensor fascia latae (TFL), biceps femoris, vastus lateralis.

Relax contracted muscles. Soft tissue release, foam roller, static or dynamic stretching.

Identify, reactivate and strengthen inhibited or weak muscles. Gluteus medius, transversus, multifidus, gluteus maximus, vastus medialis obliques (VMO).

Treat synergistic dominance and reciprocal inhibition. Synergistic dominant muscle could be the biceps femoris, which is overactive because the gluteus maximus is inhibited from the psoas muscle, which could be short and tight. So we need to incorporate softening and lengthening (pliability) of the psoas, release the biceps femoris and isolate strengthening of the glute muscles.

Implement a core and lumbopelvic stability programme. Transversus activation with dead bugs, bird–dog, bridging, bear-crawls, standing clam with band and other key foundational exercises for targeting lumbopelvic control.

Treat the movement pattern with functional exercise (locally then globally). In this case of dynamic knee valgus, the focus will be on the transversus, multifidus, internal oblique, gluteus maximus, gluteus medius in terms of strengthening, to then progress to double leg squat, split squats, lunges, and single squats, etc.

Let us take look at another example:

An overactive TFL (a hip flexor, internal rotator of the femur and an abductor) may result in reciprocal inhibition of gluteus maximus or lateral hamstrings. In such cases, unconscious movement practice will only reinforce a pattern of TFL dominance. The retraining will need to include reducing TFL activation and/or increasing activation of gluteus maximus and gluteus medius in motion.

- Utilize exercises with a higher gluteus medius activation than TFL, such as prone hip extension or bridges with a band around the knees to enhance abduction forces.
- An extra tip is to take advantage of the potential of gluteus maximus to reciprocally inhibit TFL by combining hip abduction with hip extension.
- Reducing the degrees of freedom of movement (i.e., by reducing the range of motion of the exercises) can also help. For instance, if the range of the hip abduction is 0–90 degrees, lay down in a side position and with the leg straight one can work in a range between 20 and 60 degrees. In this range the gluteus medius fibres become increasingly active.

Synergistic dominance is the process by which the main agonist muscle of a movement is inhibited or weak and the synergist (a helper muscle) becomes the main contributor to the movement.

An example of synergistic dominance is when the inhibition of the gluteus maximus muscle precipitates the overlying dominance of the lateral hamstrings (biceps femoris in particular) for external rotation of the femur and hip extension (Billiet et al., 2018). This may be identified by electromyography, if available, or through muscle palpation techniques. Of course, it is always important to note that muscles are not mutually exclusive in relation to contraction. There is often partial or cocontraction of antagonists, tightness or weakness of the psoas and/or rectus femoris muscle. These will all play a role in gluteus maximus recruitment, or inhibition in this case.

Synergistic dominance may be a contributory factor to an ACL injury (Box 38.2). The hamstrings may overwork as a hip external rotator rather than as a hip extensor, which is their prime movement. This can be assessed by means of standard manual muscle testing. When they work in this manner they no longer act efficiently as knee flexors and, more importantly, as stabilizers. This dominance needs to be addressed if present, before unconscious movement control is carried out, otherwise tissue fatigue and a cumulative injury cycle could follow.

How do we perform movement analysis?

Movement analysis is an assessment of an individual's motion. It may combine the assessment of biomechanics by a trained individual or the use of technology such as video analysis.

Neurophysiology should also be considered in movement analysis. Its contribution is difficult to measure but theories from Isokinetic Medical Group suggest that to understand and eliminate a deficit it is important to stimulate the conscious learning process through education and review of video analysis.

An analysis of specific sports-relevant movements is made based on set criteria in order to carry out a qualitative assessment (prevailing deficit) and a quantitative evaluation. This is based on a scoring system.

Here is an example of the movements and criteria focused on within the movement analysis test (MAT) used by Isokinetic Medical Group. It is important to bear in mind that this is one strategy to test movement.

Biomechanical measures during landing and postural stability predict second ACL injury after ACL reconstruction and RTP (Paterno et al., 2010). The MAT involves examining six specific movements: single leg squat, deceleration, drop jump, frontal hop, side hop and a change of direction. Five criteria are used to quantify deficits; these include:
- limb stability
- pelvis stability
- trunk stability
- shock absorption
- movement strategy

Box 38.2 Post-ACLR gait biomechanics and their implications

What do the experts say about the consequences of abnormal movement?

Estimated lifetime risk of symptomatic knee osteoarthritis (OA) following anterior cruciate ligament (ACL) injury (regardless of management) is 34% compared to 14% in noninjured individuals and the risk of having a total knee replacement is 22% vs. 6% (Suter et al., 2017). The prevalence of both tibiofemoral and patellofemoral OA in patients following ACL injury and subsequent reconstruction has been related to specific changes in landing mechanics, walking and running gait (Culvenor and Crossley, 2016).

ACL-reconstructed (ACLR) patients land, run and walk with decreased knee flexion angles and internal knee extensor moments (Kline et al., 2016; Roewer et al., 2011). This change in movement may have implications for long-term function and joint loading stresses. Erhart-Hledik et al. (2017) found the presence of these changes in walking gait (decreased knee flexion angle and internal extensor moments) at 2 years postoperation and predicted KOOS questionnaire score (functional outcome) at 8 years. The changes in walking gait appear to have occurred by as early as 4 weeks postoperation (Hadizadeh et al., 2016). These distinct changes in kinematic and kinetic parameters (decreased knee flexion, internal knee extension moment) also occurred during a higher load landing tasks (forward hop landing) in ACLR patients who were showing radiological signs of patellofemoral joint OA in the first 2 years postoperation (Culvenor et al., 2016). These changes when seen in running appear to be associated with increased patellofemoral joint loads and stress (Herrington et al., 2017), which may be the precursor to the development of patellofemoral joint pain and OA (Culvenor and Crossley, 2016). These changes when seen in running gait at 6 months appear to be related to quadriceps strength at 3 months postoperation (Kline et al., 2016).

Current research appears to show that postoperatively ACLR patients fail to appropriately both flex their knees and generate appropriate internal joint moments during landing, walking and running; this may be related to poor quadriceps strength. The presence of this movement pattern appears to increase loads on the patellofemoral joint, which may predispose this joint to degeneration. The presence of this movement pattern appears to have significant implications for long-term functional outcomes.

With grateful acknowledgement to Dr. Lee Herrington for this section.

Culvenor, A., Crossley, K., 2016. Patellofemoral osteoarthritis: are we missing an important source of symptoms after anterior cruciate ligament reconstruction? Journal of Orthopaedic and Sports Physical Therapy 46 (4), 232–234.

Culvenor, A., Perration, L., Guermazi, A., Bryant, A., Whitehead, T., Morris, H., et al., 2016. Knee kinematics and kinetics are associated with early patellofemoral osteoarthritis following anterior cruciate ligament reconstruction. Osteoarthritis & Cartilage 24, 1548–1553.

Erhart-Hledik, J., Chu, C., Asay, J., Andriacchi, T., 2017. Gait mechanics 2 years after anterior cruciate ligament reconstruction are associated with longer-term changes in patient-reported outcomes. Journal of Orthopaedic Research 5 (3), 634–640.

Hadizadeh, M., Amri, S., Mohafez, H., Roohi, S., Mokhtar, A., 2016. Gait analysis of national athletes after anterior cruciate ligament reconstruction following three stages of rehabilitation program: symmetrical perspective. Gait & Posture 48, pp. 152–158.

Herrington, L., Alarifi, S., Jones, R., 2017. Patellofemoral joint loads during running at the time of return to sport in elite athletes with ACL reconstruction. American Journal of Sports Medicine 45, 2812–2816.

Kline, P., Johnson, D., Ireland, M., Noehren, B., 2016. Clinical predictors of knee mechanics at return to sport after ACL reconstruction. Medicine and Science in Sports and Exercise 48 (5), 790–795.

Roewer, B., Di Stasi, S., Synder-Mackler, L., 2011. Quadriceps strength and weight acceptance strategies continue to improve two years after ACL reconstruction. Journal of Biomechanics 44 (10), 1948–1953.

Suter, L., Smith, S., Katz, Englund M., Hunter, D., Frobell, R., et al., 2017. Projecting lifetime risk of symptomatic knee osteoarthritis and total knee replacement in individuals sustaining a complete ACL tear in early adulthood. Arthritis Care & Research 69 (2), 201–208.

Limb stability

This centres on the ability to stabilize the leg and avoid motions that may cause damage to joints. Biomechanical issues such as knee valgus, knee varus, tibial rotation, foot pronation and foot supination are all important movement characteristics that need to be picked up on in order to fully understand where excessive or insufficient loading could be occurring for an individual (Khayambashi et al., 2016).

As an example, if a knee is in a valgus position this could lead to excessive compression forces across the lateral knee compartment contrasting to shearing or stretching forces medially; this could precipitate an injury to the medial collateral ligament of the knee amongst other issues.

Pelvis stability

This largely refers to the ability to stabilize the pelvis in the frontal plane. A role of the gluteus medius is to stabilize the pelvis and prevent one side falling past the other when walking, known as a 'Trendelenburg gait'. The gluteus medius works like the external rotator cuff muscles of the shoulder joint. When this happens, it can influence motion through the rest of the body and influence force dissipation through the hip by overloading one side more than the other.

Trunk stability

This refers to the ability to maintain control of the torso in motion. ACL injuries typically involve a trunk lateral drop, which shifts the centre of mass.

Shock absorption

Shock absorption is visually estimated through examining landing mechanics and in particular the extent to which the athlete can effectively land softly, dissipating the force throughout the muscles. A highlighted risk factor of ACL injuries is known as ligament dominance (Myer et al., 2004, 2011). This is when force is absorbed via the ligament and/or joint as opposed to being absorbed eccentrically by the muscle tendon unit. 'Softening' the joints by flexion at the hip and knee joints will help dissipate loads at the knee significantly.

Movement strategy

Movement strategy details the adoption of movement patterns by the patient in which they favour certain muscle groups in the sagittal plane over others. As an example, weakness of the gluteus maximus could result in the patient leaning forward, with greater loading on their knees, thus adopting a 'knee strategy' in place of a more correct 'hip strategy' whereby loading is through the posterior hip muscles initially. This relates to the centre of mass, muscle strength and the production of torque. To decrease the required muscle force production or to avoid pain, one can adopt certain positions in movements to preferentially use or avoid certain muscle groups. This can be termed quad dominance or knee avoidance.

Other areas that one must look at include:

Hip muscle strength

This is key in reducing potential knee injuries, as shown by the work done by Khayambashi et al. (2014) . Reduced hip external rotator strength (<20% bodyweight) and reduced hip abduction strength (<35% bodyweight) is associated with predicting noncontact ACL injuries.

Anterior or posterior tilting of the pelvis also influences pelvic stability in the sagittal plane of motion. A key factor in core training should be training the ability to resist unwanted motion (e.g., improving activation and timing of gluteus medius in single leg landing to have the strength to stabilize and prevent the pelvis from falling to one side). The ability to resist gravity's hip adduction torque is crucial.

This can be targeted in many ways. Here are some examples:

In a resisted slide-board back lunge the pull of the cable creates a hip flexion force against which the gluteus maximus has to stabilize. The movement also mimics the hip action of running and climbing stairs. Akin to running, the body has to be pulled over the foot by a powerful hip extension. The single leg stance emphasizes the gluteus medius and the upper fibres of the gluteus maximus (Billiet et al., 2018).

Other exercises that elicit a high gluteus maximus and gluteus medius activity that can help translate to improved single leg landing are the single leg squat and the single leg Romanian deadlift (Stastny et al., 2016).

These single leg exercises require concentric or eccentric hip extension throughout a large range of motion and frontal plane pelvic stability in conjunction with a control of the stance leg in the frontal and transverse planes. This leads to a high neural drive to the gluteus maximus, gluteus medius and the posterior chain in its entirety. Practicing single leg landing whilst holding a light dumbbell on the contralateral side is likely to help with gluteus medius firing and pelvic stabilization, as this is a great way to counter rotational forces and create lumbopelvic pillar strengthening.

Muscle function

Muscle function is largely determined by muscle architecture; understanding this anatomy is important for training movement control well. For example, the gluteus medius is a very strong muscle given its relatively small cross-sectional area due to packing many short muscle fibres in parallel. Due to this makeup, it cannot produce very large forces over large ranges of motion; essentially, it stabilizes the pelvis and femur, and should be trained and assessed in such a manner.

An example of an exercise for this could be the clam exercise in isolation: Lay down on a side, hips and knees bent at a 45-degree angle, heels close to each other; then perform hip abduction without rolling the pelvis, staying still with heels together. This exercise isolates the gluteus medius. One can then move to the step-up or standing clam in order to train it globally.

Postmovement analysis: targeted neuromotor training

Movement is produced via the neuromuscular system; this system involves muscles contracting via neural signals from the central nervous system and producing force via tendon connections to bone (Hamill et al., 2015). Developing movement coordination is not just as simple as getting patients to move. Antalgic movement patterns (i.e., those that develop to avoid pain) may be challenging to correct. Additionally, underlying muscle imbalances, from either before the injury or because of injury, can alter the way the body moves to 'compensate' for weakness.

Therefore, when there is movement dysfunction, correct movement patterns need to be redeveloped by the patient through an individualized corrective programme of *neuromotor training* (NMT) that targets the neuromuscular system in its entirety. Having ascertained the movement dysfunction, specific NMT must take place to address the issues identified from the movement analysis test.

NMT involves targeting motor skills such as coordination, agility and proprioception. Specific, effective and sensitive NMT can help restore full function and expedite a RTP. An athlete may move efficiently after an injury but they must also learn to move correctly using NMT.

Optimal motor patterning is imperative after an injury to the ACL. Once the ACL has been torn, there is decreased somatosensory input (Grooms et al., 2015) and altered movement quality bilaterally (Goerger et al., 2014). The connection between the brain and the muscles needs to be retrained.

This NMT emphasizing movement control quality should help reduce the potential for reinjury or secondary injuries upon RTP. As well as helping prevent reinjury, performance enhancement can occur as NMT helps sharpen the feedforward loop mechanism, and this is a key component to keeping athletes fit and playing.

Neuroplasticity theory and practical application

Having considered all the factors that can influence motor pattern quality (Fig. 38.13) it is important to understand that neuroplasticity plays an important role after the movement analysis when addressing issues practically. Neuroplasticity can be defined as the brain's ability to change, remodel and reorganize for purpose of better ability to adapt to new situations (Demarin et al., 2014).

Doyon and Benali (2005) described a model of learning a new motor sequence and a new motor adaptation in response to a change. Upon initially being taught a new exercise, cognitive processes govern the phase called 'fast learning'. Other neural pathways are involved in the second step, which is known as the 'slow learning' phase. The final

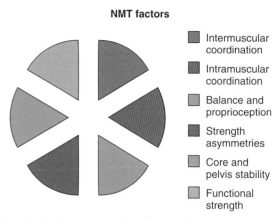

NMT factors

- Intermuscular coordination
- Intramuscular coordination
- Balance and proprioception
- Strength asymmetries
- Core and pelvis stability
- Functional strength

Fig. 38.13 Movement pattern factors that may contribute to an incorrect motor pattern. One must develop an individualized holistic programme that tackles all or some of these aspects. A focus on rate of force development (how quickly force can be produced), rapid neural activation and overall muscular coordination is imperative.

Feedforward motor mechanism

The role of the feedforward motor mechanism is to preactivate certain muscles and tendons needed for motor tasks to provide optimal movement control. These include activating the correct muscles prior to landing, changing direction or slowing down.

---

phases of learning a new motor sequence are called 'consolidation', 'automation' and 'retention', when the movement pattern becomes ingrained in the brain. Once each new adaptation takes place a new 'correct' motor sequence is created.

This theoretical model has been translated into clinical practice for more practical application. To learn a new basic movement identified from movement analysis it is imperative to follow a phased approach to learn a new habit. This can take anywhere from 18 to 254 days (Lally et al., 2010). Table 38.1 describes a model for teaching the drop jump as an example.

The goal of this training is to achieve long-term retention of new motor patterns, which should be associated with better clinical and functional results, especially with movement analysis retesting for all injuries.

Conclusion

Life requires movement.

Aristotle (384–322 BCE), Greek philosopher and scientist

Table 38.1 Motor learning process for practical application

Phase rationale	Process
Cognitive phase	
Deconstruct dysfunctional movement	Verbal cueing of what the patient is doing wrong (may include 'absorb load softly, bend through your hips then knees, do not lean forward') Video revealing correct movement of how to execute the drop jump properly Few, high-quality repetitions Feedforward (e.g., video and cueing during execution helps understanding of incorrect movement of the drop jump for the patient's education)
Associative phase	
Reconstruct new movement task	Fewer instructions (only one or two now, such as 'keep chest upward') More repetition, more practice Immediate biofeedback in real time continues (Seeing each jump prior to the next jump) Self-correction strategies begun (patient starts to recognize faulty habits and addresses on their own)
Automatic phase	
Progressive automation of the movement	No cueing External focus points (such as 'push floor away from you') Delayed biofeedback (video and show after) Self-correction more regular and rigorous by patient

A holistic approach is required to retrain movement prior to RTP and various factors influence movement competency. Movement dysfunction is a significant factor in ACL injuries as well as the many other entities that we see each and every day.

Movement incompetency may have been the contributor to the original injury or could have developed because of the injury; thus, movement reeducation should form an aspect of all bespoke rehabilitation programmes. The goal here is to coach patients to be able to move efficiently and safely before they return to sport-specific movements.

Movement analysis and correcting a movement profile using selectively distilled NMT, aiming for long-term movement retention, is the cornerstone of understanding how to analyse and train movement better. This can significantly help with improving outcomes from rehabilitation and help reduce reinjury rates.

Acknowledgement

A special thanks to Dr. Matthew Buckthorpe of Isokinetic Medical Group who really helped with the development of my education in this field and this chapter.

References

Ardern, C., Taylor, N., Feller, J., Webster, K., 2014. Fifty-five percent to competitive sport following anterior cruciate ligament reconstruction surgery: an updated systematic review and meta-analysis including aspects of physical functioning and contextual factors. British Journal of Sports Medicine 48 (21), 1543–1552.

Bartlett, R., 2007. Introduction to Sports Biomechanics. Routledge, London.

Billiet, L., Swinnen, T., De Vlam, K., Westhovens, R., Van Huffel, S., 2018. Recognition of physical activities from a single arm-worn accelerometer: a multiway approach. Informatics 5, 20.

Buckthorpe, M., Roi, G.S., 2018. The time has come to incorporate a greater focus on rate of force development training in the sports injury rehabilitation process. Muscles, Ligaments and Tendons Journal 7 (3), 435–441.

Claiborne, T.L., Armstrong, C.W., Gandhi, V., Pincivero, D.M., 2006. Relationship between hip and knee strength and knee valgus during a single leg squat. Journal of Applied Biomechanics 22 (1), 41–50.

Clark, M., Lucett, S., Sutton, B., 2013. NASM Essentials Of Corrective Exercise Training. Jones & Bartlett Learning/National Academy of Sports Medicine, Burlington, MA.

Demarin, V., Morovic, S., Bene, R., 2014. Neuroplasticity. Periodicum Biologorum 116 (2), 209–211.

Di Stasi, S., Myer, G.D., Hewett, T.E., 2013. Neuromuscular training to target deficits associated with second anterior cruciate ligament injury. The Journal of Orthopaedic & Sports Physical Therapy 43 (11), 777–A11.

Doyon, J., Benali, H., 2005. Reorganization and plasticity in the adult brain during learning of motor skills. Current Opinions in Neurobiology 15 (2), 161–167.

Goerger, B., Marshall, S., Beutler, A., Blackburn, J., Wilckens, J., Padua, D., 2014. Anterior cruciate ligament injury alters pre-injury lower extremity biomechanics in the injured and uninjured leg: the JUMP-ACL study. British Journal of Sports Medicine 49 (3), 188–195.

Grooms, D., Appelbaum, G., Onate, J., 2015. Neuroplasticity following anterior cruciate ligament injury: a framework for visual–motor training approaches in rehabilitation. Journal of Orthopaedic Sports Physical Therapy 45 (5), 381–393.

Hamill, J., Knutzen, K., Derrick, T.R., 2015. Biomechanical Basis of Human Movement, fourth ed. Lippincott Williams & Wilkins, Philadelphia, PA.

Hewett, T.E., Myer, G.D., Ford, K.R., Heidt Jr., R.S., Colosimo, A.J., McLean, S.G., et al., 2005. Biomechanical measures of neuromuscular control and valgus loading of the knee predict anterior cruciate ligament injury risk in female athletes: a prospective study. American Journal of Sports Medicine 233 (4), 492–501.

Imwalle, L.E., Myer, G.D., Ford, K.R., Hewett, T.E., 2009. Relationship between hip and knee kinematics in athletic women during cutting manoeuvres: a possible link to noncontact anterior cruciate ligament injury and prevention. Journal of Strength Conditioning Research 23 (8), 2223–2230.

Jamison, S.T., Pan, X., Chaudhari, A.M., 2012. Knee moments during run-to-cut maneuvers are associated with lateral trunk positioning. The Journal of Biomechanics 45 (11), 1881–1885.

Khayambashi, K., Fallah, A., Movahedi, A., Bagwell, J., Powers, C., 2014. Posterolateral hip muscle strengthening versus quadriceps strengthening for patellofemoral pain: a comparative control trial. Archives of Physical Medicine and Rehabilitation 95 (5), 900–907.

Khayambashi, K., Ghoddosi, N., Straub, R.K., Powers, C.M., 2016. Hip muscle strength predicts noncontact anterior cruciate ligament injury in male and female athletes: a prospective study. American Journal of Sports Medicine 44 (2), 355–361.

Lally, P., van Jaarsveld, C.H.M., Potts, H.W.W., Wardle, J., 2010. How are habits formed: modelling habit formation in the real world. European Journal of Social Psychology 40, 998–1009.

Leppänen, M., Pasanen, K., Kujala, U.M., 2017. Stiff landings are associated with increased ACL injury risk in young female basketball and floorball players. The American Journal of Sports Medicine 45 (2), 386–393.

Myer, G.D., Ford, K.R., Hewett, T.E., 2011. New method to identify athletes at high risk of ACL injury using clinic-based measurements and freeware computer analysis. The British Journal of Sports Medicine 45 (4), 238–244.

Myer, G.D., Ford, K.R., Hewett, T.E., 2004. Rationale and clinical techniques for anterior cruciate ligament injury prevention among female athletes. Journal of Athletic Training 39 (4), 352–364.

Paterno, M., Schmitt, L., Ford, K., Rauh, M., Myer, G., Huang, B., et al., 2010. Biomechanical measures during landing and postural stability predict second anterior cruciate ligament injury after anterior cruciate ligament reconstruction and return to sport. American Journal of Sports Medicine 38 (10), 1968–1978.

Peh, S.Y., Chow, J.Y., Davids, K., 2011. Focus of attention and its impact on movement behaviour. The Journal of Science and Medicine in Sport 14 (1), 70–78.

Pollard, C.D., Sigward, S.M., Powers, C.M., 2010. Limited hip and knee flexion during landing is associated with increased frontal plane knee motion and moments. Clinical Biomechanics 25 (2), 142–146.

Sigward, S.M., Powers, C.M., 2007. Loading characteristics of females exhibiting excessive valgus moments during cutting. Clinical Biomechanics 22 (7), 827–833.

Stastny, P., Tufano, J.J., Golas, A., Petr, M., 2016. Strengthening the gluteus medius using various bodyweight and resistance exercises. Journal of Strength and Conditioning Research 38 (3), 91–101.

Tran, A.A., Gatewood, C., Harris, A.H.S., Thompson, J.A., Dragoo, J.L., 2016. The effect of foot landing position on biomechanical risk factors associated with anterior cruciate ligament injury. The Journal of Experimental Orthopaedics 3, 13.

Zazulak, B.T., Hewett, T.E., Reeves, N.P., Goldberg, B., Cholewicki, J., 2007. Deficits in neuromuscular control of the trunk predict knee injury risk: a prospective biomechanical–epidemiologic study. American Journal of Sports Medicine 35 (7), 1123–1130.

Chapter | **39** |

Conditioning efficacy: a road map for optimizing outcomes in performance-based rehabilitation

Claire Minshull

Introduction

Whether we are dealing with the high-performance professional athlete or the recreational sports performer, injury can mean the undesirable cessation of training or performance, or both. The aim of any subsequent sports rehabilitation programme is to enable the performer to return to sports, safely, effectively and, ideally, as quickly as possible.

The development and deployment of a successful rehabilitation plan often requires the rehabilitation professional to have the knowledge and command of several different disciplines from kinesiology to strength and conditioning, behavioural psychology to imagery and diagnostics. With all of these requirements, coupled with the pressures of getting the athlete back to sport quickly, one can be forgiven for letting something drop off the list. Unfortunately, this can sometimes mean overlooking some of the basic principles that fundamentally drive adaptation and thus successful recovery.

Outside the realms of well-funded elite sport, with plentiful resources and multidisciplinary teams, there are often shortages of time, expertise, personnel, equipment and funding. Often rehabilitation professionals are limited to a single session per week with an athlete, yet the goal remains the same: to get the athlete back to sport as soon as possible.

In this chapter we introduce the concept of *conditioning efficacy* and a process to follow to provide best opportunity to achieve the desired outcomes from your intervention. We address how to structure rehabilitation to enhance favourable neuromuscular adaptation, and explore how to leverage science to optimize the efficacy of rehabilitation and end-stage conditioning. The aim is to equip you with more tools to achieve the best results, even under some of the most demanding of conditions.

Before we delve into conditioning efficacy, we will look at the fundamental factors that determine dynamic joint stability and, thus, the factors that we want to influence in our rehabilitation endeavours, using the knee as an example.

Dynamic knee joint stability

Joint stability is determined by the complex interaction of contributions from both 'passive' and 'active' structures. The passive structures represent the osseous geometry, menisci, ligaments, tendons, etc. Whilst we recognize that they are not truly passive, i.e., they have sensory tissue that modulates reflex responses (Çabuk and Çabuk, 2016; Solomonow, 2006), the musculature, which represents the 'active' side of the model, has a greater role in joint stabilization under dynamic conditions and thus protects these vulnerable joint structures (Fig. 39.1). Dynamic activities of increasing intensity and complexity require increasing contributions from the active structures (i.e., the musculature). For example, standing still, we can maintain stability at the knee by 'locking' out the knees via the 'screw home' mechanism (Box 39.1). However, during strenuous activities involving rapid accelerations, decelerations and directional changes, mechanical joint loading has the potential to exceed the tensile capacities of connecting tissue; these

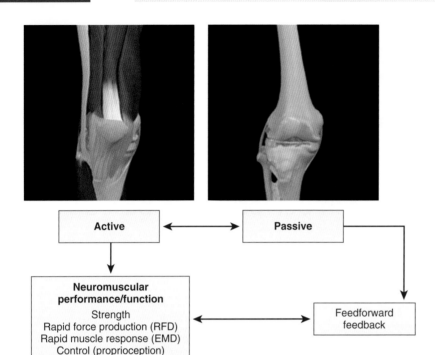

Active ←→ Passive

Neuromuscular
performance/function
Strength
Rapid force production (RFD)
Rapid muscle response (EMD)
Control (proprioception) ←→ Feedforward feedback

Fig. 39.1 A conceptual model
for knee joint stability. *EMD*,
Electromechanical delay; *RFD*, rate
of force development.

Box 39.1 The 'screw home' mechanism

This is the rotation between the tibia and femur occurring
at the end of knee extension, between full extension
(0 degrees) and 20 degrees of knee flexion. External
rotation of the tibia occurs during the terminal degrees of
knee extension and results in tightening of both cruciate
ligaments, which locks the knee. The tibia is then in the
position of maximal stability with respect to the femur.

---

forces must be counteracted effectively by contributions
from the surrounding musculature (Blackburn et al., 2008;
Minshull et al., 2012a)

The importance of neuromuscular capabilities to the
maintenance of dynamic joint stability and the avoidance of noncontact injuries is widely recognized (Hannah et al., 2014; Hewett et al., 2013). Neuromuscular
performance parameters that have been used to estimate injury risk include: muscle strength, defined as
the maximal amount of force that can be exerted in a
single effort; rate of force development (RFD), defined
as rate of rise in contractile force; and preceding all is
the response time of the musculature, termed electromechanical delay (EMD). EMD is defined as the time delay
between the onset of electrical activity and the onset of
muscle force production and is determined by a number

of physiological processes to get the muscle into a state
of 'readiness' to produce substantial force. The faster
these processes occur, the faster muscle force can be initiated and produced. Of course, the resulting patterning
of muscular responses must be performed in a controlled
manner that is appropriate for the situation. Review of
this sensorimotor performance (also called proprioception) constitutes a chapter in itself and is outside the
scope of our focus here on neuromuscular activation and
force production.

Injuries typically happen very quickly, often within milliseconds (Krosshaug et al., 2007). Thus successful dynamic
joint stabilization during sudden loading is dependent on
the temporal parameters related to the initiation, development and magnitude of the muscle force response
(Blackburn et al., 2008; Minshull et al., 2012a), i.e., the
production of sufficient force to harness these harmful
joint forces very quickly. This posits the question: What is
the relative importance of muscle strength? Whilst muscle
strength, or peak torque, is easy to measure and has been
the primary index used in several return-to-sport criteria,
such as the limb symmetry index (Zwolski et al., 2015), we
might be missing a trick if we solely focus on 'the maximum amount of force that can be produced in a single
contraction'.

Let us conceptually explore this using a simple illustration of a force–time curve of a maximal voluntary isometric
contraction (MVIC).

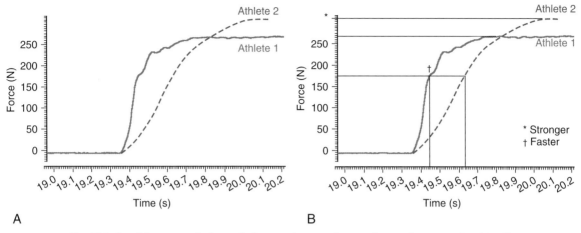

Fig. 39.2 Quadriceps muscle force during maximum voluntary isometric contraction *(MVIC)*.

Fig. 39.2 illustrates that Athlete 2 is stronger than Athlete 1 (see * on the curve) during this maximal knee extension test. However, if we consider the rate of force production, even though Athlete 1 is weaker they are able to 'produce' force much more quickly, as evidenced by a steeper gradient of the force–time curve. Measured against an arbitrary amount of muscle force of, for example, 175 N, we can see that it takes Athlete 2 almost 200 ms longer to produce this compared to Athlete 1 (see † on the curve). The emergency response, i.e., the neuromuscular response during critical threats to the stability of the joint system (Minshull et al., 2007), is a coordinated response from multiple muscle groups. If we consider that anterior cruciate ligament (ACL) injuries may happen within 50 ms of foot contact with ground (Koga et al., 2010), and that it typically takes >300 ms to achieve maximal force during an isometric contraction (Hannah et al., 2014), we can see the importance of speed of the first neuromuscular response to resist mechanical threats to musculoskeletal integrity.

Now that we have covered the basics of neuromuscular performance, let us address the topic of conditioning efficacy (CE).

Conditioning efficacy for performance-based rehabilitation

What do we mean by *conditioning efficacy*? Efficacy is 'the ability to produce a desired or intended result'. Therefore, we are talking about ability to achieve the performance or rehabilitation outcomes through the conditioning prescribed – and of course adhered to (see Chapter 43 on patient 'buy in'). A single generic programme will not deliver all the desired outcomes discussed thus far, such as

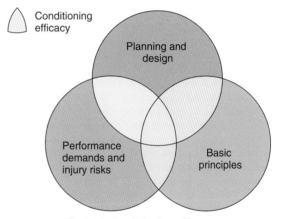

Fig. 39.3 Conditioning efficacy.

strength, rate of force development, muscle response times and sensorimotor performance; neither will managing athletes 'on the fly' – although the temptation can be great when short on time. Without a progressive systematic plan to achieve specific outcomes, incremental improvements in performance will start to diminish, as will your returns on investment.

Achieving conditioning efficacy (Fig. 39.3) requires upfront preparation and the determination of goals (see Programme planning and design). It also requires an understanding of the basic principles that underpin adaptation and methods that ensure you are delivering the right stimulus to elicit the desired physiologic adaptation (see Addressing basic principles). Finally, to achieve a successful return to sport, we need deployment of the newly formed neuromuscular capacities in relevant and unpredictable performance-based situations to build resilience against future injury (see Performance demands and injury risks).

Programme planning and design

As acknowledged above, a single generic programme will not deliver multiple desired outcomes. Different neuromuscular stimuli, and thus adaptations, will be produced by manipulation of the number of repetitions, sets, load/intensity and periods of rest within an exercise programme.

To deliver the most effective sports rehabilitation programme we need a clear vision of its ultimate aim. Multiple short-term goals will be established in the planning phases that enable a systematic and progressive approach towards achieving this aim. The programme can then be optimally designed for each of the component parts, such that efforts can be invested accordingly to achieve these goals. Decisions such as how important absolute muscle strength is compared to fast muscle response times (EMD) or cardiovascular fitness will need to be made within each phase to hone the focus.

Muscle strength is important to dynamic joint stability and shock-absorption capabilities; therefore, in individuals where strength capacity has been dramatically depleted, for example in the frail and elderly, or following prolonged injury, surgical intervention and immobilization, muscle strength might form a principal focus of the preliminary phases of rehabilitation. However, in a high-performance athlete who has suffered a less severe injury and only limited absence from training, their strength capacity may be depleted to a lesser degree and restored much more quickly. The principal focus here may be on establishing a quick speed of muscle response (EMD) and ability to produce some of their strength very quickly (RFD). Indeed, compromised temporal neuromuscular capabilities may have constituted a risk factor for the initial injury!

Threats to conditioning efficacy

The threats to conditioning efficacy here are improper design and planning. This can simply be due to lack of time or, crucially, thinking that we do not have enough time to devote to planning. This means that the chance of diminishing returns increases, whereby the benefits gained continually diminish for the amount of effort invested. Some of the controllable negative effects resulting from improper planning that threaten conditioning efficacy are given below.

Fatigue

Repeated high-intensity muscle contractions or bouts of exercise can cause progressive losses to performance (Minshull et al., 2012a); for example, a progressive reduction in muscle strength of up to 15% was reported following a basketball match simulation (Ansdell and Dekerle, 2020). The

underpinning mechanisms are likely to mean that training in a fatigued state will have a negative impact on the potential for adaptation.

Consider the sequencing of exercise and, more importantly, rest periods within each session to maximize the opportunity for recovery and thus for conditioning efficacy. For example, if time dictates that your session must involve a muscle strengthening component as well as match agility training, how will you sequence these exercises? Intrasession exercise order may influence the magnitude of physiological adaptations. Performing strength training prior to endurance type exercise may minimize the intrusion of muscle fatigue and optimize the opportunity for both neuromuscular and cardiovascular gains and vice versa (Coffey and Hawley, 2017). Likewise, challenging sensorimotor performance exercises on unstable surfaces, requiring pivoting, directional changes and challenges to balance requires significant contributions from the fast twitch motor unit capacity. Preceding fatiguing exercise with insufficient rest may compromise the ability for fast twitch motor unit activation and present an increased risk for injury as well as suboptimal opportunity for adaptation.

Carry-over effects – exercise-induced muscle damage

Skeletal muscle is susceptible to ultrastructural damage following unaccustomed high-intensity eccentric exercise. This may be evident in the athlete who commences training, match play or rehabilitation following a prolonged period of inactivity or injury-related deconditioning (Minshull et al., 2012b). Exercise-induced muscle damage (EIMD) is predominantly caused by eccentric muscle activity whereby the muscle lengthens whilst under load, such as downhill running, the lowering phase during resistance exercise, landing from a jump, etc. Major functional consequences of EIMD include prolonged reductions in muscle strength, rate of force development, power and balance of between 15% and 70% (Power et al., 2012; Sayers and Clarkson, 2001) that peak 24–48 hours postexercise (Hyldahl et al., 2014).

Eccentric muscle training should form an important component of any rehabilitation programme, since most sporting activities require high-level performance under these conditions (e.g., decelerations, direction changes) and the resulting microtrauma and remodelling is important for neuromuscular gains and morphological changes. However, as with the case of muscle fatigue, it is important to consider the sequencing of exercise, particularly within-day sequencing. Due to preferential damage to the fast twitch muscle fibres (Hyldahl et al., 2014), it is plausible that an RFD or muscle strength training intervention is unlikely to elicit the same gains in a muscle symptomatic of damage compared with an undamaged muscle, particularly

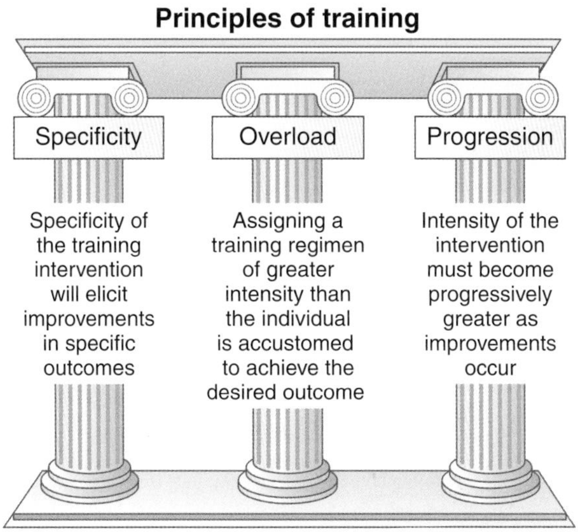

Principles of training

Fig. 39.4 Principles of training.

where soreness might cue reduced levels of volitional effort. In the absence of complex dynamometry systems, simple assessments of delayed-onset muscle soreness (DOMS) on a visual analogue scale and functional vertical jumping tests may help the practitioner monitor recovery.

Techniques to enhance conditioning efficacy

Basic principles of training will determine the efficacy of your intervention (i.e., achieving the outcomes that you want to achieve). These are: specificity, overload and progression (Kraemer and Ratamess, 2004) (Fig. 39.4). These fundamental pillars are well established in the performance literature, but unfortunately do not appear as frequently within rehabilitation research (Minshull and Gleeson, 2017). Application of these principles will ensure that your intervention is likely to elicit the desired outcome, whether that be increased muscle strength, sprint speed or cardiovascular fitness.

Specificity

Specificity of the training intervention will elicit improvements in specific outcomes. Following injury an aim might be to 'increase the strength of the knee muscles'. However, a far more specific and measurable aim would be to 'increase the strength of the hamstrings by 20%'.

Overload

This term refers to assigning a training regimen of greater physical demand than the individual is accustomed to in

order to achieve the desired outcome. This is determined by the training intensity, volume, repetitions, sets, rest and frequency, which will be addressed in the next section.

Progression

This means that the physical demand of the intervention must become progressively greater as improvements occur. If an aim is to promote a strength adaptation, we need to plan how to maintain this strengthening stimulus as adaptation occurs. Incidentally, this does not mean increase the number of repetitions.

Addressing basic principles

In a recent systematic review of resistance training (compared to a nonexercise control) for the management of knee osteoarthritis, we found that the basic principles of specificity, overload and progression were inconsistently applied and inadequately reported across all studies eligible for review (Minshull and Gleeson, 2017).

Let us say you have determined that a major goal for your athlete is to increase muscle strength of the quadriceps. An exercise that is commonly prescribed, for any joint, might be: 3 sets of 10–12 repetitions of knee extensions with a resistance band. Is this *really* a strength training exercise?

Here are a few further questions:
- Why the 10–12 repetition range?
- What happens when 12 repetitions can be easily achieved?
- Relating to the above, do you increase to 20 repetitions?
- What determines exercise cessation?

This series of simple questions really challenges the rationale for the intervention. If the efficacy of conditioning has been properly considered and the programme planned to achieve the outcomes intended, they will stand up to scrutiny. However, this type of exercise is *not* a muscle strength exercise *per se*. It will condition muscle endurance. Whilst some changes in muscle strength may be achieved in the very early phases of rehabilitation, where the athlete has experienced significant muscle atrophy or they are new to resistance training, these effects will quickly plateau. Thereafter larger muscle forces are required to optimally elicit changes in maximal muscle strength.

To optimally condition muscle we refer to the strength–endurance continuum of resistance training (Peterson et al., 2005) (Fig. 39.5). This describes how programmes using low repetitions and high resistance (3–5 repetitions maximum; RM) will elicit optimal adaptation of strength, whereas training with high repetitions and low resistance (≥12RM) promotes muscular endurance (Fleck and Kraemer, 2014). There

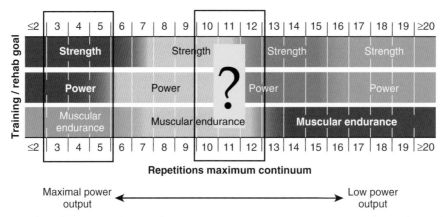

Fig. 39.5 The strength–endurance continuum of resistance training. 'Repetitions maximum' refers to the number of repetitions that can be performed (with correct form) against a resistance; 5RM means a failure to perform the sixth repetition. (Adapted from Baechle, T., Earle, R., 2008. Essentials of Strength Training and Conditioning, third ed. Human Kinetics, Champaign, Ill; Fleck, S.J., Kraemer, W.J., 2014. Designing Resistance Training Programmes. fourth ed. Human Kinetics, Champaign, Ill.)

are other ways to measure and ensure that the muscle receives sufficient overload, such as using a calculated percentage of 1RM. However, this requires a maximal 1RM test that the patient may not be able to tolerate and it is difficult to progress the load in the absence of supervision and repeat testing. By assigning a number of RMs (e.g., 3–5), the individual is able to individually determine what that represents in terms of load and progress it independently as adaptation occurs.

A classic study by Campos et al. (2002) illustrated this very nicely. Thirty-two participants were divided into four groups: a low repetition group performing 3–5RM for four sets of leg press, squat and knee extension; an intermediate repetition group performing 9–11RM for three sets (same exercises); a high repetition group performing 20–28RM for two sets (same exercises); and a nonexercising control group. All exercising groups performed the same volume of training. Maximal dynamic strength (leg press 1RM) improved significantly more for the low repetition group (61%) compared to the other training groups (36% and 32%). Not surprisingly, the greatest gains in muscle endurance, measured as the number of repetitions performed at 60% 1RM (leg press), was shown in the high repetition group (94% vs. a 20% loss in the low repetition group).

It is probably not wise to suddenly load up muscles unaccustomed to resistance training in this manner. However, this does show that proper planning and design enable a progressive approach to efficacious muscle strengthening. Incidentally, exactly the same basic principles apply to interventions to condition other neuromuscular parameters.

Rehabilitating rate of force development

As we have already established, RFD is the ability to rapidly develop muscular force. The determinants of RFD include the recruitment of fast twitch motor units, the rapidity of cross-bridge cycling and the stiffness of muscle and connective tissue (Maffiuletti et al., 2016). Accordingly, improvements in any of these factors are likely to bring about a positive adaptation in RFD. Whilst studies have suggested numerous modalities can elicit improvements in RFD, in individuals accustomed to exercise, high-load resistance, and ballistic training have been shown to improve RFD (Bogdanis et al., 2018; Farup et al., 2014).

Rehabilitating electromechanical delay

Electromechanical delay – the time lag between the onset of electrical activity and the onset of force production – is determined by the recruitment of motor units, the propagation of the action potential through the muscle and the stretch of the series elastic component (the viscoelastic structures including tendon, aponeurosis and muscle fibres) (Nordez et al., 2009). Under most circumstances the delay is principally determined by how 'stretchy' this connective tissue is: the stretchier it is, the longer it takes to transmit muscle force to bone. Therefore, efficacious conditioning of EMD will involve interventions to promote fast twitch motor unit activation and, perhaps more importantly, connective tissue stiffness. Exercise modalities include heavy resistance training (Stock et al., 2016).

Threats to conditioning efficacy

The consequences of disuse when managing an injured athlete include losses to muscle strength, cross-sectional area and changes to neural drive (Farthing and Zehr, 2014). These can be exacerbated in the injured limb by pain and effusion

(Fitzgerald, 2005) and are driven by arthrogenic muscle inhibition (AMI). AMI is an ongoing neural inhibition that prevents the central nervous system from fully activating the musculature. This means that maximal muscle activation is not achievable and, as such, the efficacy of any associated conditioning requiring this will likely achieve suboptimal outcomes. Below are three evidence-based techniques to mitigate influence of AMI.

Techniques to enhance conditioning efficacy

Mode and range of muscle activation

Consider mode of muscle activation. Typically it follows a concentric–eccentric pattern as muscles contract and get shorter to lift a resistance and then lengthen under load to control the deceleration of the load. What are your options if an inhibitory pain response is elicited? Can you identify when in the movement pain is elicited? If it relates to the concentric part, is it possible to focus solely on the lowering (eccentric) part? Eccentric strength training protocols, when tailored to eccentric capacity, can elicit greater gains in muscle strength compared to concentric training (Roig et al., 2009). If any forceful dynamic contraction is not possible, consider isometric contractions. You can manipulate the range to identify a comfortable joint position. As well as inducing neuromuscular changes at the selected joint position, maximal isometric training at long muscle lengths has been shown to confer changes to concentric strength, i.e., under dynamic conditions (Noorkõiv et al., 2015).

Speed of muscle activation

Pain is perceived in just less than a second after the stimulus is applied and repetition of that stimulus within 3 seconds increases the intensity of the pain sensation (Barrell and Price, 1975). Therefore, very short duration efforts of ≤1 s may be sufficient to bypass the pain response and its inhibitory effects. Combined with the technique of modulating the type of muscle activation, you have opportunity to induce heavy loads for a very short time. With sufficient rest, this might provide an efficacious stimulus for developing muscle force- and speed-generating capacities.

Cross-education

What happens if the pain, effusion or dysfunction is just too much to overcome? Perhaps the limb is in a cast or there are clinical constraints that prevent heavy resistance exercise. The cross-education phenomenon describes the strength gain in the opposite, untrained limb following unilateral resistance training of the 'trained' limb. In practice this means that properly designed strength training in the noninjured limb can elicit gains, or attenuate decline,

in the injured limb. Under certain circumstances, strength gains may be as much as 50% of that observed for the trained side (Farthing and Zehr, 2014).

The cross-education effect is a well-documented phenomenon in sports performance and physiology literature. However, it is a little-used technique in rehabilitation where, arguably, there are the greatest opportunities for impact. This phenomenon is thought, in part, to be due to a neural adaptation and 'spill-over' of unintended motor activity from the trained to the untrained motor cortex during forceful unilateral contractions. For a comprehensive review of the cross-education effect see Hendy and Lamon (2017). In order to maximize strength gains in the untrained side, the resistance training intervention on the trained side must be of sufficiently high intensity and volume, and adhere to the principles of specificity, overload and progression. A personal and qualitative review of the relevant literature shows that a minimal dose of 300+ repetitions, adhering to a strength training focus (high load, low reps), is likely required. Further, a recent meta-analysis reported the potential for a slightly greater effect via eccentric training (Manca et al., 2017).

Performance demands and injury risks

The rehabilitation practitioner should understand the demands of the sport for both performance needs and to build resilience against future injury. This makes possible the design of appropriate exercises to promote the deployment of newly formed neuromuscular capacities in unpredictable performance-based situations. In planning return to play, the practitioner must establish which factors are most important at what stage of the rehabilitation and then ensure the programme is designed to achieve this. Here we are balancing restoration of function, performance needs and muscle capacity, coupled with the understanding of the threats imposed by sport-specific competition and training-based exercise stress.

For example, common performance demands of sprinting and team sports are fast accelerations and straight-line speed. However, whilst sprinting involves short performance demands in a predominantly sagittal plane in a predictable environment, team sports involve multiple accelerations, decelerations, changing of direction and multiplanar performance demands in an often unpredictable environment. Accordingly, the injury risks and injury profiles are different between these sports, with the exception of a high incidence of hamstring strains, perhaps. Thus, team sports require an additional progressive approach to conditioning fast muscle response times and RFD across multiple planes to successfully attenuate dynamic loading during high-speed directional changes. Different again, consider gymnasts who are

Hierarchy of importance

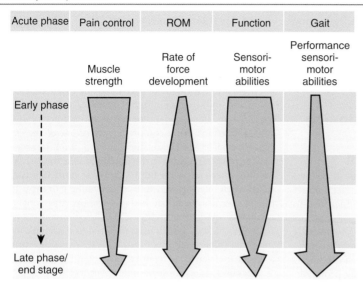

Fig. 39.6 **Rehabilitating neuromuscular performance.** Example hierarchy of importance throughout a performance-based rehabilitation programme. *ROM*, Range of motion.

exposed to many high-impact landings during apparatus dismounting, sometimes performing in excess of 200 dismounts per week (Özguven and Berme, 1988). Given that over one-third of all injuries sustained by young competitive females occur during dismounting (Caine et al., 1988), conditioning here should focus on progressively enhancing the ability to resist and to attenuate the reaction forces in a controlled manner to maintain joint stability.

A hypothetical example of the hierarchy of importance of neuromuscular factors within an ACL rehabilitation programme is shown in Fig. 39.6. After addressing the range of motion (ROM), pain and restoration of gait in the acute postoperative phase, the principal focus in the early stages of rehabilitation is strength development and sensorimotor (proprioception) abilities. As strength and control is improved, the focus shifts towards improving explosive muscle force production (RFD), finally culminating in the performance–sensorimotor abilities, whereby dynamic exercises are representative of the sports-specific demands and threats. By the time we reach the final stages of a rehabilitation programme and prepare for return to play, the athlete will have achieved the required foundations in strength, explosive force production and 'static' sensorimotor performance. The focus becomes being able to deploy it functionally through safe exposure to unpredictable, less stable scenarios – in effect, practicing for the emergency scenario. An example might be building from low-velocity directional change drills within the sports-specific environment (i.e., on the pitch, court) to high-velocity directional change drills involving performance tasks and subtle changes in surface stability.

Once return to play has been achieved, the preservation of these prophylactic gains throughout the competitive season requires a structured plan that takes account of the acute physical effects of single training sessions and performances, the carry-over effects of the seasonal training and performance timetable and the recovery required for adequate restoration of neuromuscular capacities. Clearly, each sport will differ in the volume and type of physical demands (in relation to elite rugby, see Chapter 37).

Threats to conditioning efficacy

Specific threats to conditioning efficacy here are varied and will be determined by the sport-specific situation. However, clearly a lack of understanding of the sports performance demands and injury risks will influence the effectiveness of a successful return to play. For continued preservation of prophylactic effects there are a few common factors to consider:

Cumulative effects

The cumulative effects of sports-specific training and competition can relate to intrasession effects such as acute muscle fatigue or intersession effects such as exercise-induced muscle damage. We have covered some of the deleterious effects to performance and neuromuscular capacities in the previous section.

Training load

This is a big topic, incorporating many different measures of load. However, recent research focused specifically on high-speed running proposes this as a risk factor for injury. Bear in mind that this research is still in its infancy and more high-quality investigation is required. Nevertheless, it is interesting to note that large training volumes at high speeds and large weekly changes in high-speed running have been correlated with injury risk in soccer and Australian rules football (Malone et al., 2018; Saw et al., 2018).

Techniques to enhance conditioning efficacy

The repeated bout effect

The repeated bout (RB) effect refers to the adaptation whereby a single bout of eccentric exercise protects against the consequences of subsequent eccentric bouts (Nosaka and Marcelo, 2011), meaning that compared to the first bout, a second bout of lengthening contractions is associated with a decreased loss of contractile force, less soreness, and a reduction in the amount indirect markers of damage in the blood.

We have addressed the potential detrimental effects of eccentric exercise and associated muscle damage in the previous section. However, if planned properly, you can build resilience in your athlete to future episodes. This will be beneficial for periods of congested training and match play. So, how much and when?

A single high-intensity episode of eccentric exercise can result in substantial losses to neuromuscular performance, including progressively increasing losses to hamstring muscle strength and RFD up to 36% and 65%, respectively, at 48 hours postexercise, and a prolonged DOMS response (Minshull et al., 2012b). If the athlete performed exactly the same exercise again days to weeks later, the changes to strength and soreness will be comparably less. Naturally, DOMS is not pleasant and within a competitive season it might not be feasible to degrade athletes' performance to such an extent. So how much is enough?

The dose and intensity of the initial bout determines the length of protective effect: higher intensities and doses that elicit greater muscle damage generally convey the longest protective effects. However, short-lasting effects may be achieved via low-level eccentric contractions that provoke no consequence to neuromuscular performance. For example, eccentric contractions equivalent to only 10% MVIC significantly attenuated the magnitude of muscle damage induced by a subsequent bout of maximal eccentric exercise in the knee flexors and extensors for up to 7 days (Lin et al., 2015). Therefore, with appropriate inseason planning, episodes of low-level eccentric resistance exercise could be used prophylactically to attenuate performance losses associated with epochs of condensed performance demands. There are other ways of eliciting the RB effect, such as isometric contractions at long muscle lengths. However, this is beyond the scope of this chapter and the reader is referred to Nosaka and Marcelo (2011) for an excellent review led by a highly respected authority in the field.

Conclusion

Often multiple competing demands and constraints on time and resources seek to sabotage conditioning efficacy and thus the ability to achieve a swift and safe return to play. Herein is a framework to focus your thinking and enhance your interventions – to ultimately make sure your desired aims and your rehabilitation plan are aligned. A progressive, systematic plan incorporating the basic principles of conditioning and adaptation is the foundation to achieving your rehabilitation outcomes. Thereafter, any new training methods, techniques and technologies can be dovetailed in to achieve marginal gains. Get the basics right, and the rest will follow.

References

Ansdell, P., Dekerle, J., 2020. Sodium bicarbonate supplementation delays neuromuscular fatigue without changes in performance outcomes during a basketball match simulation protocol. Journal of Strength and Conditioning Research 34 (5), 1369–1375.

Barrell, J.J., Price, D.D., 1975. The perception of first and second pain as a function of psychological set. Perception and Psychophysics 17 (2), 163–166.

Blackburn, J.T., Bell, D.R., Norcross, M.F., Hudson, J.D., Engstrom, L.A., 2008. Comparison of hamstring neuromechanical properties between healthy males and females and the influence of musculotendinous stiffness. Journal of Electromyography and Kinesiology 19, e362–e369.

Bogdanis, G.C., Tsoukos, A., Brown, L.E., Selima, E., Veligekas, P., Spengos, K., et al. 2018. Muscle fiber and performance changes after fast eccentric complex training. Medicine & Science in Sports & Exercise 50 (4), 729–738.

Çabuk, H., Çabuk, F.K., 2016. Mechanoreceptors of the ligaments and tendons around the knee. Clinical Anatomy 29 (6), 789–795.

Caine, D., Cochrane, B., Caine, C., Zemper, E., 1988. An epidemiologic investigation of injuries affecting young competitive female gymnasts. The American Journal of Sports Medicine 17, 811–820.

Campos, G.E., Luecke, T.J., Wendeln, H.K., Toma, K., Hagerman, F.C., Murray, T.F., et al. 2002. Muscular adaptations in response to three different resistance-training regimens: specificity of repetition maximum training zones. European Journal of Applied Physiology 88, 50–60.

Coffey, V.G., Hawley, J.A., 2017. Concurrent exercise training: do opposites distract? The Journal of Physiology 595 (9), 2883–2896.

Farthing, J.P., Zehr, E.P., 2014. Restoring symmetry: clinical applications of cross-education. Exercise and Sport Sciences Reviews 42 (2), 70–75.

Farup, J., Sørensen, H., Kjølhede, T., 2014. Similar changes in muscle fiber phenotype with differentiated consequences for rate of force development: endurance versus resistance training. Human Movement Science 34, 109–119.

Fitzgerald, G.K., 2005. Therapeutic exercise for knee osteoarthritis; considering factors that may influence outcome. Europa Medicophysica 41, 163–171.

Fleck, S.J., Kraemer, W.J., 2014. Designing Resistance Training Programmes, fourth ed. Human Kinetics, Champaign, Ill.

Hannah, R., Minshull, C., Smith, S.L., Folland, J.P., 2014. Longer electromechanical delay impairs hamstrings explosive force versus quadriceps. Medicine & Science in Sports & Exercise 46 (5), 963–972.

Hendy, A.M., Lamon, S., 2017. The cross-education phenomenon: brain and beyond. Frontiers in Physiology 8, 297.

Hewett, T.E., Di Stasi, S.L., Myer, G.D., 2013. Current concepts for injury prevention in athletes after anterior cruciate ligament reconstruction. The American Journal of Sports Medicine 41 (1), 216–224.

Hyldahl, R.D., Hubal, M.J., 2014. Lengthening our perspective: morphological, cellular, and molecular responses to eccentric exercise. Muscle Nerve 49 (2), 155–170.

Koga, H., Nakamae, A., Shima, Y., Iwasa, J., Myklebust, G., Engebretsen, L., et al., 2010. Mechanisms for noncontact anterior cruciate ligament injuries: knee joint kinematics in 10 injury situations from female team handball and basketball. The American Journal of Sports Medicine 38 (11), 2218–2225.

Kraemer, W.J., Ratamess, N.A., 2004. Fundamentals of resistance training: progression and exercise prescription. Medicine & Science in Sports & Exercise 36, 674–688.

Krosshaug, T., Slauterbeck, J.R., Engebretsen, L., Bahr, R., 2007. Analysis of anterior cruciate ligament injury mechanisms: three-dimensional motion reconstruction from video sequences. The Scandinavian Journal of Medicine Science in Sports 17, 508–519.

Lin, M.J., Chen, T.C., Chen, H.L., Wu, B.H., Nosaka, K., 2015. Low-intensity eccentric contractions of the knee extensors and flexors protect against muscle damage. Applied Physiology, Nutrition, and Metabolism 40, 1004–1011.

Maffiuletti, N.A., Aagaard, P., Blazevich, A.J., Folland, J., Tillin, N., Duchateau, J., 2016. Rate of force development: physiological and methodological considerations. European Journal of Applied Physiology 116 (6), 1091–1116.

Malone, S., Owen, A., Mendes, B., Hughes, B., Collins, K., Gabbebtt, T.J., 2018. High-speed running and sprinting as an injury risk factor in soccer: can well-developed physical qualities reduce the risk? The Journal of Science and Medicine in Sport 21 (3), 257–262.

Manca, A., Dragone, D., Dvir, Z., Deriu, F., 2017. Cross-education of muscular strength following unilateral resistance training: a meta-analysis. European Journal of Applied Physiology 117, 2335–2354.

Minshull, C., Eston, R., Rees, D., Gleeson, N., 2012b. Knee joint neuromuscular activation performance during muscle damage and superimposed fatigue. Journal of Sports Sciences 30 (10), 1015–1024.

Minshull, C., Gleeson, N., Walters-Edwards, M., Eston, R., Rees, D., 2007. Effects of acute fatigue on the volitional and magnetically-evoked electromechanical delay of the knee flexors in males and females. European Journal of Applied Physiology 100, 469–478.

Minshull, C., Eston, R., Bailey, A., Rees, D., Gleeson, N., 2012a. Repeated exercise stress impairs volitional but not magnetically evoked electromechanical delay of the knee flexors. Journal of Sports Sciences 30 (2), 217–225.

Minshull, C., Gleeson, N., 2017. Considerations of the principles of resistance training in exercise studies for the management of knee osteoarthritis: a systematic review. Archives of Physical Medicine and Rehabilitation 98 (9), 1842–1851.

Noorkõiv, M., Nosaka, K., Blazevich, A.J., 2015. Effects of isometric quadriceps strength training at different muscle lengths on dynamic torque production. Journal of Sports Sciences 33 (18), 1952–1961.

Nordez, A., Gallot, T., Catheline, S., Guével, A., Cornu, C., Hug, F., 2009. Electromechanical delay revisited using very high frame rate ultrasound. The Journal of Applied Physiology 106 (6), 1970–1975.

Nosaka, K., Marcelo, A., 2011. Repeated bout effect; research update and future perspective. Brazilian Journal of Biomotricity 5, 5–15.

Özguven, H.N., Berme, N., 1988. An experimental and analytical study of impact forces during human jumping. Journal of Biomechanics 21, 1061–1066.

Peterson, M.D., Rhea, M.R., Alvar, B.R., 2005. Applications of the dose–response for muscular strength development: a review of meta-analytic efficacy and reliability for designing training prescription. Journal of Strength and Conditioning Research 9, 950–958.

Power, G.A., Dalton, B.H., Rice, C.L., Vandervoort, A.A., 2012. Power loss is greater following lengthening contractions in old versus young women. Age (Dordr). 34 (3), 737–750.

Roig, M., O'Brien, K., Kirk, G., Murray, R., McKinnon, P., Shadgan, B., et al. 2009. The effects of eccentric versus concentric resistance training on muscle strength and mass in healthy adults: a systematic review with meta-analysis. The British Journal of Sports Medicine 43 (8), 556–568.

Saw, R., Finch, C.F., Samra, D., Baquie, P., Cardoso, T., Hope, D., et al. 2018. Injuries in Australian rules football: an overview of injury rates, patterns, and mechanisms across all levels of play. The Journal of Science and Medicine in Sport 21 (3), 257–262.

Sayers, S.P., Clarkson, P.M., 2001. Force recovery after eccentric exercise in males and females. European Journal of Applied Physiology 84 (1–2), 122–126.

Solomonow, M., 2006. Sensory-motor control of ligaments and associated neuromuscular disorders. Journal of Electromyography & Kinesiology 16 (6), 549–567.

Stock, M.S., Olinghouse, K.D., Mota, J.A., Drusch, A.S., Thompson, B.J., 2016. Muscle group specific changes in the electromechanical delay following short-term resistance training. The Journal of Science and Medicine in Sport 19 (9), 761–765.

Zwolski, C., Schmitt, L.C., Quatman-Yates, C., Thomas, S., Hewett, T.E., Paterno, M.V., 2015. The influence of quadriceps strength asymmetry on patient-reported function at time of return to sport after anterior cruciate ligament reconstruction. The American Journal of Sports Medicine 43 (9), 2242–2249.

Chapter | **40** |

The 'all-around' athlete: key performance considerations for managing injuries related to the ankle, trunk and tendon in female gymnasts

Jason Laird

Introduction

Managing the health and performance of elite athletes is a demanding task and involves many practitioners working in sport, including those who form part of sports science and sports medicine teams. The fact that athletes work on the edge of what is physically possible, coupled with the inherent risks in repeatedly performing certain physical tasks, makes keeping athletes injury free and available to perform a full time job for many practitioners across the globe. Due to myriad factors, there are certain sports or athletic environments that represent the most challenging end of the continuum when it comes to managing athlete health and performance. Women's artistic gymnastics (WAG) is one such environment.

One of the most important aspects of managing athletic performance and injury is to understand the athletes' 'world' and how they interact with it. Given the typical age profile of WAG athletes and the unique nature of this discipline and its training demands, it is essential that practitioners in this field are aware of the factors that may influence a female gymnast. This enables them to fully address issues that arise and helps support these athletes on their journey towards success. The aim of this chapter is to provide the reader with clear and practical information on the world of a female gymnast and to highlight and reinforce the understanding of critical factors that influence injury, rehabilitation, training and sporting performance. This should help practitioners on the road to supportive success and with it provide a fuller understanding of the 'all-around' female gymnast.

Typical age profile of elite gymnasts

A good starting point in understanding the female gymnast is to know the typical ages of elite-level performers in women's artistic gymnastics. There is a stark difference between the age of male and female gymnastic all-around Olympic champions, with women being, on average, 7 years younger than their male counterparts. The average age for women is 17 years of age and for men it is 24 years of age.

Key factors influencing athlete health in the female gymnast

The gymnast's multidisciplinary team

Holistic care provided by the multidisciplinary team (MDT) is essential when managing a female gymnast. With the variety of personal, physical and sport-related features associated with elite-level gymnastics, it is imperative that an appropriate inclusive communication policy is adopted. Indeed, as well as medical/science practitioners, parents, coaches, teachers, siblings and teammates can combine to make up the gymnast's MDT in the global sense. With the demanding nature of elite-level training and the requirement for specialist coaching, the role of the coach in providing autonomous support, encouragement after mistakes and technical/ tactical expertise plays a key role in motivating the athlete whilst having an effect on minimizing injury risk

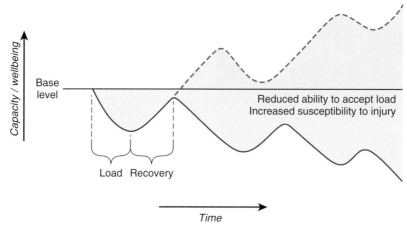

Fig. 40.1 Biological maladaptation through cycles of excessive loading and/or inadequate recovery. (From Soligard, T., Schwellnus, M., Alonso, J.M., Bahr, R., Clarsen, B., Dijkstra, H.P., et al., 2016. How much is too much? (Part 1) International Olympic Committee consensus statement on load in sport and risk of injury. British Journal of Sports Medicine 50 (17), 1030–1041.)

(Knight et al., 2010). By developing relationships with key stakeholders (perhaps most importantly the gymnast's parents and coaches), the practitioner can more successfully manage injury and performance threats by facilitation of the MDT to pull together in the same direction and ensure relevant information is understood and actioned by all.

Growth and maturation

It has been suggested that elite youth athletes are particularly vulnerable to sporting injury due to physical and physiological processes of growth (Popovic et al., 2012). Injury risk factors that are unique to the young athlete include, but are not limited to:

- growth plate vulnerability (Frank et al., 2007)
- peak height velocity, skeletal maturity and the adolescent growth spurt (Niemeyer et al., 2006)
- biologic maturity (Malina et al., 2004)
- postural control (Quatman-Yates et al., 2012)
- volume of training (Loud et al., 2005).

Given that female gymnasts are exposed to training programmes that are higher in volume and intensity than athletes of a similar age in other sports (Burt et al., 2010), it is pertinent for practitioners to be fully aware of these growth and maturation related risk factors. One of the key roles of a practitioner working with a female gymnast is to provide key stakeholders with an awareness of how these risk factors may interact with injury and performance. In addition, it is important that practitioners play a proactive role in addressing modifiable risk factors (in particular postural control and volume of training) during these stages of growth and maturation alongside the parent and coach.

Managing 'load'

In order to fully understand load and its effect on the female gymnast, it is first important to be aware of perceived time constraints commonly attributed to training within women's artistic gymnastics. With female gymnasts being eligible for Olympic selection from the age of 16 years, the time available to introduce and develop technical difficulty into routines is comparably less than for male gymnasts, who are eligible to compete at the Olympics from 18 years of age. This relatively small perceived window of opportunity to introduce and develop technical expertise can result in very high technical training volume loads for female gymnasts at young ages with the aim of maximizing performance improvement. When load is looked at in a more global sense, things such as travel load and psychological load also come into play. Given the typical age and life stage of young female elite gymnasts, they often have a variety of types of load to juggle – for example club training, overseas competitions, school work and exams. This global load concept is important and information should be sought on all these factors when trying to determine how best to affect load and its very real relationship to injury and performance decline. As indicated by a range of authors (Fry et al., 1991; Kenttä and Hassmén, 1998; Kuipers and Keizer, 1988) and represented in Fig. 40.1, a balance between load and recovery is vital; a lack of understanding of this concept can lead to prolonged fatigue, reduced ability to accept load and an increase in the risk of injury and illness.

Technical training and physical preparation

Having the correct structure and balance between technical training and physical preparation is key in developing robustness in the female gymnast. The technical mastery of routines is the desired outcome and performance goal for gymnasts. However, what is less well understood and addressed is how robust physical competencies can help to underpin these technical aspects. There is a need to provide gymnasts with the ability to tolerate the high forces they are subjected to during training and competition. Strength and conditioning training, specifically those methods aimed at improving strength and power qualities, has been a contentious issue in youth athletes and is especially controversial in aesthetic environments such as ballet and gymnastics. However, there is now a wealth of evidence to support the use of resistance training in youth populations (Faigenbaum et al., 2009). Another important consideration is the contentious view that increased muscular strength reduces the aesthetic appearance of a gymnast's routine. Research within professional ballet, however, has shown that strength training has a positive performance impact and does not alter selected thigh aesthetic components (Koutedakis and Sharp, 2004). It is also important to note that the use of appropriate strength training dosages (e.g., 1–4 reps at 80–100% of 1 repetition maximum (1RM) for 3–4 sets) can target muscular strength rather than muscular hypertrophy.

Nutrition

Gymnastics is a sport that requires a number of physical attributes including power, speed and coordination. As such, it is important that young gymnasts consume sufficient energy and nutrients to support the demands of their training and competition, as well as growth and tissue maintenance (Sundgot-Borgen et al., 2013). Due to the aesthetic nature of their sport, however, gymnasts appear to be at a higher risk of employing dieting and overtraining strategies to achieve a thinner physique (Siatras and Mameletzi, 2014). This may lead to inadequate energy and nutrient intake resulting in effects such as delayed menarche, bone growth issues and a reduction in height, weight and body fat (Sundgot-Borgen and Garthe, 2011). Recommendations from coaches and judges to improve performance by reducing weight may also exacerbate this issue (Sundgot-Borgen and Garthe, 2011). Dieting can set in train a cascade of events ultimately resulting in: low energy availability (with or without disordered eating), amenorrhea and bone mineral disorders; this is termed the 'female athlete triad' and is explained in detail elsewhere (Brown et al., 2017). In combination these conditions can predispose female athletes to a greater risk of illness and injury (Triplett and Stone, 2016). Therefore, there must be a continuous focus towards educating gymnasts, parents and coaches on optimizing energy and nutrient intake in order to support health and growth, improve performance and reduce injury and illness. All practitioners working with young gymnasts should take a proactive role in this information sharing and use the support of appropriately trained professional nutritionists should the need arise.

Psychological stressors

There are numerous psychological stressors that may play a part in the life of a female gymnast. Life-related stress is a common finding in the preinjury literature (Kerr and Minden, 1988). Significant life stress events (experiences that produce perceived strain such as starting a new school or the loss of a family member) have been shown to be highly predictive of injury in athletes (Kerr and Minden, 1988). Stress and anxiety can manifest themselves at any point along the gymnast's journey to success but can be of particular significance when the gymnast is competing. The competition floor can be a nerve-racking environment where the potential for stress and anxiety is great, especially for inexperienced individuals. Some gymnasts rise to the occasion and can produce their best performances in front of judges, spectators and under the scrutiny of TV cameras, while others are incapable of appropriately addressing their stress levels. This can lead to hostility, confusion or depression and, ultimately, performance decline (Massimo and Massimo, 2013).

There are some important techniques for coping with stress for all practitioners to be aware of when working with gymnasts as these may help prevent, or support the management of, psychological stressors. These techniques include imagery, relaxation skills, positive self-talk, concentration skills and retraining of negative thinking patterns. It is important to consider the option of referral to an appropriately trained sport psychologist (if available) to further address coping issues.

Injury and rehabilitation considerations

This section outlines the common injuries within women's artistic gymnastics as well as providing suggestions as to their management and rehabilitation.

Injury epidemiology

Epidemiological research into injuries sustained by elite-level gymnasts at the Olympic Games (Edouard et al., 2017). Table 40.1 shows the injury incidence for male and female artistic gymnasts and highlights a clear increase in the incidence at Rio 2016 when compared with the previous two Games.

These results, however, may not give us a true picture of the injury landscape. There are a few reasons to be cautious with these findings. There was an improved compliance rate in reporting injuries over this time. Furthermore, this

Table 40.1 Injury incidence per 1000 registered gymnasts in 2008, 2012, 2016 Olympic Games

Olympic Games	Total incidence	Male incidence	Female incidence
Beijing 2008	72.5	62.5	82.5
London 2012	76.9	91.8	61.9
Rio 2016	134.0	93.8	173.5

Adapted from Edouard, P., Steffen, K., Junge, A., Leglise, M., Soligard, T., Engebretsen, L., 2017. Gymnastics injury incidence during the 2008, 2012 and 2016 Olympic Games: analysis of prospectively collected surveillance data from 963 registered gymnasts during Olympic Games. British Journal of Sports Medicine 52 (7), 475–481.

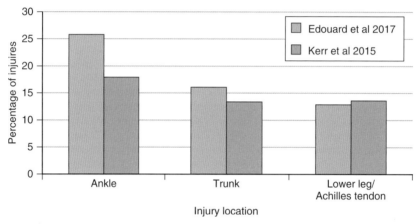

Fig. 40.2 Injury locations from women's artistic gymnastic epidemiology studies. (From Edouard, P., Steffen, K., Junge, A., Leglise, M., Soligard, T., Engebretsen, L., 2017. Gymnastics injury incidence during the 2008, 2012 and 2016 Olympic Games: analysis of prospectively collected surveillance data from 963 registered gymnasts during Olympic Games. British Journal of Sports Medicine 52 (7), 475–481; Kerr, Z.Y., Hayden, R., Barr, M., Klossner, D.A., Dompier, T.P., 2015. Epidemiology of National Collegiate Athletic Association women's gymnastics injuries, 2009–2010 through 2013–2014. Journal of Athletic Training 50 (08), 870–878.)

study was based on a relatively small number of gymnasts. Injuries were only included if they were 'newly incurred' during training or competition at the Olympic Games; as such, this type of injury surveillance does not provide information on overuse or recurrent injuries, which represent a high proportion of injuries in this athlete group.

Fig. 40.2 summarizes the most common injury locations from two recent papers (Edouard et al., 2017; Kerr et al., 2015). Injuries to the ankle, trunk and lower leg tendinopathy are the most frequently found in women's artistic gymnastics.

Ankle injuries

As well as being the most common injury, ankle injuries typically cause the greatest injury burden within women's artistic gymnastics. Ligamentous sprains are common (Kerr et al., 2015), as are injuries affecting tendons surrounding the ankle and foot such as tibialis posterior. Ankle joint issues such as osteochondral lesions and ankle impingement have also been reported in female gymnasts.

When considering ankle injuries it is important to look at the common mechanisms of injury and their relationship to the individual apparatus. With regard to vault and floor, the take-off and landing components are often the precursors to ankle injury, as is the fact that these components are repeated at high-volume loads (Marshall et al., 2007). The use of softer floor equipment (such as fast-track and tumble-track) can be used to minimize the impact forces that a gymnast is subjected to over the course of a training session or block. In addition, the types of tumbles that are included in a floor routine (and are therefore practised extensively) are important to consider when addressing ankle injuries. Increasing the technical difficulty of tumbles often means a need for increased power, jump height and somersaults/spins in the air. As the difficulty increases, the risk of not fully completing the tumble or executing it incorrectly also rises, increasing the likelihood of a poor landing.

Short landings are a major risk factor for developing an ankle injury and efforts should be made to (1) reduce the

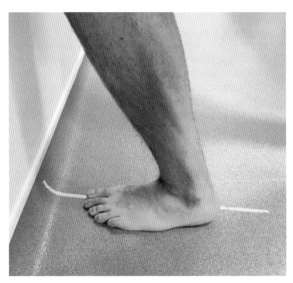

Fig. 40.3 Knee-to-wall ankle dorsiflexion measurement.

frequency of short landings, in the first instance, and (2) promote a robust reporting and management system aimed at improving medical access to those that sustain an injury related to a short landing.

Bars and beam also require a dismount from height and, therefore, are subject to a high landing force. Given the propensity for gymnasts to be subject to high jumping and landing frequencies and forces during training and competition, optimum landing mechanics as well as lower limb strength and capacity should be essential parts of a gymnast's physical preparation.

Key considerations in ankle injuries

Early reporting of ankle injury is imperative in order to allow the gymnast rapid access to suitable medical care and to help prevent any secondary complications to injury; this injury communication pathway (from the gymnast sustaining an ankle injury to the responsible medical practitioner being made aware of the incident) should be well established in advance of injury. Information regarding the mechanism of injury is key (short landings and ankle inversion/eversion mechanisms are common in this population), as is the location and severity of pain. Subjective reports of instability should be assessed as a matter of priority in the elite female gymnast. Objectively, a measure such as a knee-to-wall ankle dorsiflexion measurement (Fig. 40.3) may also help to establish any lack of range or movement and/or pain with the dorsiflexion position. As well as being used as an initial assessment marker, a knee-to-wall ankle dorsiflexion measurement may also help to guide progression through a return-to-gymnastics

programme by helping to evaluate range of motion and its relationship to load.

A key role of the gymnast's ankle is to produce force during running and jumping tasks. As a consequence, during periods of immobility or offload (such as postoperatively) it is essential that key muscle groups maintain their ability to produce force through safe ranges of movement. In order to prevent muscle wasting and possible delays in rehabilitation progressions, isometric contractions can often be utilized in the early stage. Muscle stimulation (e.g., Compex) for the calf complex, peroneals, tibialis posterior and tibialis anterior can also be of value. The use of hand-held dynamometry or isokinetic dynamometry may also help track muscle strength through the rehabilitation process, in particular for the invertors and evertors.

Typically, the mid to late stages of return to gymnastics following an ankle injury should include a variety of jumping and landing tasks, including the use of different heights, velocities and directions, as well as addressing any biomechanical flaws in landing technique. In particular, backwards landings should be readily included as this is the landing direction for the most common skills related to vault, floor and dismounts. Care should be taken to address the quality of the landings as well as just number of repetitions completed. Foot contact with the springboard is a key component of the vault apparatus and should therefore be steadily progressed throughout an ankle rehabilitation plan; progressions from standing impact jumps to running impacts and round-off impacts onto the springboard need to be factored into the rehabilitation design process. A progressive running/sprinting programme should also be designed in order to facilitate a smooth transition into a full vault sprint at the end of the rehabilitation process. Simple monitoring strategies such as quantifying impacts (number of landings per exercise or per session) and distance (how much running at which sprint intensity) will help aid progressive overload of the gymnast and prevent any unwanted spikes in training load during the rehabilitation programme.

Trunk injuries

Injuries to the trunk and lumbar spine are common in gymnastics and can affect the female gymnast in particular. Pathologies affecting gymnasts include facet joint dysfunction, stress fractures/pars defects, disc injuries and vertebral compression fractures (Kruse and Lemmen, 2009). Given the level of flexibility, force and unique body positions required for the sport, there are a variety of movement patterns and positions that need to be understood when considering trunk injuries within gymnastics, in particular with regard to landings, take-offs and hyperextension.

Studies into the biomechanics of gymnastic techniques have shown that a large amount of force is translated

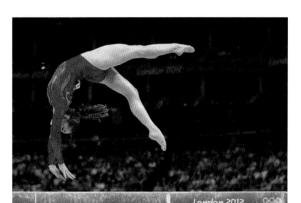

Fig. 40.4 Requirement for spinal mobility is great in gymnasts. This is seen in backward elements on beam.

along the axial spine during tasks such as take-off from the ground, rebounding and landing (Bruggeman, 1987). Vertical forces have been measured at 3.4–5.6 times body-weight during the take-off for a backward somersault skill. These high forces should be taken into consideration when managing gymnasts, in particular with adolescents who may have immature musculoskeletal systems and consequently are more susceptible to injury (Engebretsen et al., 2010).

The nature of certain skills within gymnastics requires the athlete to have a great deal of spinal mobility, particularly into hyperextension (for example backward elements on beam; Fig. 40.4). Skills such as Yurchenko vault preflights and backward tumbling elements include high-speed hyperextension (Bruggemann, 2005) and may be contributing factors to posterior spine pathologies. The repetition involved in training these hyperextension elements can lead to chronic lumbar conditions. However, the presence of pathology on investigation does not always correlate with a history of low back pain (Goldstein et al., 1991; Jackson et al., 1976). A clear understanding of the biomechanics of a gymnast's routine and training schedule is, therefore, imperative in order to effectively manage lumbar spine disorders in this population.

Key considerations in trunk injuries

The assessment of trunk and low back pain in gymnasts should be multimodal and include both subjective and objective elements. Key features to assess include subjective pain scores on extension movements and axial loading of the trunk (e.g., landings), as well as pain scores with activities of daily living (school/work, walking, etc.). Objective measurements such as lumbar spine combined movement patterns, neurodynamic testing and trunk capacity testing may also be useful. As mentioned, the presence of

pathology on investigation may or may not fit with a gymnast's current symptoms. It is important, therefore, not to use imaging in isolation. Robust discussions with the medical team are required with regard to undertaking an investigation and whether any results would change the planned management (based on subjective and objective findings).

Returning to gymnastics following trunk injuries can provide the practitioner with a number of challenges. This is due, in part, to the high functional level required at the end stage of rehabilitation where the final elements of sport-specific training include maximal hyperextension and high-force landings. Extension-related pathologies (e.g., a lumbar spine stress fracture) can be managed with an aggressive offload period in the early stage and progression to a suitable loading programme. This loading programme must include, at the end stage, a replication of gymnastic-specific positions with an emphasis on both strength and capacity of trunk musculature in order to cope with the high demand and frequency of gymnastics training. The key to this rehabilitation strategy should be an awareness of when to reintroduce lumbar extension, the speed and position of how this loading occurs and the maintenance of key communication links with coaching staff around the reintroduction of gymnastic technical elements along the rehabilitation continuum in relation to the gymnast's pain and function.

Spencer et al. (2016) highlighted and categorized modifiable spinal abilities; this information provides a framework for practitioners to use when selecting exercises for gymnasts based on the objective of the exercise and the intended physical outcomes. Fig. 40.5 shows the use of spinal exercises classified by 'physical outcome' (mobility, motor control, work capacity, strength) and 'functionality' (nonfunctional, functional). Although not an exact continuum of exercises, it may assist a practitioner's clinical reasoning in relation to spinal rehabilitation exercise selection. For example, during the early stages of rehabilitation following a lumbar spine stress fracture, there may be an emphasis on pain-free mobility work (both nonfunctional and functional) in addition to static and dynamic motor control exercises.

Leg strength and power is an important component in women's artistic gymnastics, in particular for the vault and floor apparatus. Higher difficulty elements are now requiring the gymnast to be more powerful off the floor and vault table in order to give themselves more time in the air to execute the skill. As such, the modern female gymnast now has a greater requirement to produce this strength and power in order to keep up with the difficulty level required to win at the top level. Strategies to improve leg strength and power need to take into consideration the gymnast's history of injury as well as their technical ability with regard to the exercises selected. It is important to highlight the high levels of axial spinal load inherent in a

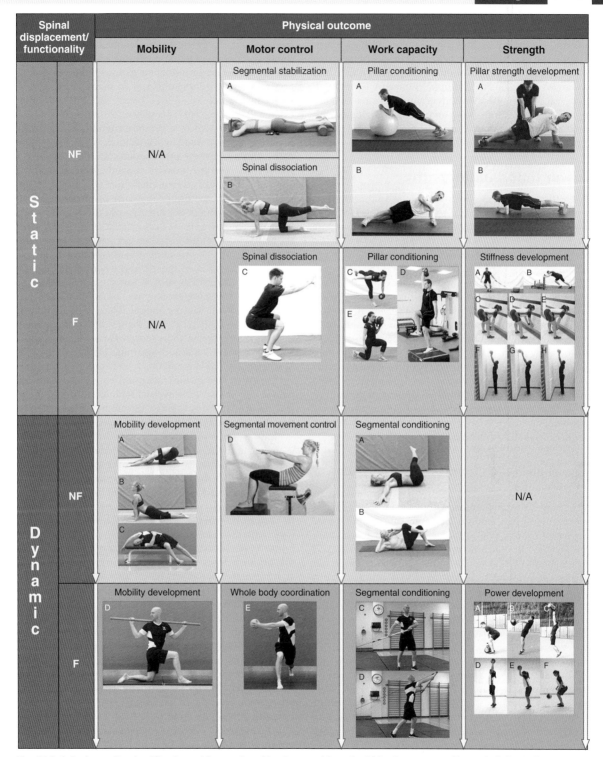

Fig. 40.5 Spinal exercise classification with exercise objectives positioned within the context of intended physical outcomes. *F,* Functional; *N/A,* not applicable; *NF,* nonfunctional). (Adapted from Spencer, S., Wolf, A., Rushton, A., 2016. Spinal-exercise prescription in sport: classifying physical training and rehabilitation by intention and outcome. Journal of Athletic Training, 51 (8), 613–628.)

jumping and landing sport (Bruggeman, 1987). Exercises utilizing equipment such as the leg press and knee extension/flexion machines may help to provide the gymnast with a suitable and safe stimulus to improve strength and power. Whichever method is used to improve leg strength and power, fitting these sessions around a gymnast's training week/block is imperative and an open dialogue with coaches is required to maximize the training and developmental opportunities.

Lower limb tendinopathy

Take-offs and landings play a key part in gymnastics performance, with jumps, leaps, rebounds, tumbles and dismounts making up the majority of a gymnast's routine. The force through an Achilles tendon during a back take-off has been measured to be as high as 16 times bodyweight (Bruggeman, 1987). Given these high forces and the frequency with which these skills are trained or performed, it is not surprising that lower limb tendinopathy (including Achilles and patella) is consistently amongst the top three most common injuries in women's artistic gymnastics. As indicated previously, the surface on which the gymnast lands can be a key factor in the development of certain injuries. For example, in the lead up to competition when gymnasts undertake a higher percentage of their routines on harder surfaces (e.g., full floor routines on the competition floor rather than with mats or partly on fast/tumble-track) there is a tendency towards a flaring up of lower limb tendon disorders such as Achilles tendinopathy.

Key rehabilitation considerations in tendon injuries

By its very definition, tendinopathy includes both pathology and pain in a tendon. This pain can inhibit energy storage utilization within the tendon and can lead to a compromise in function and performance (Cook and Purdam, 2014). Full rehabilitation of such injuries can be slow; it is common for gymnasts to continue to train and compete while having ongoing tendinopathy-related pain. It is important, however, that dialogue between the gymnast, coach and medical team is clear and open regarding tendinopathy-related pain. During periods in which the gymnast is training and competing in pain, the use of simple tendon pain–monitoring tests can be used to monitor the pattern of pain and help adjust a gymnast's training load appropriately. Using pain visual analogue scale (VAS) scores with tests such as single leg heel raise (Achilles) or decline squat (patella) may be suitable. The use of imaging to help with in-season management of tendinopathy is not commonplace. However, ultrasound tissue characterization may offer a way to monitor tendons in the future and further research is needed (Cook and Purdam, 2014).

As with tendinopathy management in other sports, the management of a gymnast's tendon must start with understanding the stage of tendinopathy and whether or not the tendon is tolerant or intolerant to load. Further information regarding tendinopathy and its management can be found in a variety of sources (Cook and Purdam, 2009; Cook and Purdam, 2012; Scott et al., 2013).

The management of a gymnast's tendinopathy within season is an important consideration, with there being many chronic tendon presentations in this population. Heavy-load eccentric exercise rehabilitation may be an appropriate strategy given a 'preseason' window of opportunity. However, the use of this type of programme may not be appropriate for the gymnast while they continue to train and compete. Heavy-load isometrics are common in the management of the in-season gymnast with tendinopathy with the aim of providing a load stimulus to the tendon without associated muscle and tendon pain (Ranson et al., 2016). Modalities such as extracorporeal shockwave therapy and strapping/bracing may be beneficial adjuncts to the traditional loading model. These modalities may help to bridge the gap between the need to continue training/performing in the short term and the undertaking of a comprehensive loading programme whose efficacy may only appear in the longer term.

The use of medications and injections to reduce tendon pain in athletes is a controversial topic and one that is outside the scope of this chapter; further information can be found in a paper by Cook and Purdam (2014).

The key to the in-season management of tendinopathy is to ensure the tendon is being subjected to appropriate loading in relation to the rest of the gymnastic-specific programme and that there is no mismatch between the tendon's load capacity and the load being placed upon it (Cook and Purdam, 2014). Being aware of the gymnast's training and competition calendar and having ongoing dialogue with the coach is important in planning certain rehabilitation phases alongside the training schedule. It may be that during periods of intense plyometric training (such as an increase in the numbers of full tumbles on the competition floor), other tendon-focused exercises can be reduced in frequency or intensity.

Given the high forces demanded of a tendon during jumping and landing tasks it is important that exercises aimed at strengthening the muscle–tendon complex (most commonly the calf–Achilles tendon or quadriceps–patella tendons) are adequately loaded. The use of relatively heavy weights (over 80% of the gymnast's 1RM) are required to produce the outcome of increasing maximal force production; this is typically done in 3–4 sets of 5–8 reps (Baker, 2014). The use of external strength equipment or a strength gym may be required in order to safely apply these loads to the gymnast (e.g., the use of a leg press machine for calf isometric or eccentric loading). Once integrated into

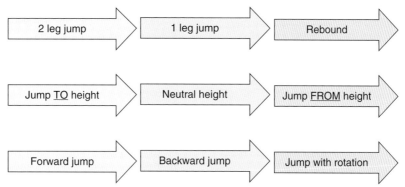

2 leg jump	1 leg jump	Rebound
Jump TO height	Neutral height	Jump FROM height
Forward jump	Backward jump	Jump with rotation

Fig. 40.6 Plyometric rehabilitation progression basics for gymnasts.

a gymnast's weekly programme, this progressive strength programme can continue throughout the season and can be tapered off in the week(s) prior to competition.

The principle of progressive overload should be used when designing return-to-jumping protocols for gymnasts. Prescription of the load, frequency and intensity of plyometric exercises must be overlaid onto the gymnast's overall training volume so that consideration is given to the summative load of plyometric activities. It is easy to overload a gymnast's programme if a joined up approach is not used. Collaboration with coaching staff is key. Plyometric exercises can be added as soon as concentric/eccentric lower limb work is pain free and the gymnast has good form. Quick tests such as the ability to perform single leg calf rising, single leg pistol squat movements and low-level running drills are a good indicator for the introduction of plyometric exercises. A basic plyometric rehabilitation progression plan is outlined in Fig. 40.6.

Summary

Working within gymnastics provides the practitioner with a unique environment in which to support sporting performance. An awareness of the age profile of female gymnasts and the relationships between growth, maturation and the physical and psychological requirements of the sport are essential for the practitioner to have a positive performance impact with this athlete group. The sport of women's artistic gymnastics is very demanding and ever-changing. There is a need for practitioners to be fully abreast of the key technical and physical requirements of the sport in order to help support the gymnast and coach to push the boundaries of human physical performance whilst minimizing the effect of injury.

References

Baker, D., 2014. Using strength platforms for explosive performance. In: Joyce, D., Lewindon, D. (Eds.), High Performance Training for Sports. Human Kinetics, Champaign, IL, pp. 127–144.

Brown, K.A., Dewoolkar, A.V., Baker, N., Docich, C., 2017. The female athlete triad: special considerations for adolescent female athletes. Translational Pediatrics 6 (3), 144–149.

Bruggeman, G.P., 1987. Biomechanics in gymnastics. Medicine and Sport Science 25, 142–176.

Bruggemann, G.P., 2005. Biomechanical and biological limits in artistic gymnastics. In: Proceedings of the XXIII International Symposium on Biomechanics in Sports. The China Institute of Sport Science, Beijing, China, pp. 22–27.

Burt, L.A., Naughton, G.A., Higham, D.G., Landeo, R., 2010. Training load in pre-pubertal female artistic gymnastics. Science of Gymnastics 2 (3), 5–14.

Cook, J.L., Purdam, C.R., 2009. Is tendon pathology a continuum? A pathology model to explain the clinical presentation of load-induced tendinopathy. British Journal of Sports Medicine 43 (6), 409–416.

Cook, J.L., Purdam, C.R., 2012. Is compressive load a factor in the development of tendinopathy? British Journal of Sports Medicine 46 (3), 163–168.

Cook, J.L., Purdam, C.R., 2014. The challenge of managing tendinopathy in competing athletes. British Journal of Sports Medicine 48 (7), 506–509.

Edouard, P., Steffen, K., Junge, A., Leglise, M., Soligard, T., Engebretsen, L., 2017. Gymnastics injury incidence during the 2008, 2012 and 2016 Olympic Games: analysis of prospectively collected surveillance data from 963 registered gymnasts during Olympic Games. British Journal of Sports Medicine 52 (7), 475–481.

Engebretsen, L., Steffen, K., Bahr, R., Broderick, C., Dvorak, J., Janarv, P., et al., 2010. The International Olympic Committee Consensus statement on age determination in high-level young athletes. British Journal of Sports Medicine 44, 476–484.

Faigenbaum, A.D., Kraemer, W.J., Blimkie, C.J., Jeffreys, I., Micheli, L.J., Nitka, M., et al., 2009. Youth resistance training: updated position statement paper from the national strength and conditioning association. The Journal of Strength & Conditioning Research 23 (5), 60–79.

Frank, J.B., Jarit, G.J., Bravman, J.T., Rosen, J.E., 2007. Lower extremity injuries in the skeletally immature athlete. Journal of the American Academy of Orthopaedic Surgeons 15 (6), 356–366.

Fry, R.W., Morton, A.R., Keast, D., 1991. Overtraining in athletes. An update. Sports Medicine 12, 32–65.

Goldstein, J.D., Berger, P.E., Windler, G.E., Jackson, D.W., 1991. Spine injuries in gymnasts and swimmers. An epidemiologic investigation. The American Journal of Sports Medicine 19, 463–468.

Jackson, D.W., Wiltse, L.L., Cirincoine, R.J., 1976. Spondylolysis in the female gymnast. Clinical Orthopaedics and Related Research 117, 68–73.

Kenttä, G., Hassmén, P., 1998. Overtraining and recovery. A conceptual model. Sports Medicine 26, 1–16.

Kerr, G., Minden, H., 1988. Psychological factors related to the occurrence of athletic injuries. Journal of Sport & Exercise Psychology 10 (2), 167–173.

Kerr, Z.Y., Hayden, R., Barr, M., Klossner, D.A., Dompier, T.P., 2015. Epidemiology of National Collegiate Athletic Association women's gymnastics injuries, 2009–2010 through 2013–2014. Journal of Athletic Training 50 (8), 870–878.

Knight, C.J., Boden, C.M., Holt, N.L., 2010. Junior tennis players' preferences for parental behaviors. Journal of Applied Sport Psychology 22, 377–391.

Koutedakis, Y., Sharp, N.C., 2004. Thigh muscles strength training, dance exercise, dynamometry, and anthropometry in professional ballerinas. The Journal of Strength & Conditioning Research 18 (4), 714–718.

Kruse, D., Lemmen, B., 2009. Spine injuries in the sport of gymnastics. Current Sports Medicine Reports 8 (1), 20–28.

Kuipers, H., Keizer, H.A., 1988. Overtraining in elite athletes. Review and directions for the future. Sports Medicine 6, 79–92.

Loud, K.J., Gordon, C.M., Micheli, L.J., Field, A.E., 2005. Correlates of stress fractures among preadolescent and adolescent girls. Pediatrics 115 (4), 399–406.

Malina, R.M., Bouchard, C., Bar-Or, O., 2004. Growth, Maturation and Physical Activity. Human Kinetics, Champaign, IL.

Marshall, S.W., Covassin, T., Dick, R., Nassar, L.G., Agel, J., 2007. Descriptive epidemiology of collegiate women's gymnastics injuries: national collegiate athletic association injury surveillance system, 1988– 1989 through 2003–2004. Journal of Athletic Training 42 (2), 234–240.

Massimo, J., Massimo, S., 2013. Psychological health and well-being. In: Gymnastics Psychology: The Ultimate Guide for Coaches, Gymnasts and Parents. Morgan James Publishing, New York, pp. 134–162.

Niemeyer, P., Weinberg, A., Schmitt, H., Kreuz, P.C., Ewerbeck, V., Kasten, P., 2006. Stress fracture in the juvenile skeletal system. International Journal of Sports Medicine 27 (3), 242–249.

Popovic, N., Bukva, B., Maffulli, N., Caine, D., 2012. The younger athlete. In: Brukne, P., Khan, K., et al. (Eds.), Brukner and Khan's Clinical Sports Medicine, fourth ed. McGraw-Hill Education, Australia, pp. 888–909.

Quatman-Yates, C.C., Quatman, C.E., Meszaros, A.J., Paterno, M.V., Hewett, T.E., 2012. A systematic review of sensorimotor function during adolescence: a developmental stage of increased motor awkwardness? British Journal of Sports Medicine 46 (9), 649–655.

Ranson, C., Joyce, D., McGuiggan, P., 2016. Tendon injuries. In: Joyce, D., Lewindon, D. (Eds.), Sports Injury Prevention and Rehabilitation. Routledge, London, pp. 199–211.

Scott, A., Docking, S., Vicenzino, B., Alfredson, H., Murphy, R., Carr, A.J., et al., 2013. Sports and exercise-related tendinopathies: a review of selected topical issues by participants of the second International Scientific Tendinopathy Symposium (ISTS) Vancouver 2012. British Journal of Sports Medicine 47, 536–544.

Siatras, T., Mameletzi, D., 2014. The female athlete triad in gymnastics. Science of Gymnastics 6 (1), 5–22.

Soligard, T., Schwellnus, M., Alonso, J.M., Bahr, R., Clarsen, B., Dijkstra, H.P., et al., 2016. How much is too much? (Part 1) International Olympic Committee consensus statement on load in sport and risk of injury. British Journal of Sports Medicine 50 (17), 1030–1041.

Spencer, S., Wolf, A., Rushton, A., 2016. Spinal-exercise prescription in sport: classifying physical training and rehabilitation by intention and outcome. Journal of Athletic Training 51 (8), 613–628.

Sundgot-Borgen, J., Garthe, I., 2011. Elite athletes in aesthetic and Olympic weight-class sports and the challenge of body weight and body composition. Journal of Sport Sciences 29 (1), 101–114.

Sundgot-Borgen, J., Garthe, I., Meyer, N., 2013. Energy needs and weight management for gymnasts. In: Caine, D.J., Russell, K., Lim, L. (Eds.), Gymnastics. John Wiley & Sons, Ltd, Chichester, UK, pp. 51–59.

Triplett, N.T., Stone, M., 2016. The female athlete. In: Joyce, D., Lewindon, D. (Eds.), Sports Injury Prevention and Rehabilitation. Routledge, London, pp. 429–435.

Chapter | **41** |

Introduction to dance medicine

Nick Allen

Introduction

While there are many similarities between sport and dance, and even more with certain aesthetically driven sports, there are numerous differences as well. Understanding the specificity of dance may enhance injury management and rehabilitation outcomes through an understanding of the various demands placed on dancers.

Extrinsic demands on dancers

Surfaces

Evidence from sports suggest the impact arises from a change in surface. Dance is typically performed in theatres; however, the nature of dance, particularly contemporary dance, means that a variety of surfaces may be encountered. For large companies, classes and rehearsals may take place in custom-built studios. The ideal force-reduction properties for a dance floor have been suggested to be 60% (Hopper et al., 2013). Dancers who take classes or rehearse in community-based halls are less likely to find surfaces that demonstrate these properties. Similarly, floors with force-reduction properties are less likely to be available in larger theatres when it comes to performances. Many theatres serve multiple uses and have floors constructed to serve a range performance types including opera, pantomime, etc., as well as coping with a great deal of scenery.

The floor surface is also an influence on risk of injury. Ballet is largely performed on lino surfaces. These can vary considerably in friction coefficient, affecting risk. The friction coefficient may be affected by cleaning products or transfer from dancers' skin (creams, massage oils, etc.) creating inconsistency on top of slippery surfaces. Some dancers, particularly in ballet, will use rosin to assist with pointe shoes on slippery surfaces.

Working with the industry, clinicians can look at stage and floor construction to reduce this risk. Working with individual dancers, it is important to create elements of unanticipated control within their training. Typically, dancers' movements are choreographed so that there are little or no unexpected movements. The use of reactionary drills as part of a proprioception programme will help support dancers in this area.

Costumes/shoes

Dancers will typically undertake class and most rehearsals in tights/leotards or tracksuits with ballet flats, jazz or character shoes or trainers. Depending on the performance, their costume may be heavy, restrictive or impede their vision (in the case of masks and head pieces). Dancers will typically have dress rehearsals prior to performances, but these may only be in the immediate build-up to a show, reducing the training impact of working within their costume.

Footwear in dance may also differ considerably. In ballet, female dancers may be expected to dance en pointe (Fig. 41.1A) or even single leg en pointe (Fig. 41.1B). In this position, weight-bearing will typically occur through the tips of the first and second toes. Aesthetically some dancers may strive to create an extended longitudinal arch through the midfoot and increased plantarflexion through the talocrural joint. The impact on key areas like the navicular and posterior talocrural joint is notable. The construction of a pointe shoe is based around aesthetics and offers reduced support. Driven by aesthetics, some dancers will also 'break' their pointe shoes to help achieve these extended positions. Dancers may also use shoes that are narrow as part of their aesthetic drive. In the presence of a Morton's neuroma this needs to be considered. When not in pointe shoes, females may wear 'ballet flats', also worn by male dancers. These

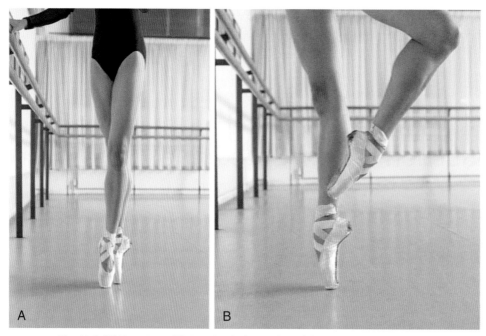

Fig. 41.1 (A) En pointe. (B) Cou-de-pied en pointe. (Photographer: Ty Singleton.)

offer little or no structural support. Dancers may also wear jazz shoes that have some heel and forefoot soles but little arch support, allowing dancers to still achieve their aesthetic of pointing their foot. Character shoes in dance can vary considerably from sandals to knee-length boots, all of which dancers will be expected to perform in.

Contemporary dancers' footwear may range from barefoot to trainers to heavy boots. Female ballroom dancers often perform in positive heels, while for male ballroom dancers, footwear resembling jazz shoes are worn; these offer some support but are designed around facilitating movement through the midfoot.

Props/equipment/lighting

Due to the variety in choreography and roles presented to dancers, there are numerous additional challenges that may impact on injuries. Due to the demands and costs associated with access to main theatre stages, many rehearsals for productions will take place in separate studio spaces. There is sometimes no capacity to include scenery in studios, so dancers will rehearse in the absence of the scenery they will need to account for during performances. Certain performances – often seen with contemporary dance – will have dancers performing at heights and this may result in an increase in traumatic injuries. Typically lighting in studios is very good, while lighting during performances is focused on presenting the performance; this may change the visual cues

available to a dancer (and what he/she has been accustomed to in rehearsals). The use of props in certain choreographies also requires competency and skill acquisition, such as the use of swords in productions like *Romeo and Juliet*.

Intrinsic demands on dancers

Workload

Dance training is designed to support the highly skilled and efficient movement observed in the professional dancers. Training for professional ballet dancers starts in earnest at vocational schools, when students enter what could be viewed as a full-time training position from the age of 11 years, but many having danced since the age of 3 or 4 in local dance schools. Fig. 41.2 is an example of the relative distribution of the different aspects of training undertaken at a vocational dance school. As can be seen throughout the dancer's development, dance-specific training is the primary focus, increasing exponentially when scholastic commitments end. Throughout their dance development, physical preparation may only consist of between 1 and 3 hours a week.

It is important to understand the nature of the training and development of a dancer and not to make assumptions around key physiological variables like strength and fitness, even for elite dancers.

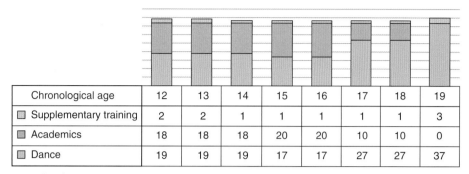

Chronological age	12	13	14	15	16	17	18	19
☐ Supplementary training	2	2	1	1	1	1	1	3
☐ Academics	18	18	18	20	20	10	10	0
☐ Dance	19	19	19	17	17	27	27	37

Fig. 41.2 An example of the weekly workload in a vocational dance school. (From Injuries and adolescent ballet dancers: Current evidence, epidemiology, and intervention, PhD Thesis, Nico Kolokythas, 2019.)

The development and training process responsible for creating the efficient movement pattern that makes movement in dance aesthetically pleasing may also create potential challenges for those looking to support dancers in their conditioning and rehabilitation. This may include a lack of exposure to the typical complementary training programmes like strength training, core stability, etc., seen in other sports. Time spent educating dancers on the objectives and expected positive outcomes from rehabilitation can be an important part of the process and improves understanding and compliance. Part of that education may need to centre on expected aesthetic changes. It is not unusual for dancers to be cautious around strength training for fear of hypertrophy or loss of flexibility. It is important that these areas are discussed to improve compliance. The lack of typical complementary training may also explain why research into physiological variables such as $\dot{V}O_{2max}$ and strength have demonstrated lower than expected results (Wyon et al., 2016). The remarkable functional outputs required in dance illustrate that lessons can be learned from dance around achieving extraordinary outcomes through efficient biomechanics and movement patterns despite lower than expected physiological indicators. However, it also means that improving certain physiological performance measures is an avenue that can be pursued in providing dancers with greater resilience against injury.

Large ballet companies may have what looks like a typical season cycle seen in premiership football or rugby. The season begins in August and runs until the start of the next summer. They may typically have a period off (up to 5 weeks) during the summer with a further week in the middle of the season. Smaller companies may not have as consistent a format and dancers may struggle to plan their conditioning in the same way. Independent dancers who work from contract to contract are challenged further, as financial pressures may mean that dancers accept contracts in lieu of recovery of training periods.

A typical schedule in a large ballet company may entail undertaking class 6 days a week. Class may take around an hour to hour and a half. The format of class may vary but will largely consist of three key areas: barre, centre and jumps. During barre, dancers will use the wall barre (or occasionally free-standing barre) to support and stabilize themselves as they undergo what may be described as a systematic warm-up and neuromuscular activation session by building up movement and intensity using balletic movements (pliés, relevés, etc.). During centre, they will no longer use the barre for support and begin to travel and turn. Finally, it will progress to jumps, again incrementally from petit (small) to grand (big) jeté (jumps). Class serves to support and develop technique and efficiency of movement synonymous with dance. Through its incremental build up, it can be used as a warm-up and support strength and power endurance.

Depending on the time of the season class may be followed by up to 6 hours of rehearsals. A dance company may rehearse more than one piece at a time due to time constraints later in the season. Rehearsals will still take place during performance periods, but they will be reduced due to shows. A large-scale production may perform between seven and nine shows a week, for periods that extend from weeks to months depending on contracts, with 150 shows a year typically performed by a large-scale ballet company. A West End or Broadway production may perform all year round and for many years, with the same dancers repeating the same movements year on year. Depending on the size of the company and length of show, there may be multiple casts for a show.

If there is only one cast, then there is pressure on the dancer as they will be involved in all relevant rehearsals as well as have the psychological pressure of knowing there is no replacement should they be unable to perform due to injury. If there are multiple casts it may mean that most of the work is done with the first cast and other casts may not have the same level of preparation. The better prepared a dancer is, the lower the risk of injury. Additionally, dancers may fulfil more than one role in a show, with some dancers undertaking numerous roles in a single performance. The variation of load and exposure this creates may increase the risk of injury if the dancer is not sufficiently prepared. There is also a variation in intensity of workload between different roles, as well as between different shows or choreographies.

Some sports have used epidemiological data to guide decisions about rule changes to help reduce injuries in their sport. For example, Australian rules football have changed the start/tip-off and thus reduced the incidence of posterior cruciate ligament injuries, while rugby union is constantly examining the correlation between injuries and the scrum and contact areas to reduce the prevalence of injuries. Those working in dance have an obligation to build epidemiological data to enhance choreographers' understanding of potential correlations between performance planning and injury rates so that they can make suitable decisions that minimize injury occurrence. The combination of intensity and volume gives dance-related workload and is an important consideration for dancers in terms of both enhancing performance and building resilience to injury.

In sport, athletes will typically warm up immediately prior to competition, often in the same kit they then compete in. However, due to the costume, hair and make-up requirements of dance performances, physical preparation may take place earlier than expected. Ballet dancers may undertake class many hours before a show due to the nature of their rehearsal schedule. Dancers supporting West End–type shows may undertake the dance captain's session prior to a show as part of their preparation for performance but, again, there can be timing constraints. The timing of performance preparation may also affect the timing of meals, with dancers often unable to eat at what is considered an optimal time before performance (3 hours preshow). Given the dynamic nature of dance, many are reluctant to eat closer to a show when their schedule allows. The use of homemade smoothies may be one way of improving nutritional intake preperformance that is better tolerated.

Injury in dance

Although there are methodological challenges, systematic reviews have indicated injury incidence in dance to be 1.3 injuries per 1000 hours of dance (Table 41.1) (Allen et al., 2014). Injury rates in ballet are reported to be higher, with up to 4.4 injuries per 1000 dance hours given in a prospective injury audit (Table 41.2) (Allen et al., 2012).

Bronner and colleagues (2003) have conducted extensive research into the injury incidence in modern and contemporary dance. Their research has shown the benefit of dance-specific medical care as well as a good appreciation of injury patterns in modern dance. They report an

Table 41.1 Musculoskeletal injury incidence in dance: a systematic review

Type of studies (design)	Overall injury incidence (observational)
No. of studies	29
Limitations	Serious limitations
Inconsistency	Serious inconsistency
Indirectness	No serious indirectness detected
Imprecision	No imprecision
Publication bias	Undetected
Quality	Very low
Injury incidence per dance hours	
Average incidence/1000 h	1.33
Range of incidence/1000 h	0.18–4.7
95% confidence interval	0.20–4.35*
Injuries per dancer/year	
Average no. of injuries/ dancer/year	1.93
Range of injuries/dancer/ year	0.05–6.83
95% confidence interval	0.29–4.5

*Based on 12 studies.
Source: Allen, N., Ribbans, W.J., Nevill, A.M., Wyon, M.A., 2014. Musculoskeletal injuries in dance: a systematic review. International Journal of Physical Medicine & Rehabilitation 3 (1), 1–8

incidence of injuries in a modern dance company at 0.41 injuries per 1000 hours of dance. They report that lower extremity injuries account for 60% of the total injuries. Of these, 52% were at the foot and ankle, 24% at the knee, and 8% each at the leg, thigh, and hip.

Modern dance can be further categorized into different genres, hip hop being one of the more popular styles. The work by Ojofeitimi et al. (2012) into hip hop dance has demonstrated that this is a discipline that dance medicine practitioners need to be aware of, with lower extremity injuries accounting for more than half of the total injuries (55%), with foot and ankle (20%) the most commonly injured of all body areas, as for ballet. Of all injuries to the foot and ankle, 48% were ankle sprains. In contrast to ballet injuries, upper extremity injuries represented 29% of total injuries. Here, the most common injuries to the hand were finger dislocations (27%), fractures (22%), and ligament ruptures (12%). The most common tissues injured were muscle–tendon (29%), followed by

Table 41.2 Injury incidence in dancers in a professional ballet company over 1 year

	FEMALE DANCERS		MALE DANCERS	
	No. of injuries (% of all injuries)	Injury incidence/ 1000 h dancing (95% CI)	No. of injuries (% of all injuries)	Injury incidence/ 1000 h dancing (95% CI)
Restricted dance activity	150 (87)	3.6 (3.1–4.2)	147 (80)	3.8 (3.3–4.5)
Complete withdrawal from dance*	22 (13)	0.53 (0.35–0.81)	36 (20)	0.94 (0.68-1.30)
All injuries	172 (100)	4.1 (3.6–4.8)	183 (100)	4.8 (4.1–5.5)

*Injuries that required the full withdrawal of dance-related activity as part of the overall severity.
Source: Allen, N., Nevill, A., Brooks, J., Koutedakis, Y., Wyon, M., 2012. Ballet injuries: injury incidence and severity over 1 year. Journal of Orthopaedic Sports Physical Therapy 42 (9), 781–790.

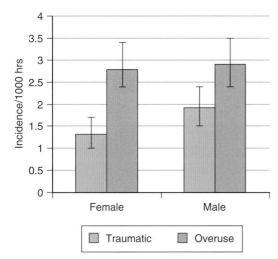

Fig. 41.3 Incidence of traumatic and overuse injuries by gender in professional ballet dancers. (Allen et al., 2012)

joint–ligament (nonbone) (25%), and bone stress/fracture (11%).

Dancers often record higher exposure levels in comparison to sports, with dancers known to undertake 35 hours of dance-related activity a week. Coupled with the high number of performances, it is not surprising that there is a higher prevalence of overuse injuries in dance (Fig. 41.3).

Given dancers' reliance on optimal biomechanics and technically proficient movement patterns for injury protection, the high exposure rates are an important consideration when developing rehabilitation programmes for this population. Dancers, through their typically high exposure rates, have less tolerance to deviations from the norm before risking the development of overuse injuries. Therefore, what

may seem like a subtle biomechanical anomaly may be detrimental through repeated loading over a prolonged period (Allen et al., 2013).

Dance terminology

Part of the assessment and successful management of a dancer will be through understanding the specificity of their needs. Part of this involves understanding the nature of movement and terminology used to describe these movements.

From ballet terminology you may come across any number of these terms. Many will develop from the five standard positions used in ballet that relate to the position of the legs and/or arms (Figs 41.4 and 41.5).

Alongside this, dancers will describe performing movements like a plié (squat-type movement, Fig. 41.6), relevé (heel raise, Fig. 41.7), développés (Fig. 41.8A,B), battements including tendu and glissés (dynamic leg movements) and port de bras cambre (trunk movements into flexion or extension with arms) or arabesques (Fig. 41.8C).

More dynamic or ballistic movements include pirouettes and fouettés (turning), jeté and sissonnes (jumps, Fig. 41.9) and pas de deux (partnering /lifting/lifted).

From contemporary perspective you may encounter more movement-based descriptions; while many movements have their origins on balletic movement, they have evolved and may no longer be easily described using the same terminology. Contemporary dance may involve more 'floor work', where dancers utilize the contact with the floor to a greater extent than in ballet, with 'crashing' to the floor not uncommon. This aspect of contemporary work can increase the incidence of upper limb and even concussion

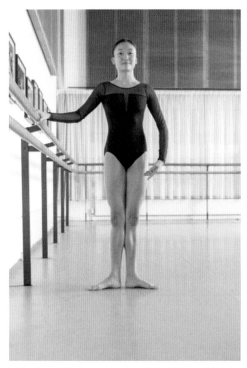

Fig. 41.4 First position arms bras bas. (Dancer: Yaoqian Shang; photographer: Ty Singleton.)

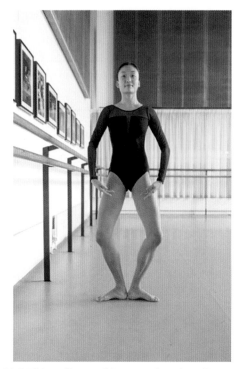

Fig. 41.6 Plié on first position arms bras bas. (Dancer: Yaoqian Shang; photographer: Ty Singleton.)

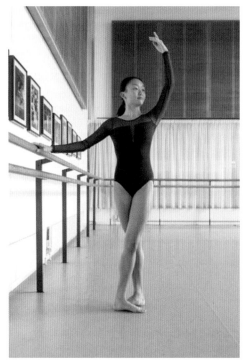

Fig. 41.5 Fifth position arms in fifth. (Dancer: Yaoqian Shang; photographer: Ty Singleton.)

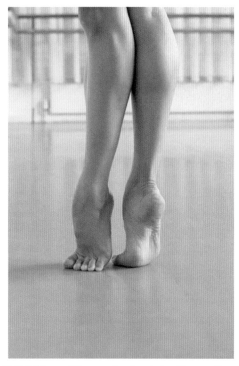

Fig. 41.7 Fifth position en demi-pointe. (Dancer: Yaoqian Shang; photographer: Ty Singleton.)

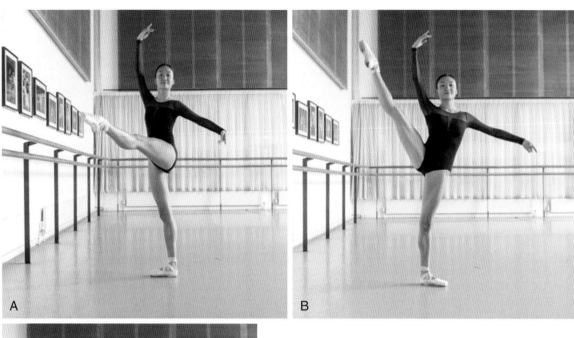

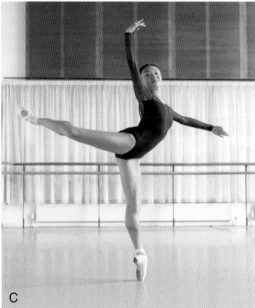

Fig. 41.8 (A) Développé devant en croisé. (B) Développé à la seconde. (C) Attitude derrière efface en pointe, arms in fourth. (Dancer: Yaoqian Shang; photographer: Ty Singleton.)

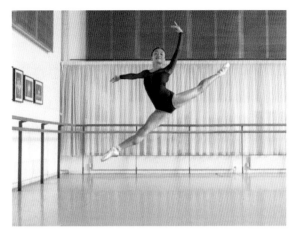

Fig. 41.9 Sissonne with arms in fourth. (Dancer: Yaoqian Shang; photographer: Ty Singleton.)

injuries. Partnering in contemporary dance may also differ. Rather than executing some of the cleaner lines exhibited in ballet, contemporary dancers are known to engage in momentum-based lifts using rotation and angles. This enables them to create lifts where smaller partners can execute lifts with larger partners. While this supports the artistic ambition, if it is not executed well it introduces a disproportionate load and increased risk of injury.

Rehabilitation of a dancer

Rehabilitation of any athlete is a multifactorial process with numerous considerations including the nature and severity of injury, predisposing factors, time in season and career, previous injury, etc. When applying dance specificity to traditional aetiological models it allows the attending clinician to formulate a strategy around the rehabilitation process to account for some areas not necessarily seen in other sporting populations.

When examining a patient, the clinician formulates ideas around the injury diagnosis, possible causative factors, as well as the functional outcomes required by the athlete or dancer for a safe return, including reducing the risk of recurrence.

Establishing a clear diagnosis with an understanding of the origin of symptoms is important. Differentiation of the origin of symptoms as chemical (inflammatory), mechanical (tissue loading) or both will assist in the management process and rehabilitation design. In the traumatic injuries there may be an expectation of a chemical origin due to tissue trauma from an inciting event. In overuse injuries, the influence of biomechanical loading in the development of symptoms is most likely, with a combined presentation of

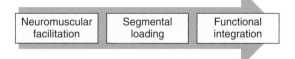

Fig. 41.10 The hybrid interventional model.

chemical and mechanical. In dancers there is a larger prevalence of overuse injuries. This requires the examining clinician to undertake a thorough biomechanical assessment to establish origin and causation.

Injury management programmes, including rehabilitation, are centred on an evaluation of what is stopping the patient from undertaking all that they would normally do. Is it the acute injury and associated pain/limitation? Are there any underlying strength or power deficits? Is there a limited functional capacity due to lack of appropriate training?

The hybrid interventional model (HIM) is a theoretical model designed to allow clinicians to plan the strategies employed through the injury and rehabilitation process (Allen et al., 2013) (Fig. 41.10). The model proposes the implementation of three stands, namely: neuromuscular foundation training, segmental loading (including strength or power endurance), and functional integration. The key to the implementation of the HIM is the sequence (neuromuscular followed by strength followed by functional integration) and the relative ratios of the different components at each stage of the injury episode. The relative ratios are influenced by the clinician's assessment of the current limiting factor.

In the early stage of an acute injury the likely limiting factor is the injury itself and any associated pain, and thus forms the focus of the management programme,. One notable result of pain in acute injury is the impact on muscle inhibition. Within the HIM, neuromuscular facilitation would form the greatest component of the rehabilitation programme to restore and support muscle activation during this key time. Neuromuscular exercise is typically well tolerated in the presence of pain and so fits well in the early stages.

As a patient progresses through the injury stages, the next limiting factor and management focus may be the cause of the injury. Here the identification and addressing of any potential strength or power deficits may be the largest proportion of the programme design. Within this stage the programme will still begin with muscle activation drills but also include some functional activation drills at the end of the session.

In the final stages of an injury, the focus and management shifts towards the functional requirements of the athlete for their safe return to performance or competition. A shorter muscle activation and strength-based programme will be followed by an extended functionally driven component. In the rehabilitation of dancers, it is important to optimize loading as part of this preparation and resilience training. This is a key part of the functional integration component of the HIM. It enables the creation of suitable chronic load through the rehabilitation programme to build resilience for the inevitable spikes in acute workload typically seen in professional dance. It takes into account the impact of career loading, the previous seasons' loading, as well as chronic training load from the previous 4 weeks. Research has suggested that younger athletes may be at increased risk of injury due to a lack of suitable chronic training load and older athletes may be more at risk due to either excessive accumulative chronic loading or previous injury affecting training load. Research also suggests spikes in acute workload may result in increased bone stress injury; this may be of particular relevance to younger dancers who do not yet possess the chronic workload to support against these spikes. In contrast, accumulative excessive chronic workload may result in increased risk of pathological changes to joint surfaces, a problem associated with older, more experienced dancers. These issues all need to be taken into consideration when designing rehabilitation programmes for dancers.

Return-to-dance criteria

When determining the return-to-play suitability in the sporting population, it is usually clear what physical criteria are required for full return, as the nature of the sport in question, although affected by the opposition, provides a relative degree of consistency. In dance, due to the vast potential for variation in physiological demands of different choreographies and roles, the decision for a dancer to return to performance is more nuanced. It requires a full understanding of what is required in the role that the dancer will be returning to. A graded return may be considered if the role involved does not require full physical capacity; in this case, the return to full-level performance commitment at a later point must be contingent on the completion of the rehabilitation process. As in sports, 'return to play' needs a team decision that involves the dancer, artistic staff, clinical and conditioning staff. The artistic staff can shed light on the physical requirements needed from the dancer for upcoming rehearsal and performance roles. It is important to understand the dancer's perspective; an awareness of their views around contracts, career development and performance pressure is important.

From a clinical perspective, adaptation of a commonly used sports model may guide the healthcare practitioner in the decision process. In the absence of preseason baseline data, the use of limb symmetry index testing can provide a useful reference point for lower and upper limb injuries.

A limb symmetry index of ≤25% gives some suggestion of a reduced injury risk based on the literature from anterior cruciate ligament rehabilitation and return-to-play protocols and ≤10% gives even stronger confidence that there will not be a performance deficit. The tests can be adjusted to suit particular pathologies but for the lower limb may include the following.

- Normal movement:
  - functional movement testing to assess movement competency and neuromuscular control
- Range of movement:
  - hip range of motion (particularly internal rotation as an indicator of how the external rotators of the hip are coping)
  - knee to wall – an indicator of symmetry for functional positions like plié and the ability to get the heels down during jumps
- Balance/proprioception:
  - star excursion balance test
  - Biodex – single leg athletic test
  - Hop and hold – assessment of control
- Muscle power:
  - jumping – height, distance, stamina, symmetry (distance on single hop, distance on repeated hops, cross-overs, speed over distance, etc.)
  - jumping – OptoJump/force plate (if available)
- Muscle strength:
  - knee, ankle extension/flexion isokinetics (if available)

Further functional testing includes the incremental participation in the stages of class (barre, centre and jumps) with additional work on lifting/partnering, as relevant, but should be included with all dancers who are required to lift as part of their role to ensure they are safe to proceed.

A challenging part of the return-to-dance decision is around strength and power endurance assessment. The nature of dance may involve prolonged bouts of high-intensity intervals against longer, lower intensity work. Using repeated strength (repeated lifts or rises) and power drills (jump box plyometric drills) with short recovery sessions can help assessment and preparedness. Additionally, evaluating chronic training load of a role (a result of combined exposure and training intensity) will help to establish suitability for return to a performance period rather than just whether the dancer can perform the technical requirements for a single show.

Role of screening in dance

The role of screening in injury prediction is an area of debate. There is a lack of consensus as to its value in injury prediction and, furthermore, what screening should entail.

Screening in dance can include an appreciation of the baseline stage of conditioning of the dancer, on which performance enhancement and injury prevention programmes may be based.

Medical screening

Standard medical screens used in sport, as advocated by the International Olympic Committee as a Periodic Health Evaluation, will assist those managing dancers (Ljungqvist et al., 2009). Questioning around menstrual cycle frequency and dietary intake may provide insight as to potential risk associated with relative energy deficits. With the exception of the competitive ballroom environment, dancers are not subject to World Anti-Doping Agency regulations and testing. The role of the healthcare professional must include educating dancers around the risks of performance-enhancement drugs and this can be covered through the medical screen.

Cardiac screening in sport is a growing area, with many sports advocating a resting electrocardiogram (ECG) and family history prior to participation at the elite level. There is a lack of research into cardiac risk in dancers. Following on from our own research that included ECG, echocardiogram and family history, until additional research shows otherwise we advocate the need for at least a family history and resting ECG for adult dancers.

Musculoskeletal screening

Musculoskeletal assessments of joint range of movement and muscle strength have been employed in various sports. Research in sports has suggested that reduced internal rotation at shoulders and hips may be linked to increased risk of injury. Similarly, increased or excessive range of movement has been associated with injury risk through decreased stability. Generalized joint hypermobility has been found in sports where acquired range of movement exceeds the normal physiological range. Dancers may typically exceed range of movements seen in most sporting populations. Additionally, research has demonstrated a higher prevalence of hypermobility spectrum disorders (HSD; formally known as benign hypermobility joint syndromes) in vocational schools and the lower ranks of professional ballet companies (below principal level) compared to the general population. However further analysis shows a lower prevalence of HSD in the upper ranks of professional ballet companies compared to the general population. A suggestion has been made that the talent identification in younger dancers has focused on greater flexibility or 'facilities' as seen in people with HSD, but the ability to withstand the physical demands of top-tier ballet requires greater stability. Nevertheless, recognizing the impact and applying appropriate

management strategies for dancers with increased mobility is important. The use of the Brighton criteria (Grahame et al., 2000) as an evaluation of HSD and may assist in management decisions around the nature of support programmes needed.

The differentiation between HSD and acquired hypermobility is important from a medical model perspective as HSD may impact on autonomic function, fatigue, pain, postural orthostatic tachycardia, gastrointestinal, bladder or pelvic functions. Additionally, the impact of excessive range of movement is considerable with regard to injury risk. Research has demonstrated notable postural differences and increased pain in 35 subjects with HSD compared to matched controls. The knee joint has been shown to be the joint with the greatest risk of hypermobility (Booshanam et al., 2011). A relationship between generalized joint hypermobility and a history of glenohumeral instability ($P = 0.23$) in military recruits has been found (Cameron et al., 2010). Furthermore, hypermobility patients have a higher incidence of recurrent shoulder dislocations (60% vs. 39%) (Muhammad et al., 2013). Finally, positive correlations between HSD and lumbar disc herniations have also been reported (Aktas et al., 2011).

Movement testing

Movement competency through normal movement testing like the Functional Movement Screen (FMS) can help elucidate where dancers struggle to control certain 'normal' movements while achieving remarkable skill levels in dance-specific movements. However, the higher level of flexibility needs to be factored into the interpretation of normal movement testing rather than employing generic evaluations and analysis taken from other sport populations.

The evaluation of some dance-specific movements may add value but require good technical appreciation. For example, it may be noted that in a plié position in second position a dancer is achieving their turn out through excessive tibial rotation rather than hip external rotation, thereby increasing the risk of injury to knee or tibia. Furthermore, symmetry may be assessed by observing a shift in alignment through the lower limbs.

Fitness tests provide a challenge in the dance environment. Within sports, improving technology has seen an increase in field-based testing that shows good correlations with recognized physiological variables like $\dot{V}O_{2max}$. The use of a dance-specific test, such as the Dance Aerobic Fitness Test designed by Professor Wyon, can assist in providing an appreciation of dance-specific fitness levels; it shows good correlations with $\dot{V}O_{2max}$ for both contemporary and ballet dancers (Wyon et al., 2003).

Summary

The term 'artistic athlete' is well suited to dance; it is the result of artistic aptitude against a background of physiological demands. A key to successfully supporting these remarkable athletes is understanding the specificity of their discipline. This includes applying risk modifiers through understanding intrinsic and extrinsic risk. Utilizing a rehabilitation model like the HIM allows healthcare practitioners to plan programmes that incorporate the fundamental aspects of neuromuscular control, strength and functional capacity needed for dance. Returning to dance from injury holds similar challenges to sport, and systematic testing and exit strategies can reduce the risk of reinjury and performance deficits. With injury prevention a key objective, utilizing information gained from dance screening can increase the basis upon which injury-prevention programmes can be based.

References

Aktas, I., Ofluolu, D., Akgün, K., 2011. Relationship between lumbar disc herniation and benign joint hypermobility syndrome. Turkish Journal of Physical Medicine and Rehabilitation 57, 85–88.

Allen, N., Nevill, A., Brooks, J., Koutedakis, Y., Wyon, M., 2012. Ballet injuries: injury incidence and severity over 1 year. Journal of Orthopaedic & Sports Physical Therapy 42 (9), 781–790.

Allen, N., Ribbans, W.J., Nevill, A.M., Wyon, M.A., 2014. Musculoskeletal injuries in dance: a systematic review. International Journal of Physical Medicine & Rehabilitation 3 (1), 1–8.

Allen, N., Nevill, A.M., Brooks, J.H., Koutedakis, Y., Wyon, M.A., 2013. The effect of a comprehensive injury audit program on injury incidence in ballet: a 3-year prospective study. Clinical Journal of Sport Medicine 23 (5), 373–378.

Booshanam, D.S., Cherian, B., Joseph, C.P., Mathew, J., Thomas, R., 2011. Evaluation of posture and pain in persons with benign joint hypermobility syndrome. Rheumatology International 31 (12), 1561–1565.

Bronner, S., Ojofeitimi, S., Rose, D., 2003. Injuries in a modern dance company. Effect of comprehensive management on injury incidence and time loss. The American Journal of Sports Medicine 31 (3), 365–373.

Cameron, K.L., Duffey, M.L., DeBerardino, T.M., Stoneman, P.D., Jones, C.J., Owens, B.D., 2010. Association of generalized joint hypermobility with a history of glenohumeral joint instability. Journal of Athletic Training 45 (3), 253–258.

Grahame, R., Bird, H.A., Child, A., 2000. The revised (Brighton 1998) criteria for the diagnosis of benign joint hypermobility syndrome (BJHS). Journal of Rheumatology 27 (7), 1777–1779.

Hopper, L.S., Allen, N., Wyon, M., Alderson, J.A., Elliott, B.C., Ackland, T.R., 2013. Dance floor mechanical properties and dancer injuries in a touring professional ballet company. Journal of Science and Medicine In Sport / Sports Medicine Australia 17 (1), 29–33.

Ljungqvist, A., Jenoure, P.J., Engebretsen, L., Alonso, J.M., Bahr, R., Clough, A.F., et al., 2009. The International Olympic Committee (IOC) consensus statement on periodic health evaluation of elite athletes March 2009. British Journal of Sports Medicine 43 (9), 631–643.

Muhammad, A.A., Jenkins, P., Ashton, F., Christopher, M.R., 2013. Hypermobility – a risk factor for recurrent shoulder dislocations. British Journal of Sports Medicine 47, e3.

Ojofeitimi, S., Bronner, S., Woo, H., 2012. Injury incidence in hip hop dance. Scandinavian Journal of Medicine & Science in Sports 22 (3), 347–355.

Wyon, M., Redding, E., Abt, G., et.al., 2003. Development, reliability and validity of a multistage dance specific aerobic fitness test (DAFT). Journal of Dance Medicine and Science, 7 (3), 80–84.

Wyon, M., Allen, N., Cloak, R., Needham-Beck, S., 2016. Assessment of maximum aerobic capacity and anaerobic threshold of elite ballet dancers. Medical Problems of Performing Artists 31 (3), 145–150.

Chapter | **42** |

Emergency aid preparation

Natalie Shur, Paulina Czubacka, Jim Moxon, Rohi Shah, Tom Hallas and Johnny Wilson

Emergency action preparation

Medical department staff members working in professional sport have seconds to make the decision that may have a significant bearing on a player's health. Exposure to traumatic and life-threatening events may not be a common occurrence in sport, but when they arise, the medical staff on site need to be ready to react immediately and in a coordinated manner to manage the emergency situation. Clinicians must possess the right tools for the job – whether that is an ankle sprain or a cardiac arrest. The Emergency Action Protocol must be constantly under review; exposure to certain events should lead to reflection and, where appropriate, implementation of changes, to drive practice forward. Sports medicine is evolving on a daily basis, driven by discussion, the sharing of practices and through the cooperation of opposing medical teams in the event of serious trauma on the field of play. This chapter's aim is to provide an insight into the day-to-day work of the medical department in professional sport, where we will discuss the following aspects:

- the Emergency Action Protocol
- the equipment and consumables used daily by medical care providers in professional sport
- considerations for prescribing and administering medication in sport settings
- the extrication process for emergency scenarios
- the handover process
- the debrief, which will drive the practice forward
- necessary emergency first aid qualifications.

The Emergency Action Protocol

Background

The Emergency Action Protocol (EAP) embodies a notion that any emergency aid provider, given adequate practice and

preparation, should be able to safely assess and deal with most emergency clinical scenarios. They are a critical part of ensuring athlete safety during training and competition. However, when circumstances arise that are out of the conventional norm, utilizing a systematic *airway, breathing, circulation, disability, exposure* (A–E) approach will help assess, identify and treat athletes with potentially life-threatening injuries. These are the fundamental principles taught in any prehospital-based emergency aid course and this training is often a prerequisite to working in the sporting environment.

It is well known that sports practitioners do not deal with limb- or life-threatening injuries on a daily basis, as athletes are normally considered the healthiest cohort of the general population. When emergency situations do arise, there is usually a causative traumatic event as opposed to an underlying pathological issue. Therefore, when dangerous clinical pathologies unexpectedly occur, panic, incompetent personnel and training, inadequate equipment or simply poor planning and preparation can lead to abysmal outcomes. Often, the underlying cause is multifactorial, i.e., the Swiss cheese model (Reason, 2000). This highlights the importance of having a systematic, well-practised routine for dealing with any emergency.

Emergency courses may provide a foundation and delineate a system for management. However, unless practised, utilized and updated on a routine basis, this foundation is easily lost. The chaotic nature of match days, compounded by player and managerial pressures, often leads to the EAP being a quick verbal agreement between providers and, at times, the visiting team may be completely excluded from this plan. Most sporting environments are highly visible and publicized activities with the management of every incident under scrutiny. Failures are often emphasized in the media, highlighting the need for emergencies to be dealt with systematically and efficiently.

A guide to the EAP

One attempt at addressing the EAP in the dynamic environment of sporting events is the implementation of the

Match Day Protocol

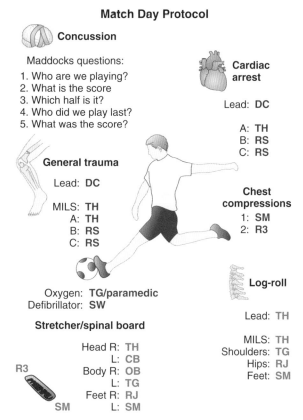

Concussion

Maddocks questions:
1. Who are we playing?
2. What is the score
3. Which half is it?
4. Who did we play last?
5. What was the score?

General trauma

Lead: **DC**

MILS: **TH**
   A: **TH**
   B: **RS**
   C: **RS**

Oxygen: **TG/paramedic**
Defibrillator: **SW**

Stretcher/spinal board

Head R: **TH**
      L: **CB**
Body R: **OB**
      L: **TG**
Feet R: **RJ**
      L: **SM**

R3

SM

Cardiac arrest

Lead: **DC**

A: **TH**
B: **RS**
C: **RS**

Chest compressions

1: **SM**
2: **R3**

Log-roll

Lead: **TH**

MILS: **TH**
Shoulders: **TG**
Hips: **RJ**
Feet: **SM**

Fig. 42.1 Example Emergency Action Protocol board for reference when conducting medical team briefing prior to sports events.

'EAP board' (Fig. 42.1) by Shah et al. (2018). This purpose-designed board defines team member roles in the event of an emergency. A dedicated time-out session should occur prior to every home match, where individual roles are clearly designated and reviewed. This ranges from general trauma scenarios where a single member manages the airway with cervical spine stabilization, to more life-threatening scenarios where team members are allocated specific roles for airway, breathing and circulation. This follows down to isolated limb management in trauma or log-rolling a patient prior to extrication. A designated team lead should be hands-off to oversee the scenario.

Routine simulation training prior to a match that replicates probable real-life emergency scenarios allows the team to practice working in sync and become time efficient. This also allows the team members to reflect on their performance and identify areas to improve upon (Fig. 42.2).

With increasing awareness of cardiac pathologies, including sudden cardiac arrest (SCA), having a strict protocol with designated A–E roles allows for time-critical interventions. In the event of a nontraumatic collapse, SCA must be presumed and therefore early application of a defibrillator and performing effective chest compressions is critical, effectively changing the classical A–B–C (airway–breathing–circulation) approach to a C–A–B (circulation–airway–breathing) approach. The EAP board accounts for a designated role to commence chest compressions, apply a defibrillator and obtain venous access for drug administration. The designated time-out session prior to a sporting event is an important time to communicate and involve the paramedic teams, away team leads or any personnel providing emergency care on the day, to designate their specific

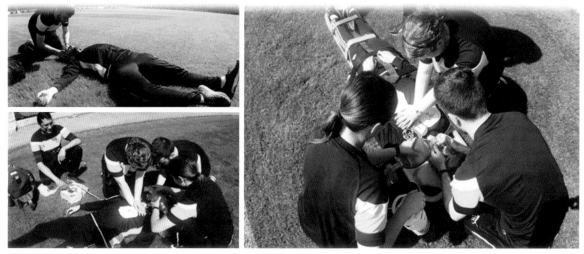

Fig. 42.2 Emergency practice scenario: cardiac arrest.

role during an emergency. Ambulance availability should be known prior to the event, including time to arrival on scene, or if on-site where their designated location should be.

Printed material highlighting on-site equipment availability and location, emergency exits, emergency contact details and the nearest accident and emergency hospital department should be readily available and distributed to visiting team leads. Whilst the EAP board provides a simple visual reminder of preassigned roles, simply by having a time-out session prior to any sporting event to discuss and allocate roles, ensures a team can work efficiently and as a unit.

Match day preparation in many ways reinforces and adapts core principles taught in emergency aid courses. However, unless practised on a routine basis, key aspects of providing emergency care can be easily overlooked and performed poorly. Creating a simple organizational step with a dedicated time-out session prior to a sporting event can help create a systematic approach to effectively dealing with medical emergencies.

Contents of kit bag and away travel bag

Doctor's kit

The equipment a doctor carries pitch-side must be sufficient to deal with any emergency should it arise. Communication with the paramedics and wider medical team prior to any event is paramount to identify what equipment each person carries and is responsible for. Table 42.1 sets out the essential equipment, with justification, a doctor should carry on match days for sporting events.

Physiotherapist's kit

Every clinician should be aware of what is required in their 'run-on' bag. It is common practice now to have large run-on bags containing nonessential equipment when attending to a player pitch-side.

The primary concern when attending the player pitch-side is management of the athlete's airway, breathing and circulation and this should be reflected by the contents of the clinician's run-on bag. Fig. 42.3 presents an example of content for a physiotherapist's run-on bag and Table 42.2 lists the equipment that adequately prepares the clinician for these emergency scenarios. All pieces of equipment within a bag should be reasoned and contain pieces of equipment required by the clinician's governing body of the relevant sport.

During the course of a sporting calendar year most sports medicine practitioners travel away from their regular venue.

It requires meticulous planning to allow the practitioner to carry out regular treatments as well as deal with emergency scenarios while away. If travelling long distances abroad, it may be necessary to source certain pieces of equipment (e.g., compressed gases and automated external defibrillator; AED) prior to travel as they may not be allowed to be transferred on a plane. Climate also plays an important role when preparing for an away trip, as the athletes may be exposed to extreme temperatures. If players require certain types of medication, the clinician should make sure to take enough for the duration of the travel. An example of an equipment list for an away travel bag is presented in Fig. 42.4 and Table 42.3.

Match days can be busy days in the medical department. Therefore certain consumables can be placed in the dressing room to allow players to self-manage taping, blister care, foam rolling and stretching for prematch preparation (Fig. 42.5).

Prescribing

When providing medical support during sporting events, clinicians will need to have access to an extensive list of medications to manage most medical situations should they arise. A practitioner should be able to justify everything in their kit bag. If you do not know why it is in your bag, or you are not comfortable prescribing it, get rid of it. Table 42.4 represents a guide to recommended medications to have access to; however, this list will be influenced by the medical history of your athletes.

The use of medications in athletes has gained attention in recent years. Evidence suggests elite athletes use antiasthmatic medications, antihistamines, nonsteroidal antiinflammatory drugs (NSAIDs) and oral antibiotics significantly more frequently than age-matched controls (Alaranta et al., 2008). It is vital to prescribe these medications judiciously in order to reduce the risk of side effects, which may adversely affect performance. Clinicians must become acquainted with the World Anti-Doping Agency (WADA) prohibited list, which is updated every January. Encourage players to check with an experienced team doctor before self-administering supplements or when prescribed anything by another professional, as not all clinicians are aware of the WADA list. Care should be taken to note not only prohibited medications but those that have a dose limit, e.g., salbutamol. If prohibited medications are required in an emergency situation, an application for a therapeutic use exemption (TUE) must be made at the first available opportunity.

Prescribing in a high-performance environment presents several challenges. Players will often request analgesia. Frequently analgesia is taken prophylactically by players, despite

Table 42.1 Recommended equipment required in a pitch-side doctor's kit

System	Equipment	Justification
Airway and breathing	Oropharyngeal and nasopharyngeal airways, selection of sizes	Airway adjuncts
	Pocket mask	Personal protective equipment
	Bag-valve-mask	Ventilation
	Non-rebreather mask	For delivery of high-flow oxygen
	Portable suction kit	Remove secretions
	Pulse oximeter	Oxygen saturation measurement
	Oxygen tank	Hypoxia
	Magill's forceps	Obstructing foreign body
	Lubricating jelly	Lubricate airway adjuncts prior to insertion
Circulation	Automated external defibrillator	Cardiac arrest
	Stethoscope	Auscultation
	Sphygmomanometer	Blood pressure measurement
	Intravenous cannula and giving sets	Establish intravenous access for fluids/medications
	Pelvic binder	Pelvic fracture
	Sharps bin	Disposal of sharps
	Sterile gauze	Haemostasis for cuts/abrasions
Dysfunction	Blood glucose monitor	Rapid assessment of blood glucose
	Pen torch	Pupil size assessment/oropharyngeal assessment
Wound management	Steristrips	Wound closure
	Wound glue	Wound closure
	Sutures	Wound closure
	Nasal tampons	Epistaxis
Other	Intraosseous access	If unable to establish IV access
	Cricothyroidotomy kit	If unable to secure airway using adjuncts
	Gloves	Personal protective equipment
	Thermometer	Temperature measurement
	Nebulizer chamber for nonrebreather mask	Deliver nebulized salbutamol for wheeze

them having no current pain or injury; some may be dependent on this as a psychological support prior to matches. Players may ask for inappropriate strength or formulations of analgesia for minor pain issues. In general, we would advocate avoiding NSAIDs in the first 48 hours after an injury as it may encourage more bleeding (Lippi et al., 2006).

Players may request sleeping tablets due to insomnia or nerves prior to a big match. Sedatives are very addictive and can remain in the system for 48 hours after ingestion, which may affect performance and reaction times. Good education on proper sleep hygiene and conservative measures should be encouraged wherever possible. Healthcare professionals should explore the reasons behind why players request certain sedatives or strong analgesics, counselling the patient on alternatives. There is a duty of care not to create dependence.

When players present with symptoms of an upper respiratory tract infection (URTI), there may be a perceived pressure to treat with antibiotics; this is also a common expectation among the general population. One compromise in this situation may be to prescribe high-dose vitamin C and zinc, given most URTIs are viral in origin (NICE, 2008). This way one can reduce unnecessary antibiotic prescribing, meanwhile the players and coaches feel that the symptoms are being taken seriously and are being treated appropriately.

Clinicians are often approached by non-playing staff for medications or treatment. Whilst it may be tempting to help colleagues, if medical treatment of non-playing staff is not a contractual obligation, is it ethical to provide care to individuals on an informal basis? Some would consider that clinicians should not, under any circumstance, prescribe medications outside their contractual obligations. Others

may perhaps restrict it to providing over-the-counter medications. It would be prudent to involve the sports club's Human Resources Department to clarify contractual agreements prior to prescribing for any non-playing staff. Physiotherapy staff may also be approached for medications. Unless they are registered physiotherapy prescribers, physiotherapists are not permitted to prescribe drugs. However, in a supportive team environment, it is permissible for the doctor to lead on prescriptions with clear protocols for medication administration by other staff with precise note keeping. Finally, all medications should be safely stored in a suitable locked cupboard with access limited to appropriate staff members.

Extrication

Equipment essential to different types of extrication should be available pitch-side and include a long back board/spinal board with head blocks and straps, a cervical collar, a scoop stretcher with head block system and straps, a basket stretcher, a selection of fracture splints and a Kendrick splint (Fig. 42.6).

Extrication for non-spinal injuries and cardiac arrest

In the event of a soft tissue injury the player should be asked if they can walk off from the field of play. If the player believes they are not able to walk off the field of play, the medical team will support the player with the use of the

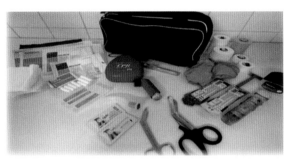

Fig. 42.3 Example of equipment for a physiotherapist's run-on bag.

Table 42.2 Recommended equipment required in a pitch-side physiotherapist's kit		
Airway and breathing	**Circulation**	**Other**
Oropharyngeal airway adjunct: used to open and maintain athlete's airway	*Trauma dressing*: used for large bleeds	*Gloves*: used for reducing risk of infection
Airway lubricant: aids in application of the airway adjunct	*Nasal buds*: used for nasal bleeds	*Razor*: to remove hair for application of AED
CPR mask: creates a seal for more effective breaths and prevents direct athlete–clinician contact	*Vaseline*: used to help stop/prevent bleeding from small cuts	*Tuff-cut scissors*: to remove clothing/boots/tape to expose the area
IV cannula: used for decompression of a suspected tension pneumothorax	*Gauze*: used for compression to help to stop bleeding	*Tape*: EAB, zinc oxide: finger splinting, joint taping
Asthma inhaler (if needed): carried in the bag if asthmatic players are in the squad; used to relieve the symptoms	*Alcohol wipes and saline*: used to clean wounds	*Epipen*: used to administer adrenaline in case of anaphylactic shock
	Dressings: applied to wounds to maintain compression and reduce risk of infection.	*Saline*: used to clean an eye/ remove dirt from eye
	Tape: EAB to apply extra compression and hold the dressing applied on the wound in place	*Contact lenses (if needed)*: when athletes wear lenses during sporting events
CPR, Cardiopulmonary resuscitation; *EAB*, elastic adhesive bandage. *IV*, Intravenous.		

appropriate extrication technique. For example, with suspected fracture or ligamentous injury, the hands-on lead can support the affected limb with/without immobilization (dependent on injury) and may be helped by other members of the medical team to ensure safe transfer into the extrication device.

In the event of a suspected concussion, the medical personnel will need to give consideration to the suitability of removal from play, with the health and safety of the player in mind. However, it is only in circumstances when the player has no capacity to make a decision about his/her care that this decision is taken by the attending clinician.

In the event of a cardiac arrest, for time efficiency the player can be transferred straight into the scoop/split device when transferring the player onto an ambulance trolley. The athlete can be lifted onto the scoop/split device by the medical team who will be placed at the head, shoulders, hips and feet. The player will be lifted enough to provide clearance for the device to slide underneath, and the athlete is then lowered into the device. Spider straps are then used to secure the

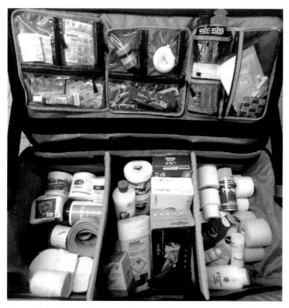

Fig. 42.4 Example of equipment in an away travel bag.

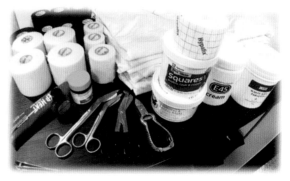

Fig. 42.5 Consumables placed in the dressing room.

Table 42.3 Example of equipment for a sports clinician's away travel bag

Match day consumables	Deep Heat, Vicks Vaporub, tweezers, nail scissors, tuff-cut scissors, blister bandage scissors, toe protectors
Wound care	Nasal buds, adhesive plasters, military field dressing, iodine dressings, Jelonet dressings, steristrips, eye patch, finger bandage, triangular bandage, assorted size adhesive dressings, wound cleansing wipes, saline pods
Consumables	TubiGrip (various sizes), surface cleansing wipes, toe dividers, second-skin blister care, Hypafix, massage wax, massage cream, sharps box, nonsterile gauze, acupuncture needles assorted sizes, Vaseline, nitrile gloves S/M/L, suncream, aftersun cream, iodine spray, pretape spray, tape-removal spray, wound-congealing spray, insect repellent, talcum powder
Emergency aid/consumables	OPAs, NPAs, airway lubricant, AED batteries, CPR mask, BVM, nonrebreather mask, nebulizer, IV cannula, foil blanket, razor
Tape	Underwrap, zinc oxide 2.5/3.5/5 cm, elastic adhesive bandage tape 5/7.5 cm, kinesiology tape
Other	Ice bags, clinical waste bags, seat belts straps, foam padding, tape measure, TheraBands, In Case of Emergency Forms (I.C.E), forms, SCAT5 forms, emergency incident forms, EAP for a venue, pen, permanent marker, blood pressure cuff

AED, Automated external defibrillator; *BVM,* bag valve mask; *CPR,* cardiopulmonary resuscitation; *IV,* intravenous; *NPAs,* nasopharyngeal airway adjuncts; *OPAs,* oropharyngeal airway adjuncts.

Table 42.4 Suggested medications for clinicians to have pitch-side

Group	Medication	Indication
Emergency	Adrenaline 1:1000 500 micrograms Epipen 1:1000 300 micrograms IM	Anaphylaxis
	Adrenaline 1:10,000 1 mg IV	Cardiac arrest
	Amiodarone	Cardiac arrest
	Benzodiazepines – buccal midazolam	Seizure
	Hydrocortisone	Anaphylaxis
	Glucagon	Hypoglycaemia
	Concentrated glucose gel – Hypostop	Hypoglycaemia
	Oxygen	Cardiac arrest, hypoxia, severe injury
	Aspirin 300 mg	Myocardial infarction
	Glyceryl trinitrate (GTN) sublingual spray	Angina
	Antihistamine – chlorpheniramine	Anaphylaxis
	Short-acting inhaled β_2 agonists – salbutamol + aerochamber	Asthma/bronchoconstriction
General	Antibiotics – including penicillin, nonpenicillin broad spectrum, topical	Infection
	Analgesia – paracetamol, NSAIDs, aspirin, parenteral	Pain
	Anaesthesia – lidocaine (including topical), bupivacaine	Procedures, e.g., suturing
	Sterile water	Wound irrigation
	Prochlorperazine (parenteral)	Vomiting
Respiratory/ENT	Inhaled steroids	Asthma
	Antibiotic ointment – chloramphenicol	Conjunctivitis
	Naseptin	Recurrent epistaxis
Gastrointestinal	Antacids	Dyspepsia
	Loperamide	Diarrhoea
	Laxatives, e.g., senna	Constipation
	Antispasmodic, e.g., mebeverine	Bowel spasm

ENT, Ear, nose and throat; *IM*, intramuscular; *IV*, intravenous; *NSAIDs*, nonsteroidal antiinflammatory drugs.

player on the scoop; the top of the strap (Y-strap) is not used in the cardiac arrest scenario as it will obstruct the defibrillator pads and chest compressions. The person supporting the head is to lead the scenario, so that coordinated extrication with minimal disturbance of injuries occurs.

Extrication for spinal injuries

We have two spinal immobilization devices – long board and scoop. Personal experience has led to the assessment of their relative advantages/disadvantages shown in Table 42.5.

A player will be rolled with four people, led by the first pitch-side responder who will provide manual in-line stabilization (MILS). Three members will roll at shoulders, hips and feet (three arms over, three under). A nominated member will then insert the board or scoop to the player's back and player is lowered upon command from lead. If a long board is being used the player will then be repositioned again with command from the lead. Head blocks and straps will then be inserted while the lead is in MILS until head blocks are fitted. If possible, nominate another person not involved with the log roll to prepare the spider or seatbelt straps for a quick and easy application. Strap from shoulders down to the feet, ensuring that straps are level on both sides and tension is equal while applying the straps. Spider straps may not reach a player's feet depending on height (Hanson and Carlin, 2012).

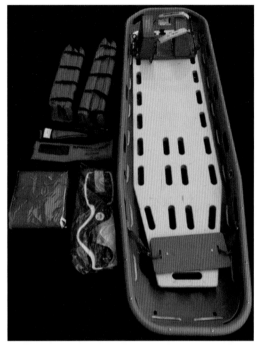

Fig. 42.6 Pitch-side extrication equipment including (clockwise from top-left) fracture splints, long board and scoop with head blocks and straps, cervical collar, blanket and spider straps.

Handover

An effective handover is vital in the sport and exercise medicine setting, where transfer of care often occurs. However, this is a difficult skill to master. In this setting, handover may occur when the first responder on the field of play (FOP) is joined by members of the medical team, if a player is transferred from FOP to ambulance, or on admission to hospital. The length of the handover will depend on the situation, but should generally include enough information for the new caregiver to safely take over care.

There are several tools that have been designed to ensure effective handover. These provide a standardized structure for concise factual communication between healthcare providers ensuring that all important information is relayed (Leonard et al., 2004). These include SBAR (Fig. 42.7), often used in the secondary care setting, and ATMIST, proposed in the football medicine setting.

Whilst one is not necessarily superior to another, what is important is to have a system that you use consistently. Communication and collaboration problems have been shown to be the strongest predictors of health-related harm (Leonard et al., 2004). Therefore, an effective handover is essential to ensure critical information is not omitted. The benefits of an accurate handover include better decision making by receiving staff, prioritization of tasks, improved patient experience and improved time management (Eggins and Slade, 2015).

Key information that should be communicated in a sports medicine environment include:

1. basic patient details
2. information about the injury or illness
3. signs and symptoms

Table 42.5 Advantages and disadvantages of long board and scoop devices

Equipment	Long board	Scoop
Advantages	Rigid for increased support Can be used to carry over further distances Can better accommodate variety of player sizes Can attach seatbelt/spider straps Player only log rolled once X-ray compatible	Adjustable length Can be split in two so player can be log 'tilted' rather than rolled X-ray and MRI compatible, therefore player does not need to be transferred to another device and can go straight for imaging
Disadvantages	Usually readjustment of position of a player on the board needed prior to immobilization Not MRI compatible so player will need be transferred	May be too short for taller players even at maximum length Narrow Should only be used for transfer into the bucket stretcher as is not as rigid as a long board Forms a large gap from base of torso support to the foot support when on maximum length

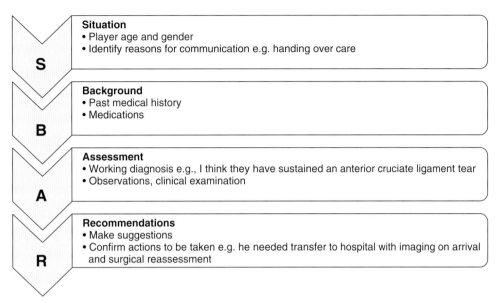

Fig. 42.7 SBAR algorithm for structuring handover.

4. background such as any past medical history that may be relevant
5. clinical assessment information, e.g., vital signs, clinical impression
6. any intervention you have provided.

If there is any injury to a limb, neurovascular status should always be communicated, and the time that pulses, etc., were lost if initially present. Players may require surgery on admission to hospital, so other important information to hand over should include when they last ate and drank as this will be important for anaesthesia planning.

Debriefing

A team debriefing is a facilitated or guided dialogue that takes place between team members to review and reflect on team performance (Lyons et al., 2015). Debriefing is a useful tool to evaluate events in order to identify areas of good practice and areas for practice improvement. However, it has also been employed as a method to reflect on events after a critical incident such as a cardiac arrest. Indeed, much of the literature relating to debriefing is around critical incidents. In these circumstances, the debriefing process allows individuals to discuss individual and team-level performance, identify errors made and develop a plan to improve their next performance (Salas et al., 2008). Several tools have been developed to provide a framework for debriefing. One of these is SHARP, a five-step feedback tool

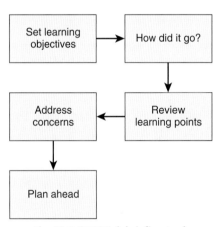

Fig. 42.8 SHARP debriefing tool.

(Ahmed et al., 2013). The five elements are shown in Fig. 42.8.

In the elite sports setting, there is often the additional burden of decision making under the scrutiny of fans and TV cameras. Furthermore, there may be conflicts between an individual's health interests and those of the club, for example with return-to-play decisions. There may be additional complexity when covering away matches or working abroad, having to cope with a new environment with different staff or facilities. All these aspects make it even more important to engage in debriefing, to process the complex decision-making skills and improve planning for

521

similar scenarios in the future. In addition, debriefing can identify areas that may benefit from auditing – to reevaluate and improve the emergency action plan for a particular scenario.

Emergency aid qualifications

Most healthcare professionals enter the sporting environment with a background of working within a hospital, general practice or community clinics. When faced with emergency situations in these environments there is usually good access to the support of fellow healthcare workers, medical equipment and a controlled environment away from the gaze of the general public, media and other patients.

This contrasts sharply when working with sports professionals, where you may be faced with managing life- and limb-threatening situations, often in poor weather conditions, with limited medical support and equipment, under the scrutiny of the media and general public. Whist working alongside individuals who have a vested interest in the outcome of your actions and decisions, these colleagues often have no medical understanding and may seek to influence medical decisions in the interests of winning a game.

Emergency care training in sport is designed to protect the players and also the healthcare practitioners. In these situations, doctors and physiotherapists do not act under the 'good Samaritan' principle, but under common law. Therefore the standard of medical care must be higher when delivered by a medically trained individual (Advanced Trauma Medical Management in Football, 2017).

The Football Association insists that any healthcare professional working with age groups above 16 years in the Premier League, English Football League and the Women's Super League should complete the Advanced Trauma Medical Management in Football (ATMMiF) course. Candidates are required to complete precourse reading and a precourse multiple choice question paper. This is followed by an intensive 2-day course composed of a mixture of didactic teaching, interactive and practical scenario-based sessions on a number of competencies such as airway management in football (Advanced Trauma Medical Management in Football, 2017). The course also provides teaching on emergency action planning, audit cycles and standard operating procedures such as managing unconscious players.

There are a variety of other sports-based emergency aid courses that have been endorsed by the Royal College of Surgeons Edinburgh's Faculty of Pre-Hospital Care and the Faculty of Sport and Exercise Medicine, which are regarded as an equivalent to the ATMMiF. These are:
- Emergency Medical Management in Individual and Team Sports (EMMITS)
- Standard Principals of Resuscitation and Trauma in Sports (SPORTS)
- Immediate Medical Management on the Field of Play (IMMFP)
- Immediate Care in Sport (ICS)
- Medical Cardiac and Pitch Side Skills (SCRUMCAPS)

Emergency aid courses are a vital component of training for healthcare providers. Not only do they provide the practical-based medical competencies, but they also provide valuable guidance on clinical governance and an opportunity to network with others working in sporting environments.

Conclusion

Emergency action planning is critical to provide safe and effective medical care and first aid in a sport setting. To ensure an efficient working environment where each member of the medical team is aware of their roles and responsibilities the 'EAP board' presented in this chapter can be implemented and serve as a visual reminder. To maintain the skillset developed on courses and CPD events, clinicians should practise scenarios on a regular basis. Having an EAP and practising the trauma scenarios and extrication will help reduce the risk of errors and will minimize delay in providing care. Good communication is vital for EAP. It is essential to have a handover system in place for the first aid responder to communicate their findings and diagnosis to the rest of the team. Moreover, reflection on each scenario on the field should be undertaken to allow for peer-to-peer learning in a constructive manner. To provide appropriate standard of care, the contents of the run-on bag, trauma bag and away travel bag should adhere to guidelines available for certain sports and also satisfy the medical needs of the player or playing squad. Equipment used should be regularly checked, serviced and documented.

Acknowledgements

We would like to thank Dean Chatterjee, Stephanie Makin and Rebecca Johnston for their helpful contributions, insight and expertise in the putting together of this chapter.

References

Ahmed, M., Arora, S., Russ, S., Darzi, A., Vincent, C., Sevdalis, N., 2013. Operation debrief: a SHARP improvement in performance feedback in the operating room. Annals of Surgery 258 (6), 958–963.

Alaranta, A., Alaranta, H., Helenius, I., 2008. Use of prescription drugs in athletes. Sports Medicine 38 (6), 449–463.

Eggins, S., Slade, D., 2015. Communication in clinical handover: improving the safety and quality of the patient experience. Journal of Public Health Research 4 (3), 666.

Hanson, J.R., Carlin, B., 2012. Sports prehospital-immediate care and spinal injury: not a car crash in sight. British journal of sports medicine, 46 (16), 1097–1101.

Leonard, M., Graham, S., Bonacum, D., 2004. The human factor: the critical importance of effective teamwork and communication in providing safe care. Quality and Safety in Health Care 13 (Suppl. 1), i85–i90.

Lippi, G., Franchini, M., Guidi, G.C., Kean, W.F., 2006. Non-steroidal anti-inflammatory drugs in athletes. British Journal of Sports Medicine 40 (8), 661–662;discussion 2-3.

Lyons, R., Lazzara, E.H., Benishek, L.E., Zajac, S., Gregory, M., Sonesh, S.C., Salas, E., 2015. Enhancing the effectiveness of team debriefings in medical simulation: More best practices. The Joint Commission Journal on Quality and Patient Safety, 41 (3), 115–125.

NICE Short Clinical Guidelines Technical Team, 2008. Respiratory Tract Infections – Antibiotic Prescribing. Prescribing of Antibiotics for Self-Limiting Respiratory Tract Infections in Adults and Children in Primary Care. National Institute for Health and Clinical Excellence, London.

Reason, J., 2000. Human error: models and management. British Medical Journal 320 (7237), 768–770.

Salas, E., Klein, C., King, H., Salisbury, M., Augenstein, J.S., Birnbach, D.J., et al., 2008. Debriefing medical teams: 12 evidence-based best practices and tips. Joint Commission Journal on Quality and Patient Safety / Joint Commission Resources 34 (9), 518–527.

Shah, R., Chatterjee, A.D., Wilson, J., 2018. Creating a model of best practice: the match day emergency action protocol. British Journal of Sports Medicine 52 (23), 1535–1536.

The Football Association, FA Level 5. Advanced Trauma Medical Management in Football (ATMMiF) course. http://www.thefa.com/learning/courses/the-fa-level-5-advanced-trauma-medical-management-in-football.

Chapter | **43** |

What's rehabilitation without patient buy in? The importance of psychology in sport injury rehabilitation

Anna Waters

Introduction

When injured athletes first meet with their sports medicine practitioners (SMP), the first question usually asked is: 'How soon can I get back to my sport and compete again?' The answer depends not only on the athlete's injury, but on their unique response to their injury, their ability to deal with the potential emotional impact of the injury, their trust in and communication with their rehabilitation team, and how much they buy into the rehabilitation programme and adhere to it. Finally, at the point of return to play, the athlete's confidence in their ability, trust in their injured body part and ability to manage reinjury concerns are all crucial factors in determining an athlete's readiness to return to sport.

A few years ago, I knew a jockey who sustained a fractured tibia and fibula during a fall from a horse. Throughout his rehabilitation he was doing things way ahead of his rehabilitation programme and was back on a horse a long time before his SMP or consultant advised him that he was fit to do so. He pushed everything to speed up his recovery time to be fit enough to return to race riding. Interestingly, when his consultant passed him fit to race ride again a few days later, he called me up and booked in to see me. It transpired that he had suddenly completely lost his confidence to race. When faced with the reality of race riding again, he went from having pushed himself to break all records in terms of recovery times, to being overwhelmed by fears of reinjury and doubts about his ability to ride. He kept picking up his phone to call his agent and cancel his comeback race. Instead we worked through his fears and concerns.

This is a relatively common scenario. It is usually a result of not processing and addressing the psychological issues early on and during the rehabilitation process, so that when the athlete is deemed medically fit to return to sport, they are not psychologically ready. For this jockey, everyone (including his rehabilitation team) thought he was coping remarkably well with his rehabilitation. However, by focusing so intently on speeding up his rehabilitation, he had avoided dealing with his emotional and psychological response, and had to deal with it when faced with the reality of returning to race riding.

Following on from this, how important do you believe sport psychology is in the field of sports medicine? As an SMP reading this, how much do you understand about the role of psychology in your work with patients daily? How well equipped do you believe you are to deal with the psychological aspects of sports injury rehabilitation and return to sport?

Research findings suggest that whilst sport psychology has been identified as important by SMPs, most believe themselves to be unprepared and lacking the training to address psychological factors in sports injury rehabilitation. Let us explore a summary of the key findings in this area.

Mann et al. (2007) examined sports medicine physicians' understanding of psychological issues in patient-athletes. They found that physicians frequently encounter psychological issues with this patient group. There is therefore a need for SMPs to have tools to facilitate assessment of these problems, and a need for greater communication between sport psychologists and sports medicine practitioners.

Arvinen-Barrow and her colleagues have conducted several research studies examining UK physiotherapists' understanding and use of sport psychology in their work. In particular, they noted that despite a general belief by SMPs that psychosocial strategies are important to increase effectiveness of injury rehabilitation (Arvinen-Barrow et al., 2007; 2014; Hemmings and Povey, 2002; Larson et al., 1996) and evidence that such approaches are effective (Beneka et al., 2007; Flint, 1998a; Ievleva and Orlick, 1991), many do not believe that they have the understanding and training necessary to be able to implement such strategies (Hamson-Utley et al., 2008; Stiller-Ostrowski and Hamson-Utley, 2010). In line with other researchers, Arvinen-Barrow et al. (2007) recommend that greater collaboration between sport psychologists and physiotherapists in this clinical setting would be beneficial.

Over the past 30 years, research has examined and identified the importance of psychological factors in sports injury and rehabilitation. This body of research highlights the psychological impact injury can have on athletes (Heil, 1993; Ray and Wiese-Bjornstal, 1999; Taylor and Taylor, 1997). Models have been developed to account for athletes' psychological responses to injury (Walker et al., 2007; Wiese-Bjornstal et al., 1998). Alongside this, psychological skills and interventions have been developed to facilitate the speed of recovery and athletes' successful return to play (Ievleva and Orlick, 1991; Kamphoff et al., 2010; Williams and Scherzer, 2010).

Recent sport psychology research has begun to identify some interesting results of particular relevance to SMPs. For example, Ardern et al. (2013) found that certain key psychological responses measured presurgery and at 4 months postsurgery significantly predicted return to play at 12 months post–anterior cruciate ligament reconstruction. This finding, together with previous research findings (Brand and Nyland, 2009; McCullough et al., 2012), provides evidence to suggest that psychological factors are important for returning to sport and that they may have been underrecognized to date.

Whilst these research findings are interesting, how does it impact on clinical practice? Frequently there appear to be gaps between significant sport psychology research findings and their application to real world settings. From the literature conducted to date, this seems to be particularly true about the link between sport psychology research and sports medicine teams.

Despite the importance of psychological factors in sports medicine, there remains a lack of theoretical understanding in many clinical settings, insufficient structured ways for SMPs to work with sport psychologists and an absence of clear practical ways to integrate sport psychology into a sports medicine team. This chapter will begin to address these areas and will:

- provide insight into athletes' psychological responses to injury
- examine adherence to injury rehabilitation
- introduce methods to enhance rehabilitation adherence in athletes
- introduce some of the sport psychology skills and tools that can be integrated into SMPs' work with injured athletes.

The content set out here relates well to Chapter 39 on conditioning efficacy. The reader is referred to that chapter as an excellent road map to the fundamentals of neuromuscular adaptation and basic training principles when structuring rehabilitation sessions. Combined with the suggestions made here in this chapter, it may provide a holistic foundation on which to develop intervention plans for your clients.

Psychological responses to injury

Athletes display a wide range of psychological responses to injury and multiple factors impact this response. For example, their level of sport participation, severity of the injury, time in the season and previous injury experience. It is important for SMPs to gain insight and understanding of helpful and unhelpful psychological responses athletes can display and to bear these in mind when developing and delivering intervention programmes for injured athletes.

Positive response

Discussion around psychological response to sports injury often focuses on the negative response. However, injury can in fact be a positive event for some athletes; for example, if an athlete has been having a difficult season and underperforming, the injury can offer a welcome escape, or break from intensive training.

Many athletes experience positive emotional benefits emerging from sport injury. Udry (1997) examined the positive consequences of injury by conducting retrospective interviews with 21 injured athletes from the US ski team. She found that 95% of the athletes reported one or more positive consequences from their injuries. These were coalesced into three general categories: personal growth (e.g., 'I learned how to help other injured skiers', 'I learned different sides of myself'); psychologically based performance enhancements (e.g., 'I became mentally tougher', 'It (injury) gave me a greater work ethic'); and physical-technical development (e.g., 'I learned to ski technically better', 'I learned what my body can handle').

Udry (1999) adds that not all injured athletes will experience positive benefits from injuries, and that SMPs working with injured athletes can help facilitate the process by which athletes derive positive consequences from their injuries and suggested five recommendations for how this can be done (Box 43.1).

Models of athletes' psychological response to injury

Theoretical models have been developed to demonstrate and offer insight into the psychological reactions athletes experience when injured. It is helpful for SMPs to consider the individual athlete's response to injury and then reflect on how these responses fit with a validated model. Kolt (2004a) suggests that this process allows the SMP to interpret why many reactions are occurring and how these reactions may impact on the rehabilitation process. In particular, the grief response models and cognitive appraisal models have been widely adopted.

Grief response models

Grief response models or stage models have been taken from other areas of research such as death and dying and applied to the context of sports injury (Mueller and Ryan, 1991). The Kübler Ross (1969) model was developed to explain significant loss (such as the death of a family member or loved one) and suggests that people progress through five stages of grieving: denial, anger, bargaining, depression and acceptance. This model has been suggested to relate to sports injuries, as athletes can experience a sense of loss of self because of the injury (Gordon, 1991; Macci and Crossman, 1996).

The sports injury literature demonstrates some support for the grief models (McDonald and Hardy, 1990; Mueller and Ryan, 1991). Criticism includes that the models assume that the injury represents a form of loss to the athlete and therefore requires grieving (Walker and Heaney, 2013). Secondly, these models fail to pick up on a key element of sports injury which is the individual differences in response to injury (Evans and Hardy, 1995; Harris, 2003; Walker et al., 2007). In the sport psychology world, it is generally accepted that responses to injury are viewed in a flexible way, recognizing each athlete's uniqueness. Weinberg and Gould (2011) suggest that athletes all have a typical response to injury, but the speed and ease with which they progress through varies widely.

The integrated model of response to sport injury and rehabilitation

The second major category of psychological response to injury models are cognitive appraisal models, which are based around stress, coping and emotional responsivity theories. The integrated model of response to sport injury and rehabilitation is arguably the most accepted and well-developed model within the sports psychology literature (Anderson et al., 2004; Kolt and McEvoy, 2003; Walker et al., 2007).

The integrated model (Fig. 43.1) suggests that an athlete's response to a sports injury is influenced by both pre-injury variables such as personality, history of stressors, coping resources and preventative interventions, as well as postinjury variables (Wiese-Bjornstal et al., 1998). As can be seen in Fig. 43.1, during the postinjury phases, the way that the athlete appraises the injury influences their behavioural response (e.g., their use of social support, psychological skills and rehabilitation adherence), their emotional responses (e.g., fear of unknown, frustration or positive attitude) and the psychosocial and physical outcomes. The model acknowledges the interaction among the cognitive appraisal and emotional and behavioural responses as a dynamic and bidirectional cyclic process, which in turn has an effect on both physical and psychological recovery outcomes. In this model, characteristics of the personal (e.g., injury history, pain tolerance, coping skills) and situational factors (e.g., type of sport, coach influences, family dynamics, rehabilitation environment) are suggested to have direct impact on the cognitive appraisals.

This model offers SMPs a helpful framework for understanding the psychological aspects of sports injury and rehabilitation and it can be used to help develop individualized intervention plans for each unique athlete.

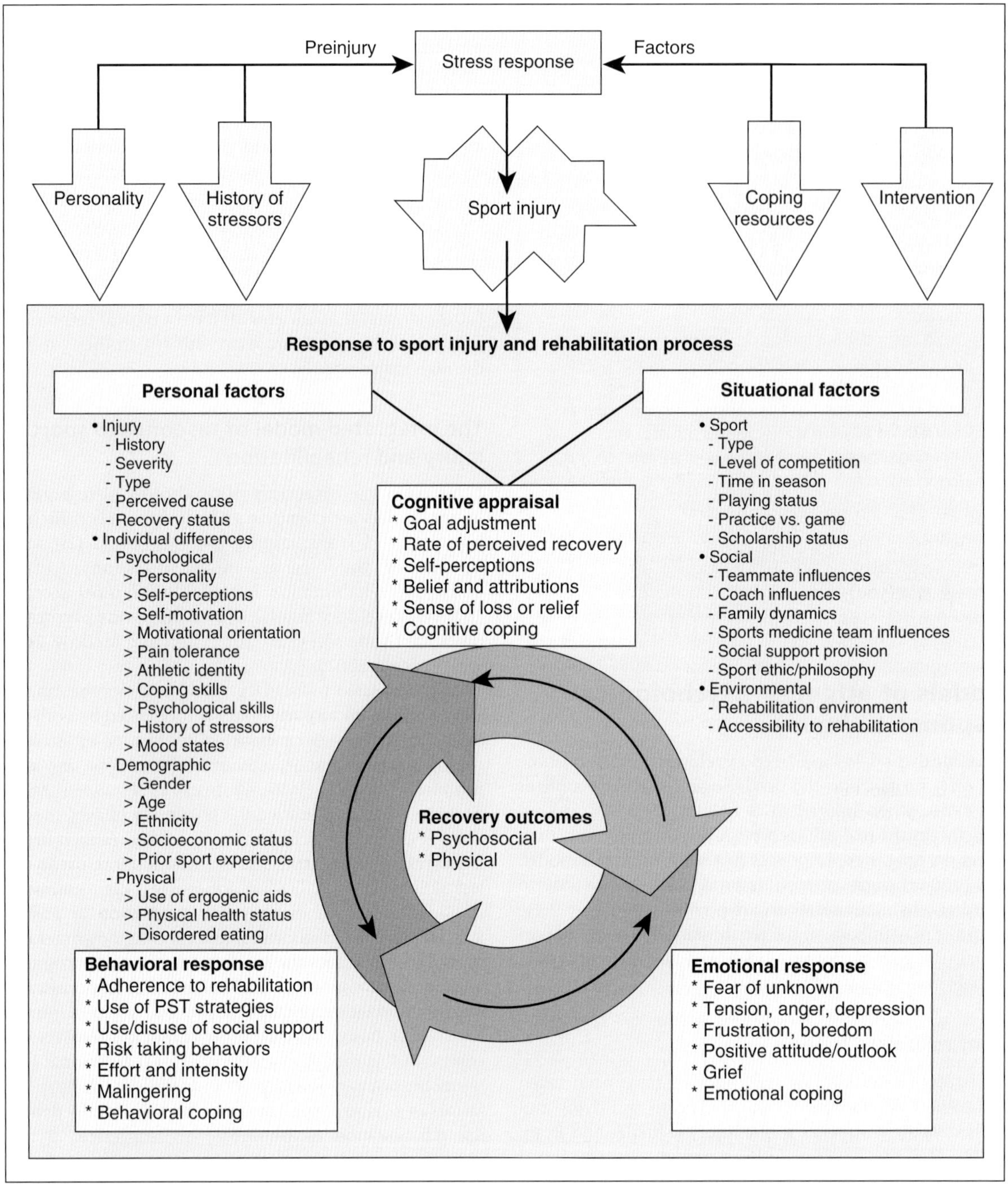

Fig. 43.1 Integrated model of response to stress injury. *PST*, Psychological skills training. (Adapted from Wiese-Bjornstal, D.M., Smith, A.M., Shaffer, S.M., Morrey, M.A., 1998. An integrated model of response to sports injury: psychological and sociological dynamics. Journal of Applied Sport Psychology 10, 46-69.)

Limbic system

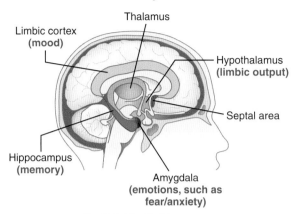

Fig 43.2 The limbic system.

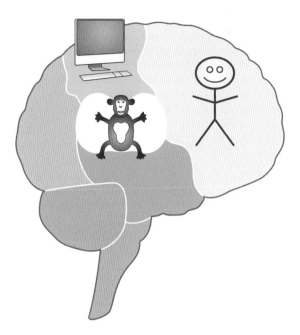

Fig. 43.3 The chimp brain. (© Steve Peters and Jeff Battista).

The Chimp Model

For the past 3 years I have been working with Professor Steve Peters using his Chimp Model (Peters, 2012). The Chimp Model greatly simplifies the neuroscience and explains how the mind can be seen as having three teams, each with their own agenda and way of working.

The *human* (you) is mainly based in the frontal lobe, is associated with logical thinking and works with facts and truth. The *chimp*, mainly based in the limbic system, is an independent emotional thinking machine that works with feelings and impressions. The limbic system is found on the underside of the cerebrum; it combines higher mental functions and primitive emotion into a single system often referred to as the emotional nervous system. It is not only responsible for our emotional lives but also learning and memory. The limbic system includes the amygdala, hippocampus, thalamus, hypothalamus and the basal ganglia (Figs 43.2 and 43.3).

There is also the *computer*, spread throughout the brain, which is a storage area for programmed thoughts and behaviours. It is important to note that a model is not pure scientific fact or a hypothesis. It is just a simple representation to aid understanding and help us to use the science. Professor Peters developed the model based on his 30-year experience of working as a psychiatrist and teaching neuroscience to medical students at Sheffield University. Despite the model's huge popularity across a wide spectrum of fields and disciplines, the value of the model has yet to be proven through scientific research.

In my work using the Chimp Model with injured sports people, I have found that it allows people to understand how their mind works and how their unique brain is responding to the injury and rehabilitation process. Learning to distinguish between emotional thinking and logical/rational thinking about the injury can be a helpful way to start to manage individual responses. The *chimp* part of

the brain finds it hard to deal with reality and expresses emotional thinking about the injury ('Why did it happen to me?' 'I'm never going to get back to where I was', 'It's not fair'), whereas the *human* part of the brain accepts and understands the injury relatively quickly and can then start to work on coping plans, rehabilitation plans and processes.

In the example of the horse racing jockey at the beginning of this chapter, the *human* part of his brain accepted the injury, but his *chimp* became fixated on getting back to race riding as quickly as possible and this distracted his *chimp* away from processing his emotional response to the injury. Breaking records to recover as quickly as possible became an exciting challenge for his *chimp*. However, when faced with the reality of having to race ride again, his *chimp* panicked and all the emotion that had not been expressed at the onset and during the rehabilitation came out and had to be processed and addressed at that point.

Adherence to injury rehabilitation

As defined by Meichenbaum and Turk (1987) adherence is an 'active voluntary collaborative involvement of the patient in a mutually acceptable course of behaviour to produce a desired preventative or therapeutic result' (p. 20). For SMPs, adherence may involve behaviours such as complying with practitioner instructions, attending and actively being involved in rehabilitation sessions, avoiding potentially harmful behaviours, completing home rehabilitation exercises, completing home cryotherapy and medical prescriptions.

Despite it seeming obvious that adherence is crucial to successful rehabilitation of injured athletes, there is a lack of empirical evidence to support this notion. One study by Brewer (1998) indicated that depending on how adherence to sports injury rehabilitation programmes was measured, rates ranging from 40% to 91% have been recorded. Findings from Taylor and May (1996) indicate that nonadherence for home-based activities are 54–60%. Relatively few studies have provided evidence that higher levels of adherence were related to better sports injury outcomes (Brewer et al., 2000; Kolt and McEvoy, 2003; Schoo, 2002).

Methods to enhance rehabilitation adherence in athletes

The integrated model demonstrates how various situational, personal, emotional factors can impact on rehabilitation adherence. The model provides a useful way of understanding the importance of treating each athlete as an individual and how vital it is to gain insight of a variety of factors across all aspects of the athlete's life, all of which could impact on their ability to adhere to their rehabilitation programme.

For SMPs it might be interesting to note that several contextual factors have been found to be related to greater adherence. These include higher belief in the efficacy of the treatment (Duda et al., 1989; Taylor and May, 1996), comfort of the rehabilitation setting (Brewer et al., 1999), convenience of rehabilitation scheduling (Fields et al., 1995), perceived exertion during rehabilitation exercises (Brewer et al., 1999), and rehabilitation practitioner expectancy of patient adherence (Taylor and May, 1996). A study by Fisher and Hoisington (1993) found that patients reported that having practitioners who were caring, honest and encouraging helped them through the rehabilitation process.

In a review of the literature on adherence to sports injury rehabilitation programmes, Levy et al. (2006) concluded that SMPs should employ various strategies to enhance rehabilitation behaviour. These included goal setting, use of diaries, development of action plans, enhancing beliefs and capabilities towards rehabilitation modalities and use of decisional balance sheets.

Kolt (2004b) outlines a variety of methods to enhance rehabilitation adherence in athletes, six of which are summarized in Box 43.2.

Sport psychology skills to integrate into your practice

Kolt and Andersen (2004) have found that for psychological interventions to be well received by an athlete, they need

---

> **Box 43.2 Methods to enhance rehabilitation adherence in athletes**
>
> 1. *Education* – taking time to educate clients about their injuries, the rationale behind treatment approaches and injury management, and establishing realistic expectations.
> 2. *Communication and rapport building* – very important to establish a rapport and communicate in ways suitable for everyone. This needs to be learned through experience, not textbooks.
> 3. *Social support* –through injury support groups and peer modelling recommended for sports injury rehabilitation. Peer modelling involves linking a currently injured athlete with an athlete who has undergone successful rehabilitation and returned to preinjury functioning.
> 4. *Goal setting and attainment* – setting specific rehabilitation goals has been found to result in greater time spent doing rehabilitation exercise and greater understanding of the rehabilitation programme. See further suggestions on goal setting later in this chapter.
> 5. *Treatment efficacy and tailoring of rehabilitation programmes* – important to tailor the programme to the needs of the individual. To build treatment efficacy in clients, SMPs need to ensure client can perform assigned rehabilitation tasks and that tasks are meaningful and worthwhile to the individual.
> 6. *Athlete responsibility* – athletes like to feel responsible for their rehabilitation, and this sense of control can increase commitment and adherence. SMPs could use approaches that encourage some level of independence for clients.

to be delivered by the SMP in a such a way that they appear as an expected and integral part of the rehabilitation. It is important for the SMP to be confident in the effectiveness of the skills and their own ability to teach the skills. The key word here is 'skill'. The following are sport psychology *skills* and like any physical rehabilitation skill, they take time and practice to be of benefit. Some athletes may already have been using sport psychology skills prior to their injury, in which case they simply need to be guided in adapting them for use in rehabilitation. For athletes who are not familiar with these skills, the SMP will need to educate the athlete on the benefits of the skills and teach the skill using a structured intervention plan.

Goal setting

Goal setting is a technique pioneered by Locke (1968) and is one of the most popular psychological interventions in sport. Is often used by athletes to promote performance (Weinberg and Gould, 2011) and for many athletes goal setting forms an integral part of their daily training. The goal setting process can help athletes understand where they are currently and also where they want to get to. Locke (1968) suggested that goal setting impacts performance in four ways: it focuses attention, mobilizes effort in proportion to the demands of the task, enhances persistence, and encourages the individual to develop strategies for achieving their goals. Sports injury rehabilitation literature has identified goal setting to have several benefits to the athlete. Three types of goals have been identified and become popular in the sports psychology literature. These are: outcome goals, performance goals and process goals (Hardy et al., 1996).

Outcome goals. These focus on the outcome of an event such as winning a gold medal or a specific result of a competition, and as such involve interpersonal comparison. An outcome goal is not in the athlete's control. An example of an outcome goal in rehabilitation could be:

- successful return to previous level of sporting performance
- to win a gold medal at the next Olympics.

Performance goals. These are related to personal statistical goals related to the athlete's own personal previous performance. As such they are more within the athlete's control than outcome goals, but still not under complete control. For example, a performance goal in rehabilitation could be being able to regain a 50% range of motion in an injured limb. Other examples could be:

- regaining stability in a body part with specific percentage increments
- regaining confidence in an injured body part with specific percentage increments
- being able to squat a specific amount of weight at the gym
- being able to run a certain distance and/or speed.

Process goals. These are related to performance goals and are focused on the actions or tasks that the athlete needs to engage in to achieve the desired performance outcome. Process goals should be tasks or actions that are within the athlete's control. In rehabilitation, examples of process goals could be:

- completing specific exercises to improve range of motion
- attending all five rehabilitation sessions at the gym each week
- focusing on a specific movement during a rehabilitation exercise
- doing the stretches recommended by the SMP.

According to Cox (2007), when outcome goals, performance goals and process goals are employed in conjunction, athletes have far greater chance of experiencing performance improvements and psychological development than when one is employed in isolation (e.g., outcome goals). For example, you initially set an outcome goal, then set performance goals to help move you towards

---

> ### Box 43.3 **Key points for goal setting**
>
> - Start the goal setting process in conversation together with the athlete
> - Set specific goals (the common tendency is to set vague goals)
> - Include outcome, performance and process goals
> - Set performance and process goals with the athlete around psychological parameters such as: confidence in the injured body part, motivation, commitment, adherence, anxiety, etc.
> - Ensure agreement between the SMP and athletes on goal achievement strategies
> - Write goals down 'Ink it, don't think it'
> - Provide goal support to the athletes
> - Incorporate goals into the rehab sessions
> - Remember to review and modify goals regularly

---

achieving your outcome goal, and then process goals to focus on the processes you need to engage in to achieve your performance goals.

Short-term goals were the most widely used sport psychology technique reported by the physiotherapists in the study by Arvinen-Barrow et al. (2007). However, the study identified that whilst the physiotherapists set daily physical goals as well as overall recovery goals, these goals were very much mandated by the physiotherapist; as a result the athletes had little or no ownership of the goals. For goal setting to be effective, it is vital for the athlete to be involved in the goal setting process. Arvinen-Barrow et al. (2010) suggest that as physiotherapists are experts to the physical aspects of the healing process, their opinion should be the primary one to consider; however, it is imperative that the athlete is actively part of the process (Box 43.3).

Relaxation

Simply inhaling, exhaling and relaxing for a few minutes can have a significant impact on performance. Watching some well-known sporting individuals, it is easy to see Johnny Wilkinson for example, taking a few deep breaths, relaxing and focusing before taking a penalty kick. Christiano Ronaldo is another good example of a player who, when taking a penalty, lines up his strike, takes a deep breath and waits until he is focused and ready before kicking the penalty. Being able to relax and focus does not happen overnight, but it can be practised and developed effectively over time.

The sports psychology literature has identified two types of relaxation, both of which are applicable to healthy athletes and those with injury (Box 43.4). These are physical (somatic) and mental (cognitive) relaxation (Flint, 1998b). The key aim of physical relaxation is to release tension from the body and the most commonly used technique in sport

Box 43.4 **Key points for relaxation**

- Relaxation is helpful throughout all of the injury process
- Relaxation can help athletes deal with pain and the stress and anxiety associated with the injury process
- Relaxation can help athletes gain a sense of control over their pain and their rehabilitation
- It is helpful to educate the athlete on the benefits of relaxation
- Ensure that there is a structure to the relaxation training
- Measure relaxation effectiveness

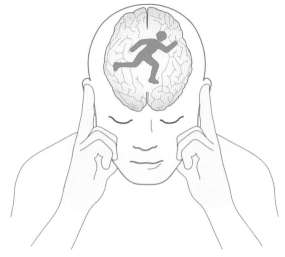

Fig. 43.4 Mental imagery.

is progressive muscle relaxation (Jacobson, 1938). The aim of mental relaxation is to focus on the mind, rather than the body, with the idea that a relaxed mind can lead to a relaxed body and the most common techniques include autogenic training (Schultz and Luthe, 1969), breath control and the relaxation response (Benson, 2000). Relaxation training can be used to relieve pain and stress, which can often be prominent during injury rehabilitation.

Progressive muscle relaxation

Progressive muscle relaxation (PMR) aims to teach the individual what it feels like to relax the muscles by contrasting tensing the muscle groups in turn, followed by relaxing them. In this way, athletes learn to be aware of how the muscles feel when they are tense, and then what they can do to relax them. Through practice athletes can learn to recognize the difference between a tensed and relaxed muscle.

PMR is a good exercise to do initially when an athlete is injured, because muscle tension contributes to increased experience of pain. Actively tensing and relaxing the muscles gives the athletes a sense of control over their pain and injury management. The first sessions of PMR can take up to 30 minutes and it is recommended that the athletes follow a script for 16 muscle groups. Studies have demonstrated a variety of benefits of PMR including reducing somatic anxiety (Kolt et al., 2002; Maynard et al., 1995), rheumatic pain (Stenstrom et al., 1996) and muscle tension (Lehrer, 1982).

The relaxation response

Benson (2000) popularized a scientific way of relaxing based on meditative relaxation, but without the spiritual element and called it 'the relaxation response'. There are four key elements to the relaxation response:
1. A quiet place to minimize distractions.
2. A comfortable position that can be maintained.

3. Choosing a single thought or word to focus attention on, e.g., 'calm' or 'relax', that does not stimulate thoughts; the word is repeated on exhalation.
4. A passive attitude; this means allowing thoughts and images to pass through your mind without engaging with them.

The relaxation response teaches athletes to quiet the mind, concentrate and reduce muscle tension. The relaxation response can help athletes to gain a greater sense of control over their pain and the rehabilitation process (Taylor and Taylor, 1998).

Mental imagery

Mental imagery, or visualization, is one of the most useful skills to use during rehabilitation. Imaging refers to creating or recreating an experience in the mind (Weinburg and Gould, 2011) (Fig. 43.4). There is a huge amount of evidence to support imagery use by healthy athletes (Arvinen-Barrow et al., 2008), and its application to sports injury recovery is well documented in the literature. Despite this, mental imagery seems to be the least favoured by SMPs. This may be due to a lack of understanding as to its benefits and possibly an erroneous perception of what an imagery intervention entails (Arvinen-Barrow et al., 2010).

Research studies have found that four types of imagery may be helpful during the rehabilitation process (Box 43.5).

Healing imagery. The athlete images the injured body part healing (e.g., imaging ruptured tissue healing together, imaging a break in a bone healing to a strong healthy bone).

Pain management. The athlete distracts themselves from the pain by imaging lying on a beach, for example. Ievleva and Orlick (1991) suggest imaging the pain being

Box 43.5 **Key points for mental imagery/visualization**

- Encourage use of healing and pain management imagery in the early part of the rehabilitation process
- Encourage use of rehabilitation process imagery during the rehabilitation/recovery phase
- Encourage use of performance imagery throughout the rehabilitation process, but in particular during the return to full activity phase
- Measure athletes imagery ability and effectiveness

Box 43.6 **Key points for social support**

- Initially, informational support is really important for the athlete to understand the nature of their injury. It is also important to provide listening and emotional support.
- During the rehabilitation phase, the need for social support is greatest when the recovery is slow. The athlete may also benefit from emotional challenge, technical support and motivational support.
- During the return to full activity phase, the social support may need to focus on building the athlete's confidence and motivation towards return to play.
- Research findings suggest that athletes turn to SMPs for informational support and family and friends for emotional support.

washed away, or seeing cool colours running through the pain to reduce it (e.g., seeing cool blues running through the area, imaging the pain leaving the body).

Rehabilitation process. The athlete images themselves undertaking the processes they need to complete in order to fully recover (e.g., specific exercises at the gym, overcoming challenges and setbacks, adhering to the rehabilitation programme).

Performance. The athlete images undertaking sport specific-skills (e.g., imaging training drills, or a competition performance).

Social support

Social support facilitates coping. According to Weinberg and Gould (2011) it can help to reduce stress, enhance mood, increase motivation for rehabilitation, and improve treatment adherence. Within the sport psychology literature, social support is believed to be an integral part of the coping process for injured athletes (Bianco, 2001; Podlog and Eklund, 2007). Box 43.6 outlines some key aspects of this process.

Family, friends and team mates can find it difficult to understand the impact an injury can have on the athlete. If the injury is career threatening, support members may feel uncomfortable talking about the sport to the injured athlete (Petitpas and Danish, 1995). Similarly, it can be easier for support team members to talk about the physical and practical aspects of the injury rehabilitation, rather than the athlete's feelings. When this happens, the athlete might not have the opportunity to discuss how they are feeling about their injury and may miss out on an important part of their psychological adjustment to their injury (Petitpas and Danish, 1995).

In working with injured athletes, it is important to consider the type of social support that the athlete might be receiving. A variety of forms of social support exist including listening support, emotional support, emotional challenge, task appreciation, task challenge, reality confirmation, material assistance and personal assistance (Richman et al., 1993).

The athletes in a 2014 study by Arvinen-Barrow and colleagues, 2014 reported that they assumed that SMPs know how they feel, so they did not feel the need to explain. In reality, only the athlete knows their individual pain or how they are feeling. Therefore, it is vital for SMPs to initiate an open line of communication about feelings and psychological pain with the athletes they work with by asking about it.

Understanding when to refer

A key skill for an SMP is to know when it is time to refer an athlete on to the sport psychologist or another mental health advisor. Harris (2005) highlights the importance of physiotherapists being mindful of personal competence with regard to use of psychological interventions and knowing when it is time to refer on. SMPs who establish a rapport with an athlete are in a good position to spot the warning signs if that individual is struggling to cope with their injury. Generally when athletes feel understood they are much more likely to speak about their fears, concerns and anxieties. Box 43.7 shows areas identified by Petitpas and Danish (1995) as signs of poor adjustment and if you see one or several of these, it would be advisable to refer the athlete on.

Conclusion

This chapter has taken you on a journey through the psychology of sports injury rehabilitation, beginning with noting its role in sports medicine, then moving on to exploring psychological responses to sports injury, then examining adherence and practical strategies to enhance adherence;

Box 43.7 **Signs of poor adjustment**

- Feelings of anger, confusion or apathy
- Lack of engagement with rehabilitation
- Obsessively asking, 'When will I be able to play again?'
- Lack of belief in the rehabilitation process
- Denial, e.g., 'This injury isn't serious'
- A history of coming back too soon from an injury
- Bragging about accomplishments
- Withdrawal from significant others
- Dwelling on minor physical complaints
- Dependence on the physiotherapist
- Guilt about letting the team down
- Rapid mood swings or sudden changes in behaviour
- Feelings of helplessness to impact the injury

From Petitpas, A., Danish, A., 1995. Caring for injured athletes. In: Murphy, S., (Ed.), Sport Psychology Interventions. Human Kinetics, Champaign, IL, pp. 255–281.

finally, we looked at four psychological skills that can be taught to aid injured athletes. The key message I would like to leave you with is the importance of treating each athlete as a unique individual, whom you can get to know and help through their rehabilitation journey. No two athletes will respond to and deal with the same injury in the same way. Each time a new client walks through my door, my job is to gain insight into that person's unique brain. Remember the jockey at the beginning of the chapter; it appeared he was coping exceptionally well with his rehabilitation, but the emotional impact hit him at the point of return to sport. Never take things at face value. Take time to listen to your clients, ask the right questions and develop individual intervention plans to suit each person.

References

Anderson, A.G., White, A., McKay, J., 2004. Athletes' emotional response to injury. In: Lavallee, D., Thatcher, J., Jones, M. (Eds.), Coping and Emotion in Sport. Nova Science, New York, pp. 207–221.

Ardern, C.L., Taylor, N.F., Feller, J.A., Whitehead, T.S., Webster, K.E., 2013. Psychological responses matter in returning to pre-injury level of sport after anterior cruciate ligament reconstruction surgery. The American Journal of Sports Medicine 41 (7), 1549–1558.

Arvinen-Barrow, M., Hemmings, B., Weigand, D., Becker, C.A., Booth, L., 2007. Views of chartered physiotherapists on the psychological content of their practice: a national follow-up survey in the UK. Journal of Sports Rehabilitation 16 (2), 111–121.

Arvinen-Barrow, M., Massey, W.V., Hemmings, B., 2014. Role of sport medicine professionals in addressing psychosocial aspects of sport-injury rehabilitation: professional athletes views. Journal of Athletic Training 49 (6), 764–772.

Arvinen-Barrow, M., Penny, G., Hemmings, B., Corr, S., 2010. UK chartered physiotherapists' personal experiences in using psychological interventions with injured athletes: an interpretative phenomenological analysis. Psychology of Sport and Exercise 11 (1), 58–66.

Arvinen-Barrow, M., Weigand, D.A., Thomas, S., Hemmings, B., Walley, M., 2008. The use of imagery across competitive levels and time of season: a cross-sectional study amongst synchronized skaters in Finland. European Journal of Sport Sciences 8 (3), 135–142.

Beneka, A., Malliou, P., Bebetsos, E., Gioftsidou, A., Pafis, G., Godolias, G., 2007. Appropriate Counselling Techniques for Specific Components of the Rehabilitation Plan: A Review of the literature. Physical Training, August 2012. Available at: https://ejmas.com/pt/2007pt/ptart_beneka_0707.html.

Benson, H., 2000. The Relaxation Response. HarperCollins, New York.

Bianco, T., 2001. Social support and recovery from sport injury: elite skiers share their experiences. Research Quarterly for Exercise & Sport 72, 376–388.

Brand, E., Nyland, J., 2009. Patient outcomes following anterior cruciate ligament reconstruction: the influence of psychological factors. Orthopedics 32, 335–341.

Brewer, B.W., 1998. Adherence to sport injury rehabilitation programs. Journal of Applied Sport Psychology 10, 70–82.

Brewer, B.W., Daly, J.M., Van Raalte, J.L., Petitpas, A.J., Sklar, J.H., 1999. A psychometric evaluation of the rehabilitation adherence questionnaire. Journal of Sport & Exercise Psychology 21, 167–173.

Brewer, B.W., Van Raalte, J.L., Cornelius, A.E., Petitpas, A.J., Sklar, J.H., Pohlman, M.H., et al., 2000. Psychological factors, rehabilitation outcome following anterior cruciate ligament reconstruction. Rehabilitation Psychology 45, 20–37.

Cox, R.H., 2007. Sport Psychology: Concepts and Application, sixth ed. McGraw-Hill, Boston, MA.

Duda, J.L., Smart, A.E., Tappe, M.L., 1989. Predictors of adherence in the rehabilitation of athletic injuries: an application of personal investment theory. Journal of Sport & Exercise Psychology 11, 367–381.

Evans, L., Hardy, L., 1995. Sport injury and grief response: a review. Journal of Sport & Exercise Psychology 17, 227–245.

Fields, J., Murphey, M., Horodyski, M., Stopka, C., 1995. Factors associated with adherence to sport injury rehabilitation in college-age athletes. Journal of Sport Rehabilitation 4, 172–180.

Fisher, A.C., Hoisington, L.L., 1993. Injured athletes' attitudes and judgments towards rehabilitation adherence. Journal of Athletic Training 28 (1), 48–53.

Flint, F.A., 1998a. Integrating sports psychology and sports medicine in research: the dilemmas. Journal of Applied Sport Psychology 10, 83–102.

Flint, F.A., 1998b. Specialized psychological interventions. In: Flint, F.A. (Ed.), Psychology of Sports Injury. Human Kinetics, Leeds, UK, pp. 29–50.

Gordon, S., Milios, D., Grove, R., 1991. Psychological aspects of the recovery process from sport injury: the perspective of sport physiotherapist. Australian Journal of Science and Medicine in Sport 23 (2), 53–60.

Hamson-Utley, J.J., Martin, S., Walters, J., 2008. Athletic trainers' and physical therapists' perceptions of the effectiveness of psychological skills within sport injury rehabilitation programs. Journal of Athletic Training 43 (3), 258–264.

Hardy, L., Jones, G., Gould, D., 1996. Understanding Psychological Preparation for Sport: Theory and Practice for Elite Performers. Wiley, Chichester, UK.

Harris, L., 2005. Perceptions and attitudes of athletic training and students toward a course addressing psychological issues in rehabilitation. Journal Of Allied Health 34, 101–109.

Harris, L.L., 2003. Integrating and analysing psychosocial and stage theories to challenge the development of the injured collegiate athlete. Journal of Athletic Training 38 (1), 75–82.

Heil, J., 1993. Psychology of Sport Injury. Human Kinetics, Champaign, IL.

Hemmings, B., Povey, L., 2002. Views of chartered physiotherapists on the psychological content of their practise: a preliminary study in the United Kingdom. British Journal of Sports Medicine 36 (1), 61–64.

Ievleva, L., Orlick, T., 1991. Mental links to enhanced healing: an exploratory study. The Sport Psychologist 5, 25–40.

Jacobson, E., 1938. Progressive Relaxation. University of Chicago Press, Chicago, IL.

Kamphoff, C., Hamson-Utley, J.J., Antoine, B., Knutson, B., Thomae, J., Hoenig, C., 2010. Athletic training students perceptions of the importance and effectiveness of psychological skills within sport injury rehabilitation. Athletic Training Education Journal 5 (3), 109–116.

Kolt, G.S., 2004a. Psychology of injury and rehabilitation. In: Kolt, G.S., Snyder-Mackler, L. (Eds.), Physical Therapies in Sport and Exercise. Churchill Livingstone, London, pp. 165–183.

Kolt, G.S., 2004b. Injury from sport, exercise and physical activity. In: Kolt, G.S., Andersen, M.B. (Eds.), Psychology in the Physical and Manual Therapies. Churchill Livingstone Inc., Philadelphia, PA, pp. 247–267.

Kolt, G.S., Andersen, M.B., 2004. Psychology in the Physical and Manual Therapies. Churchill Livingstone Inc, Philadelphia, PA.

Kolt, G.S., McEvoy, J.F., 2003. Adherence to rehabilitation in patients with lower back pain. Manual Therapy 8, 110–116.

Kolt, G.S., Gill, S., Keating, J., 2002. An examination of the multi-process theory: the effects of two relaxation techniques on state anxiety. [Abstract]. Australian Journal of Psychology 54 (Suppl.), 39.

Kübler-Ross, E., 1969. On Death and Dying. MacMillan, London.

Larson, G.A., Starkey, C., Zaichkowsky, L.D., 1996. Psychological aspects of athletic injuries as perceived by athletic trainers. The Sport Psychologist 10, 37–47.

Lehrer, P.M., 1982. How to relax and how not to relax: a re-evaluation of the work of Edmund Jacobson. Behaviour Research and Therapy 20, 417–428.

Levy, A.R., Pullman, R.C.J., Clough, P.J., McNaughton, L.R., 2006. Adherence to sports injury rehabilitation programmes: a conceptual review. Research in Sports Medicine 14, 149–162.

Locke, E.A., 1968. Towards a theory of task motivation incentives. Organizational Behavior & Human Performance 3, 157–189.

Macci, R., Crossman, J., 1996. After the fall: reflections of injured classical ballet dancers. Journal of Sport Behaviour 19, 221–234.

Mann, B.J., Grana, W.A., Indelicato, P.A., O'Neill, D.F., George, S.Z., 2007. A survey of sports medicine physicians regarding psychological issues in patient-athletes. The American Journal of Sports Medicine 35 (12), 2140–2147.

Maynard, I.W., Hemmings, B., Warwick-Evans, L., 1995. The effects of a somatic intervention strategy on competitive state anxiety and performance in semi-professional soccer players. The Sport Psychologist 9, 51–64.

McCullough, K.A., Phelps, K.D., Spindler, K.P., Matava, M.J., Dunn, W.R., Parker, R.D., et al., 2012. Return to high school and college-level football after anterior cruciate ligament reconstruction. The American Journal of Sports Medicine 40, 2523–2529.

McDonald, S.A., Hardy, C.J., 1990. Affective response patterns of the injured athlete: an exploratory analysis. The Sport Psychologist 4, 261–274.

Meichenbaum, D., Turk, D.C., 1987. Facilitating Treatment Adherence. Plenum, New York.

Mueller, F.O., Ryan, A. (Eds.), 1991. The Sports Medicine Team and Athletic Injury Prevention. Davis, Philadelphia, PA.

Peters, S., 2012. The Chimp Paradox. Random House, London.

Petitpas, A., Danish, A., 1995. Caring for injured athletes. In: Murphy, S. (Ed.), Sport Psychology Interventions. Human Kinetics, Champaign, IL, pp. 255–281.

Podlog, L., Eklund, R.C., 2007. Psychosocial consideration of the return to sport following injury. Journal of Applied Sport Psychology 19, 207–225.

Ray, R., Wiese-Bjornstall, D.M., 1999. Counseling in Sports Medicine. Human Kinetics, Champaign, IL.

Richman, J.M., Rosenfeld, L.B., Hardy, C.J., 1993. The Social Support Survey: a validation study of a clinical measure of the social support process. Research on Social Work Practice 3, 288–311.

Schoo, A.M., 2002. Exercise Performance in Older People with Osteoarthritis: Relationships between Exercise Adherence Correctness of Exercise Performance and Associated pain. Unpublished Doctoral Dissertation. La Trobe University, Bundoora, Australia.

Schultz, L., Luthe, W., 1969. Autogenic Methods, 1. Grune and Stratton, New York.

Stenstrom, C.H., Arge, B., Sundbom, A., 1996. Dynamic training versus relaxation training as home exercise for patients with inflammatory rheumatic diseases: a ransomised controlled study. Scandinavian Journal of Rheumatology 25, 28–33.

Stiller-Ostrowski, J.L., Hamson-Utley, J.J., 2010. Athletic trainers' educational satisfaction and technique use within the psychosocial intervention and referral content area. Athletic Training Education Journal 5 (1), 4–11.

Taylor, A.H., May, S., 1996. Threat and cooing appraisals as determinants of compliance with sports injury rehabilitation: an application of protection motivation theory. Journal of Sports Science 14, 471–482.

Taylor, J., Taylor, S., 1997. Psychological Approaches to Sports Injury Rehabilitation. Aspen, Gaithersburg, MD.

Taylor, J., Taylor, S., 1998. Pain education and management in the rehabilitation from sports injury. The Sport Psychologist 12, 68–88.

Udry, E., 1997. Coping and social support among injured athletes following surgery. Journal of Sport & Exercise Psychology 19, 71–90.

Udry, E., 1999. The paradox of injuries: Unexpected positive consequences. In: Pargman, D. (Ed.), Psychological Bases of Sport Injuries, second ed. Fitness Information Technology, Morgantown, WV, pp. 79–88.

Walker, N., Heaney, C., 2013. Psychological response to injury. In: Arvinen-Barrow, M., Walker, N. (Eds.), The Psychology of Sport Injury and Rehabilitation. Routledge, London, pp. 23–40.

Walker, N., Thatcher, J., Lavallee, D., 2007. Psychological responses to injury in competitive sport: a critical review. Journal of the Royal Society for the Promotion of Health, the 127 (4), 174–180.

Weinberg, R.S., Gould, D., 2011. Foundations of Sport and Exercise Psychology, fifth ed. Human Kinetics, Champaign, IL.

Wiese-Bjornstal, D.M., Smith, A.M., Shaffer, S.M., Morrey, M.A., 1998. An integrated model of response to sports injury: psychological and sociological dynamics. Journal of Applied Sport Psychology 10, 46–69.

Williams, J.M., Scherzer, C.B., 2010. Injury risk and rehabilitation: psychological considerations. In: Williams, J.M. (Ed.), Applied Sport Psychology: Personal Growth to Peak Performance. McGraw-Hill, New York, pp. 512–541.

Index

Page numbers followed by "*f*" indicate figures, "*t*" indicate tables, and "*b*" indicate boxes.

Index

Index

Index